MW01268931

Genetic Epidemiology of Cancer

Editors

Henry T. Lynch, M.D.
Professor and Chairman
Department of Preventive Medicine and Public Health
and
Creighton University School of Medicine
Omaha, Nebraska

Takeshi Hirayama, M.D.
Director
Institute of Preventive Medicine
Tokyo, Japan

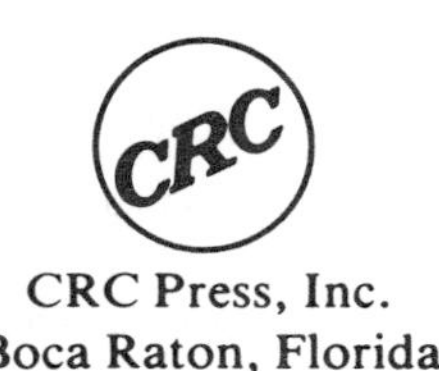

CRC Press, Inc.
Boca Raton, Florida

Library of Congress Cataloging-in-Publication Data

Genetic epidemiology of cancer.

Includes bibliographies and index.
1. Cancer—Genetic aspects. 2. Cancer—Epidemiology.
3. Genetic epidemiology. I. Lynch, Henry T.
II. Hirayama, Takeshi, 1923- . [DNLM: 1. Neoplasms
—familial & genetic. 2. Neoplasms—occurrence.
QZ 202 G3312]
RC268.4.G446 1989 616.99'4042 88-16669
ISBN 0-8493-6756-5

Direct all inquiries to CRC Press, Inc., 2000 Corporate Blvd., N.W., Boca Raton, Florida, 33431.

International Standard Book Number 0-8493-6756-5

Library of Congress Number 88-16669
Printed in the United States

PREFACE

The discipline of cancer genetic epidemiology has shown rapid progress worldwide. This is timely in that, heretofore, cancer geneticists have investigated patients almost exclusively within the confines of basic genetic methodologies without consideration of environmental effects on the phenotype; similarly, cancer epidemiologists have focused their primary attention upon environmental factors, and often totally ignored host factors. As a consequence, with the exception of certain rarely occurring genetic precancerous diseases, such as xeroderma pigmentosum, we have a paucity of knowledge about genetic/environmental interaction in the etiology of the more than 100 hereditary cancer syndromes.

This book has been written to focus upon the urgent need of researchers to integrate more closely the disciplines of genetics and epidemiology in the quest for answers to etiology and carcinogenesis. The study of cancer-prone families is ideally suited for genetic epidemiology investigations. For example, one can often identify cancer-*free* lineages and compare them with cancer-*prone* lineages wherein cancer of specific anatomic sites will show a high predictability of occurrence. Occasionally, certain hereditary cancer syndromes, such as multiple endocrine neoplasia type II, will harbor a biomarker(s); namely, calcitonin excess. Others may show premonitory clinical signs such as multiple adenomatous polyps of the colon and/or congenital hypertrophy of the retinal pigment epithelium in familial polyposis coli, thereby enabling designation of genotypic status *early* in life. Thus, one can frequently identify, within the same family and early in life, ''normal'' individuals and individuals who are extremely susceptible to cancer of a particular site. These natural groupings provide unparalleled opportunities for the study of environmental and genetic effects and their interaction.

ACKNOWLEDGMENT

This book is dedicated to our families, patients, and medical centers: without their help, this effort would not have been possible.

THE EDITORS

Dr. Henry T. Lynch is Professor and Chairman of the Department of Preventive Medicine and Public Health and Professor of Medicine at Creighton University School of Medicine. He is President of Creighton's Hereditary Cancer Institute and Director of the Hereditary Cancer Consultation Center. He is a graduate of the Univeraity of Oklahoma (B.S.) and Denver University (M.A. in clinical psychology), worked toward his Ph.D. in genetics, and then entered medical school at the University of Texas Medical Branch, Galveston (M.D., 1960). He completed a residency in internal medicine, followed by a 2-year fellowship in medical oncology at the University of Nebraska College of Medicine, Omaha. He is a member of Alpha Omega Alpha Honor Medical Society and a winner of the Billings Silver Medal from the American Medical Association (1966), the Distinguished Service Award from Creighton University (1985), the Distinguished Research Career Award from Creighton University (1986), and the Ungerman-Lubin Lecture Prize for Outstanding Cancer Research (1987). Dr. Lynch has published more than 275 scientific papers and 10 books. The majority of these have related to cancer genetics. He was a short-term consultant in oncology to the World Health Organization, and is a consultant to and has been a member of several study groups at the National Cancer Institute. He is currently a consultant to the Food and Drug Administration. His most current book is *Cancer Genetics in Women,* published by CRC Press in 1987.

Dr. Takeshi Hirayama is Director of the Institute of Preventive Oncology and the Institute for Healthy Aging and Visiting Professor of Public Health at Tokai University School of Medicine. He is the former chief of epidemiology, National Cancer Center Research Institute (1965 to 1985). Before that, he was chief of theoretical epidemiology, Epidemiology Division, Institute of Public Health (1947 to 1965).

He holds a M.D. degree, is a graduate of the Manchuria Medical College (1946), and received the degree of Doctor of Medical Science at Medical Faculty, Kyoto University (1951).

He received the degree of Master of Public Health at the School of Health, Johns Hopkins University, 1952. He was a research associate, Sloan Kettering Institute, Memorial Cancer Center, New York, 1959 and 1960.

He served as a WHO medical officer, Geneva, mainly stationed at New Delhi for the epidemiological study of oral-pharyngeal cancer, 1963 to 1965.

He served as a member of Scientific Council, IARC for 8 years and also served as chairman, UICC Epidemiology and Prevention programs, for 8 years. He served as a WHO consultant/advisor over ten times in southeast Asia and western Pacific regions. He has been Secretary General, Asia and Pacific Federation of Organizations for Cancer Research and Control, 1973 to date. He was a member of the Standing Committee, Japan Cancer Society and is currently an advisor of the Society. He is also affiliated with many medical societies in Japan.

CONTRIBUTORS

Robert P. Bolande, M.D.
Professor
Department of Pathology
East Carolina School of Medicine
Greenville, North Carolina

Bruce M. Boman, M.D., Ph.D.
Director
Creighton Cancer Center
and
Associate Professor of Medicine
Creighton University School of Medicine
Omaha, Nebraska

Theresa A. Conway, B.S.N.
Nursing Research Associate
Department of Preventive Medicine
Creighton University School of Medicine
Omaha, Nebraska

Giuseppe Cristofaro, M.D.
Gastroenterologist
Department of Medicine
Hereditary Gastrointestinal Cancer Prevention Center
Brindisi, Italy

Robert C. Elston, Ph.D.
Professor and Head
Department of Biometry and Genetics
Louisiana State University Medical Center
New Orleans, Louisiana

Mary Lee Fitzsimmons, M.A.
Nurse Coordinator
Department of Preventive Medicine
Hereditary Cancer Consultation Center
St. Joseph Hospital
Creighton University School of Medicine
Omaha, Nebraska

Ramon M. Fusaro, M.D., Ph.D.
Sections of Dermatology
University of Nebraska Medical Center
Creighton University Medical School
Omaha, Nebraska

Varghese T. George, Ph.D.
Assistant Professor
Department of Biometry and Genetics
Louisiana State University Medical Center
New Orleans, Louisiana

Robert E. Grier, Ph.D.
Assistant Professor
Department of Pediatrics
University of Texas Medical School
Houston, Texas

Takeshi Hirayama, M.D.
Director
Institute of Preventive Oncology
Tokyo, Japan

R. Rodney Howell, M.D.
David R. Park Professor of Pediatrics
Department of Pediatrics
University of Texas Medical School
Houston, Texas

Nan Hu, Ph.D.
Research Associate
Department of Cell Biology
Cancer Institute, CAMS
Beijing, China

John A. Johnson, Ph.D.
Associate Professor
Departments of Internal Medicine (Dermatology) and Biochemistry
University of Nebraska Medical Center
Omaha, Nebraska

Henry T. Lynch, M.D.
Professor and Chairman
Department of Preventive Medicine and Public Health
and
Professor of Medicine
Creighton University School of Medicine
Omaha, Nebraska

Jane F. Lynch, B.S.N.
Instructor
Department of Preventive Medicine and Public Health
Creighton University
Omaha, Nebraska

Joseph N. Marcus, M.D.
Assistant Professor
Department of Pathology
Creighton University School of Medicine
Omaha, Nebraska

Ei Matsunaga, M.D., D.Sc.
Director
National Institute of Genetics
Mishima, Japan

Motoi Murata, Ph.D.
Head
Division of Epidemiology
Chiba Cancer Center
Chiba, Japan

Chikako Nishigori
Department of Experimental Radiology and Dermatology
Faculty of Medicine
Kyoto, Japan

Olavi Pelkonen, M.D.
Professor
Department of Pharmacology and Toxicology
University of Oulu
Oulu, Finland

Yoshiaki Satoh
Department of Dermatology
Tokyo Medical and Dental University
Tokyo, Japan

Takashi Takahashi, M.D.
Chief of Colon and Rectal Services
Surgical Department
Cancer Institute Hospital
Tokyo, Japan

Hiraku Takebe
Department of Experimental Radiology
Kyoto University
Kyoto, Japan

Margaret A. Tempero, M.D.
Associate Professor
Department of Internal Medicine
University of Nebraska Medical Center
Omaha, Nebraska

Joji Utsunomiya, M.D.
Professor and Chairman
Second Department of Surgery
Hyogo College of Medicine
Nishinomiya, Japan

Kirsi Vahakangas, M.D.
Acting Assistant Professor
Department of Pharmacology and Toxicology
University of Oulu
Oulu, Finland

Xiuqin Wang
Senior Technician
Department of Cell Biology
Cancer Institute, CAMS
Beijing, China

Patrice Watson, Ph.D.
Assistant Professor
Department of Preventive Medicine
Creighton University School of Medicine
Omaha, Nebraska

Min Wu, D.Med.Sc.
Chairman and Professor
Department of Cell Biology
Cancer Institute, CAMS
Beijing, China

TABLE OF CONTENTS

Chapter 1

INTRODUCTION

Henry T. Lynch and Takeshi Hirayama

TABLE OF CONTENTS

I. GROWING IMPORTANCE OF GENETIC EPIDEMIOLOGY

What has the genetic epidemiologic approach to cancer, the subject of this book, to offer to cancer geneticists, epidemiologists, basic cancer researchers, medical and surgical oncologists, family physicians, and the public at large? If one could look into a "crystal ball" to assess future developments in the etiology and ultimate cure of cancer, one would see those rapidly emerging advances in molecular biology and genetic engineering providing important clues to many mysteries of cancer. Cytogenetics have been providing promising leads to etiology and carcinogenesis, and are integrally related to biomolecular investigations in cancer. For example, chromosomal translocations may suggest the identity of oncogene sites. Translocations have been identified in renal cell carcinoma — t(3;8)(p1;g24)(constitutional); Burkitt's lymphomas — t(8;14)(g24;g32) and t(8;22)(g24;g11)100%; nodular lymphomas — t(14;18)(g32;g21.3); and in diffuse lymphomas — t(11;14)(g13;g32). Somatic loss of heterozygosity of normal alleles in human tumors suggests the presence of recessive oncogenes. Cytogenetic examples include retinoblastoma — deletion 13q14 (constitutional); Wilms' tumor — deletion 11p13 (constitutional); MEN-2 — deletion 20p120 (constitutional); and small cell lung cancer — deletion 3(p14-p23)(all).

A primary objective of this book is to view problems of cancer genetic epidemiology in the perspective of an interaction between those primary genetic contributions of the host in concert with the myriad exogenous events which are etiologic in the multistep process of carcinogenesis. This is obviously a matter of extreme complexity. Ferreting out the specific details of those endogenous and exogenous events, and the manner in which they interact, will be essential for a more full comprehension of the mechanisms contributing to carcinogenesis. Future biomolecular/genetic technology, particularly when integrated with informative cancer-prone families as investigatory models, may enable us to derive answers to cancer etiology and carcinogenesis more fully. Thus, genetic epidemiology — particularly the study of familial cancer clusters resulting from the interaction of genetic and environmental factors — will provide invaluable models and methods for investigation.

II. HEREDITARY DISORDERS AS COMMON BACKGROUNDS FOR INVESTIGATION OF CANCER OF ANY SITE

One may refer to any chapter in this book and immediately learn that cancer of any specific anatomic site may occur in a plethora of etiologically distinctive, cancer-associated hereditary disorders.[1-5] They may have only one thing in common: the organ and tissue in which the tumor arises. For example, in the case of colorectal[3] or breast cancer,[4] it is clear that we are dealing with many heterogeneous forms of these disorders wherein each variant may be attributable to differing gene loci, primary or secondary cytogenetic events, and variable environmental interactions. However, the researcher may become blinded to these facts if he pursues investigations of colon or breast cancer patients/families as if each etiologic variety represented a disease resulting from an inborn genetic mutation acting in isolation on the one hand, or on the other, was due exclusively to a stream of commonly occurring carcinogenic events. Rather, a greater assurance of success in revealing the factual details of carcinogenesis would be achievable through focusing meticulous attention upon those individual attributes of each distinctive heterogeneous form of the respective cancers acting in concert with its primary endogeneous (genetic) and exogenous (environmental carcinogens) exposures.

III. PROBLEM AREAS

In spite of prodigious worldwide documentation of the importance of primary genetic factors in the etiology of cancer, particularly among such common sites as the breast, colon, and skin, coupled with the fact that more than 100 hereditary cancer syndromes have now been identified, only a paucity of attention has been given to the application of this knowledge toward cancer prevention and control in the clinical practice setting. Even less systematic research has been devoted toward the investigation of the responsible pathogenetic mechanisms involved when environmental factors perturb primary genetic factors in the course of carcinogenesis in humans. Thus, the basic elements of genetic epidemiology methodologies are given insufficient attention in the study of the etiology of carcinogenesis in man.

The compilation of the cancer family history remains notoriously neglected in the workup of patients. In turn, physicians frequently fail to consider the natural history of hereditary cancer in their surveillance of patients at increased genetic cancer risk. Undoubtedly, these shortcomings are a product of the traditional medical education wherein environmental factors are often considered as being the *sole* cause of cancer. Medical attention is often restricted to the single patient, with neglect of potential relatives at risk for cancer.

Only a fraction of patients exposed to a given carcinogen develop cancer. Why is it then that so many patients with heavy carcinogenic exposure remain cancer-free? A plausible explanation of this phenomenon is that the genotype controlling cancer *expression* variably predisposes to host *resistance* as well as *susceptibility* to cancer. This phenomenon had been clearly recognized at the infrahuman level since the turn of the century and has been only recently appreciated in humans, where an extraordinary interhuman variability in susceptibility to carcinogens, consonant with the concept of ecogenetics has been identified. For example, research in the laboratories of Harris and associates[6,7] at the National Cancer Institute in the U.S. have shown that binding levels of benzo(a)pyrene to DNA vary from 50- to 100-fold in cultured human cells. This enormous variation in carcinogen interaction with human cells may be attributed to the fact that the majority of chemical carcinogens require enzymatic activation, and herein, host factors play a major role in determining variation in such enzyme capability.

IV. HETEROGENEITY, GENETICS, AND ENVIRONMENTAL INTERACTION: CLINICAL VIGNETTES

There are several clinical models which, descriptively, have provided us with insights about cancer etiology that are testable, given present clinical/laboratory expertise. We therefore present several clinical models in this chapter, some of which are exceedingly rare (xeroderma pigmentosum) and others which are common (urinary bladder cancer). These disorders clearly depict the significance of our treatise for encompassing genetic and environmental events for elucidation of etiology in virtually all forms of human cancer.[1-5]

A. Xeroderma Pigmentosum

An excellent, contemporary, genetic-epidemiological, clinical example of the line of reasoning employed throughout this book is that of xeroderma pigmentosum (XDP). Until the pioneering works of Cleaver on DNA repair in skin fibroblasts, we considered this as a *single* disease entity, although it was recognized that there was at least one possible variant of XDP that was associated with neurological abnormalities: xerodermic idiocy of DeSanctis-Cacchione.[2] However, utilizing cultured skin fibroblasts from patients with XDP and exposing them to UV light, it became apparent that there were significant differences in these fibroblasts with respect to their capacity for repair of UV-damaged DNA. Cell-fusion studies subsequently disclosed that complementation can take place between the fibroblasts from specific pairs of XDP patients. Complementation groups based upon correlations with DNA repair rate were then established and assigned letters from the alphabet. For example, group A showed less than 2% of normal repair, while group B had 3 to 7%, and group C had 10 to 25% DNA repair replication, with variable gradations so that there are now at least eight and possibly as many as ten different XDP complementation groups. A specific complementation group characterizes those patients within a specific XDP family. There is no overlap within kindreds, i.e., all affected members of an XDP kindred will be classified as belonging to a single complementation group. Thus, XDP in fact represents a genetically heterogeneous group of diseases which, on the surface, have many phenotypic features in common. Nevertheless, investigations may eventually disclose clinical subtleties based upon differing environmental interactions which may further distinguish one complementation category from another.

Jung et al.[8] have shown that the clinical and biochemical features of XDP affecteds are relatively constant within each complementation group. However, minor variations do occur from one sibling to another, suggesting that this may be a function of the lifelong influence of the amount of UV light exposure as well as the degree of sunlight protection. Variations between families and complementation groups are larger, indicating that the gene activity and its product(s) as well as the residual repair activity show variation from one mutation to another. For example, of interest is the finding of an apparent excess of malignant melanomas in complementation group D, with severe and early squamous cell carcinoma of the skin in group A, both squamous cell carcinoma and basal cell carcinomas of the skin of moderate to severe activity in complementation group C, and basal cell carcinoma of the skin of mild to late onset in complementation group E and in the variant.

Capitalizing upon problems of genetic heterogeneity, Lynch et al.[9] have postulated that patients with XDP of the complementation group C variety may be at *greater* risk for manifesting malignant melanoma than patients with XDP and any of the other complementation groups. These observations also fit well with our unifying hypothesis of genetic epidemiology in that it shows that even in such a rarely occurring hereditary disorder as XDP, heterogeneity exists. Furthermore, patients with a certain genetic subset (complementation group C) may be at increased susceptibility to malignant melanoma.

Therefore, when studying environmental interaction in cancer occurrence in this rare disease(s), it is mandatory that one consider each complementation group as a distinctive entity with its own potential uniqueness for genetic-environmental carcinogenesis. Thus, XDP patients may vary with respect to their carcinogenic expression dependent upon their specific underlying complementation group.

B. Bloom's Syndrome

Bloom's syndrome is a rare, autosomal recessively inherited cancer-associated genodermatosis. This disorder is characterized by dwarfism of the "low birth weight" type, which is associated with a cutaneous photosensitivity to sunlight. Chromatid breaks occur characteristically in this disorder. Bloom's syndrome is of interest because of the finding by Aurias et al.[10] showing that cells from affected patients are exquisitely sensitive to gamma ray irradiation when this is performed immediately prior to adding bromodeoxyuridine (BrdU) to lymphocyte cultures when compared to a control. Cells from patients with Bloom's syndrome were more sensitive to irradiation when compared to control cells at the end of the S and at G_2 phases. In addition, chromosome breaks as well as chromatid breaks and exchanges were increased. The authors concluded that their findings were compatible with the existence of a cell subpopulation in this disorder which was characterized by a slow cycle in concert with a high spontaneous chromosome aberration rate and high gamma-radiation sensitivity. Bloom's syndrome cells were also highly sensitive to the long wave of UV light, a finding which was comparable to electrons emitted by X- and gamma-radiation, as evidenced by investigations of Zbinden and Cerutti.[11]

C. Retinoblastoma

Draper et al.[12] discuss second primary neoplasms in patients with retinoblastoma (RB). They studied a series of 882 RB patients, of whom 384 were known to have the genetic form of the disease. In this series, 30 patients developed second primary tumors. The cumulative incidence rates of second tumors in the entire series was 2% at 12 years after diagnosis and 4.2% at 18 years postdiagnosis. Among the patients with the genetic form of RB, the cumulative incidence rate after 18 years was 8.4% for all second neoplasms, and 6% for osteosarcomas alone. These investigators noted that the inherent risk among the genetic RB survivors for developing osteosarcoma, with exclusion of possible effects of treatment, was estimated to be 2.2% after 18 years. When consideration was given to the field of radiation treatment, the cumulative incidence rate for all second neoplasms after 18 years was 6.6%, with 3.7% of these being osteosarcomas.

There was evidence that patients with the hereditary form of RB were particularly sensitive to the carcinogenic effects of radiation. Of further interest was the suggestion that the use of cyclophosphamide may also increase the risk of second primary neoplasms among those patients with genetic RB. Finally, evidence from this study as well as those reported from the literature suggested an association between RB and malignant melanoma.[13] Studies of this type clearly depict the importance of investigating susceptibility to differing environmental factors, including those clearly identified as carcinogens, among patients afflicted with *all* forms of hereditary cancer.

It is reasonable to conclude that with greater accumulation of knowledge, we may have to tailor our treatment plans in accord with the specific carcinogenic risk that patients with different forms of hereditary cancer may manifest. For example, there is abundant evidence that patients with ataxia telangiectasia show severely untoward effects to radiation therapy.[14] This evidence has also been documented at the *in vitro* level. Other examples include a highly prolific occurrence of basal cell carcinomas in the radiation zone of patients with the multiple nevoid basal cell carcinoma syndrome who have been treated with radiation for medulloblastoma.[13]

D. Familial Atypical Multiple Mole Melanoma (FAMMM) Syndrome

Smith et al.[15] studied cultured skin fibroblasts (*cfs*) from patients with the FAMMM syndrome, also known as the dysplastic nevus syndrome (DNS), a disorder characterized by hereditary cutaneous malignant melanoma (HCMM) and, in our own experience, a susceptibility to intraocular malignant melanoma (IOM) as well as a variety of visceral malignant neoplastic lesions.[16,17] Smith et al.[15] showed *in vitro* UV sensitivity in patients who were genetically predisposed to the FAMMM syndrome. Specifically, the *cfs* tissues derived from the FAMMM patients exhibited an enhanced UV sensitivity. It was of interest that this abnormal UV response showed a wide range, starting at the lower limit of the normal range and extending to one which was more than a twofold increase in sensitivity. Also of interest was the fact that this *in vitro* phenotype was similar to that reported for XDP variant cell strains as observed by Lehmann et al.[18] Thus, the authors concluded that "UV-radiation seems to play a role in CMM pathogenesis, although the precise nature of this causal pathway has yet to be defined. Members of melanoma-prone families with the DNS are at increased risk for HCMM, which almost always arises from a dysplastic nevus . . . although melanoma patients are not generally considered 'sunlight sensitive' in the manner of patients with XP, the limited epidemiologic data consistently indicate that, in comparison with controls, melanoma patients burn and freckle more readily and tan less well on sun exposure."

The data are of considerable cogency when seen in a clinical investigation of dysplastic nevi patients performed by Kopf et al.[19] These investigators studied 104 consecutive Caucasian individuals who had histologic evidence of atypical moles. They measured the number and diameter of these nevocytic nevi into equally sized contiguous rectangles in a specific anatomic area of the body, namely, the lumbosacral region, wherein the cephalad or superior portion of the rectangle would be a relatively sun-exposed site, while in constrast, the caudad or inferior portion of the rectangle would be in a relatively sun-protected area. The nevocytic nevi which were identified in these rectangles had the clinical features of atypical moles. It was therefore of interest that a significantly greater number of nevi were located in the cephalad rectangle as opposed to the caudad rectangle. There was a sex difference in that men greater than or equal to age 40 had significantly larger nevi in the cephalad as opposed to the caudad rectangle. These investigators concluded that their data were consistent with the hypothesis that " . . . sunlight promotes development of more and larger nevocytic nevi in individuals afflicted with the dysplastic nevus syndrome."

These observations should be extended to a larger number of individuals with the FAMMM syndrome, including multiple members of individual families. We mention such studies within and between families since there may well exist considerable heterogeneity in this syndrome so that in certain FAMMM individuals, there may be a greater or lesser susceptibility to the effects of sunlight in the production of FAMMM moles. Furthermore, it will be of value to determine whether sunlight has a role in the neoplastic progression of FAMMM moles during the course of their evolution to cutaneous malignant melanoma. Finally, given the propensity to an excess of visceral cancer in the FAMMM syndrome, one wonders about the possibility that these patients may have a genetic susceptibility to other environmental exposures such as food, alcohol, cigarette smoking, and countless other potential incriminating factors in the environment.

Given the interesting findings of Kopf et al.[19] relevant to greater sun exposure in the cephalad vs. the caudad portions of the lumbosacral region and its correlation with sunlight, one remains perplexed about the fact that the face shows a general sparing of atypical moles in patients with the FAMMM syndrome. This is a paradox in that the face receives heavy sunlight exposure.

Finally, in a effort to elucidate the role of host/environmental interactions in the etiology of the FAMMM syndrome, Smith et al.[20] studied *cfs* in a manner similar to their UV *in vitro* exposure studies mentioned above.[15] In this particular investigation, these authors examined " . . . the *in vitro* responses to a model environmental carcinogen, 4-nitroquinolone 1-oxide (4NQO), of six non-tumour skin fibroblast strains from HCMM/DNS patients representing five families. Three of the six HCMM/DNS strains showed enhanced cell killing with sensitivities greater than that of a xeroderma pigmentosum (XP) variant strain but less than those of ataxia telangiectasia and XP Group D cell strains. The inhibition and recovery of *de novo* DNA synthesis, together with the expression of repair synthesis, following 4NQO exposure appeared to be normal in HCMM/DNS strains, irrespective of their subsequent clonogenic potential. Our data point to a metabolic anomaly which may contribute to the carcinogenic risk of the melanoma prone preneoplastic state presented by some DNS patients."

E. Testicular Carcinoma

Familial testicular carcinoma, while rare, provides a cogent model for the study of genetic-environmental interaction, including a propensity for cancer of differing anatomic sites in testicular cancer-prone families. Lynch et al.[21] recently reviewed the subject of familial testicular carcinoma and provided a detailed family study. This family manifested an unusual cancer spectrum that included the infantile form of embryonal carcinoma of the testis in the son of a cancer-free, but putative obligate gene carrier mother, and the adult form of embryonal carcinoma in this woman's maternal half-brother (their mutual mother had malignant melanoma and urinary bladder carcinoma) (Table 1 and Figure 1). Urologic cancer was present in three generations, with possible transmission through a putative obligate gene carrier mother to her son (Figure 1). The spectrum of tumors in this family (Figure 1 and Table 1) clearly indicates the necessity of studying cancer of *all* anatomic sites in extended kindreds. Note also on the pedigree findings of renal cell carcinoma in the paternal lineage of the proband. The hereditary significance of this pedigree remains enigmatic. Nevertheless,

Table 1
FAMILY TUMOR REGISTRY

Pedigree number	Sex	Age at diagnosis	Basis of diagnosis[a]	Diagnosis
I-1	M	72	PA	Squamous cell carcinoma, lung
I-2	F	67	MR	Carcinoma, gall bladder
I-3	M	77	MR	Carcinoma, prostate
I-4	F	65	PA	Clear cell carcinoma, probable primary of kidney
II-1	F	45	PA	Squamous cell carcinoma, uterine cervix
II-2	M	62	PA	Papillary transitional cell carcinoma, kidney
II-4	F	53	PA	Malignant melanoma
II-4	F	60	PA	Epithelial cell carcinoma urinary bladder
II-7	M	45	DC	Adenocarcinoma, pancreas
III-8	F	47	PA	Adenocarcinoma, breast
III-11	M	23	PA	Embryonal cell carcinoma, right testicle
IV-2	M	1	PA	Embryonal cell carcinoma, right testicle

[a] PA = Pathologic diagnosis, MR = Medical records, and DC = Death certificate.

sufficient information is at hand to indicate the need for genetic counseling and highly targeted surveillance/management programs for these patients who are at increased risk by virtue of their position in the pedigree. Families such as these also provide an invaluable model for environmental-genetic interaction investigations as well as the search for biomarkers.

F. Urinary Bladder Cancer

Kantor et al.[22] performed a population-based study of 2982 bladder cancer patients and 5782 controls from 10 geographic areas of the U.S. Their purpose was to evaluate the role of environmental risk factors in this disease and to determine whether or not an interaction existed between these and the history of urinary tract cancer in first-degree relatives. Of keen interest was the finding that a family history of urinary tract cancer significantly elevated the risk of bladder cancer. Specifically, a relative risk (RR) equal to 1.45 was observed. Even higher risks were found among patients under the age of 45 years. In general, the bladder cancer risk associated with positive family history was found to be higher among persons with suspected environmental exposures; in the case of heavy cigarette smokers (those who smoked more than three packs per day), the RR was 10.7.

These studies have an outgrowth of anecdotal family studies emanating from a report by Fraumeni and Thomas[23] which showed four members of a family to be afflicted with bladder cancer. Similar reports of familial aggregations of bladder cancer followed this initial observation.[24-31]

Kantor et al.[22] draw a striking similarity between their results and those of Cartwright et al.[32,33] which showed an overall increased risk of 45% in association with a positive family history of urinary tract cancer.

The highest risks observed among cigarette smokers suggested that there was an interaction between smoking and familial predisposition to urinary tract cancer.

Attention was called to variations in *N*-acetyltransferase activity, which had been theoretically linked to the development of some bladder tumors. The authors quoted the work of Lower[34] who reasoned that the level or concentration of acetylatable arylamine bladder carcinogens, including β-naphthylamine, benzidine, and phenacetin, would be higher in individuals who were slow to inactivate them. Kantor et al.[22] also reviewed other studies of bladder cancer patients which suggested putative associations with slow acetylator phenotype.[35,36] They also reviewed associations alleged to occur between tryptophan metabolism

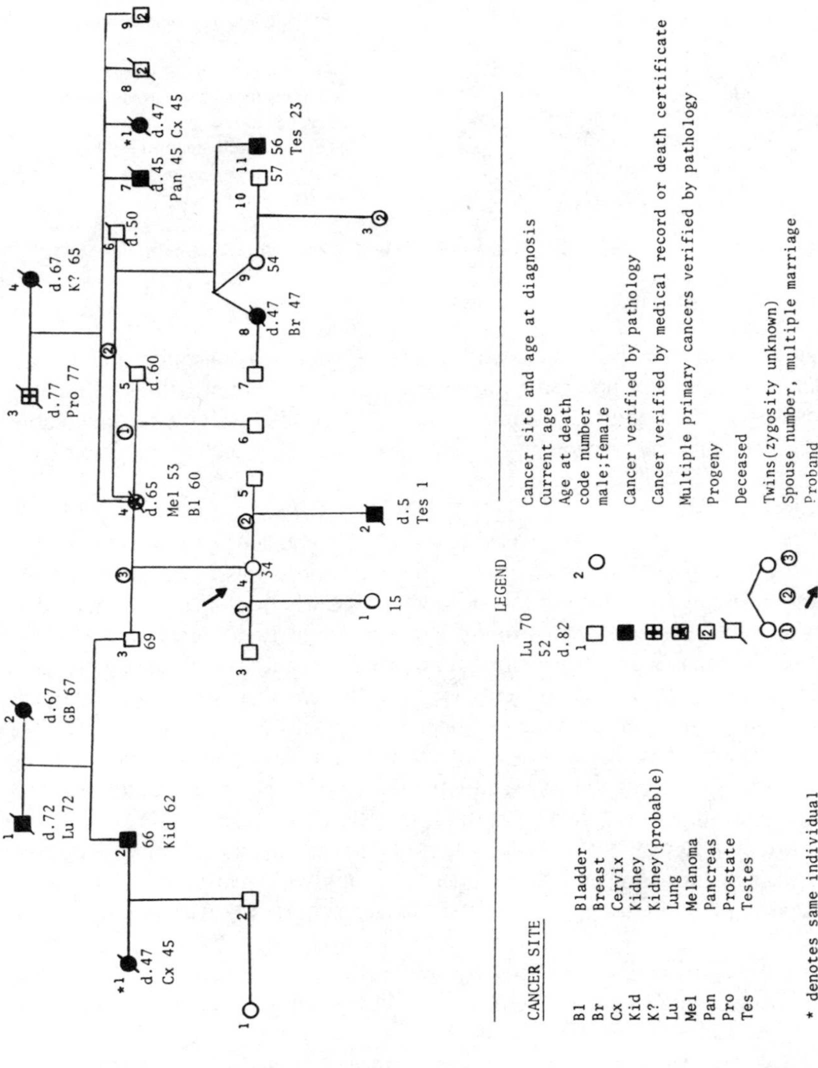

FIGURE 1. Pedigree of a cancer-prone family showing a wide spectrum of tumors, including embryonal cell carcinoma of the testicle. (From Lynch, H. T., Katz, D., Bogard, P., Voorhees, G. J., Lynch, J., and Wagner, C., *Am. J. Med.*, 78, 891, 1985. With permission.)

and bladder cancer, with particular attention being called to observations reported by Leklem and Brown[25] in a single high-risk family. However, these observations were not confirmed by Fraumeni and Thomas[23] or by Friedlander and Morrison.[37]

In summary, Kantor et al.[22] have provided an excellent case/control study showing significant (45%) increased risk for bladder cancer among persons with a family history of urinary tract cancers. Most interestingly, however, they further observed that this risk was enhanced by heavy cigarette smoking and possibly by other forms of environmental factors. While they conceded that potential differences in recall between cases and controls could have produced some bias, they nevertheless reasoned that " . . . it is unlikely that such bias would explain the interactions found between family history and environmental factors, such as cigarette smoking. Future epidemiologic studies of bladder cancer incorporating biological markers, such as the acetylator genotype, may be useful in characterizing mechanisms of familial susceptibility and interactions with environmental risk factors."[22]

We recently evaluated family history and cigarette smoking history on 49 consecutively ascertained patients with urinary bladder carcinoma and compared them with 956 consecutively ascertained patients with histologically verified cancer (all sites), all of whom were being treated in the same oncology clinics.[38] Data was collected through interviews, questionnaires, and primary medical and pathology documents. Cancer risks were compared on the basis of anatomic sites involved and with cumulative risk estimated from data in the Third National Cancer Survey. A permutation test was also employed. Significant heterogeneity of risk ($Z = 4.85$; $p < 0.02$) for bladder cancer was found in relatives of probands with bladder cancer. Significant heterogeneity or increase in risk of bladder cancer was not observed when families with lung, other smoking related cancers, and nonsmoking related cancers were analyzed. Though based on a limited number of verified bladder cancer patients, we have provided statistical evidence in support of our hypothesis that bladder cancer may have a stronger familial etiologic component than heretofore recognized.

V. OTHER HUMAN MODELS

Other human models abound for the employment of genetic epidemiology methodologies. For example, the highest known risk for cancer is that which involves a patient whose first-degree relative manifests cancer in the context of an autosomal dominantly inherited cancer syndrome. Such a first-degree relative would become a prime candidate for the study of genetic/environmental interactive processes wherein the clinician would then be armed with a high degree of precision in the predictability of the particular hereditary cancer syndrome natural history, namely, anatomic site of predilection, age of cancer onset, pattern of multiple primary cancer, and its autosomal dominant inheritance pattern.

A common theme of genetic epidemiology of cancer is that all exposed patients are not equal with respect to their cancer risk. The basic premise of heterogeneity in cancer etiology is that some patients are at higher risk for cancer than others, given any specific environmental exposure. The converse also applies, namely, given the same exposure, certain individuals have greater host resistance to cancer. An example of genetic/environmental interaction, based upon a dose-response curve (cumulative frequency distribution) relevant to quantitative aspects of cigarette smoking exposure and host susceptibility, is provided in Figure 2.

Thus, it is clear from this figure that lung cancer risk is a function of both genetic susceptibility and level of cigarette exposure wherein light smokers with strong susceptibility are more vulnerable to lung cancer development on the one hand, while on the other hand, those with low susceptibility require an inordinately greater amount of cigarette exposure for development of lung cancer. In Figure 3, we see three examples, namely, carcinoma of the stomach, breast, and childhood leukemia, wherein specific parameters in concert with family history appear to significantly modulate the risk for the respective cancers. This figure

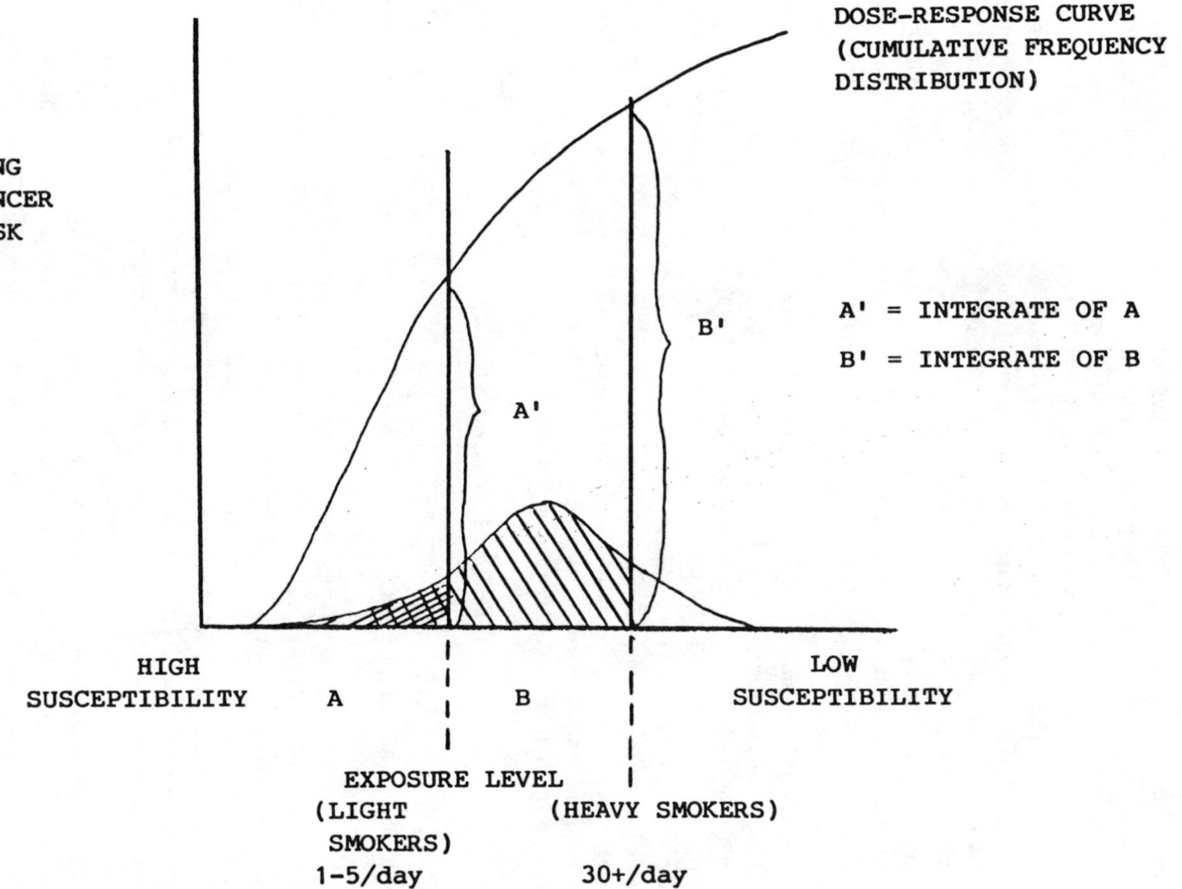

FIGURE 2. Genetic/smoking history interaction with respect to the development of lung cancer. A: Lung cancer from individuals with high genetical handicap and B: lung cancer from individuals with low genetical handicap.

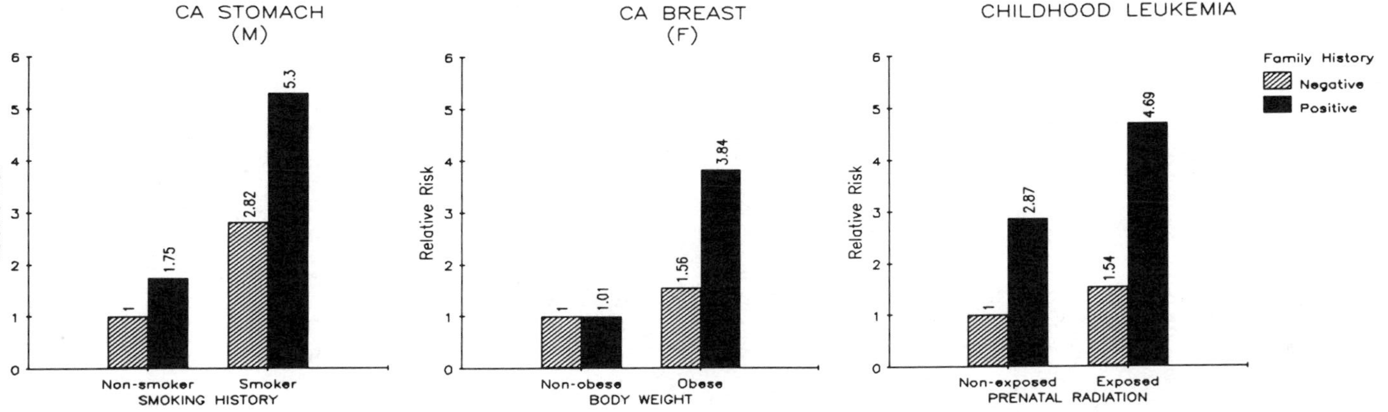

FIGURE 3. Risk for developing specific cancers based upon family history and certain risk factors. (M) = male and (F) = female.

clearly decries the need for an eclectic approach to the study of cancer risk through the embracement of as many significant intervening variables as we can possibly integrate in the search for the elucidation of cancer etiology.

VI. INDIVIDUAL VARIATION IN THE EFFECT OF SAME ENVIRONMENTAL EXPOSURES OR SAME THERAPY

This same heterogeneity can be inferred for all forms of cancer. Thus, genetic epidemiology may be able to pinpoint differing environmental and genetic factors and their interaction. Within a given patient with a specific form of cancer, a certain environmental exposure may be advantageous, while in another individual with the same histologic form of cancer, but one which is due to differing etiology, this exposure may be harmful. Extending this line of reasoning to the therapeutic arena, there may be certain forms of chemotherapy which in a given patient may be harmful, while in another, it may have potential for remission or even cure. This line of thinking will not be perceived as impossible to those knowledgeable about pharmacogenetics.

VII. GENETIC EPIDEMIOLOGY-BASED STRATEGY FOR CANCER CONTROL

Given the premise espoused in this chapter, it follows that cancer control programs must utilize genetic epidemiology as a central base since preventive measures may need to be tailored to the inherent needs of certain individuals. Looking toward the horizon, it therefore is logical that common public health measures will not be applicable to *all* members of society. Differences in susceptibility to cancer among individuals are evident; their study requires the methodologies which constitute the science of genetic epidemiology.

In conclusion, the primary objectives of genetic epidemiology of cancer pertain to the elucidation of etiology, comprehension of the mechanisms involved in the multistep process of carcinogenesis, and ultimately, cancer prevention and control. Advances in biomolecular technology are making each of these objectives realistic, as evidenced by recent developments in mapping genes, sequencing them, and identifying their products. This knowledge should then enable a better grasp upon pathogenesis, treatment design, and ultimately, understanding the manner in which environmental carcinogens perturb and alter gene expression.

We are therefore hopeful that this first book of its kind devoted to genetic epidemiology of cancer will pique the interest of our readers and elicit new information which will elucidate cancer etiology and abet its control. If this can be achieved, this book will have met its primary purpose.

VIII. NEW DEVELOPMENTS IN BIOMOLECULAR GENETICS: IMPLICATIONS FOR CANCER GENETIC EPIDEMIOLOGY

Advances in biomolecular genetics have capitalized upon the employment of DNA probes which have enabled the detection of linkage between RFLPs and a mutated locus. These efforts have led to success in the mapping of several hereditary disorders, including polycystic kidney disease, cystic fibrosis, Huntington's chorea, Duschenne's muscular dystrophy, and several heritable precancer diseases to be discussed. These advances also harbor the potential for providing clues which could lead to the elucidation of some of the most formidable problems in cancer genetic epidemiology, namely, the manner in which environmental carcinogens perturb the cancer-prone genotype.

A major concern of the clinically oriented cancer geneticist pertains to problems of heterogeneity in differing hereditary cancer syndromes, e.g., the several complementation groups in XDP, the several syndromes characterized by multiple adenomatous polyps of the colon (with or without extracolonic signs such as osteomas, epidermoid cysts, and subcutaneous fibromas), and a variable tumor spectra with problems of overlap for all of these phenotypic aspects. Many other hereditary cancer and precancer syndromes could be listed. However, it is within this very framework that biomolecular genetic technologies might be able to ''sort out'' those disorders which are heterogeneous with genotypically distinct forms vs. those with a single genotype which is etiologic for a variety of so-called overlap features of the particular syndrome.

A. Von Recklinghausen's Neurofibromatosis

Neurofibromatosis (NF) is a multisystem disease which poses an enormous challenge to the geneticist, cancer epidemiologist, oncologist, neurologist, dermatopathologist, general physician, and to society because of its immense spectrum of problems, including disfigurement. The recognizable stigmata of this disease, including cases of gross disfigurement, poses a variety of psychosocial/economic problems to the patient and society. NF is inherited as an autosomal dominant. The full spectrum of benign and malignant neoplastic lesions integral to this disorder remains elusive. Malignant degeneration of the neurofibromas occurs in 3 to 15% of cases. Sarcomas, intracranial and optic nerve gliomas, acoustic neurinomas, optic neuromas, meningiomas, and pheochromocytomas are well known to be associated lesions in this disease. Bilaterality of paired organs, i.e., acoustic neurinomas and pheochromocytomas, occur excessively in this disease.[2]

With respect to these kinds of problems, Barker et al.[39] performed linkage analysis on 15 Utah kindreds characterized by von Recklinghausen's NF. The findings showed that the gene responsible for NF is located near the centromere on chromosome 17. These kindreds did not show any significant evidence for heterogeneity. Thus, these investigators concluded that a significant portion of the NF cases were due to mutations at a single locus. They now plan additional genetic analysis in order to refine this localization with the hope that they may then be able to eventually identify and clone the defective gene responsible for NF.

Hereditary disorders such as NF must constantly be investigated in the search for new clinical or biomolecular variations consonant with syndromes which may be etiologically distinctive and which could serve as important models for genetic epidemiology research. An example is that of ''intestinal neurofibromatosis''.

B. Intestinal Neurofibromatosis

Several chapters in this book deal with hereditary colorectal cancer. These forms include those associated with polyps as well as those with an absence or paucity of polyps, namely, hereditary nonpolyposis colorectal cancer (Lynch syndromes I and II).[40] However, it is important to note that a variety of polyps may occur in the colon wherein the etiology for the majority remains elusive.

It has been well established that patients with von Recklinghausen's NF may manifest neurofibromas in the GI tract as well as in other viscera.[2,41,42] Lipton and Zuckerbrod[43] described a remarkable occurrence of neurofibromas restricted to the intestinal tract in a family. No other signs of von Recklinghausen's NF were observed in this family. The findings were present in two sisters and a daughter of one of these sisters. The investigators postulated that these cases were consistent with a new syndrome which has been previously unreported.

Heimann et al.[44] have recently described a second family wherein intestinal NF occurred in the absence of other manifestations of von Recklinghausen's. These findings were observed through three generations with only females manifesting the trait. A male was an obligate gene carrier in that his sister and mother showed isolated intestinal neurofibromas, as did his three daughters. So far as can be determined, the family reported by Lipton and Zuckerbrod[43] and the one by Heimann et al.[44] are the only ones described in the literature to date. These two families show possible differences with respect to the extent of the intestinal neurofibromas. Specifically, in the family of Lipton and Zuckerbrod,[43] neurofibromas were documented in the stomach, small intestine, and proximal large intestine. In the family reported by Heimann et al.,[44] neurofibromas were documented only in the small intestine, although the stomach and large intestine had not been investigated for detection of neurofibromas. Neurofibromas presented symptomatically with intestinal obstruction due to neurofibroma-induced intussusception. Because of the similarities between these families, Heimann et al.[44] considered these as being manifestations of the same disease, namely, ''intestinal neurofibromatosis''.

Cancer predisposition remains uncertain in intestinal NF. In the family of Lipton and Zuckerbrod,[43] members of the family showing cancer of the stomach and bowel may conceivably have had intestinal NF, although this had not been documented. However, none of the individuals with documented intestinal NF in that family manifested cancer. Cancer has not occurred, as yet, in the Heimann et al.[44] kindred.

The pattern of inheritance in these kindreds is consistent with a Mendelian dominant wherein the gene could be located on one of the autosomal chromosomes or the X chromosome. Male-to-male transmission had not been observed. The female predominance could be due to chance. On the other hand, the female predominance could be meaningful and consistent with sex influence or limitation relevant to expression with an autosomal trait or X-linkage.

Heimann et al.[44] conclude that '' . . . intestinal neurofibromatosis is of importance in that it probably represents a distinctive type of neurofibromatosis. It is of genetic importance because it would appear to reflect a different allele or a different gene locus; it is of medical and surgical importance because it predisposes to intestinal bleeding, intussusception, and intestinal obstruction; and it is of importance to cancer genetics because there is no current evidence that intestinal neurofibromatosis is associated with an increased risk of malignancy, although this is a distinct possibility.''

However, the importance of discussing this relatively ''new'' disease is the fact that NF is one of the most commonly occurring cancer genetic predisposing disorders affecting humans. Nevertheless, we know very little about the manner in which environmental factors influence genetic susceptibility in this disease. It becomes of keen interest when one finds patients/families wherein a single component of any disease, in this example, neurofibromas, may occur exclusively in a single organ system of the body, such as the GI tract.

C. An Animal Model for Human Neurofibromatosis: Transgenic Mice

Hinrichs et al.[45] discuss the human T-lymphotropic virus type I (HTLV-1) which has been associated with the development of lymphoma and leukemia in humans as well as with tropical spastic paresis and possibly multiple sclerosis. It was therefore of keen interest that the *tat* gene of HTLV-1, under control of its own long terminal repeat, has been shown to induce tumors in transgenic mice. The morphology and biologic properties of these tumors show a close resemblance to NF. This phenomenon is of particular interest when considering the high spontaneous incidence of NF, including its differing clinical and pathologic phenotypic aspects, since an unknown fraction of NF may be due to environmental factors (many of these spontaneous occurrences are undoubtedly the result of fresh germinal mutations).

In the transgenic *tat* mice, multiple tumors developed simultaneously at about 3 months of age. Furthermore, the phenotype was successfully transmitted through three generations. In addition, '' . . . the tumors arise from the nerve sheaths of peripheral nerves and are composed of perineural cells and fibroblasts. Tumor cells from these mice adapt easily to propagation in culture and continue to express the *tat* protein in significant amounts. When transplanted into nude mice, these cultured cells effectively induce tumors. Evidence of HTLV-1 infection in patients with neural and other soft tissue tumors is needed in order to establish a link between infection for this human retrovirus and von Recklinghausen's disease and other nonlymphoid tumors.''[45] Thus, we see an example of a relationship between an important virus in humans (HTLV-1) which is associated with several disorders affecting man and the production of tumors in mice which may mimic the lesions found in the most common single gene disorder (NF) which involves the nervous system of man.

D. Multiple Endocrine Neoplasia Type IIa

In the case of multiple endocrine neoplasia type IIa (MEN-IIa), an autosomal dominantly inherited syndrome characterized by medullary carcinoma of the thyroid, pheochromocytoma, and hyperparathyroidism, one is now able to screen and thereby identify carriers of this disorder by utilizing calcintonin assays with pentagastrin stimulation prior to age 40. Nevertheless, the nature and localization of the gene predisposing to MEN-IIa has heretofore been elusive. However, Mathew et al.[46] have reported linkage between the MEN-IIa locus and the interstitial retinol-binding gene which has been identified on chromosome 10p11.2-q11.2.

E. Biomolecular Facets of Retinoblastoma

In a review of recent biomolecular literature on RB, Cavanee et al.[47] discuss findings which place the retinoblastoma locus on human chromosome 13 at band q14. Karyotype investigations of individuals with RBs have revealed occasional deletion of parts of chromosome 13 wherein the common overlap occurs at band q14. They note that deletions and/or rearrangements involving 13q14 have also been demonstrated by karyotypic investigations of tumors from patients with normal constitutional karyotypes. Evaluation of the activity levels of the enzyme esterase-D in cells from patients with constitutional chromosome 13 deletion has also enabled the mapping of the structural gene for this enzyme to band q14. The evidence at the biomolecular and cytogenetic level has now become substantial for localization of the RB gene to 13q14.

These biomolecular advances are particularly cogent, given the integral genetic relationship between RB and sarcoma, as shown by Abramson et al.[48] These investigators showed that survivors of heritable RB (but not of the spontaneous variant of RB) were at markedly increased risk for the occurrence of osteosarcoma as a second primary malignant neoplastic lesion. Cavanee and Hansen[49] have proposed that this stated association between heritable RB and osteosarcoma is " . . . due to the presence of a germinal mutant allele at the RB1 locus that predisposes retinoblasts and osteoblasts to a mechanistically similar second transforming event, such as that observed in retinoblastoma. Further, we hypothesize that sporadic osteosarcoma would also share the same mechanistic route for revealing initial predisposing somatic mutations.''

Matsunaga,[50] in discussing the heritable form of RB as being caused by a point mutation or deletion at a locus on 13q14 wherein tumorigenesis is due to the loss or inactivation of both alleles at this locus, suggested that additional events may be required for carcinogenesis. However, it is clear that knowledge about environmental risk factors for the occurrence of the heritable or nonheritable RB remains elusive. It is possible that viral etiology may be responsible for nonheritable RB. Nevertheless, a thorough and extensive epidemiologic investigation showed an absence of seasonal variation in the births of some 675 patients with sporadic or unilateral cases, the majority of which may be construed as somatic mutations. In addition, there was no evidence for paternal age effect on the occurrence of some 225 sporadic bilateral cases. Paternal exposure to ionizing radiation or chemical mutagens which, conceptually, should have a cumulative effect with advancing age, also did not seem to play a major role so far as the production of the germinal mutation at the RB locus was concerned. However, family studies, as mentioned, did suggest that host resistance to genes at other loci may modify the process of tumor development upon the primary genetic change and that this phenomenon was already present in all targeted cells. Thus, unaffected gene carriers may be regarded as inherently resistant to tumor formation as opposed to those individuals who present early onset bilateral RB, and thereby are designated as most susceptible. In certain kindreds, nonexpression in the carriers may be due to chromosomal rearrangement in a balanced state. Given the presence of the germinal mutation (first hit) and the somatic mutation (second hit), in accord with Knudson's hypothesis,[51] the probability of cancer expression becomes a highly significant likelihood.

F. Familial Polyposis Coli (FPC): Biomolecular Aspects

Herrera et al.[52] observed two possible sites on chromosome 5; namely, 5q13-q15 vs. 5q15-q22, as a constitutional deletion in an FPC patient. Following this observation, Bodmer et al.[53] observed close linkage of FPC to a genetic marker mapped to the 5q21-q22 region of an alternative site for this putative deletion. Of further interest is the work of Solomon et al.,[54] who observed tumor-specific allele loss in 20% of sporadic colon cancers through analysis of two loci which were mapped to the terminal third of 5q (5q31 and 5q34-qtr). Further detail is provided in Chapter 20.

G. Lessons from Animals with Implications for Carcinogenesis in Humans: The Estrogen/DES Story

There is little doubt about the etiologic role of estrogen and diethylstilbestrol (DES) in the production of specific forms of cancer in man; i.e., estrogen and its link to endometrial carcinoma, and DES in the case of clear cell adenocarcinoma of the vagina and/or uterine cervix.[55] DES is of especial importance in that it is the first example of transplacental carcinogenesis in humans, a phenomenon which has been evidenced by an excess of clear cell adenocarcinoma of the vagina and cervix in exposed women. This association was first reported in 1970[56] and 1971.[57] The subject was more extensively reviewed in 1977[58] and in 1985.[55]

Soberingly, this tragedy could have been prevented had the pharmaceutical industry and governmental regulatory bodies paid greater attention to the voluminous documentation of DES carcinogenesis at the infrahuman level.[55] With specific relevance to the treatise of this book, the prodigious work on both estrogen and subsequently DES in animals was shown to clearly involve genetic epidemiologic strategies. As will be seen, research into estrogen and DES carcinogenesis became more efficient and productive when highly inbred animal strains were utilized for these voluminous experiments.[55] Thus, following these efforts, it became clear that the study and comprehension of etiology and carcinogenesis mandated the embracing of *both* genetic and environmental events. Their orchestration is at the heart of the discipline of cancer genetic epidemiology.

Hertz[59] has reviewed the history dealing with the relationship between estrogens, with particular attention given to DES, and cancer association. This review disclosed a long-standing documentation of the etiologic relationship of estrogen to cancer. This knowledge emanated from the work of Beatson[60] in 1896, in which he showed that ovariectomy ameliorated the clinical manifestations of breast cancer in women. In 1919, Loeb[61] identified the ovarian dependence of breast cancer in mice. Subsequently, estrogen administration was found to be etiologically linked to cancer involving eight organ sites (breast, cervix, endometrium, ovary, pituitary, testicle, kidney, and bone marrow) in five species of animals (mice, rats, rabbits, hamsters, and dogs).[59] This background clearly indicated prolific activity in experimental carcinogenesis in the 1930s and 1940s. It was necessarily restricted to estrogen compounds during that time frame since DES was first synthesized by Dodds and his associates in 1938.[62] The history of DES was reviewed by Dodds in 1965.[63]

In commenting on all available evidence at the infrahuman level, Hertz stated that he knew of " . . . no other pharmacological effect so readily reproducible in such a wide variety of species which had been generally regarded as potentially inapplicable to man."[59]

It is important that the estrogen-cancer link in animals be cast in proper historical perspective since it clearly should have provided important clues to the potential carcinogenicity of DES. Indeed, on the strength of these early estrogen studies, the search for carcinogenic effect of DES should have been given the highest possible priority when one considers the pharmacologic, biochemical, and physiologic similarities between estrogen and DES.[59]

Some of the earliest investigators to pursue this line of reasoning were Shimkin and Grady,[64] who began their carcinogenesis studies of DES the same year that the compound was discovered (1938) and published their findings in 1940. They identified the carcinogenic potency of both estrone and DES in C3H mice, a strain known to have been prone to mammary cancer. They also reviewed numerous papers on DES, uniformly confirming its estrogenic activity and affirming that it was similar to the natural estrogens in all its diverse effects. In demonstrating the carcinogenic potency of DES and estrone in susceptible (C3H) mice, they concluded that " . . . stilbestrol possesses the property common to all estrogens of eliciting mammary carcinoma in mice of susceptible strains . . . "[64] They also discussed the development of mammary carcinogenesis in mice which were treated with massive doses of natural estrogens. While documenting the carcinogenicity of estrogens in mice, Shimkin[65] also defined experimental procedures and emphasized the importance of host factors in the process.

In 1939, Gardner[66] reviewed mammary carcinogenesis in genetically susceptible mice. In mice strains with low incidences of spontaneous mammary cancer, few mammary tumors were produced by estrogen administration, while the converse held in strains (C3H) susceptible to mammary cancer. Of interest was the occurrence of mammary cancer in 11 of 12 *male* mice from a susceptible strain following estrogen administration. On the other hand, tumor development following estrogen administration occurred in excess in males and females from two strains where the incidence of spontaneous neoplasms in the untreated females was less than 2%.

Carcinogenicity of stilbestrol had been concurrently advanced by Lacassagne[67] and Geschickter[68] who produced mammary cancer in C3H mice and in rats, respectively. These investigators were also interested in the genital tract. However, no definite invasive lesions were observed in the cervix or vagina. However, in both stilbestrol- and estrone-treated mice, the epithelium was hyperplastic, well-stratified, and usually heavily keratinized when compared with that in untreated animals. Mitotic figures were numerous and there were many defined prickle cells. The cells of the basal layers were usually hyperchromatic, and frequently some disturbance of polarity was noted. The cervical and vaginal stroma in treated animals was usually edematous and, in two mice receiving large doses of stilbestrol, there were large hyaline areas similar to those noted in uterine horns.

In 1938, Gardner et al.[69] described uterine cervical carcinoma following estrogen administration in mice. In 1956, Gardner and Ferrigno[70] described unusual varieties of cancers of the uterine horns among estrogen-treated mice. These included subserosal uterine adenomas, adenocarcinomas, and epidermoid carcinomas. The subserosal neoplasms were believed to have arisen either from proliferation of Mullerian rests persisting along the serosa, possibly from the serosa per se, or from endometriosis. In 1959, Gardner[71] observed a high incidence of uterine cervical carcinoma, and more frequently, vaginal epidermoid carcinomas, in mice who had been exposed to intravaginal pellets of stilbestrol-cholesterol. Placebos did not incite vaginal cancers in these mice.

Another classic paper on the subject of estrogens and cancer in animals was that of Loeb published in 1940.[72] Again, the importance of heredity was stressed, but drug dosage effect was also clearly recognized, i.e., " . . . a strain possessing a strong tendency to the development of mammary gland cancer shows a reaction to a relatively small amount of estrogen similar to that which a strain with a lesser hereditary tendency shows to a larger quantity of estrogen. An added amount of stimulation by estrogens can compensate for a certain difference in hereditary predisposition.'' This is a crucial commentary supporting our stated hypothesis, since by using larger doses in less susceptible strains, the same carcinogenic endpoint can be achieved. This observation clearly counters the claims of those investigators who found extrapolations from inbred animal strains to be inappropriate. Loeb[72] also reviewed data dealing with estrogen administration to specific strains leading to the production of carcinoma of the cervix. In addition to carcinoma or precancerous lesions in the cervix, he also noted that corresponding changes may be induced over wide areas of the vagina. ''The formation or lack of formation of cancerous changes depends upon quantitative differences in tissue response, and these differences may apply to individuals, strains, and species. In the latter, they are, as a rule, greater than between different strains of the same species, and these species differences apply to tissue reactions in general.''[72]

In summary, Loeb[72] provided an extensive review of the literature supporting a direct association between hormone administration (estrogens and stilbestrol) and cancer production in susceptible strains. While emphasis was given to mammary carcinoma, carcinoma of the cervix and vagina in susceptible strains was also discussed. These findings therefore show a spectrum of estrogen and DES-induced tumors in animals.

Hertz[59] noted that substantial skepticism was raised about the extrapolation of carcinogenesis studies in nonprimate species to primates (and ultimately, humans) because of the failure to induce malignant transformation by estrogen in monkeys. However, Gardner[66] noted that while cancer had not been observed in monkeys, there were changes in the tissues of monkeys following estrogen administration: (1) many mitotic figures in the breast of one monkey following prolonged estrogen treatment, (2) proliferation of the mammary ducts and epithelium occurred in a Rhesus monkey after injection of small amounts of estrone. The ductal epithelium was described as being hyperplastic and poorly organized and was compared to clinical gynecomastia, (3) cystic hyperplasia of the endometrium was described following daily estrogen injections in monkeys, and (4) epithelial metaplasia of the uterine cervical glands occurred in monkeys following daily administration of estrogen for 16 to 90 days. '' . . . Histologically, precancerous areas developed when the cervix was subjected to trauma at the same time.'' Attention was also given to the morphologic similarity of the cervix of the monkey to that of the human being.[66]

These points regarding estrogen effects in the breasts, endometrium, and cervix of monkeys, noted as early as the 1930s, are extremely cogent. The fact that these data were extensively reviewed[66] suggests that physicians and scientists, particularly those connected with the FDA and pharmaceutical firms producing estrogens, and subsequently DES, should have been cognizant of these facts. The phylogenetic closeness of monkeys to humans should have fueled immediate concern with respect to DES and its potential cancer association in humans.

Many years later, investigations of squirrel monkeys with DES administration resulted in malignant uterine mesotheliomas.[73] These findings are remarkable in that seven of ten squirrel monkeys (*Saimiri sciureus*) developed malignant uterine mesotheliomas following prolonged DES administration. It was of interest that the degree of development of the lesions was in direct proportion to the duration of treatment. Another finding of interest was the short latency period on tumor induction. Specifically, malignant lesions occurred in one animal only 5 months after implantation of DES, while extensive lesions were observed in animals treated for 11 and 14 months. The three remaining animals manifested extragenital serosal lesions involving the adrenal glands, spleen, and mesentery. It was concluded that DES is carcinogenic in the squirrel monkey, although the mechanism of DES carcinogenicity could not be proven to be due to its estrogenic activity.

The animal studies of estrogen and subsequently, DES, carcinogenesis focused heavily on breast and uterine cervical carcinoma, although other lesions were identified in several differing animal strains. In context with this information, Lynch and Reich,[55] with due consideration to latency effects, have postulated that the tumor spectrum in man will be more extensive than the documented examples of DES-induced clear cell carcinoma of the vagina and uterine cervix. For example, Greenberg et al.[74] have shown an excess of carcinoma of the breast among a cohort of mothers who had taken DES for antiabortifacient purposes. The potential carcinogenic effects of this drug experience in humans, involving both females and males, is legion.[55]

We have attempted to address a spectrum of genetic epidemiology cancer problems in this introductory chapter in order to provide the reader with an appreciation of the approach to this discipline which we are expounding throughout this book. We are deeply grateful to our colleagues who have focused upon individual problems which, in many cases, have formed the basis of their entire research careers.

ADDENDUM

While this manuscript was in press, three important papers were published involving studies on the retinoblastoma (Rb) gene in human breast cancer and small cell lung cancer (SCLC).[75-77] These studies showed that SCLC and breast cancer have internal structural changes in the Rb gene and abnormalities in Rb gene expression. The finding of abnormalities of the Rb gene in SCLC and breast cancer suggest that this gene may be involved in the pathogenesis of some nonocular cancers. Both of these common adult malignancies carry other genetic changes, such as chromosome 3p deletions in SCLC, suggesting that several genetic alterations are involved in expression of the malignant phenotype.

There is no established clinical association between Rb and SCLC or breast cancer. This suggests therefore that mutations at the Rb locus in these common adult cancers occur as somatic events. SCLC and breast cancer are associated with environmental factors such as cigarette smoking and dietary intake, suggesting that carcinogen exposure from environmental sources may generate and increased mutation rate in the bronchus or breast. Some genes, such as the Rb gene locus, may be susceptible to mutation and thus may become inactivated from carcinogen exposures in these organ sites. Future molecular studies indicating genetic changes, such as at the Rb locus in SCLC and in breast cancer, should be excellent model systems for studying the interaction of genetic and environmental factors that collectively result in expression of human cancers.

REFERENCES

1. **Lynch, H. T.,** *Cancer Genetics,* Charles C Thomas, Springfield, IL, 1976.
2. **Lynch, H. T. and Fusaro, R. M.,** *Cancer-Associated Genodermatoses,* Van Nostrand Reinhold, New York, 1982.
3. **Lynch, P. M. and Lynch, H. T.,** *Colon Cancer Genetics,* Van Nostrand Reinhold, New York, 1985.
4. **Lynch, H. T.,** *Genetics and Breast Cancer,* Van Nostrand Reinhold, New York, 1981.
5. **Guirgis, H. A. and Lynch, H. T.,** *Genetics, Biomarkers, and Cancer,* Van Nostrand Reinhold, New York, 1985.
6. **Harris, C. C.,** *Genetic Differences in Chemical Carcinogenesis,* CRC Press, Boca Raton, Fl., 1980.
7. **Harris, C. C., Autrup, H., and Stoner, G.,** Metabolism of benzo(a)pyrene by cultured human tissues and cells, in *Polycyclic Hydrocarbons and Cancer: Chemistry, Molecular Biology, and Environment,* Ts'O, P. O. and Gelboin, H. V., Eds., Academic Press, New York, 1980, 331.
8. **Jung, E. G., Bohnert, E., and Fischer, E.,** Heterogeneity of xeroderma pigmentosum (XP): variability and stability within and between the complementation groups C, D, E, I, and variants, *Photodermatology,* 3, 125, 1986.
9. **Lynch, H. T., Fusaro, R. M., and Johnson, J. A.,** Xeroderma pigmentosum: complementation group C and malignant melanoma, *Arch. Dermatol.,* 120, 175, 1984.

10. **Aurias, A., Antoine, J. L., Assathiany, R., Odievre, M., and Dutrillaux, B.,** Radiation sensitivity of Bloom's syndrome lymphocytes during S and G_2 phases, *Cancer Genet. Cytogenet.*, 16, 131, 1985.
11. **Zbinden, I. and Cerutti, M.,** Near-ultraviolet sensitivity of skin fibroblasts of patients with Bloom's syndrome, *Biochem. Biophys. Res. Commun.*, 98, 579, 1981.
12. **Draper, G. J., Snader, B. M., and Kingston, J. E.,** Second primary neoplasms in patients with retinoblastoma, *Br. J. Cancer,* 53, 661, 1986.
13. **Strong, L. C.,** Theories of pathogenesis: mutation and cancer, in *Genetics of Human Cancer,* Mulvihill, J. J., Miller, R. W., and Fraumeni, J. F., Eds., Raven Press, New York, 1977, 401.
14. **Taylor, A. M. R.,** Cytogenetics of ataxia telangiectasia, in *Ataxia-Telangiectasia — A Cellular and Molecular Link Between Cancer Neuropathology and Immune Deficiency,* Bridges, B. A. and Harnden, D. G., Eds., John Wiley & Sons, New York, 1982, 53.
15. **Smith, P. J., Greene, M. H., Devlin, D. A., McKeen, E. A., and Paterson, M. C.,** Abnormal sensitivity to UV-radiation in cultured skin fibroblasts from patients with hereditary cutaneous malignant melanoma and dysplastic nevus syndrome, *Int. J. Cancer,* 30, 39, 1982.
16. **Lynch, H. T., Fusaro, R. M., Pester, J., Oosterhuis, J. A., Went, L. N., Rumke, Ph., Neering, H., and Lynch, J. F.,** Tumor spectrum in the FAMMM syndrome, *Br. J. Cancer,* 44, 553, 1981.
17. **Oosterhuis, J. A., Went, L. N., and Lynch, H. T.,** Primary choroidal and cutaneous melanomas, bilateral choroidal melanomas, and familial occurrence of melanomas, *Br. J. Ophthalmol.*, 66, 230, 1982.
18. **Lehmann, A. R., Kirk-Bell, S., Arlett, C. F., Paterson, M. C., Lohman, P. H. M., deWeerd-Kasteleini, E. A., and Bootsma, D.,** Xeroderma pigmentosum cells with normal levels of excision repair have a defect in DNA synthesis after UV-irradiation, *Proc. Natl. Acad. Sci. U.S.A.*, 72, 219, 1975.
19. **Kopf, A. W., Gold, R. S., Rogers, G. S., Hennessey, N. P., Friedman, R. J., Rigel, D. S., and Levenstein, M.,** Relationship of lumbosacral nevi to sun exposure in dysplastic nevus syndrome, *Arch. Dermatol.*, 122, 1003, 1986.
20. **Smith, P. J., Greene, M. H., Adams, D., and Paterson, M. C.,** Abnormal responses to the carcinogen 4-nitroquinolone 1-oxide of cultured fibroblasts from patients with dysplastic nevus syndrome and hereditary cutaneous malignant melanoma, *Carcinogenesis,* 4, 911, 1983.
21. **Lynch, H. T., Katz, D., Bogard, P., Voorhees, G. J., Lynch, J., and Wagner, C.,** Familial embryonal carcinoma in a cancer-prone kindred, *Am. J. Med.*, 78, 891, 1985.
22. **Kantor, A. F., Hartge, P., Hoover, R. N., and Fraumeni, J. F.,** Familial and environmental interactions in bladder cancer risk, *Int. J. Cancer,* 35, 703, 1985.
23. **Fraumeni, J. F. and Thomas, L. B.,** Malignant bladder tumors in a man and his three sons, *JAMA,* 201, 507, 1967.
24. **Benton, B. and Henderson, B. E.,** Environmental exposure and bladder cancer in young males, *J. Natl. Cancer Inst.*, 51, 269, 1973.
25. **Leklem, J. E. and Brown, R. R.,** Abnormal tryptophan metabolism in a family with a history of bladder cancer, *J. Natl. Cancer Inst.*, 56, 1101, 1976.
26. **Lynch, H. T., Walzak, M. P., Fried, R., Domina, A. H., and Lynch, J. F.,** Familial factors in bladder carcinoma, *J. Urol.*, 122, 458, 1979.
27. **Mahboubi, A. O., Ahlvin, R. C., and Mahboubi, E. O.,** Familial aggregation of urothelial carcinoma, *J. Urol.*, 126, 691, 1981.
28. **Marchetto, D., Li, F. P., and Henson, D. P.,** Familial carcinoma of ureters and other genitourinary organs, *J. Urol.*, 130, 772, 1983.
29. **McCollough, D. L., Lamm, D. L., McLaughlin, A. P., and Gittes, R. F.,** Familial transitional cell carcinoma of the bladder, *J. Urol.*, 113, 629, 1975.
30. **Purtilo, D. T., McCarthy, B., Yang, J. P. S., and Friedell, G. H.,** Familial urinary bladder cancer, *Semin. Oncol.*, 6, 254, 1979.
31. **Sharma, S. K., Bapna, B. C., and Singh, S. M.,** Familial profile of transitional cell carcinoma, *Br. J. Urol.*, 48, 442, 1976.
32. **Cartwright, R. A.,** Genetic association with bladder cancer, *Br. Med. J.*, 2, 792, 1979.
33. **Cartwright, R. A., Glasham, R. W., Rogers, H. J., Ahmad, R. A., Barham-Hall, D., Higgins, E., and Kahn, M. A.,** Role of *N*-acetyltransferase in bladder carcinogenesis: a pharmacogenetic epidemiological approach to bladder cancer, *Lancet,* ii, 842, 1982.
34. **Lower, G. M.,** Concepts in causality: chemically-induced human urinary bladder cancer, *Cancer,* 49, 1056, 1982.
35. **Lower, G. M., Nilsson, T., Nelson, C. E., Wolf, H., Gamsky, T. E., and Bryan, G. T.,** *N*-Acetyltransferase phenotype and risk in urinary bladder cancer: approaches in molecular epidemiology. Preliminary results in Sweden and Denmark, *Environ. Health Perspect.*, 29, 71, 1979.
36. **Evans, D. A. P., Eze, L. C., and Whibley, E. J.,** The association of the slow acetylator phenotype with bladder cancer, *J. Med. Genet.*, 20, 330, 1983.
37. **Friedlander, E. and Morrison, A. S.,** Urinary tryptophan metabolites and cancer of the bladder in humans, *J. Natl. Cancer Inst.*, 67, 347, 1970.

38. **Lynch, H. T., Kimberling, W. J., Lynch, J. F., and Brennan, K.,** Familial bladder cancer in an oncology clinic, *Cancer Genet. Cytogenet.*, 27, 161, 1987.
39. **Barker, D., Wright, E., Nguyen, K., et al.,** Gene for von Recklinghausen's neurofibromatosis is in the pericentromeric region of chromosome 17, *Science*, 236, 1100, 1987.
40. **Lynch, H. T., Kimberling, W. J., Schuelke, G. S., et al.,** Hereditary nonpolyposis colorectal cancer. I and II, *Cancer*, 56, 934, 1985.
41. **Riccardi, V. M.,** Von Recklinghausen's neurofibromatosis, *N. Engl. J. Med.*, 305, 1617, 1981.
42. **Sivak, M. V., Sullivan, B. H., and Farmer, R. G.,** Neurogenic tumors of the small intestine: review of the literature and report of a case with endoscopic removal, *Gastroenterology*, 68, 374, 1975.
43. **Lipton, S. and Zuckerbrod, M.,** Familial enteric neurofibromatosis, *Med. Times*, 94, 544, 1966.
44. **Heimann, R., Verhest, A., Verschraegen, J., Grosjean, W., Draps, J. P., and Hecht, F.,** Hereditary intestinal neurofibromatosis. I. A distinctive genetic disease, in press.
45. **Hinrichs, S. H., Nerenberg, M., Reynolds, R. K., Khoury, G., and Jay, G.,** A transgenic mouse model for human neurofibromatosis, *Science*, 237, 1340, 1987.
46. **Mathew, C. G., Chin, K. S., Easton, D. F., et al.,** A linked genetic marker for multiple endocrine neoplasia type 2A on chromosome 10, *Nature*, 328, 527, 1987.
47. **Cavanee, W. K., Murphree, A. L., Shull, M. M., et al.,** Prediction of familial predisposition to retinoblastoma, *N. Engl. J. Med.*, 314, 1201, 1986.
48. **Abramson, D. H., Ellsworth, R. M., Kitchin, F. D., and Tung, G.,** Second nonocular tumors in retinoblastoma survivors: are they radiation-induced?, *Ophthalmology*, 91, 1351, 1984.
49. **Cavanee, W. K. and Hansen, M. F.,** Molecular genetics of human familial cancer, *Cold Spring Harbor Symp. Quant. Biol.*, 51, 829, 1986.
50. **Matsunaga, E.,** Genetics and epidemiology of retinoblastoma, *Gan No Reinsho*, 33 (Suppl. 5), 507, 1987 (in Japanese with English abstract).
51. **Knudson, A. G., Hethcote, H. W., and Brown, B. W.,** Mutation and childhood cancer: a probablistic model for the incidence of retinoblastoma, *Proc. Natl. Acad. Sci. U.S.A.*, 72, 5116, 1975.
52. **Herrera, L., Kakati, S., Gibas, L., et al.,** Gardner's syndrome in a man with an interstitial deletion of 5q, *Am. J. Med. Genet.*, 25, 473, 1986.
53. **Bodmer, W. F., Bailey, C. J., Bodmer, J., et al.,** Localization of the gene for familial adenomatous polyposis on chromosome 5, *Nature*, 328, 614, 1987.
54. **Solomon, E., Voss, R., Hall, V., et al.,** Chromosome 5 allele loss in human colorectal carcinomas, *Nature*, 328, 616, 1987.
55. **Lynch, H. T. and Reich, J. W.,** Diethylstilbestrol, genetics, teratogenesis, and tumor spectrum in humans, *Med. Hypoth.*, 16, 315, 1985.
56. **Herbst, A. L. and Scully, R. E.,** Adenocarcinoma of the vagina in adolescence: a report of seven cases including six clear cell carcinomas (so-called mesonephromas), *Cancer*, 25, 745, 1970.
57. **Herbst, A. L., Ulfelder, H., and Poskanzer, D. C.,** Adenocarcinoma of the vagina, association of maternal stilbestrol therapy with tumor appearance in young women, *N. Engl. J. Med.*, 284, 878, 1971.
58. **Herbst, A. L., Cole, P., Colton, T., Robboy, S. J., and Scully, R. E.,** Age-incidence and risk of diethylstilbestrol-related clear cell adenocarcinoma of the vagina and cervix, *Am. J. Obstet. Gynecol.*, 128, 43, 1977.
59. **Hertz, R.,** The estrogen-cancer hypothesis with special emphasis on DES, in *Origins of Human Cancer*, Vol. 4, Hiatt, H. H., Watson, J. D., and Winsten, J. A., Eds., Cold Spring Harbor Conference on Cell Proliferation, Cold Spring Harbor Laboratory, Cold Spring Harbor, N.Y., 1977, 1665.
60. **Beatson, G. T.,** On the treatment of inoperable cases of carcinoma of the mammae, *Lancet*, ii, 104, 1896.
61. **Loeb, L.,** Further investigations on the origin of tumors in mice, *J. Med. Res.*, 40, 477, 1919.
62. **Dodds, E. C., Goldberg, L., Lawson, W., and Robinson, R.,** Oestrogenic activity of certain synthetic compounds, *Nature*, 141, 247, 1938.
63. **Dodds, E. C.,** Stilboestrol and after, *Sci. Basis Med. Annu. Rev.*, 1, 1965.
64. **Shimkin, M. B. and Grady, H. G.,** Carcinogenic potency of stilbestrol and estrone in strain C3H mice, *J. Natl. Cancer Inst.*, 1, 119, 1940.
65. **Shimkin, M. B.,** Biologic testing of carcinogens. I. Subcutaneous injection technique, *J. Natl. Cancer Inst.*, 1, 211, 1940.
66. **Gardner, W. U.,** Estrogens in carcinogenesis, *Arch. Pathol.*, 27, 138, 1939.
67. **Lacassagne, A.,** Apparition d'adenocarinomes mammaires chez des souris males traitees par une substance oestrogene synthetique, *C. R. Soc. Biol.*, 129, 641, 1938.
68. **Geschickter, C. T.,** Mammary carcinoma in rat with metastasis induced by estrogen, *Science*, 89, 35, 1939.
69. **Gardner, W. U., Allen, E., Smith, G. M., and Strong, L. C.,** Carcinoma in the cervix of mice receiving estrogens, *JAMA*, 110, 1182, 1938.
70. **Gardner, W. U. and Ferrigno, M.,** Unusual neoplastic lesions of the uterine horns of estrogen-treated mice, *J. Natl. Cancer Inst.*, 17, 601, 1956.

71. **Gardner, W. U.,** Carcinoma of the uterine cervix and upper vagina: induction under experimental conditions in mice, *Ann. N.Y. Acad. Sci.*, 75, 543, 1959.
72. **Loeb, L.,** The significance of hormones in the origin of cancer, *J. Natl. Cancer Inst.*, 1, 169, 1940.
73. **McClure, H. M. and Graham, C. E.,** Malignant uterine mesotheliomas in squirrel monkeys following diethylstilbestrol administration, *Lab. Anim. Sci.*, 23, 493, 1973.
74. **Greenberg, E. R., Barnes, A. B., Ressebuie, L., et al.,** Breast cancer in mothers given diethylstilbestrol in pregnancy, *N. Engl. J. Med.*, 311, 1393, 1984.
75. **Harbour, J. W., Lai, S. L., Whang-Peng, J., Gazdar, A. F., Minna, J. D., and Kaye, F. J.,** Abnormalities in structure and expression of the human retinoblastoma gene in SCLC, *Science,* 241, 353, 1988.
76. **T'Ang, A., Varley, J. M., Chakraborty, S., Murphree, A. L., and Fung, Y. K. T.,** Structural rearrangement of the retinoblastoma gene in human breast carcinoma, *Science,* 242, 263, 1988.
77. **Lee, E. Y. H. P., To, H., Shew, J. Y., Bookstein, R., Scully, P., and Lee, W. H.,** Inactivation of the retinoblastoma susceptibility gene in human breast cancers, *Science,* 241, 218, 1988.

Chapter 2

BIOSTATISTICAL METHODS FOR THE FAMILIAL STUDY OF CANCER

Varghese T. George and R. C. Elston

TABLE OF CONTENTS

I. INTRODUCTION

Unlike diseases that are largely environmental in causation such as tuberculosis, or diseases that have a simple genetic etiology such as phenylketonuria, many of the common cancers exhibit a familial aggregation, or familiality, for which the underlying mechanism is not yet known. Familiality can be caused by common environmental risk factors and/or by susceptibility genes segregating in particular families, with different implications for disease control and prevention. The variable age of onset of the disease adds further complexity to the method of analysis. We require statistical models that incorporate this variable age of onset as well as both genetic and nongenetic types of variation, familial and nonfamilial, to investigate hereditary factors in the etiology of cancer.

In this chapter we shall first discuss how logistic regression, which is now a standard statistical tool in epidemiological studies,[15] can be used to detect familial aggregation, and how it can be adapted to incorporate information on age of onset. We shall describe two classes of age of onset distributions that are very flexible in that they can accommodate a wide range of skewness and kurtosis, and that allow the easy incorporation of environmental covariates into the model. Finally we shall indicate how logistic regression analysis can be extended to allow for the segregation of major genes, following the regressive logistic models of Bonney,[3] and its relation to previously proposed methods of segregation analysis for diseases with variable age of onset.

Families that are sampled for a study of familial aggregation, or to undergo genetic segregation analysis, are usually ascertained via probands. In other words, we first obtain a sample of probands (persons with the disease of interest) and, together with each proband, we sample a predetermined set of his or her relatives. Thus, each family comes into the sample because it contains at least one proband, and this must be taken into account in the analysis. We shall assume that each family contains exactly one proband, this being a situation that simplifies the analysis of familial aggregation. The presence of more than one proband in a family due to "multiple ascertainment" necessitates special methods.[8]

II. LOGISTIC REGRESSION

Consider all the individuals in the data who are not probands, the phenotype of the i-th individual being denoted y_i. We shall assume the phenotype is classified by a simple dichotomy, "affected" or "unaffected", so that y_i can take on only one of two values, say 1 and 0, respectively. On each individual i we also have a set of k predictor variables, say $\mathbf{x}_i = (x_{i1}, x_{i2}, \ldots, x_{ik})$, which may include sex, relationship of the individual to the proband, and other covariates such as age at examination.

Because of the dichotomous nature of the phenotype y_i, a logistic regression model can be used to analyze the relationship of the predictor variables to cancer incidence. Define

$$p_{1i} = \Pr(y_i = 1|\mathbf{x}_i) \quad \text{and} \quad p_{0i} = 1 - p_{1i}$$

In logistic regression analysis this conditional probability is modeled by the logistic function as

$$p_{1i} = \frac{\exp\left(\beta + \sum_{j=1}^{k} \beta_j x_{ij}\right)}{1 + \exp\left(\beta + \sum_{j=1}^{k} \beta_j x_{ij}\right)}$$

and the log odds of the disease, given $\mathbf{x}_i$, is

Table 1
DEFINITION OF SEVEN VARIABLES TO ALLOW FOR SEX-SPECIFIC RELATIONSHIPS (SPOUSE AND FIRST DEGREE) TO PROBAND

Relationship to proband	Variable						
	x_1	x_2	x_3	x_4	x_5	x_6	x_7
Father	1	0	0	0	0	0	0
Mother	0	1	0	0	0	0	0
Son	0	0	1	0	0	0	0
Daughter	0	0	0	1	0	0	0
Brother	0	0	0	0	1	0	0
Sister	0	0	0	0	0	1	0
Male spouse	0	0	0	0	0	0	1
Female spouse	0	0	0	0	0	0	0

$$\log\left(\frac{p_{1i}}{p_{0i}}\right) = \beta + \sum_{j=1}^{k} \beta_j x_{ij}$$

Thus β is the log odds of the disease for an individual with a baseline (i.e., $\mathbf{x}_i = 0$) set of predictor variables, and β_j measures the change in log odds for one unit change in x_{ij}.

In usual logistic regression analysis it is assumed that all the observed y_i are independent conditional on x_i, so that the likelihood is of the form ${}_i\Pi p_{1i}\ {}_h\Pi h p_{0h}$, where i indexes an affected individual and h indexes an unaffected individual. This likelihood is maximized to obtain maximum likelihood estimates of the parameters β and β_j. We shall comment later on the implicit assumption that, conditional on the $\mathbf{x}_i$, the y_i are independent.

To illustrate how logistic regression can be used to analyze familial aggregation, let us suppose that we have pedigrees of three generations, each comprising (apart from the proband) the proband's parents, sibs, spouse, and children. Then for each nonproband individual in the sample we can build a "full" model that allows for an interaction between relationship to proband and sex by incorporating the seven sex-specific variables indicated in Table 1. Thus, for the father of a proband, we have $x_1 = 1$ and all the other seven x's are zero; for the mother of a proband, $x_2 = 1$ and all the other x's are zero, and so on. Note, however, that for the female spouse of a proband all the x's are zero, so that this is taken to be the baseline relationship. The parameter β is thus the log odds of the disease for a female spouse of a proband, $\beta + \beta_1$ is the log odds of the disease for the father of a proband, $\beta + \beta_2$ is the log odds for the mother of a proband, and so on. The model may include other covariates as well, but we shall not concern ourselves here with other such variables.

We might start the analysis by testing the hypothesis of no interaction between sex and relationship to proband. Under this hypothesis sex can be specified by a single variable (e.g., x_1), which takes on the value 1 or 0 depending on whether the person is male or female, and relationship to proband can be specified by the three variables indicated in Table 2. The hypothesis of no interaction between relationship to the proband and sex can then be tested by calculating the likelihood ratio statistic 2(maximum $\log_e$ likelihood of the full model minus maximum $\log_e$ likelihood of the restricted model), and comparing it to the chi-square distribution with three degrees of freedom.

To test whether the parental effect is the same as the child effect, (which, in the absence of specific environmental, age, or secular effects, would be the case for a genetic etiology), we combine parent and children in Table 2 into one category, defining variables x_2 and x_3 appropriately. Twice the difference in maximum $\log_e$ likelihoods under this hypothesis and that defined by the variables in Table 2 would then be compared to the chi-square distribution

Table 2
DEFINITION OF THREE VARIABLES TO ALLOW FOR SPOUSE AND FIRST-DEGREE RELATIONSHIPS TO PROBAND

Relationship to proband	Variable		
	x_2	x_3	x_4
Parent	1	0	0
Child	0	1	0
Sib	0	0	1
Spouse	0	0	0

with one degree of freedom. One can similarly test whether the risk to a sib is the same as that to a parent or child, by combining all three categories into a single variable, and comparing the maximum $\log_e$ likelihood to one of the previous $\log_e$ likelihoods. This test would not be expected to be significant if there is an underlying additive genetic mechanism on the logistic scale (whether single gene or polygenic), provided any environmental and/or age effects are nonexistent or properly allowed for by other covariates. More generally, for larger pedigree structures, a genetic mechanism that is additive on the logistic scale is modeled by a single x-variable that is equal to the individual's coefficient of relationship to the proband. For example, $x = 1/2$ for a first degree relative (parent, child, or sib), $x = 1/4$ for a second degree relative (grandparent, grandchild, half sib, uncle, aunt, nephew, or niece) and $x = 0$ for a spouse.

Ooi et al.[18] used logistic regression analysis in a manner similar to that described here to compare the odds of lung cancer for relatives of probands to the odds for the same type of relatives of controls. Thus, they obtained odds ratios for parents of probands vs. parents of controls, and for sibs of probands vs. sibs of controls. Such a study design is an ideal one if there is no systematic difference in the quality of the data gathered on the two sets of relatives, proband relatives vs. control relatives.

In large samples, any hypothesis regarding the effects of a set of predictor variables can be tested by comparing the test statistic $2(l_1 - l_0)$ with the appropriate percentile of a chi-square distribution, where l_0 is the maximum $\log_e$ likelihood under the given null hypothesis and l_1 is the maximum $\log_e$ likelihood under a model that subsumes the null hypothesis as a special case. The degrees of freedom of the chi-square distribution is equal to the difference between the number of functionally independent parameters estimated under the hypothesis and the number estimated under the model.

As noted above, this analysis assumes that under the full model the residuals are independent, whereas it may be that, because of the familial dependencies, the residuals are correlated. Under the null hypothesis of no familial segregation, however, the residuals are uncorrelated, so the method of analysis that we have described will not lead to spuriously significant results (provided the sample size is large enough for the chi-square approximation to hold).

III. VARIABLE AGE OF ONSET

An important extension of the dichotomous phenotypic distribution is the incorporation of a variable age of onset distribution into the analysis. In the previous section, we indicated that age at examination could be included as one of the covariates. If, for affected individuals, age of onset is also available, use of such data can provide much more information.

Let the random variable a denote age of onset and let a' denote age at examination. The information available on each individual in the sample may be one of three kinds: affected by age a', unaffected by age a', or affected at age a. Let $f(a)$ denote the density function of a and $F(a)$ the cumulative distribution function of a. Then the corresponding three likelihoods are given by

$$L(\text{affected by age } a') = F(a')$$

$$L(\text{unaffected by age } a') = 1 - F(a')$$

and

$$L(\text{affected at age } a) = f(a)$$

Now let **x** denote the set of predictor variables excluding age at examination, and let α be the change in log odds for one unit change in a'. Then if the age of onset distribution is logistic, we can equate p_{1i} and p_{0i}, respectively, to

$$F(a') = \frac{\exp\left(\beta + \sum_{j=1}^{k} \beta_j x_j + \alpha a'\right)}{1 + \exp\left(\beta + \sum_{j=1}^{k} \beta_j x_j + \alpha a'\right)}$$

and

$$1 - F(a') = \frac{1}{1 + \exp\left(\beta + \sum_{j=1}^{k} \beta_j x_j + \alpha a'\right)}$$

Furthermore, for an individual whose age of onset is known, we have

$$f(a) = \frac{\alpha \exp\left(\beta + \sum_{j=1}^{k} \beta_j x_j + \alpha a\right)}{\left\{1 + \exp\left(\beta + \sum_{j=1}^{k} \beta_j x_j + \alpha a\right)\right\}^2}$$

and this can be incorporated into the likelihood instead of p_{1i}. This simple extension to logistic regression analysis is not available in the usual packages of statistical programs, but is available as an option in (SAGE).[7]

Now let us suppose that age of onset has a normal distribution, so that, defining $\phi(a\text{-}\mu,\sigma^2)$ to be the ordinate at a of a normal density function with mean μ and variance σ^2, and

$$\Phi(t) = \frac{1}{\sqrt{2\pi}} \int_{-\infty}^{t} \exp(-u^2/2)du$$

we have

$$F(a') = \Phi\left(\frac{a' - \mu}{\sigma}\right)$$

$$1 - F(a') = 1 - \Phi\left(\frac{a' - \mu}{\sigma}\right)$$

and

$$F(a) = \phi(a - \mu, \sigma^2)$$

Then this distribution and the above logistic distribution are approximately equal if we set

$$\mu = -\left(\beta + \sum_{j=1}^{k} \beta_j x_j\right) \Big/ \alpha$$

and

$$\sigma = 1/\alpha$$

It should be pointed out that under these conditions the means of the two distributions are equal, but the variances are not. The variance of the logistic distribution is $\pi^2/3$ times the variance of the corresponding normal distribution.[14]

Rather than restricting ourselves to normal or logistic distributions for age of onset it is possible to use more general classes of distributions based on the generalized modulus power transformation proposed by George and Elston.[12] The generalized modulus power normal density is a four-parameter density function given by

$$f(a) = \frac{(|a - \kappa| + 1)^{\lambda - 1}}{\sqrt{2\pi}\sigma} \exp\left[\frac{-1}{2\sigma^2}\left\{\operatorname{sgn}(a - \kappa)\frac{(|a - \kappa| + 1)^{\lambda} - 1}{\lambda} - \mu\right\}^2\right]$$

where $\operatorname{sgn}(a - \kappa)$ denotes the sign of $(a - \kappa)$. The parameters of this density function are $\lambda \geq 0$, $-\infty < \kappa < \infty$, $-\infty < \mu < \infty$ and $\sigma^2 > 0$. Notice that the normal distribution is the special case in which $\lambda = 1$ and $\kappa = 0$. The limiting distribution of a as $\lambda \to 0$ is a lognormal distribution shifted by an amount $\kappa - 1$ from zero. One major advantage of using this generalized normal density is that it allows the age of onset distribution to be skewed and/or kurtotic, and even bimodal. Assuming such a distribution is equivalent to assuming that a power transformation of a is normally distributed, the particular power transformation being given by

$$a^* = \begin{cases} \operatorname{sgn}(a - \kappa)\left\{\dfrac{(|y - \kappa| + 1)^{\lambda} - 1}{\lambda}\right\} & \text{if} \quad \lambda > 0 \\[2ex] \operatorname{sgn}(a - \kappa)\log(|a - \kappa| + 1) & \text{if} \quad \lambda = 0 \end{cases}$$

The same principle can be applied to obtain a generalized logistic density for age of onset, given by

$$f(a) = \frac{\alpha(|a - \kappa| + 1)^{\lambda - 1} \exp\left(\beta + \sum_{j=1}^{k} \beta_j x_j + \alpha a^*\right)}{\left\{1 + \exp\left(\beta + \sum_{j=1}^{k} \beta_j x_j + \alpha a^*\right)\right\}^2}$$

where a^* is the power transformed a defined above. Again, similar to the previous case, $f(a)$ is logistic when $\lambda = 1$ and $\kappa = 0$, and the limiting distribution as $\lambda \rightarrow 0$ is a shifted log logistic distribution.

An advantage in assuming a generalized logistic distribution for age of onset, rather than a generalized normal distribution, is that we then have an explicit expression for $F(a')$, the probability of being affected by age a'; in the case of a generalized normal distribution we need to refer to a cumulative normal probability table or use a series approximation. Whether logistic or normal, the generalized distribution can fit a wide range of skewness and kurtosis in the age of onset distributions, thereby allowing much more flexibility in modeling.

IV. SEGREGATION ANALYSIS

So far we have only allowed for familial effects in a general way, without modeling any specific genetic mechanism. Segregation analysis of family data is a statistical methodology used to detect segregation at a single locus and to determine the mode of inheritance of a particular phenotype at that locus. Elston and Stewart[10] described a general model in which arbitrary phenotypic distributions could be assumed for each genotype, and an algorithm for calculating the corresponding likelihood for an arbitrarily large pedigree structure, provided only that it goes back to a single pair of original ancestors and does not include consanguineous mating or marriage loops. This algorithm was later extended to pedigrees of arbitrary structure by Lange and Elston[17] and by Cannings et al.[5]

Elston and Yelverton[11] developed general models for segregation analysis that incorporated normally distributed ages of onset, and these were reviewed in detail by Elston.[6] Recently, Bonney[3] has proposed using regressive logistic models for segregation analysis. In this section we extend the discussions of the previous sections by including the possibility of a major gene effect in the model. In this way we arrive at the class A regressive logistic model of Bonney,[3] but extended to incorporate age of onset information.

Consider an autosomal locus with two alleles, A and a, the major genotypes being denoted g = AA, Aa, or aa. Letting the gene frequency of allele A be q, under Hardy-Weinberg equilibrium we have the population probabilities

$$\Pr(g) = \begin{cases} q^2 & \text{if} \quad g = AA \\ 2q(1 - q) & \text{if} \quad g = Aa \\ (1 - q)^2 & \text{if} \quad g = aa \end{cases}$$

Let g_F and g_M denote the genotypes of the father and mother of the i-th individual, who has genotype g_i. Elston and Stewart[10] showed how the transition probabilities $\Pr(g_i|g_F,g_M)$ could be written in terms of parameters they called transmission probabilities. For the simple two-allele case, there are basically three transmission probabilities, defined by τ_g = Pr(genotype g transmits A to offspring), together with the three complementary probabilities of transmitting a to offspring. We can then write

$$\Pr(g_i = AA|g_F = h, \quad g_M = j) = \tau_h\tau_j$$

$$\Pr(g_i = Aa|g_F = h, \quad g_M = j) = \tau_h(1 - \tau_j) + \tau_j(1 - \tau_h)$$

$$\Pr(g_i = aa|g_F = h, \quad g_M = j) = (1 - \tau_h)(1 - \tau_j)$$

where under Mendelian transmission $\tau_{AA} = 1$, $\tau_{Aa} = 1/2$, and $\tau_{aa} = 0$. In order to test the null hypothesis of Mendelian transmission, Elston and Stewart[10] suggested using a model in which the transmission probabilities are generalized, letting τ_g (g = AA, Aa, or aa) take on any value in the interval [0,1]. Under such a model g is no longer necessarily a genotype, but rather a "type"[13] or "ousiotype".[5]

Now suppose we have n individuals in a pedigree ordered so that ancestors always precede their descendants, and the ordered types of these individuals are given by the vector $\mathbf{g} = (g_1, g_2, \ldots, g_n)$. Consider $\Pr(\mathbf{g}) = \Pr(g_1) \cdot \Pr(g_2|g_1) \ldots \Pr(g_n|g_1, g_2, \ldots g_{n-1})$. An individual i with no parents in the pedigree can be preceded by a spouse, but not by a blood relative. So, for such an individual,

$$\Pr(g_i|g_1, g_2, \ldots, g_{i-1}) = \Pr(g_i)$$

provided that mating is independent of types and the pedigree is randomly sampled from the population. For an individual i whose parents are in the pedigree, the individual's type is derived only from his/her father and mother. Therefore, for such an individual,

$$\Pr(g_i|g_1, g_2, \ldots, g_{i-1}) = \Pr(g_i|g_F, g_M)$$

Hence

$$\Pr(\mathbf{g}) = \prod_{i=1}^{n} p_i$$

where

$$p_i = \begin{cases} \Pr(g_i) & \text{if the parents of i are not in the pedigree} \\ \Pr(g_i|g_F, g_M) & \text{if the parents of i are in the pedigree} \end{cases}$$

As we have seen, $\Pr(g_i)$ can be expressed as a function of q (which is the frequency of gene *A* if the types are genotypes), and $\Pr(g_i|g_F, g_M)$ is simply a function of the transmission probabilities.

Now suppose, as before, that on each individual i we have the dichotomous disease outcome y_i, an age at examination a_i', and other predictor variables $\mathbf{x}_i = (x_{i1}, x_{i2}, \ldots, x_{ik})$. Assume in addition that, conditional on a_i', $\mathbf{x}_i$, and g_i, the y_i are independent. It follows that the likelihood of a random pedigree can then be expressed as

$$\sum \prod_{i=1}^{n} p_i \Pr(y_i|a_i', \mathbf{x}_i, g_i)$$

where the p_i are as just given above and the summation is over all possible vectors of types, **g**. Information on age of onset can of course be incorporated as indicated in the previous section, replacing $\Pr(y_i|a_i', \mathbf{x}_i, g_i)$ by the corresponding density function. The problem we shall now address is how to model $\Pr(y_i|a_i', \mathbf{x}_i, g_i)$, it being implicitly understood that age of onset information, when available, is to be incorporated by using the corresponding density function.

There are basically two ways in which dependence on type can be modeled, and these were termed models I and II by Elston et al.[9] in the context of a normally distributed age of onset. In model I, we let $F(a')$ depend on type. For convenience, let us define

$$\text{antilogit}(\theta) = \frac{\exp\theta}{1 + \exp\theta}$$

Then for a logistic distribution of age of onset, for example, we can set

$$\Pr(y_i|a_i', \mathbf{x}_i, g_i) = \begin{cases} F(a_i') & \text{if i is affected} \\ 1 - F(a_i') & \text{if i is unaffected} \end{cases}$$

with the definition

$$F(a_i') = \text{antilogit}\left[\beta_{g_i} + \sum_j \beta_j x_{ij} + \alpha a_i'\right]$$

This is the same as the previous definition of $F(a')$ for a logistic distribution, except that now the baseline β is dependent on type. However, such a model assumes that all individuals, if only they could live to an infinite age, would eventually succumb to the disease. We therefore introduce a new parameter, γ, the susceptibility to disease. It is assumed that a proportion γ of the population is susceptible and will eventually (by age infinity) become affected, whereas a proportion $1 - \gamma$ will never become affected (for these individuals there is no age of onset distribution). We thus define model I as

$$\Pr(y_i|a_i', \mathbf{x}_i, g_i) = \begin{cases} \gamma F(a_i') & \text{if i is affected} \\ 1 - \gamma F(a_i') & \text{if i is unaffected}, \quad 0 < \gamma \leq 1 \end{cases}$$

$F(a_i')$ being dependent on type as indicated. The corresponding density for a person affected with age of onset a_i is $\gamma f(a_i)$. In model II we let the susceptibility γ, rather than $F(a_i')$, depend on type. It is thus defined by the same formulation, except that γ now becomes γ_{g_i} and the baseline β is no longer dependent on type.

These segregation analysis models that incorporate age of onset were first proposed in the context of normal distributions, rather than logistic distributions, and there is no difficulty in extending them to the generalized distributions described above. They have a distinct disadvantage, however, in that the only familial dependence among pedigree members that they allow is that due to the transmission of type from one generation to the next. This can be overcome by incorporating a polygenic component into the model,[10,16] but this greatly increases the complexity of calculating the corresponding likelihood. The regressive models introduced by Bonney[2,3] achieve the same purpose by a very simple means, which will now be described. In particular, we shall describe Bonney's class A regressive model, in which it is assumed that any dependencies in a sibship, over and above that due to the $\mathbf{x}_i$ or the types g_i, can be accounted for by the sibs' common parentage. Bonney[2] also described other classes of models that allow for further dependencies, but these will not be described here.

Let the subscripts F, M, and S denote, respectively, the father, mother, and spouse of individual i. Then in class A regressive models we simply alter $F(a_i')$ to include the phenotype of the father, mother, and spouse as covariates (but not including as covariates the parents of those who do not have parents in the pedigree). In other words, we now have

$$F(a_i') = \begin{cases} \text{antilogit}\left[\beta + \sum_j \beta_j x_{ij} + \alpha a_i' + \delta_F y_F + \delta_M y_M + \delta_S y_S\right] & \\ \qquad\qquad \text{if } y_S \text{ precedes } y_i \text{ in the data} & \\ \text{antilogit}\left[\beta + \sum_j \beta_j x_{ij} + \alpha a_i' + \delta_F y_F + \delta_M y_M\right] & \\ \qquad\qquad \text{if } y_i \text{ precedes } y_s \text{ in the data,} & \end{cases}$$

with three new regression coefficients, δ_F, δ_M, and δ_S, to estimate. (In the case of model I, β is type dependent.) Missing data on spouses or parents cause a problem that Bonney[3] resolved by defining a new variable that is a linear function of y_i. This new scaling is equivalent to defining

$$y_i = \begin{cases} 1 & \text{if affected} \\ {}^1/_2 & \text{if missing} \\ 0 & \text{if unaffected} \end{cases}$$

However, it may not be appropriate to assign a missing value weight corresponding to the halfway point between affected and unaffected individuals.[19]

So far we have developed the likelihood, under a general model that allows for both major gene segregation and other residual familial effects, for a randomly selected pedigree. As already noted, however, pedigrees are usually selected for analysis because they include probands, and the likelihood needs to be multiplied by a correction factor to allow for this mode of ascertainment. Provided there is single ascertainment, which results in only one proband in each pedigree, this correction factor is quite simple to specify. Basically, it is the reciprocal of an analogous likelihood for the whole pedigree, but in which one assumes that the phenotypes for all individuals other than the proband are missing, and one assumes an age at examination (rather than age of onset) for the proband. For those special cases in which the distribution of types is constant from generation to generation (i.e., the case of Mendelian transmission and the case of no transmission with $\tau_{AA} = \tau_{Aa} = \tau_{aa} = q$), the correction factor is equal to the population likelihood that an individual, examined at the same age as the proband, should be affected. The correction factor must be expressed in terms of the parameters of the model, and so changes as these parameters change.

The joint likelihood of several independent pedigrees can be computed by multiplying together the individual likelihoods, and maximized numerically to obtain maximum likelihood estimates of the various parameters. Different hypotheses such as Mendelian transmission, no transmission, dominance, and codominance can be tested using the likelihood ratio criterion, as described above. In addition, Akaike's[1] AIC criterion can be used to choose the best-fitting model among several alternatives. The AIC criterion is $-2(\log_e$ likelihood$)$ $+ 2$(number of estimated parameters) and the model with smallest AIC is considered to be the best-fitting one. Table 3 indicates examples of the many specific hypotheses that can be tested under the general model I developed above. In each case the likelihood is maximized under a set of constraints and the $\log_e$ likelihood can be compared to the maximized $\log_e$ likelihood of the most general model with no constraints. The rightmost column in Table 3

Table 3
EXAMPLES OF HYPOTHESES THAT CAN BE TESTED BY SEGREGATION ANALYSIS UNDER A TWO-ALLELE (*A*, *a*) SYSTEM USING MODEL 1 (β DEPENDS ON TYPE)

Hypotheses: Mode of transmission	Hypotheses: Residual familial effects	Constraints	Degrees of freedom
Three types			
General	Present	None	—
Mendelian	Present	$\tau_{AA} = 1, \tau_{Aa} = 1/2, \tau_{aa} = 0$	3
No Transmission	Present	$\tau_{AA} = \tau_{Aa} = \tau_{aa} = q_A$	3
General	Absent	$\delta_F = \delta_M = \delta_S = 0$	3
Mendelian	Absent	$\delta_F = \delta_M = \delta_S = 0, \tau_{AA} = 1, \tau_{Aa} = 1/2, \tau_{aa} = 0$	6
No transmission	Absent	$\delta_F = \delta_M = \delta_S = 0, \tau_{AA} = \tau_{Aa} = \tau_{aa} = q_A$	6
Two types			
General	Present	$\beta_{AA} = \beta_{Aa}$ or $\beta_{Aa} = \beta_{aa}$	1
Mendelian	Present	$\beta_{AA} = \beta_{Aa}$ or $\beta_{Aa} = \beta_{aa}, \tau_{AA} = 1, \tau_{Aa} = 1/2, \tau_{aa} = 0$	4
No transmission	Present	$\beta_{AA} = \beta_{Aa}$ or $\beta_{Aa} = \beta_{aa}, \tau_{AA} = \tau_{Aa} = \tau_{aa} = q_A$	4
General	Present	$\beta_{AA} = \beta_{Aa}$ or $\beta_{Aa} = \beta_{aa}, \delta_F = \delta_M = \delta_S = 0$	4
Mendelian	Absent	$\beta_{AA} = \beta_{Aa}$ or $\beta_{Aa} = \beta_{aa}, \delta_F = \delta_M = \delta_S = 0, \tau_{AA} = 1, \tau_{Aa} = 1/2, \tau_{aa} = 0$	7
No transmission	Absent	$\beta_{AA} = \beta_{Aa}$ or $\beta_{Aa} = \beta_{aa}, \delta_F = \delta_M = \delta_S = 0, \tau_{AA} = \tau_{Aa} = \tau_{aa} = q_A$	7
One type			
General	Present	$\beta_{AA} = \beta_{Aa} = \beta_{aa}$	6
	Absent	$\beta_{AA} = \beta_{Aa} = \beta_{aa}, \delta_F = \delta_M = \delta_S = 0$	9

gives the number of degrees of freedom for each of these tests. With a minor change, Table 3 is also applicable to analyses under model II; it is only necessary to substitute γ for β, i.e., γ_{AA} for β_{AA}, γ_{Aa} for β_{Aa}, and γ_{aa} for β_{aa}.

Finally, it should be noted that these models are very flexible and only some of the hypotheses of interest are indicated in Table 3. Unlike the unified model of Lalouel et al.,[16] which is a modification of the mixed model to incorporate transmission probabilities, the regressive models introduced by Bonney[2,3,19] allow one to test the significance of predictor variables and to test whether residual transmission from the father (δ_F) is equal to that from the mother (δ_M). Current versions of the program package SAGE[7] allow implementation of many of these models, and an example of their use if provided by Bonney et al.[4]

ACKNOWLEDGMENTS

This work was supported in part by U.S. Public Health Service Research Grants CA28198 from the National Cancer Institute and GM28356 from the National Institute of General Medical Sciences, and Training Grant HL07567 from the National Heart, Lung and Blood Institute.

REFERENCES

1. **Akaike, H.,** On entropy maximization principle, in *Applications of Statistics,* Krishnaiah, P. R., Ed., North-Holland, Amsterdam, 1977, 27.
2. **Bonney, G. E.,** On the statistical determination of major gene mechanisms in continuous human traits: regressive models, *Am. J. Med. Genet.,* 18, 731, 1984.
3. **Bonney, G. E.,** Regressive logistic models for familial disease and other binary traits, *Biometrics,* 42, 611, 1986.
4. **Bonney, G. E., Elston, R. C., Correa, P., Haenszel, W., Zavala, D. E., Zarama, G., Collazos, T., and Cuello, C.,** Genetic etiology of genetic carcinoma. I. Chronic atrophic gastritis, *Genet. Epidemiol.,* 3, 213, 1986.
5. **Cannings, C., Thompson, E. A., and Skolnick, M. H.,** Probability functions on complex pedigrees, *Adv. Appl. Probab.,* 10, 26, 1978.
6. **Elston, R. C.,** Segregation analysis, *Adv. Hum. Genet.,* 11, 63, 1981.
7. **Elston, R. C., Bailey-Wilson, J. E., Bonney, G. E., Keats, B. J., and Wilson, A. F.,** S.A.G.E. — A package of computer programs to perform statistical analysis for genetic epidemiology, presented at the 7th Int. Cong. Human Genetics, Berlin, September 22 to 26, 1986.
8. **Elston, R. C. and Bonney, G. E.,** Sampling considerations in the design and analysis of family studies, in *Genetic Epidemiology of Coronary Heart Disease,* Rao, D. C., Elston, R. C., Kuller, L., Carter, C., and Havlik, R., Eds., Alan R. Liss, New York, 1984, 349.
9. **Elston, R. C., Namboodiri, K. K., Spence, M. A., and Rainer, J. D.,** A genetic study of schizophrenia pedigrees. II. One-locus hypotheses, *Neuropsychobiology,* 4, 193, 1978.
10. **Elston, R. C. and Stewart, J.,** A general model for the genetic analysis of pedigree data, *Hum. Hered.,* 21, 523, 1971.
11. **Elston, R. C. and Yelverton, K. C.,** General models for segregation analysis, *Am. J. Hum. Genet.,* 27, 31, 1975.
12. **George, V. T. and Elston, R. C.,** Generalized modulus power transformations, *Commun. Stat.,* A17, 2933, 1988.
13. **Go, R. C. P., Elston, R. C., and Kaplan, E. B.,** Efficiency and robustness of pedigree segregation analysis, *Am. J. Hum. Genet.,* 30, 28, 1978.
14. **Johnson, N. L. and Kotz, S.,** *Distributions in Statistics: Continuous Univariate Distributions,* Vol. 2, Houghton Mifflin, Boston, 1970, 1.
15. **Kleinbaum, D. C., Kupper, L. L., and Morgenstern, H.,** *Epidemiologic Research — Principles and Quantitative Methods,* Lifetime Learning, Belmont, Ca., 1982, 419.
16. **Lalouel, J.-M., Rao, D. C., Morton, N. E., and Elston, R. C.,** A unified model for complex segregation analysis, *Am. J. Hum. Genet.,* 35, 816, 1983.
17. **Lange, K. and Elston, R. C.,** Extensions to pedigree analysis. I. Likelihood calculations for simple and complex pedigrees, *Hum. Hered.,* 25, 95, 1975.
18. **Ooi, W. L., Elston, R. C., Chen, V. W., Bailey-Wilson, J. E., and Rothschild, H.,** Increased familial risk for lung cancer, *J. Natl. Cancer Inst.,* 76, 217, 1986.
19. **Bonney, G. E.,** Logistic regression for dependent binary observations, *Biometrics,* 43, 951, 1987.

Chapter 3

HOST VARIATIONS IN CARCINOGEN METABOLISM AND DNA REPAIR

Kirsi Vähäkangas and Olavi Pelkonen

TABLE OF CONTENTS

I. INTRODUCTION

Chemical carcinogens must be in reactive form or they must produce other reactive radicals to be able to initiate the oncogenic process, most probably by binding covalently to, or otherwise damaging, the DNA.[1] There may be other mechanisms for the initiation of the carcinogenic process, and almost certainly some of the mechanisms behind later stages of carcinogenesis are different, but the concept of metabolic activation of chemical carcinogens into reactive intermediates has provided a unified framework for understanding the mechanism of action of numerous structurally unrelated carcinogenic compounds.[2]

Because *metabolic activation* or *toxification* as well as *detoxication* or *inactivation* are catalyzed by the enzymes of the body, it would be of utmost importance to elucidate the factors which modify the activity of enzymes participating in the activation and detoxication of these carcinogenic chemicals. A highly schematic depiction of chemical carcinogenesis is presented in Figure 1. This scheme shows the central role of xenobiotic-metabolizing enzymes in the initial phase of action of a carcinogenic substance. However, it is not known when (or whether) toxification is rate limiting to the overall carcinogenic process. The multistep nature of carcinogenesis makes it also very difficult to obtain convincing evidence about the possible causal link between an early process, initiation, and the significance of metabolic processes in it, and the final outcome, clinically manifest cancer.

As in almost any other complex attribute of an organism, interindividual differences in the metabolism of carcinogens are due to three types of factors, genetic or inherited host factors, nongenetic or acquired host factors, and environmental factors (Figure 2). These determinants are usually interdependent to such an extent that it is difficult to elucidate the contribution of any one singly. The genetic background represents only the potential of an individual and sets the limits to the response, but the current potential to respond is revealed as a consequence of acquired host factors and environmental influences.

Despite intensive research of 2 to 3 decades we are still uncertain as to how significant host variation is in the overall causality of human carcinogenesis. We still have more questions than answers. Consequently, it may be useful to list some of the more important questions we will try to deal with in this review, although we do not yet know the exact answers.

1. Why study enzyme activities and/or DNA-bound products in connection with chemical carcinogenesis? The second section tries to answer this question and also tries to give a view on our possibilities to detect the end result in human situations.
2. The third section tries to answer the question: What causes the variations in *in vitro* enzyme activities of carcinogen metabolism and DNA repair?
3. Do we have useful animal models to study genetic variations in enzymes associated with chemical carcinogenesis? This question is dealt with in the fourth section.
4. Is there a link between *in vitro* enzyme activities, polymorphisms of metabolism in human populations, and chemically induced cancer? Answering this question is the topic of the fifth section.

II. FACTORS CONTROLLING CARCINOGEN-INDUCED DNA DAMAGE

A. Enzymes Activating and Inactivating Carcinogens

Enzymes participating in the metabolism of foreign substances (''xenobiotics''), including carcinogens, are usually divided into phase I (functionalization) and phase II (conjugation) enzymes.[3,4] The most important group of enzymes in the first category is the family of cytochrome P-450 isozymes, which catalyze different oxidative reactions with numerous endogenous and exogenous substances. P-450 enzymes are also regarded as the most im-

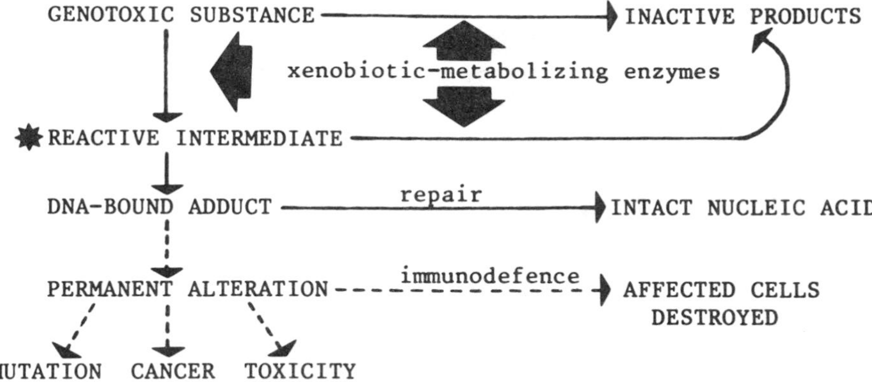

FIGURE 1. Schematic presentation of the sequence of events leading from exposure to a carcinogenic substance to biological consequences.

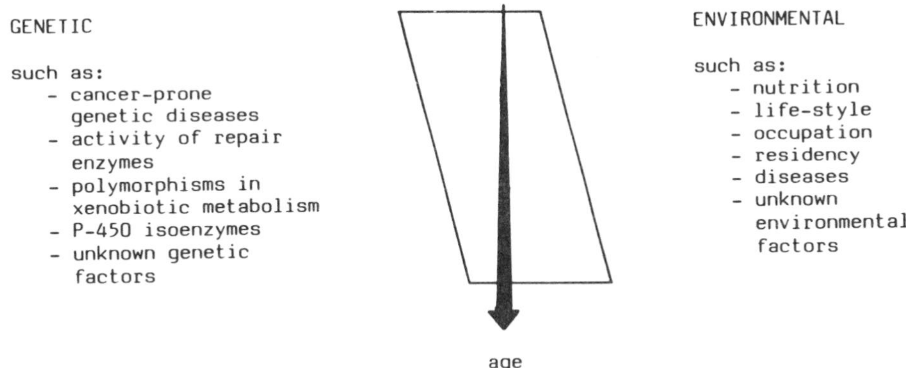

FIGURE 2. The proportions of genetic and environmental determinants in affecting the susceptibility to cancer in relation to age.

portant group in the metabolic activation of carcinogens. Conjugative enzymes consist of a more variable group of enzymes, mainly in the cytoplasmic compartment of the cell, which catalyze the linkage of various endogenous groups — glucuronic acid, sulfate and glutathione as examples — with the foreign compounds. Conjugation reactions are often regarded as true detoxication reactions, although this notion is not entirely correct.[5]

Although the liver is the main site of xenobiotic-metabolizing enzymes, other tissues contain variable amounts and variable patterns of these enzymes.[6] With respect to carcinogen activation it is speculated that tissue-specific enzyme composition is of prime importance in the determination of target-specific activation of chemical carcinogens.[7] Furthermore, it is the balance between activating and detoxicating reactions, which determines the level of reactive intermediates in the cell and the availability of the reactive species to covalent binding with DNA.

B. DNA Repair

Once active metabolites of carcinogens are bound to DNA, they must be removed by enzymatic repair mechanisms, if permanent damage is to be prevented. DNA-repair pathways in human cells, although less well known than in bacterial systems, seem to be as abundant and even more complicated than in bacteria.[8,9] DNA repair is dynamic in nature and individual events can proceed very quickly, as is demonstrated for instance by the very short half-life of DNA strand breaks in cultured human fibroblasts.[10] O^6-methylguanine-DNA methyltransferase (O^6-MT), which removes the putative precarcinogenic DNA lesions caused by a number of N-nitroso compounds, is one of the best known repair enzymes in human tissues.[11] It has been found in all of the tissues studied, but in different amounts. A correlation between sister chromatid exchange (SCE)-induction with the amount of N^3-alkyl-adenine and also with lack of O^6-MT suggests SCE to be a measure of the repair capacity.[12]

There are several lines of evidence supporting the importance of DNA repair processes in human cancer. The development of acute nonlymphocytic leukemia in a high percentage of patients given alkylating agents is linked to low levels of O^6-MT in myeloid precursors (6.6% of the activity in liver[13]). In several genetic diseases a deficiency in DNA repair may be the basis for the increased susceptibility to cancer. The evidence for such a link is strong in xeroderma pigmentosum, but much less so in ataxia telangiectasia, Bloom's syndrome, or Fanconi's anemia.[14] Cultured lymphocytes from cancer patients display a higher number of chromosome breaks per cell induced by bleomycin than those from healthy individuals,[15] and mononuclear leukocytes from patients with colorectal cancer or persons predisposed for the disease have lower levels of *N*-acetoxy-2-acetylaminofluorene-induced UDS than individuals from the general population.[16]

C. Novel Methodology for Carcinogen-DNA Adducts

It seems to be proved that the adducts, activated carcinogen metabolites bound covalently to DNA, have a central role in the initiation. In animal studies a correlation, although not a perfect one, has been shown to occur between the total covalent binding and tumor initiation potency of selected chemical carcinogens.[17,18] This implies that only one or some of the adducts formed are important for the carcinogenicity, although on the basis of studies with alkylating agents, Swenberg et al.[19] have come to the conclusion that no single adduct alone would be responsible. In any case it is evident that in addition to DNA binding the repair of damage and cell replication are important.[19,20] For benzo(a)pyrene, the most thoroughly studied PAH, quantitatively and, according to animal studies also qualitatively, the most important adduct is a certain isomer of benzo(a)pyrene-7,8-dihydrodiol-9,10-epoxide (BPDE) bound to the exocyclic nitrogen of guanine.[4,21-24] Naturally, human studies are now largely concentrating on this adduct, because it would be difficult to directly show the relevance of any adduct in humans.

During recent years, novel analytical methods have been employed for the study of the presence of bulky carcinogen-DNA adducts formed *in vivo* after environmental exposure in human tissues.[25] It has become possible to quantitate carcinogen-DNA adducts by synchronous fluorescence spectrophotometry (SFS),[26] immunological assays,[27,28] or the so-called ^{32}P postlabeling assay[29] in different available human tissues (see also Table 1). In principle, these measurements should allow us to evaluate the end result of the combined processes of exposure to carcinogens, metabolic activation, detoxication, and DNA repair in the initiation phase of carcinogenesis. These methods fall principally into two categories: specific methods for the detection of one adduct (ELISA and USERIA immunoassays, and SFS) and fingerprint-type assays, which detect a whole range of adducts at the same time (^{32}P-postlabeling assay). Three-dimensional SFS[33,34] in which multiple synchronous scans with a range of differences between excitation and emission wavelengths are combined to give a fingerprint-type assay has also been tried, but not applied for human studies by now.

Antibodies towards many carcinogen-DNA adducts already exist.[35,36] A polyclonal antibody towards BP-DNA[37] has been used in human studies,[27,28,30,32] but unfortunately, this antibody seems to have some cross reactivity with DNA-adducts of some other polycyclic hydrocarbons.[28] There have been attempts also to develop a monoclonal antibody towards BP-DNA with promising results.[31,38]

Randerath et al.[29,39] have developed a very sensitive assay, where the damaged DNA

Table 1
HUMAN STUDIES ON CARCINOGEN-DNA ADDUCTS AFTER ENVIRONMENTAL EXPOSURES

Probable source of exposure	Tissue studied[a]	DNA adduct measured	Method[b]	Number of positives/number of studied	Ref.
Smoking/passive exposure to smoke (lung cancer patients)	Lung	BPDE-DNA	ELISA	5/15	27
Work exposure, smoking	PBL	BPDE-DNA	ELISA	16/50	30
Aluminum plant, smoking	PBL	BPDE-DNA	SFS	1/30	26
Coke oven, smoking	PBL	BPDE-DNA	SFS	10[c]/41	28
			USERIA	18/27	
Smoking	Placenta	Not known	^{32}P-postlabeling	16/17 (smokers) 3/14 (nonsmokers)	31
	Placenta	BPDE-DNA	ELISA	nm[d]	
Coke oven, smoking	PBL	BPDE-DNA	SFS	4/38	32
			USERIA	13/38	

[a] PBL, peripheral blood lymphocytes.
[b] Announced sensitivities of the methods: ELISA 0.1 femtomoles of adducts DNA; SFS 0.2 femtomoles of adducts DNA; USERIA 0.1 femtomoles of adducts DNA.
[c] In addition to sharp peaks, in some cases a more hill-like increase of the fluorescence at the region for BPDE-DNA was found. These are not included, because the explanation for the phenomenon is not known so far.
[d] nm means not mentioned (higher mean adduct level found in smokers compared to nonsmokers).

bases are labeled radioactively after DNA isolation, and separated from unmodified bases by the means of chromatography. The chemical identity of the adducts need not be known for the DNA binding to be detected. On the other hand, many carcinogens seem to give spots on the same areas of the TLC plates. This possible overlap between adducts might interfere with the identification, especially after multiple exposures (which most human exposures are), and even more so with the quantitation. By the ^{32}P postlabeling method carcinogen-DNA adducts have been detected in human tissues from smokers.[29,31]

Highly sensitive fluorescence assays to measure PAH-DNA adducts have been pursued by several groups.[33] Because the sensitivity of fluorescence methods is very much dependent on the sensitivity of the equipment, it has not been possible earlier to apply fluorometry for human *in vivo* studies. New interesting developments include fluorometric HPLC-assay,[40] fluorescence line narrowing spectrometry,[41,42] and SFS,[26,34,43] of which only the SFS for benzo(a)pyrene diolepoxide-DNA adducts has been applied for human studies to date.[26] The correlation between different assays, which would be badly needed, has not been systematically studied. Thus far, only BPDE-DNA adducts have been measured and quantitated by several assays from same human samples (see Table 1). Even if, by these assays, we were not measuring the most relevant adducts for carcinogenicity, they might be useful as a better measure of exposure (taking into account the absorption and metabolism and repair) than, for example, showing carcinogens in the work atmosphere.

III. VARIATIONS IN *IN VITRO* ENZYME ACTIVITIES

A. Phenomenology: Carcinogen-Metabolizing Enzymes

One of the most conspicuous features of human xenobiotic metabolism is its extreme variability.[44-46] Several tenfold or sometimes even several hundredfold variation have been demonstrated in *in vivo* elimination rates of various drugs and other exogenous substances and in *in vitro* tissue studies in which the metabolic rates of model substances have been studied. Although in some situations the methodology used may contribute to variation, overwhelming evidence suggests that the large variability is a true phenomenon. The variability has become all the more relevant to the assessment of a carcinogenic process in man, when tissue explants and cells from different individuals have been studied with respect to carcinogen metabolism and covalent binding to DNA.[25]

Table 2 shows some examples of the variations in carcinogen metabolizing enzymes found in human tissues and cells. AHH in placenta, EH in liver, and GSH-transferase in leukocytes display a particularly wide variation. Another interesting feature is the different variation of the same enzyme in different tissues, or even different cell compartments of the same tissue (EH in liver microsomes vs. EH in liver cytosol). The differences in enzyme activities, no doubt, lead to differences in *in vivo* DNA binding. The human *in vivo* studies, however, are too few and the materials too small to say much more than that adducts are found in humans after environmental exposure, but not in all of them even after similar exposure, so there certainly is interindividual variation also in this parameter (Table 1).

B. Determinants of Variability

What are the determinants for this extreme variability? This question is of considerable importance, because it alludes to the most important problem from the predictive point of view: stability of variability. Is the carcinogen-metabolizing capacity of an individual relatively constant during most of his/her lifetime or does it exhibit wide fluctuations on a short-term or long-term basis? In other words, is it genetic background, acquired characteristics, or environment which determine primarily the ability of an individual to metabolize carcinogens? If acquired features and environment are most critical, predictions based on measurements of xenobiotic metabolism at a single time point could be meaningless.

Data on numerous exogenous and endogenous determinants affecting xenobiotic metabolism have been studied and reviewed by Vesell et al.[59,60] Some factors tend to increase, others to decrease xenobiotic-metabolizing enzymes and a very large variation (Table 2) is observed in cross-sectional studies of relatively unselected individuals[61] or of selected groups such as lung cancer patients.[62] There are, however, studies in man, which suggest that the activity of xenobiotic-metabolizing enzymes in the basal state (although sometimes this seems rather hypothetical in man) is determined to a large extent by the genetic background of the individual. For example, intrapair differences are always much larger in dizygotic twins than in monozygotic twins, implicating a strong hereditary factor.[63] A recent evaluation suggested that a hereditary contribution to debrisoquine hydroxylation in man is about 79% and an environmental contribution only 13%.[64] It must also be noted that some factors which at first sight are thought to be dependent totally on exogenous influences, e.g., induction of xenobiotic metabolism by environmental chemicals, are in fact controlled by the individual's genetic responsiveness to environmental exposure. In the induction of xenobiotic metabolism, the final result is determined by the dose of the chemical, the genetic background of the exposed person, and the acquired features of the host. The same phenomenon is probably true of most environmental influences. The level of xenobiotic biotransformations may be consequently determined by the constant interplay of host and environmental factors, which are very difficult to study separately in man.

The data reviewed above clearly shows that xenobiotic metabolism, including carcinogen activation, displays extensive interindividual variation, which is due to both host and environmental factors. The crucial question, which has not been definitely answered yet, is whether carcinogen activation is ever the rate-limiting step in human cancer.

C. Phenomenology: DNA Repair

Recent studies have shown that repair mechanisms in human tissues display a much larger variation than was earlier thought (see Table 2). Studies on parenchymal tissues and lym-

Table 2
INTERINDIVIDUAL VARIATIONS OF CARCINOGEN-METABOLIZING AND DNA-REPAIRING ENZYME ACTIVITIES AND DNA-REPAIR ASSOCIATED PHENOMENA IN HUMAN TISSUES

Function	Enzyme	Tissue	Highest variation reported	Ref.
Carcinogen activation/ deactivation	Aryl hydrocarbon hydroxylase	Liver	76	47
		Lung	20	47
		Bronchus	20	47
		Placenta	350	47
		Skin	7	47
		Kidney	12	47
		Lymphocytes	50	48
	Epoxide hydrolase	Liver, micros.	63	49
		Liver, cytosol.	539	49
		Blood cells	5	49
		Lung	4, 30[a]	58
		Bronchus	3	47
		Placenta	8	47
		Skin	3	47
	GSH transferase	Liver	57	57
		Lung	2	51
		Heart	3	51
		Brain	5	51
		Pancreas	2	51
		Rectum	7	51
		Lymphocytes	5, 27[b]	57
		Mononuclear leukocytes	100—200	52
	N-Acetyltransferase		100	53
DNA repair	O^6-methyltransferase	Liver	8	25
		Lung	10	50
		Colon	10	25
		Small intestine	42	25
		Esophagus	2	50
		Blood cells	8	56
	Uracil DNA-glycosylase	Liver	3	25
		Stomach	3	25
		Small intestine	65	25
		Colon	6	25
	UDS	Lymphocytes	5	54
	SCE	Lymphocytes	>2	55

Note: SCE: sister chromatid exchanges and UDS: unscheduled DNA synthesis.

[a] Variation for EH with BPO as a substrate was 4-fold and with TSO as a substrate 30-fold.
[b] Depending on the substrate.

phocytes have demonstrated that the activities of two DNA repair enzymes, guanine O^6-methyltransferase and uracil DNA glycosylase, are variable between individuals, although the factors behind the variation remain largely unknown.[50,65]

Carcinogen-induced damage to DNA initiates a definite response in the cell, the so-called unscheduled DNA synthesis (UDS), which is taken as representing DNA repair. Genetic background may be the most important factor in determining this response on the basis of a study on mono- and dizygotic twins.[16] Pero et al.[66] also demonstrated reduced UDS in monocytes exposed *in vitro* to *N*-acetoxy-2-acetylaminofluorene taken from individuals with colorectal cancer or a genetic predisposition to this disease. Setlow[54] has shown a fivefold interindividual variation in UDS after UV damage. A wider, even 45-fold variation in the baseline SCE frequency has been reported, but after a careful exclusion of preparative variation Carrano et al.[55] showed still a 2-fold variation in human lymphocytes.

It is conceivable therefore, that individuals differ with respect to the activity of DNA repair processes, and this variation may contribute to differences in cancer susceptibility. The variation in enzyme activities involved in carcinogen metabolism and DNA repair are reflected in variation in DNA-bound products. In both DNA and protein adducts a wide variation has been found in cultured human tissues.[47,67]

D. Isoenzymes

From animal studies it has been clear for a long time that several isoenzymes exist for many of the enzymes involved in carcinogen activation, particularly for cytochrome P-450. The basis for the isoenzymes seems to be at the genetic level, although the possibility of posttranscriptional modifications cannot be completely excluded. It has been suggested that cytochrome P-450 genes constitute a ''superfamily'', including, to date, 5 different families and a total of 30 to 200 genes.[68] Isoenzymes are also found in human tissues and by time the number of various forms may rise to the same numbers found in animals. Indirect evidence demonstrates several isoenzymes of P-450 especially in the human liver.[69,70] Evidence for several isoenzymes of EH[49,71] and GSH-transferase[72] in human liver also exists.

It seems probable that a large portion of the interindividual variability in carcinogen metabolism and activation can be explained by variable patterns of specific P-450 isozymes in tissues of different individuals. Polymorphic variation of some critical enzymes may have important implications in sensitivity to carcinogens (see Section V). Probing this variability is one of the most interesting current research areas.

E. Induction-Inhibition

Many of the enzymes in pertaining both to the activation of carcinogens and DNA repair are inducible. Because people are exposed to different amounts of inducing chemicals, this leads to different enzyme activities also in genetically similar individuals. Furthermore, interindividual differences have been shown to occur in the extent of genetically determined inducibility in man (AHH[57,73]). Exposure to alternative substrates of carcinogen-metabolizing enzymes may lead to an inhibition and the possible outcome is dependent on whether activating or detoxicating enzymes are inhibited. What seems important here is the long-lasting exposures to inducing or inhibiting chemicals. It is speculated that at least a portion of cancer-modifying effects of, for example, alcohol, coffee, or chronic drug treatment may be due to effects on carcinogen metabolism.

F. *In Vitro* Methods Used

Usually variation observed in experimental studies is regarded as reflecting the true situation, but the design of the studies as well as the actual methods used are critical when judging whether the interindividual variation found is real. The qualitative aspect is easy to judge, but with quantitative variation one ought to be careful. The importance of this aspect has been shown in connection with the AHH assay in mitogen-induced lymphocytes[74] (see also Section V.B) and baseline SCE level in lymphocytes.[55] Possibly the lowest interindividual variation, rather than the highest found in studies large enough, should be regarded as the most valid. If two or more methods are used to study the same variable and give similar or comparable results, the conclusions rest on a much firmer basis. Also, results from studies with cultured or explanted tissues and cells should never be presented without relevant measures of comparability (the measures of viability, passage number of cells, a quantitative measure of the amount of tissue used like the number of cells per plate, etc.). Many enzyme assays are based on the quantitation of the product, which, again, is dependent as much on the number of cells as on the metabolizing capacity of the cells. If we are working on a cell culture the cells can be easily counted, but for the explant cultures no such easy and unquestionable way of quantitation is currently available. These problems, as well as the interlaboratory comparisons, should be pursued much more vigorously than is currently done.

IV. ANIMAL MODELS

Ever since the Millers' group[75,76] demonstrated that susceptibility to 2-acetylaminofluorene-induced cancer in different species showed a fairly good correlation with sulfotransferase activity, attempts to delineate the contribution of genetic and environmental factors to cancer susceptibility have been pursued. However, interspecies comparisons rarely give definite information about molecular mechanisms behind differences in susceptibility, because there are a large number of gene differences between even closely related species. Species differences, while providing useful clues, do not constitute definitive information. The development of inbred strains within species has provided a much more powerful tool to study the contribution of genetic factors, because of the possibility of definitive breeding experiments.[77,78] The essential conclusion from studies with inbred animal strains has been, perhaps expectedly, that in most instances many genes contribute to cancer susceptibility.

There are some indications, although the evidence is sometimes contradictory, that single-gene differences in xenobiotic metabolism may contribute to chemical carcinogenesis. In inbred strains of mice, the Ah locus that controls the induction of certain xenobiotic-metabolizing enzymes, e.g., cytochrome P_1-450-associated aryl hydrocarbon hydroxylase (AHH), by polycyclic aromatic hydrocarbons has been shown to be of importance in cancers induced by polycyclic aromatic hydrocarbons and a number of other chemicals as well.[79] Mice which are genetically responsive to polycyclic hydrocarbons, i.e., those in which the enzymes in the liver and other tissues are increased after the exposure, are at increased risk for cancers at proximal sites, such as dermis and lung. Also mice not responsive to polycyclic aromatic hydrocarbons are susceptible to some cancers at distal sites, which are exposed to larger doses of carcinogens because of unresponsiveness of the ''protective'' enzymatic systems.[80] However, AHH induction also provides protection in certain instances. If the enzyme is induced in skin by the application of TCDD, the development of skin papillomas and carcinomas by the subsequent application of 3-methylcholanthrene is lowered.[81] Also, systemic tumorigenesis after intragastric 3-methylcholanthrene is prevented to a variable extent in responsive mice by pretreatment with β-naphthoflavone, whereas protection was not found in nonresponsive strains.[82]

On the basis of these extensive studies on murine Ah locus several potentially important conclusions can be drawn: (1) the genetic background for the inducibility of a single enzyme (AHH) activating and inactivating carcinogens is important, (2) activating and protecting roles depend upon the specific tissue, whether proximal or distal in terms of the entry of the inducer and the carcinogen to the body, and (3) there are complex consequences of even a primarily single-gene difference in carcinogen metabolism.

Recent interest in the role of debrisoquine hydroxylation polymorphism in cancer susceptibility (see Section V.C) has led to a search for possible animal models. It has been demonstrated that the Fischer rat strain is eight times more effective in metabolizing debrisoquine than the DA strain.[83,84] Fischer rats have also shown to be very sensitive to aflatoxin B_1-induced liver tumors, whereas DA rats are resistent.[85] However, rates of activation of aflatoxin to a mutagen and to a covalently bound metabolite are similar in two strains.[86] Consequently, the evidence seems to favor the interpretation that a difference in cancer susceptibility is not due to a difference in debrisoquine locus.

Table 3
THE POSSIBLE LINKS BETWEEN THE POLYMORPHISMS OF HUMAN XENOBIOTIC METABOLISM AND THE METABOLISM AND/OR CARCINOGENIC EFFECTS OF CHEMICAL CARCINOGENS

Known polymorphism	Carcinogen	Relationship	Ref.
Acetylation	Probably aromatic amines	A positive relationship between bladder cancer and the slow phenotype	87 88
Antipyrine	Benzo(a)pyrene	Metabolisms closely correlated in human liver	89
Debrisoquine 4-hydroxylation	Possibly PAH and/or nitrosamines	A positive relationship between bronchial cancer and the extensive phenotype	90
	Probably aflatoxin	A positive relationship between hepatocellular cancer and the extensive phenotype	90
	Benzo(a)pyrene	No relationship of metabolism in human liver; no relationship with AHH	91 92
Bufuralol oxidation[a]	2-Acetylaminofluorene	No relationship of metabolisms in human liver	93
AHH induction	PAH	A positive relationship between bronchial carcinoma and high induction claimed	94
GSH *S*-transferase	Probably many carcinogens	A positive relationship between lung cancer and lack of activity suggested	95

[a] The same polymorphism as debrisoquine hydroxylation.

V. GENETIC BACKGROUND OF CARCINOGEN METABOLISM

A. Genetic Polymorphisms in Man

A large number of pharmacogenetic conditions inherited as a single-gene difference are known and reviewed extensively during the recent years.[59,60,78] Both increases and decreases in the elimination and effects of drugs and other foreign chemicals have been observed in connection with these conditions. Analogously, it seems highly probable that genetically controlled differences can be found with carcinogen-metabolizing enzymes and DNA repair enzymes. Several polymorphic conditions that have been linked with differences in cancer susceptibility in man or that may be of potential significance, are listed in Table 3, and will be discussed in some detail in the next sections. There are also a number of other situations which may prove to be important in the future investigations. For example, estrogens are metabolized by the P-450 system and because there are variations between individuals in the pattern of metabolites it has been suggested that interindividual differences in estrogen oxidation are associated with cancer risk.[96] However, it is not known whether these differences are of genetic origin.

B. Aryl Hydrocarbon Hydroxylase Induction

In a kind of analogy to the Ah locus model in mice, Kellermann and co-workers[97] suggested that AHH inducibility in human peripheral lymphocytes was inherited as a single gene with two alleles showing additive inheritance. They reported that patients with lung cancer had a different distribution of AHH inducibility, with predominantly intermediate and high AHH inducibility phenotypes, and concluded that the allele for high inducibility (corresponding to the responsive Ah^b allele in the mouse) conferred an increased risk of lung cancer.[98] Later studies have provided very conflicting evidence. The authors have been relatively unanimous, that AHH induction in man is mostly genetically controlled, but the possible association with lung cancer is still unresolved. Several studies have suggested a positive correlation between high AHH activity in lymphocytes and lung cancer,[74,99] but there are also some negative findings. The situation has been repeatedly reviewed[23,100,101] and here we discuss only the basic aspects and controversies of this association.

First of all, the metabolism of benzo(a)pyrene is extremely complicated, as is the case with most chemical carcinogens. The AHH assay measures only hydroxymetabolites, predominantly 3- and 9-hydroxyderivatives. Thus, it is no wonder that studies exist, where no correlation between AHH activity and benzo(a)pyrene-DNA adducts have been found.[102] The most reproducible and consistently higher results for benzo(a)pyrene metabolism in cultured tissues or cells from cancer patients have given investigations in which DNA-binding has been measured.[103] Consequently, it is quite possible that the assay selection also determines the finding, either negative or positive.

The basic prerequisite for the use of lymphocytes to measure the genetically controlled induction of AHH is the underlying assumption that AHH induction is ''systemically'' regulated, in other words, the regulation is similarly expressed in both the target tissue and the tissue where the measurement is made. Although this condition is fulfilled in inbred strains of mice,[4] it is not that certain in man. Pelkonen et al.[104] demonstrated that AHH induction in lymphocytes from cord blood (representing fetal lymphocytes) is in a statistically significant correlation with cigarette smoke-induced AHH activity in the corresponding placentas. In a later study the pulmonary AHH activity correlated significantly with AHH induction in lymphocytes.[105] There are also studies which seem to indicate that AHH activities or inducibilities do not correlate in different cells or tissues. Consequently, the question has not been settled.

Another problem is the selection of the tissue in which to measure the activity and inducibility. In most studies lymphocytes have been used, but monocytes or pulmonary macrophages have also been suggested as more reliable alternatives. This problem is also related to the stability of the tissue. It is known that numerous factors affect the mitogen responsiveness of the lymphocytes, but it is not known how profoundly these effects are reflected in the AHH assay.[74,99,106,107] Monocytes have been recommended on the basis that they are much more stable and do not need mitogen stimulation, but on the other hand, a much larger blood sample is needed.

In addition to the question of mitogen responsiveness, other technical problems must be dealt with. What is the proper measure of the induction? Is it the ratio between induced and uninduced values or the induced value or either one standardized with a measure for the mitogen response such as thymidine incorporation or with a measure for endoplasmic reticulum such as NADH-cytochrome c reductase? Both negative and positive associations have been found with any one of these possibilities. Thus far strictly comparative studies between different assays have not been performed and at present it is impossible to say which one to select.

Recently it has been suggested that rapidly advancing molecular biology technology should be employed for the solution of these problems.[99] Potentially useful approaches include the assay of Ah receptor,[108] measurement of the specific mRNA for AHH,[109] analysis of the chromosomal genes coding for AHH,[110] including possible restriction fragment length polymorphisms (RFLPs), and determination of types of cytochrome P-450s by monoclonal antibodies.[111-113] The experiences with these techniques are still very few, although undoubtedly they will add much to our knowledge in the near future.

C. Debrisoquine Hydroxylation

Recently, another genetic polymorphism of xenobiotic metabolism, debrisoquine 4-hydroxylation capacity, has been linked with the increased risk for liver[114] and lung cancer.[115]

In both cases, the relative lack of poor metabolizers among cancer patients may suggest that extensive metabolizer phenotype is required for efficient conversion of appropriate chemical carcinogens into initiating agents. However, there are a number of problems in the interpretation of these recent studies. First, the numbers of cases and controls are rather small, especially in the study of liver cancer, and taking the incidence of the poor metabolizer phenotype into consideration, much larger populations are needed for reliable statistics. Second, in retrospective studies it is difficult to avoid the bias created by the disease itself. Furthermore, although debrisoquine hydroxylation polymorphism has been linked with variations in the metabolism of at least 20 drugs, not a single relevant carcinogen has been found to display this polymorphism. Thus far, benzo(a)pyrene,[91,92] aflatoxin B1, some nitrosamines, and aromatic amines[93] have been studied. Consequently, there is no biologically meaningful explanation for the association between the above-mentioned cancers and the genetic trait. One possibility is that debrisoquine locus is linked to a nearby locus which is of significance for the susceptibility, thus conferring an increased risk to lung or liver cancer.[90] Although this hypothesis is testable in the near future, the overall conclusion at this moment is that the suggested link between debrisoquine locus and lung and liver cancer is only an interesting ''association'' and which may not have etiological implications.

It is of interest, that both induced benzo(a)pyrene hydroxylation and debrisoquine oxidation are preferentially catalyzed by distinct, and separate, cytochrome P-450 isozymes in man.[111,112,116] Studies in experimental animals and in humans have demonstrated the presence of a number of other isozymes displaying polymorphisms, e.g., the hydroxylation of *S*-mephenytoin, oxidation of 5-carboxymethyl-L-cysteine and the production of each of the three major metabolites of antipyrine.[117,118] The last mentioned polymorphism has been linked with cancer risk in the study of Kellermann et al.,[119] which demonstrated the increased antipyrine elimination in the saliva of lung cancer patients. There are certainly interindividual differences in the isozyme compositions in any given target tissue, which may lead to comparable differences in carcinogen activation and detoxication. These interindividual differences are being investigated by different techniques, e.g., by antibodies to specific P-450 isozymes, thus making it possible to ''phenotype'' individuals.

D. Polymorphic Acetylation

N-Acetylation polymorphism is another well-known genetic trait affecting the pharmacokinetics, and consequently therapeutic efficacy and side-effects, of several drugs. There is some evidence that carcinogenic aromatic amines in occupational settings might increase bladder cancer risk more in slow acetylators than in rapid,[120,121] possibly because acetylation serves as a detoxication pathway for carcinogenic aromatic amines. This association is biologically sound, because at least some carcinogenic aromatic amines are metabolized through this polymorphic enzyme. Nevertheless, epidemiologically undisputable proof is difficult to obtain, due in part to the fact that the exposure has been drastically decreased ever since aromatic amines were established as human carcinogens. Consequently it is difficult to find populations with sufficiently differing exposures. However, Weber and Hein[87] have developed an animal model, which has shown promise in the elucidation of the above problems. A structural mutation in a single enzyme of liver is the cause of polymorphic acetylation in rabbit, and it seems that the molecular basis in human is similar, while in hamster two different *N*-acetyltransferases exist.[87,123]

E. Glutathione *S*-Transferase (GSH-Transferase) Polymorphism

Recently the first plausible human example about the potential importance of detoxication enzymes in cancer susceptibility has been suggested. Seidgård et al.[52,124] demonstrated that glutathione *S*-transferase (stilbene oxide as a substrate) displays 100- to 200-fold variation in lymphocytes. The high activity is due to a single isoenzyme, which is principally genetically controlled. Later on they demonstrated that the lack of enzyme was more common in patients with lung cancer.[95] The plausible explanation behind this finding was suggested to be the relative inability of the patients to detoxify carcinogenic intermediates formed in the body from cigarette smoke constituents.

VI. CONCLUSIONS

It is important to realize that although the DNA binding of the carcinogens followed by the fixation of the damage seems to be the most probable initiation event in chemical carcinogenesis, it still is an unproven case. However, since this appears to represent "the best-fit model", it should be tested in humans. It has only been during recent years that methods sensitive enough have emerged to enable the study of carcinogen binding in humans after environmental exposures.

Another equally important task is to find measures for the individual sensitivity to chemical carcinogens. The work being currently done in this aspect is totally based on the hypothesis mentioned above. In Figure 3 we have tried to illustrate the complexity of the whole system around carcinogen activation, DNA binding and DNA repair, and the difficulties encountered when attempting to correlate two (or more) events in the sequence. This reasoning shows that the existence of DNA damage is impossible to predict if only one factor is known. Only certain probabilities remain which are higher if more than one factor points to the same direction. The only clearcut case is the absence of the enzyme activity, in which case no products exist. Theoretically, if there is no exposure to carcinogens, the result is the same, but in practice this is never the case. Most humans are exposed to the bulk of the existing carcinogens during their lifetime. Risk is thus probably more of a quantitative than qualitative nature. Pathways which are worthwhile to study are evidently those, and maybe only those of direct significance to the carcinogenic process. Thus they ought to be found first in connection with each of the specific carcinogens. This work is far from completed.

One last point to consider: while genetic determinants of cancer susceptibility are an important area of scientific inquiry, the implications of results might have far-reaching practical and even ethical problems in everyday life. Although scientists cannot solve these problems it is however their responsibility to be aware of them.

ACKNOWLEDGMENTS

The authors thank Dr. Hannu Raunio for helpful comments. The original research from the authors' laboratory was supported by The Academy of Finland.

This review is dedicated to Professor Niilo T. Kärki, M.D., the long-time Head of the Department of Pharmacology, on the occasion of his retirement.

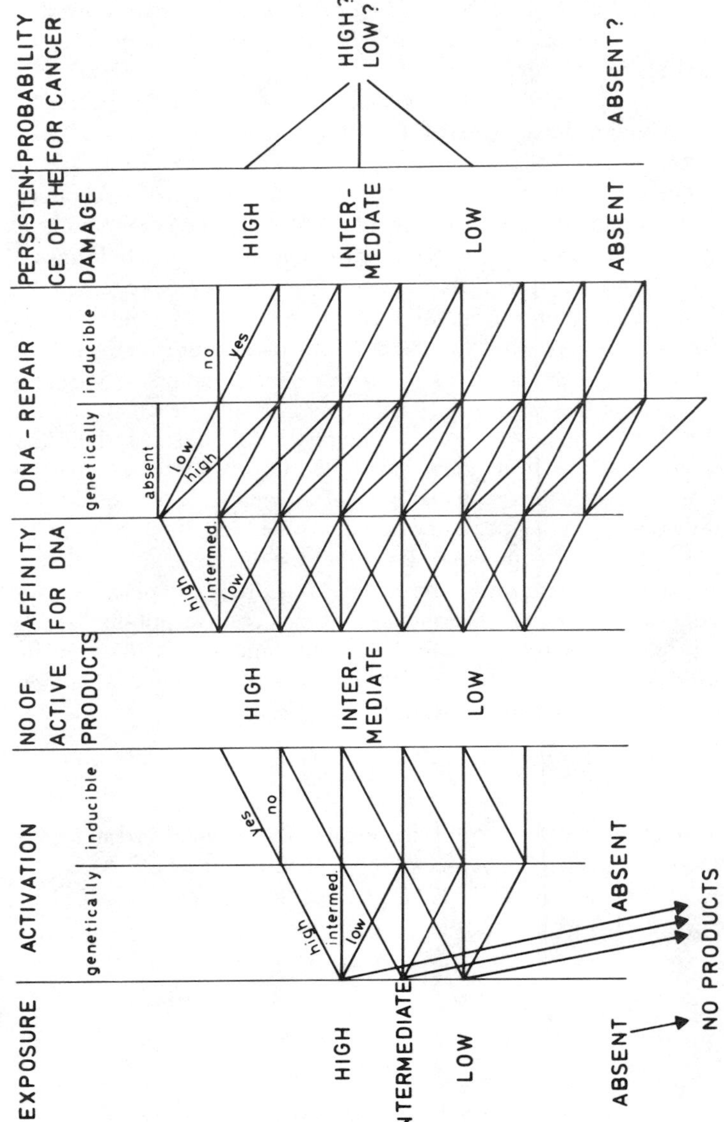

FIGURE 3. Complexity of the network of factors affecting the measurable target tissue damage (e.g., BPDE-DNA adducts) potentially initiating and leading to manifest cancer.

REFERENCES

1. **Grover, P. L., Ed.,** *Chemical Carcinogens and DNA,* Vol. 1 and 2, CRC Press, Boca Raton, Fl., 1979.
2. **Miller, E. C.,** Some current perspectives on chemical carcinogenesis in humans and experimental animals: presidential address, *Cancer Res.,* 38, 1479, 1978.
3. **Testa, B. and Jenner, P.,** *Drug Metabolism: Chemical and Biochemical Aspects,* Marcel Dekker, New York, 1976.
4. **Pelkonen, O. and Nebert, D. W.,** Metabolism of polycyclic aromatic hydrocarbons: etiologic role in carcinogenesis, *Pharmacol. Rev.,* 34, 189, 1982.
5. **Caldwell, J.,** The significance of phase II (conjugation) reactions in drug disposition and toxicity, *Life Sci.,* 24, 571, 1979.
6. **Vainio, H. and Hietanen, E.,** Role of extrahepatic metabolism in drug disposition and toxicity, in *Concepts in Drug Metabolism, Part A,* Jenner, P. and Testa, B., Eds., Marcel Dekker, New York, 1980, 251.
7. **Wolf, C. R., Hartmann, R., Oesch, F., and Adams, D. J.,** Regulation and multiplicity of drug metabolizing enzymes in tissues and cells, *Biochem. Pharmacol.,* Suppl. 1, 121, 1985.
8. **Setlow, R. B.,** DNA repair pathways, in *DNA Repair and Mutagenesis in Eukaryotes,* Generoso, W. M., Shelby, M. D., and deSerres, F. J., Eds., Plenum Press, New York, 1980, 45.
9. **Hanawalt, P. C., Cooper, P. K., Ganesan, A. K., Lloyd, R. S., Smith, C. A., and Zolan, M. E.,** Repair responses to DNA damage: enzymatic pathways in E coli and human cells, *J. Cell. Biochem.,* 18, 271, 1982.
10. **Morgan, W. F. and Cleaver, J. E.,** Effect of 3-aminobenzamide on the rate of ligation during repair of alkylated DNA in human fibroblasts, *Cancer Res.,* 43, 3104, 1983.
11. **Yarosh, D. B.,** The role of O^6-methylguanine-DNA methyltransferase in cell survival, mutagenesis and carcinogenesis, *Mutation Res.,* 145, 1, 1985.
12. **Yagi, T., Yarosh, D. B., and Day, R. S., III,** Comparison of repair of O^6-methylguanine produced by *N*-methyl-*N'*-nitro-*N*-nitrosoguanidine in mouse and human cells, *Carcinogenesis,* 5, 593, 1984.
13. **Gerson, S. L., Miller, K., and Berger, N. A.,** O^6Alkylguanine-DNA alkyltransferase activity in human myeloid cells, *J. Clin. Invest.,* 76, 2106, 1985.
14. **Arlett, C. F.,** Do defects in DNA repair contribute to cancer, in *Familiar Cancer,* Muller, Hj. and Weber, W., Eds., S. Karger, Basel, 1985, 234.
15. **Hsu, T. C., Cherry, L. M., and Samaan, N. A.,** Differential mutagen susceptibility in cultured lymphocytes of normal individuals and cancer patients, *Cancer Genet. Cytogenet.,* 17, 307, 1985.
16. **Pero, R. W., Bryngelsson, A., Bryngelsson, T., and Norden, A.,** A genetic component of the variance of *N*-acetoxy-2-acetylaminofluorene-induced DNA damage in mononuclear leukocytes determined by a twin study, *Human Genet.,* 65, 181, 1983.
17. **Lutz, W. K.,** In vivo covalent binding of organic chemicals to DBA as a quantitative indicator in the process of chemical carcinogenesis, *Mutat. Res.,* 65, 289, 1979.
18. **Pelkonen, O., Vähäkangas, K., and Nebert, D. W.,** Binding of polycyclic aromatic hydrocarbons to DNA: comparison with mutagenesis and tumorigenesis, *J. Toxicol. Environ. Health,* 6, 1009, 1980.
19. **Swenberg, J. A., Richardson, F. C., Boucheron, J. A., and Dyroff, M. C.,** Relationships between DNA adduct formation and carcinogenesis, *Environ. Health Perspect.,* 62, 177, 1985.
20. **McGormick, J. J. and Maher, V. M.,** Cytotoxic and mutagenic effects of specific carcinogen-DNA adducts in diploid human fibroblasts, *Environ. Health Perspect.,* 62, 145, 1985.
21. **Daudel, P., Duquesne, M., Vigny, P., Grover, P. L., and Sims, P.,** Fluorescence spectral evidence that benzo(a)pyrene-DNA products in mouse skin arise from diol-epoxides, *FEBS Lett.,* 57, 250, 1975.
22. **Weinstein, I. B., Jeffrey, A. M., Jennette, K. W., Blobstein, S. H., Harvey, R. G., Harris, C., Autrup, H., Kasai, H., and Nakanishi, K.,** Benzo(a)pyrene diol epoxides as intermediates in nucleic acid binding in vitro and in vivo, *Science,* 193, 592, 1976.
23. **Gelboin, H. V.,** Benzo(a)pyrene metabolism, activation, and carcinogenesis: role and regulation of mixed-function oxidases and related enzymes, *Physiol. Rev.,* 60, 1107, 1980.
24. **Hemminki, K.,** Nucleic acid adducts of chemical carcinogens and mutagens, *Arch. Toxicol.,* 52, 249, 1983.
25. **Harris, C. C., Vähäkangas, K., Trump, B. F., and Autrup, H.,** Interindividual variation in carcinogen activation and DNA repair, in *Genetic Predisposition in Responses to Chemical Exposures: Banbury Report 16,* Omenn, G. S. and Gelboin, H. V., Eds., Cold Spring Harbor Laboratory, Cold Spring Harbor, N.Y., 1984, 145.
26. **Vähäkangas, K., Haugen, A., and Harris, C. C.,** An applied synchronous fluorescence spectrophotometric assay to study benzo(a)pyrene-diolepoxide-DNA adducts, *Carcinogenesis,* 6, 1109, 1985.
27. **Perera, F. P., Poirier, M. C., Yuspa, S. H., Nakayama, J., Jaretzki, A., Curnen, M. M., Knowles, D. M., and Weinstein, I. B.,** A pilot project in molecular cancer epidemiology: determination of benzo(a)pyrene-DNA adducts in animal and human tissues by immunoassays, *Carcinogenesis,* 12, 1405, 1982.

28. **Harris, C. C., Vähäkangas, K., Newman, M. J., Trivers, G. E., Shamsuddin, A., Sinopoli, N., Mann, D. L., and Wright, W. E.,** Detection of benzo(a)pyrene diol epoxide-DNA adducts in peripheral blood lymphocytes and antibodies to the adducts in serum from coke oven workers, *Proc. Natl. Acad. Sci. U.S.A.*, 82, 6672, 1985.
29. **Randerath, K., Randerath, E., Agraval, H. P., and Reddy, M. V.,** Biochemical (postlabelling) methods for analysis of carcinogen-DNA adducts, in *Monitoring Human Exposure to Carcinogenic and Mutagenic Agents,* Berlin, A., Draper, M., Hemminki, K., and Vainio, H., Eds., IARC Sci. Publ. No. 59, International Agency for Research on Cancer, Lyon, 1984, 217.
30. **Shamsuddin, A. K. M., Sinopoli, N. T., Hemminki, K., Boesch, R., and Harris, C. C.,** Detection of benzo(a)pyrene:DNA adducts in human white blood cells, *Cancer Res.*, 45, 66, 1985.
31. **Everson, R. B., Randerath, E., Santella, R. M., Cefalo, R. C., Avitts, T. A., and Randerath, K.,** Detection of smoking-related covalent DNA adducts in human placenta, *Science,* 231, 54, 1986.
32. **Haugen, A., Becher, G., Benestad, C., Vähäkangas, K., Trivers, G. E., Newman, M. J., and Harris, C. C.,** Determination of polycyclic aromatic hydrocarbons in the urine. Benzo(a)pyrene diol epoxide-DNA adducts in lymphocyte DNA and antibodies to the adducts in sera from coke oven workers exposed to measured amounts of polycyclic aromatic hydrocarbons in the work atmosphere, *Cancer Res.*, 46, 4178, 1986.
33. **Vähäkangas, K., Trivers, G., Rowe, M., and Harris, C. C.,** Benzo(a)pyrene diolepoxide-DNA adducts detected by synchronous fluorescence spectrophotometry, *Environ. Health Perspect.*, 61, 101, 1985.
34. **Harris, C. C., LaVeck, G., Groopman, J., Wilson, V., and Mann, D.,** Measurement of aflatoxin B_1, its metabolites, and DNA adducts by synchronous fluorescence spectrophotometry, *Cancer Res.*, 46, 3249, 1986.
35. **Adamkievicz, J., Nehls, P., and Rajewsky, M. F.,** Immunological methods for detection of carcinogen-DNA adducts, in *Monitoring Human Exposure to Carcinogenic and Mutagenic Agents,* Berlin, A., Draper, M., Hemminki, K., and Vainio, H., Eds., IARC Sci. Publ. No. 59, International Agency for Research on Cancer, Lyon, 1984, 199.
36. **Wogan, G. N. and Gorelic, N. J.,** Chemical and biochemical dosimetry of exposure to genotoxic chemicals, *Environ. Health Perspect.*, 62, 5, 1985.
37. **Poirier, M. C., Santella, R., Weinstein, I. B., Grunberger, D., and Yuspa, S.,** Quantitation on benzo(a)pyrene-deoxyguanosine adducts by radioimmunoassay, *Cancer Res.*, 40, 412, 1980.
38. **Santella, R. M., Hsieh, L.-L., Lin, C.-D., Viet, S., and Weinstein, I. B.,** Quantitation of exposure to benzo(a)pyrene with monoclonal antibodies, *Environ. Health Perspect.*, 62, 95, 1985.
39. **Randerath, K., Reddy, M., and Gupta, R. C.,** ^{32}P-labeling test for DNA damage, *Proc. Natl. Acad. Sci. U.S.A.*, 78, 6126, 1981.
40. **Rahn, R. O., Chang, S. S., Holland, J. M., and Shugart, L. R.,** A fluorometric-HPLC assay for quantitating the binding of benzo(a)pyrene metabolites to DNA, *Biochem. Biophys. Res. Commun.*, 109, 262, 1982.
41. **Heisig, V., Jeffrey, A. M., McGlade, M. J., and Small, G. J.,** Fluorescence-line-narrowed spectra of polycyclic aromatic carcinogen-DNA adducts, *Science,* 223, 289, 1984.
42. **Sanders, M. J., Cooper, R. S., Jankowiak, R., Small, G. J., Heisig, V., and Jeffrey, A. M.,** Identification of polycyclic aromatic hydrocarbon metabolites and DNA adducts in mixtures using fluorescence line narrowing spectrometry, *Anal. Chem.*, 58, 816, 1985.
43. **Gill, J. H. and Holder, G. M.,** Application of synchronous luminescence to the separate determination of cochromatographing metabolites of the carcinogen, 7-methylbenz(c)acridine, *J. Pharm. Biomed. Anal.*, 4, 31, 1986.
44. **Conney, A. H., Buening, M. K., Pantuck, E. J., Pantuck, C. B., Fortner, J. G., Anderson, K. E., and Kappas, A.,** Regulation of human drug metabolism by dietary factors, in *Environmental Chemicals, Enzyme Function and Human Disease* (Ciba Foundation Symposium 76), Excerpta Medica, Amsterdam, 1980, 147.
45. **Harris, C. C., Mulvihill, J. J., Thorgeirsson, S. S., and Minna, J. D.,** Individual differences in cancer susceptibility, *Ann. Intern. Med.*, 92, 809, 1980.
46. **Bartsch, H. and Armstrong, B., Eds.,** *Host Factors in Human Carcinogenesis,* IARC Sci. Publ. No. 39, International Agency for Research on Cancer, Lyon, 1982.
47. **Vähäkangas, K., Autrup, H., and Harris, C. C.,** Interindividual variation in carcinogen metabolism, DNA damage and DNA repair, in *Methods of Monitoring Human Exposure to Carcinogenic and Mutagenic Agents,* Berlin, A., Draper, C., Hemminki, K., and Vainio, H., Eds., IARC Scientific Publications, International Agency for Research on Cancer, Lyon, 1984, 85.
48. **Kouri, R. E., Levine, A. S., Edwards, B. K., McLemore, T. L., Vesell, E. S., and Nebert, D. W.,** Sources of interindividual variations in aryl hydrocarbon hydroxylase in mitogen-activated human lymphocytes, in *Genetic Variability in Responses to Chemical Exposure,* Banbury Report, No. 16, Omenn, G. S. and Gelboin, H. V., Eds., Cold Spring Harbor Laboratory, Cold Spring Harbor, N.Y., 1984, 131.

49. **Glatt, H. and Oesch, F.,** Variations in epoxide hydrolase activities in human liver and blood, in *Genetic Variability in Responses to Chemical Exposure,* Banbury Report No. 16, Omenn, G. S. and Gelboin, H. V., Eds., Cold Spring Harbor Laboratory, Cold Spring Harbor, N.Y., 1984, 189.
50. **Myrnes, B., Gierscksky, K.-E., and Krokan, H.,** Interindividual variation in the activity of O^6-methylguanine-DNA methyltransferase and uracil-DNA glycosylase in human organs, *Carcinogenesis,* 4, 1565, 1983.
51. **Mukhtar, H., Zoetelmelk, C. E. M., Baars, A. J., Wijnen, J. Th., Blankenstein-Wijnen, M. M., Khan, P. M., and Breimer, D. D.,** Glutathione *S*-transferase activity in human fetal and adult tissues, *Pharmacology,* 22, 322, 1981.
52. **Seidegård, J. and Pero, R. W.,** The hereditary transmission of high glutathione transferase activity towards transstilbene oxide in human mononuclear leucocytes, *Hum. Genet.,* 69, 66, 1985.
53. **Carr, K., Oates, J. A., Nies, A. S., and Woolsey, R. L.,** Simultaneous analysis of dapsone and monooacetyldapsone employing high performance liquid chromatography, *Br. J. Clin. Pharmacol.,* 6, 421, 1978.
54. **Setlow, R. B.,** Variations in DNA repair among humans, in *Human Carcinogenesis,* Harris, C. C. and Autrup, H., Eds., Academic Press, New York, 1983, 231.
55. **Carrano, A. V., Minkler, J. L., Stetka, D. G., and Moore, D. H.,** Variation in the baseline sister chromatid exchange frequency in human lymphocytes, *Environ. Mutagen.,* 2, 325, 1980.
56. **Cleaver, J. E., Bodell, W. J., Gruenert, D. C., Kapp, L. N., Kaufman, W. K., Park, S. D., and Zelle, B.,** Repair and replication abnormalities in various human hypersensitive diseases, in *Mechanisms of Chemical Carcinogenesis,* Harris, C. C. and Cerutti, P., Eds., Alan R. Liss, New York, 1982, 409.
57. **Glatt, H. R., Halfer-Wirkus, H., Herborn, J., Lehrbach, E., Löffler, S., Pornn, W., Setiabudi, F., Wölfel, T., Gemperlein-Mertes, I., Doerjer, G., and Oesch, F.,** Interindividual variations in epoxide-detoxifying enzymes, in *Familial Cancer,* Muller, Hj. and Weber, W., Eds., S. Karger, Basel, 1985, 242.
58. **Guenthner, T. W. and Karnezis, T. A.,** Multiple epoxide hydrolases in human lung, *Drug Metab. Dispos.,* 14, 208, 1986.
59. **Vesell, E. S. and Penno, M. B.,** Assessment of methods to identify sources of interindividual pharmacokinetic variations, *Clin. Pharmacokin.,* 8, 378, 1983.
60. **Vesell, E. S.,** Pharmacogenetic perspectives: genes, drugs and disease, *Hepatology,* 4, 959, 1984.
61. **Sotaniemi, E. A., Pelkonen, R. O., Ahokas, J. T., Pirttiaho, H. I., and Ahlqvist, J.,** Relationship between in vivo and in vitro drug metabolism in man, *Eur. J. Drug Metab. Pharmacokin.,* 1, 39, 1978.
62. **Sabadie, N., Richter-Reichhelm, H. B., Saracci, R., Mohr, U., and Bartsch, H.,** Interindividual differences in oxidative benzo(a)pyrene metabolism by normal and tumorous surgical lung specimens from 105 lung cancer patients, *Int. J. Cancer,* 27, 417, 1981.
63. **Vesell, E. S. and Passananti, G. T.,** Genetic and environmental factors affecting host response to drugs and other chemical compounds in our environment, *Environ. Health Perspect.,* 20, 159, 1977.
64. **Steiner, E., Iselius, L., Alvan, G., Lindsten, J., and Sjöqvist, F.,** A family study of genetic and environmental factors determining polymorphic hydroxylation of debrisoquine, *Clin. Pharmacol. Ther.,* 38, 394, 1985.
65. **Pegg, A. E., Roberfroid, M., von Bahr, C., Foote, R. S., Mitra, S., Bresil, H., Likhachev, A., and Montesano, R.,** Removal of O^6-methylguanine from DNA by human liver fractions, *Proc. Natl. Acad. Sci. U.S.A.,* 79, 5162, 1982.
66. **Pero, R. W., Miller, D. G., Lipkin, M., Markowitz, M., Gupta, S., Winaver, S. J., Enker, W., and Good, R.,** Reduced capacity for DNA repair synthesis in patients with or genetically predisposed to colorectal cancer, *J. Natl. Cancer Inst.,* 70, 867, 1983.
67. **Harris, C. C., Trump, B. F., Grafström, R., and Autrup, H.,** Differences in metabolism of chemical carcinogens in cultured human epithelial tissues and cells, *J. Cell. Biochem.,* 18, 285, 1982.
68. **Nebert, D. W. and Gonzales, F. J.,** Cytochrome P450 gene expression and regulation, *Trends Pharmacol. Sci.,* 6, 160, 1985.
69. **Boobis, A. R. and Davies, D. S.,** Human cytochromes P-450, *Xenobiotica,* 14, 153, 1984.
70. **Pelkonen, O., Pasanen, M., Vähäkangas, K., and Sotaniemi, E. A.,** Multiple forms of human hepatic cytochrome P-450, in *Cytochrome P-450, Biochemistry, Biophysics and Induction,* Vereczkey, L. and Magyar, K., Eds., Akademiai Kiado, Budapest, 1985, 247.
71. **Oesch, F., Timms, C. W., Walker, C. H., Guenthner, T. M., Sparrow, A., Watabe, T., and Wolf, C. R.,** Existence of multiple forms of microsomal epoxide hydrolases with radically different substrate specificities, *Carcinogenesis,* 5, 7, 1984.
72. **Warholm, M., Guthenberg, C., and Mannervik, B.,** Molecular and catalytic properties of glutathione transferase myy from human liver: an enzyme efficiently conjugating epoxides, *Biochemistry,* 22, 3610, 1983.
73. **Pelkonen, O., Vähäkangas, K., Kärki, N. T., and Sotaniemi, E. A.,** Genetic and environmental regulation of aryl hydrocarbon hydroxylase in man: studies with liver, lung, placenta and lymphocytes, *Toxicol. Pathol.,* 12, 256, 1984.

74. **Kouri, R. E., McKinney, C. E., Slomiany, D. J., Snodgrass, D. R., Wray, N. P., and McLemore, T. L.,** Positive correlation between high aryl hydrocarbon hydroxylase activity and primary lung cancer as analyzed in cryopreserved lymphocytes, *Cancer Res.*, 42, 5030, 1982.
75. **Miller, J. A.,** Carcinogenesis by chemicals. An overview. G. H. A. Glowes memorial lecture, *Cancer Res.*, 30, 559, 1970.
76. **Thorgeirsson, S. S.,** Metabolic determinants in the carcinogenicity of aromatic amines, in *Biochemical Basis of Chemical Carcinogenesis,* Greim, H., Jung, R., Kramer, M., Marquardt, H., and Oesch, F., Eds., Raven Press, New York, 1984, 47.
77. **Heston, W. E.,** Genetics: animal tumors, in *Cancer. A Comprehensive Treatise. Etiology: Chemical and Physical Carcinogenesis,* Vol. 1, Becker, F. F., Ed., Plenum Press, New York, 1975, 33.
78. **Nebert, D. W.,** Pharmacogenetics: an approach to understanding chemical and biologic aspects of cancer, *J. Natl. Cancer Inst.*, 64, 1279, 1980.
79. **Nebert, D. W., Negishi, M., Lang, M. A., Hjelmeland, L. M., and Eisen, H. J.,** The Ah locus, a multigene family necessary for survival in a chemically adverse environment: comparison with the immune system, *Adv. Genet.*, 21, 1, 1982.
80. **Nebert, D. W. and Jensen, N. M.,** The Ah locus: genetic regulation of the metabolism of carcinogens, drugs and other chemicals by cytochrome P-450 mediated monooxygenase, *Crit. Rev. Biochem.*, 6, 401, 1979.
81. **DiGiovanni, J., Berry, D. L., Gleason, G. L., Kishore, G. S., and Slaga, T. J.,** Time-dependent inhibition by 2,3,7,8-tetrachlorodibenzo-*p*-dioxin of skin tumorigenesis with polycyclic hydrocarbons, *Cancer Res.*, 40, 1580, 1980.
82. **Anderson, L. M. and Seetharam, S.,** Protection against tumorigenesis by 3-methylcholanthrene in mice by β-naphthoflavone as a function of inducibility of methylcholanthrene metabolism, *Cancer Res.*, 45, 6384, 1985.
83. **Al-Dabbagh, S. G., Idle, J. R., and Smith, R. L.,** Animal modelling of human polymorphic drug oxidation — the metabolism of debrisoquine and phenacetin in rat inbred strains, *J. Pharm. Pharmacol.*, 33, 161, 1981.
84. **Kahn, G. C., Rubenfield, M., Davies, D. S., Murray, S., and Boobis, A. R.,** Sex and strain differences in hepatic debrisoquine 4-hydroxylase activity of the rat, *Drug Metab. Disp.*, 13, 510, 1985.
85. **Neal, G. E.,** personal communication.
86. **Boobis, A. R., Kahn, G. C., Davies, D. S., and Plummer, S.,** The metabolic activation of aflatoxin B_1 in rat and man, *Br. J. Pharmacol.*, (Suppl.), 78, 61, 1983.
87. **Weber, W. W. and Hein, D. W.,** *N*-Acetylation pharmacogenetics, *Pharmacol. Rev.*, 37, 25, 1985.
88. **Ladero, J. M., Kwok, C. K., Jara, C., Fernandez, L., Silmi, A. M., Tapia, D., and Uson, A. C.,** Hepatic acetylator phenotype in bladder cancer patients, *Ann. Clin. Res.*, 17, 96, 1985.
89. **Kapitulnik, J., Poppers, P. J., and Conney, A. H.,** Comparative metabolism of benzo(a)pyrene and drugs in human liver, *Clin. Pharmacol. Ther.*, 21, 166, 1977.
90. **Idle, J. R. and Ritchie, J. C.,** Probing genetically variable carcinogen metabolism using drugs, in *Human Carcinogenesis,* Harris, C. C. and Autrup, H. N., Eds., Academic Press, New York, 1983, 857.
91. **Wolff, T. and Strecker, M.,** Lack of relationship between debrisoquine 4-hydroxylation and other cytochrome P-450 dependent reactions in rat and human liver, *Biochem. Pharmacol.*, 34, 2593, 1985.
92. **Birgersson, C., Blanck, A., Woodhouse, K., Mellström, B., and von Bahr, C.,** Comparative metabolism of debrisoquine, 7-ethoxyresorufin and benzo(a)pyrene in liver microsomes from humans, and from rats treated with cytochrome P-450 inducers, *Acta Pharmacol. Toxicol.*, 57, 117, 1985.
93. **McManus, M. E., Boobis, A. R., Minchin, R. F., Schwarz, D. M., Murray, S., Davies, D. S., and Thorgeirsson, S. S.,** Relationship between oxidative metabolism of 2-acetylaminofluorene, debrisoquine, bufuralol, and aldrin in human liver microsomes, *Cancer Res.*, 44, 5692, 1984.
94. **Gelboin, H. V.,** Carcinogens, drugs and cytochromes P-450, *N. Engl. J. Med.*, 309, 105, 1983.
95. **Seidegård, J., Pero, R. W., Miller, D. G., and Beattie, E. J.,** A glutathione transferase in human leukocytes as a marker for the susceptibility to lung cancer, *Carcinogenesis,* 7, 751, 1986.
96. **Schneider, J., Kinne, D., Fracchia, A., Pierce, V., Anderson, K. E., Bradlow, H. L., and Fishman, J.,** Abnormal oxidative metabolism of estradiol in women with breast cancer, *Proc. Natl. Acad. Sci.*, 79, 3047, 1982.
97. **Kellermann, G., Luyten-Kellermann, M., and Shaw, C. R.,** Genetic variation of aryl hydrocarbon hydroxylase in human lymphocytes, *Am. J. Hum. Genet.*, 25, 327, 1973.
98. **Kellermann, G., Shaw, C. R., and Luyten-Kellermann, M.,** Aryl hydrocarbon hydroxylase inducibility and bronchogenic carcinoma, *N. Engl. J. Med.*, 289, 934, 1973.
99. **Kouri, R. E., McLemore, T., Jaiswal, A. K., and Nebert, D. W.,** Current cellular assays for measuring clinical drug metabolizing capacity — impact of new molecular biologic techniques, in *Ethnic Differences in Reactions to Drugs and Xenobiotics,* Kalow, W., Goedde, H., and Agarwal, S., Eds., Alan R. Liss, New York, 1986, 453.

100. **Pelkonen, O., Sotaniemi, E. A., and Kärki, N. T.,** Human metabolic variability in xenobiotic biotransformation: implications for genotoxicity, in *Mutagens in Our Environment,* Sorsa, M. and Vainio, H., Eds., Alan R. Liss, New York, 1982, 61.

101. **Bartsch, H., Aitio, A., Camus, A. M., Malaveille, C., Roberfroid, M., Vo Thi, K. O., and Sabadie, N.,** Carcinogen-metabolizing enzymes and susceptibility to chemical carcinogenesis, in *Modulators of Experimental Carcinogenesis,* Turusov, V. and Montesano, R., Eds., IARC Sci. Publ. No. 51, International Agency for Research on Cancer, Lyon, 1983, 147.

102. **Wilson, A. G. E., Kung, H.-C., Boroujerd, M., and Anderson, M. W.,** Inhibition in vivo of the formation of adducts between metabolites of benzo(a)pyrene and DNA by aryl hydrocarbon hydroxylase inducers, *Cancer Res.,* 41, 3453, 1981.

103. **Rudiger, H. W., Nowak, D., Hartmann, K., and Cerutti, P.,** Enhanced formation of benzo(a)pyrene:DNA adducts in monocytes of patients with a presumed predisposition to lung cancer, *Cancer Res.,* 45, 5890, 1985.

104. **Pelkonen, O., Kärki, N. T., and Tuimala, R.,** A relationship between cord blood and maternal blood lymphocytes and term placenta in the induction of aryl hydrocarbon hydroxylase activity, *Cancer Lett.,* 13, 103, 1981.

105. **Kärki, N. T., Pokela, R., Nuutinen, L., and Pelkonen, O.,** Aryl hydrocarbon hydroxylase in lymphocytes and lung tissue from lung cancer patients and controls, *Int. J. Cancer,* 39, 565, 1987.

106. **Pelkonen, O., Kärki, N. T., and Sotaniemi, E. A.,** Determination of carcinogen-activating enzymes in the monitoring of high-risk groups, in *Human Cancer. Its Characterisation and Treatment,* Davis, W., Harrap, K. R., and Stathopoulos, G., Eds., Excerpta Medica, Amsterdam, 1980, 48.

107. **Nebert, D. W.,** The Ah locus. A gene with possible importance in cancer predictability, *Arch. Toxicol. Suppl.,* 3, 195, 1979.

108. **Okey, A. B., Roberts, E. A., Harper, P. A., and Denison, M. S.,** Induction of drug-metabolizing enzymes: mechanisms and consequences, *Clin. Biochem.,* 19, 132, 1986.

109. **Jaiswal, A. K., Gonzalez, F. J., and Nebert, D. W.,** Human P_1-450 gene sequence and correlation of mRNA with genetic differences in benzo(a)pyrene metabolism, *Nucleic Acids Res.,* 13, 4503, 1985.

110. **Iversen, P. L., Hines, R. N., and Bresnick, E.,** The molecular biology of the polycyclic aromatic hydrocarbon inducible cytochrome P-450; the past is prologue, *BioEssays,* 4, 15, 1986.

111. **Fujino, T., Park, S. S., West, D., and Gelboin, H. V.,** Phenotyping of cytochrome P-450 in human tissues with monoclonal antibodies, *Proc. Natl. Acad. Sci. U.S.A.,* 79, 3682, 1982.

112. **Pelkonen, O., Pasanen, M., Kuha, H., Gachalyi, B., Kairaluoma, M., Sotaniemi, E. A., Park, S. S., Friedman, F. K., and Gelboin, H. V.,** The effect of cigarette smoking on 7-ethoxycoumarin *O*-deethylase and other monooxygenase activities in human liver: analyses with monoclonal antibodies, *Br. J. Clin. Pharmacol.,* 22, 125, 1986.

113. **Gelboin, H. V. and Friedman, F. K.,** Monoclonal antibodies for studies on xenobiotic and endobiotic metabolism. Cytochromes P-450 as paradigm, *Biochem. Pharmacol.,* 34, 2225, 1985.

114. **Idle, J. R., Mahgoub, A., Sloan, T. P., Smith, R. L., Mbanefo, C. O., and Bababunmi, E. A.,** Some observations on the oxidation phenotype status of Nigerian patients presenting with cancer, *Cancer Lett.,* 11, 331, 1981.

115. **Ayesh, R., Idle, J. R., Ritchie, J. C., Crothers, M. J., and Hetzel, M. R.,** Metabolic oxidation phenotypes as markers for susceptibility to lung cancer, *Nature,* 312, 169, 1984.

116. **Distlerath, L. M., Reilly, P. E. B., Martin, M. V., Davis, G. G., Wilkinson, G. R., and Guengerich, F. P.,** Purification and characterization of the human liver cytochromes P-450 involved in debrisoquine 4-hydroxylation and phenacetin *O*-deethylation, two prototypes for genetic polymorphism in oxidative drug metabolism, *J. Biol. Chem.,* 260, 9057, 1985.

117. **Kupfer, A. and Preisig, R.,** Pharmacogenetics of mephenytoin: a new drug hydroxylation polymorphism in man, *Eur. J. Clin. Pharmacol.,* 26, 753, 1984.

117a. **Mitchell, S. C., Waring, R. H., Haley, C. S., Idle, J. R., and Smith, R. L.,** Genetic aspects of the polymodally distributed sulphoxidation of *S*-carboxymethyl-L-systeine in man, *Br. J. Clin. Pharmacol.,* 18, 507, 1984.

118. **Penno, M. B. and Vesell, E. S.,** Monogenic control of variations in antipyrine metabolite formation, *J. Clin. Invest.,* 71, 1698, 1983.

119. **Kellerman, G., Jett, J. R., Luyten-Kellermann, M., Moses, H. L., and Fontana, R. S.,** Variation of microsomal mixed-function oxidase(s) and human lung cancer, *Cancer,* 45, 1438, 1980.

120. **Lower, G. M., Nilsson, T., Nelson, C. E., Wolf, H., Gamsky, T. E., and Bryan, G. T.,** *N*-Acetyltransferase phenotype and the risk of urinary bladder cancer: approaches in molecular epidemiology. Preliminary results in Sweden and Denmark, *Environ. Health Perspect.,* 29, 71, 1979.

121. **Cartwright, R. A., Glashan, R. W., Rogers, H. J., Ahmad, R. A., Barham-Hall, D., Higgins, E., and Kahn, M. A.,** Role of *N*-acetyltransferase phenotypes in bladder carcinogenesis: a pharmacogenetic epidemiological approach to bladder cancer, *Lancet,* II, 842, 1982.

122. **Weber, W. W.,** Commentary: the molecular basis of hereditary acetylation polymorphism, *Drug Metab. Disp.*, 14, 377, 1986.
123. **Seidegård, J., DePierre, J. W., and Pero, R. W.,** Hereditary interindividual differences in the glutathione transferase activity towards trans-stilbene axide in resting human mononuclear leukocytes are due to a particular isozyme(s), *Carcinogenesis*, 6, 1211, 1985.

Chapter 4

TERATOGENESIS AND ONCOGENESIS: A DEVELOPMENTAL SPECTRUM

Robert P. Bolande

TABLE OF CONTENTS

I. INTRODUCTION

Teratogenesis and oncogenesis are developmentally different reactions to special cellular injuries or events in prenatal life. The timing of these events is critical in determining the outcome. The pathologic effects of the earliest injuries are embryolethal or teratogenic. Teratogenesis is the most primitive reaction and ostensibly the most common, being manifested as congenital malformation in upwards of 3% of new born infants.[1,2] As gestation proceeds, cytoproliferative reactions appear, culminating at birth in hamartomas, benign neoplasms, or true malignancies. Neoplasia is comparatively rare. Intermediate phases in this developmental spectrum would be manifested as a concurrence of malformations and tumors in childhood. In later gestation, the more highly evolved inflammatory reactions assert themselves, typically the result of transplacental infections, e.g., rubella, toxoplasmosis, syphilis, etc. These give rise to the inflammatory deformations of previously normal fetal tissues and organs. There is no derangement of embryogenetic programming (Figure 1).

II. THE ASSOCIATION OF NEOPLASMS WITH MALFORMATIONS

Epidemologic studies have shown that important associations of tumors and malformations exist which are diverse and complex. A concurrence of anomalies with sacrococcygeal teratoma has been reported.[3] These anomalies are mainly localized to the region of the tumor and included meningomyeloceles, spina bifida, sacral defects, hypospadias, imperforate anus, genitourinary, and hindgut duplications.[4,5]

In an analysis of 371 carefully studied cases of childhood malignant disease at the University of Tokyo,[6] 41% of the children showed evidence of congenital malformation, in contrast to 13% in children without malignant neoplasms. Wilms' tumor showed the highest concurrence (58%), followed by lymphoreticular malignancies (48%), hepatoblastoma (45%), leukemia (44%), neuroblastoma and retinoblastoma (35% each), brain tumors (28%), and testicular-ovarian tumors (17%).

It has now become clear after the pioneering observations of Miller[7] at the NIH, that more-or-less specific congenital defects or teratologic syndromes predispose to the development of certain neoplasms. There is, thus, some degree of specificity of the teratologic conditions and the tumors they herald. In most instances, the neoplasms appear in infancy and childhood. Some of these teratologic conditions are sporadic, some are hereditary, while a growing number are being shown to be cytogenetically determined. These are summarized in Table 1.

Tumors, furthermore, may develop directly in developmental vestiges, heterotopias, hamartomas, and dysgenetic gonads. This is a reenunciation of the Cohnheim[8] "fetal rest" theory of cancer proposed in 1877 which held that neoplasia arises from deranged embryogenesis. This is quite evident in the hereditary hamartoses (Table 2) and in the undescended testes and dygenetic gonads associated with sex chromosomal abnormalities (Table 3).

Explanations for all these relationship are as yet speculative.[9] Rapidly dividing cells are a prerequisite for both teratogenesis and oncogeneis. During mitosis, the cell is most vulnerable to structural changes in DNA, to disruption of transcription to RNA, and to subsequent translation into protein-enzyme synthesis. The resting cell is more capable of a certain degree of repair and restoration of this system than is the dividing cell. Mitotic activity is more universally present throughout the body in intrauterine life than at any later stage in the life cycle.

Most agents, known to be carcinogenic postnatally, are teratogenic to the fetus or embryo.[10] Some agents, such as irradiation, estrogens, and the alkylnitrosoureas give both effects when administered prenatally.[9,11] Studies of Japanese survivors of atomic bomb explosions have

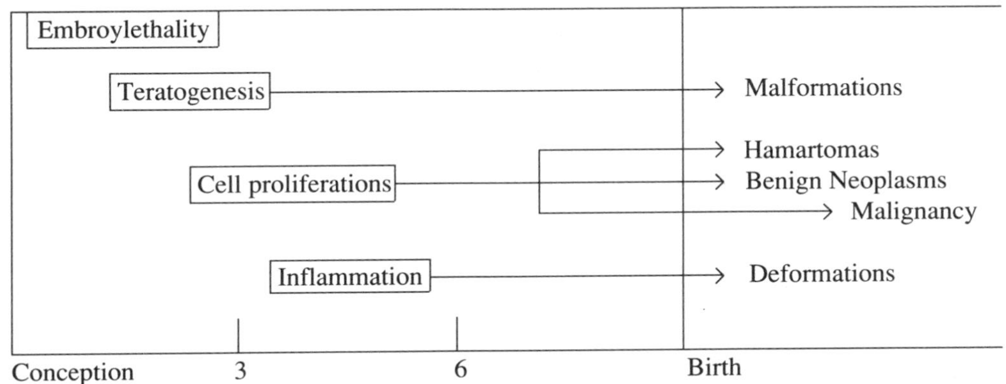

FIGURE 1. The ontogeny of reaction to injury.

Table 1
SPECIFIC TERATOLOGIC DISORDERS ASSOCIATED WITH NEOPLASM[2,3]

Anomaly	Tumor
Dysmorphic syndromes	
Hemihypertrophy	Wilms' tumor
	Hepatoblastoma
	Adrenocortical carcinoma
Beckwith syndrom	Adrenocortical carcinoma
	Wilms' tumor and nephroblastomatosis
Genitourinary tract malformation and pseudohermaphroditism (Drash syndrome)	Wilms' tumor and nephroblastomatosis
Basal cell nevus syndrome	Basal cell carcinoma
	Medulloblastoma
	Rhabdomyosarcoma
Poland syndrome	Leukemia
Chromosomal abnormalities	
Mongolism (trisomy 21)	Leukemia, retinoblastoma
Aniridia—11p⁻ syndrome	Wilms' tumor and gonadoblastoma
13q⁻ syndrome	Retinoblastoma
Chromosomal breakage syndromes	
Fanconi anemia	Leukemia
	Squamous cell carcinoma
	Hepatoma (androgen-induced)
Bloom syndrome	Leukemia
	Gastrointestinal carcinoma
Ataxia telangiectasia	Lymphoma
	Leukemia
	Others

shown that those individuals heavily exposed to radioactive fallout *in utero* have an increased incidence of microcephaly and mental retardation, but this population has not developed an excess of neoplasms. The population exposed during childhood have developed an increased incidence of leukemia and other cancers.[12] It seems clear from experimental studies with these agents that the timing of the initiating event(s) may be critical in determining the form of the outcome. Much work remains to be done in this field.

A primary event in the fetus may in some fashion predispose the organism to a secondary oncogenic influence in later life. This might explain the neoplastic transformation occurring

Table 2
HARMATOMAS AND HAMARTOSES[3,9]

Tissue of origin	Pathologic examples	Genetics	Neoplastic transformation
Vascular	Congenital hemangiomas and vascular nevi of skin		
	Lymphangiomas and cystic hygromas		
	Milroy disease	Autosomal dominant	
	Multiple glomangiomas	Autosomal dominant	
	Angiomatoses		
	Skin and viscera		
	Hereditary mucocutaneous telangiectasia (Rendu-Olser)	Autosomal dominant	
	Facial and intracranial (Sturge-Weber)	?	
	Brain and retina (von Hippel-Lindau)	Autosomal dominant	Hypernephroma, phenochromocytoma
Connective tissue	Congenital fibromatosis	Autosomal dominant?	
	Familial cervical lipodystrophy (symmetric lipomatosis)	Autosomal dominant	
Skeletal	Multiple exostosis	Autosomal dominant	Chondrosarcoma, rare
	Enchondromatosis (Ollier disease)		Chondrosarcoma, rare
	Fibrous dysplasia of bone	Autosomal dominant?	Osteogenic sarcoma, rare
Skin	Congenital melanotic nevi		Melanoma, rare
	Linear nevus sebaceous (Jadassohn)		Brain tumor
	Basal cell nevus syndrome	Autosomal dominant	Basal cell carcinomas Medulloblastoma
Intestine	Multiple familial polyposis	Autosomal dominant	Carcinoma of colon, common
	Peutz-Jegher syndrome	Autosomal dominant	Carcinoma, rare
Pleiotrophic hamartoses (sites of origin multiple)	Tuberous sclerosis	Autosomal dominant	Brain glioma
	Maffucci syndrome		Chondrosarcomas of bone, angiosarcomas of skin, rare
	Gardner syndrome	Autosomal dominant	Carcinoma of colon, fibrosarcomas of bone or soft tissue
	Cowden syndrome	Autosomal dominant	Carcinoma of breast, thyroid, bowel
Neurocristopathic hamartoses	von Recklinghausen's neurofibromatosis	Autosomal dominant	Neurogenic sarcoma, pheochromocytoma, leukemia
	Multiple mucosal neuroma syndrome	Autosomal dominant	Medullary carcinoma of thyroid, pheochromocytoma
	Sipple syndrome	—	Same as above
	Neurocutaneous melanosis		Neurogenic sarcoma Melanoma

Table 3
TUMORS IN DYSGENETIC GONADS[17]

Condition	Clinical features	Karyotype	Gonad	Tumor
Male, normal	Normal	XY	Undescended testis	Seminoma
Male, pseudo-hermaphrodite	Undescended testes, hypospadias, variable internal	XY or mosaics with Y chromosome	Undescended testes	Seminoma, gonadoblastoma
Klinefelter's syndrome	Undescended testes, hypospadias, variable internal genitalia	XXY	Undescended testes	Seminoma, breast cancer
Testicular feminization syndrome	Normal female habitus, vagina, no uterus or tubes, undescended testes	XY	Dysgenetic testes	Sertoli cell or tubular adenoma
Pure gonadal dysgenesis	Eunuchoid female habitus, uterus, and fallopian tubes	XY or mosaics	Dysgenetic testes	Gonadoblastoma-dysgerminoma-seminoma
Female pseudohermaphrodite, nonadrenal	Female habitus with variable masculinization Turner's syndrome	XY or XO/XY and other mosaics with Y chromosome	Streak ovaries or indeterminate gonads	Gonadoblastoma-dygerminoma
Mixed gonadal dysgenesis	Asymmetric gonads and internal genitalia Ambiguous external genitalia	XO/XY and other mosaics with Y chromosome	Streak or indeterminate gonad on one side Contralateral testis	Gonadoblastoma Seminoma, Sertoli cell adenoma
True hermaphrodite	Variable external and internal genitalia and secondary characteristics Usually male habitus	XX or mosaicism	Bilateral ovotestes, asymmetric testis and ovary Ovo-testis and contralateral ovary or testis	Dysgerminoma

in hamartomas and hamartoses, developmental vestiges, heterotopias, and dysgenetic tissues. It is possible that these structures might harbor a latent oncogene which may have been expressed in an attenuated form as an anomaly in intrauterine life. Environmental insults in later life, e.g., trauma, irradiation, infection, hormones, drugs, and other chemical agents, might cause a depression or activation of this cryptic genome and result in the production of cancer. For example, the heightened hormonal stimulation accompanying puberty might be largely responsible for the development of tumors in dysgenetic gonads. These anomalous tissues might respond abnormally to increasing levels or cyclic fluctuations in gonadotropins in adolescence. In effect, these hormones could exert a carcinogenic or cocarcinogenic influence. Similar mechanisms may be involved in the development of the clear-cell adenocarcinoma of the adolescent vagina, transplacentally induced by diethylstilbestrol taken by their mothers during their early gestation to prevent abortion.[13] The transplacental effects of this agent on the fetus leaves vestiges of anomalous sex duct differentiation, known as vaginal adenosis. The anomalous vestiges respond by malignant transformation in approximately 1 of 4000 exposed girls. In those teratologic conditions associated with chromosomal breakage, fragility, or imbalance, the unusual tendency to develop cancer is paralleled by a predisposition of cell cultures from these patients to be transformed by oncogenic agents. When this is associated with an immune-deficiency state, as is typical of many of the conditions in this group, a failure in the surveillance system of the host against cancer might be anticipated. This would allow for the establishment and growth of a clone of cancer cells, culminating in a frank neoplasm.

The "two-hit" hypothesis of oncogenesis as forwarded by Knudson has special relevance in these considerations. In 1971, Knudson[14] put forth the two-mutational event, or two-hit theory of carcinogenesis. It evolved primarily from his epidemiologic studies of hereditary retinoblastoma. Knudson observed that the heritable form of retinoblastoma (35 to 40% of all retinoblastomas) was usually bilateral, whereas sporadic cases were usually unilateral. The age incidence of heritable retinoblastoma described a linear regression curve, so that the heritable bilateral cases occurred in younger patients (mean age, 18 months) than did sporadic unilateral cases (mean age, 30 months). It is now axiomatic that all bilateral cases are hereditary.

Assuming *a priori,* that mutational events occur at a random and fixed rate, Knudson reasoned that at least two sequential mutational events (hits) were necessary to transform a normal cell into a neoplastic cell. These hits could result in point mutations, chromosomal deletions, inversions, or translocations. If the first hit was postzygotic, a localized population of cells was produced that was susceptible to malignant transformation by a second or subsequent hit(s). The resultant tumor was then unifocal, had a relatively late onset, and was nonhereditary. This is how the majority of common cancers of adult life are thought to develop, e.g., carcinomas of colon, breast, or lung. If the first hit was prezygotic (a germinal mutation), all bodily cells would be altered and rendered susceptible to the carcinogenic effect of a second mutagenic event. Tumors would develop bilaterally in paired organs, or multifocally, and would appear at a much younger age than sporadic cases. It would, thenceforth, be genetically transmitted as an autosomal dominant trait. Further studies of Knudson et al.[15,16] have applied this model to Wilms' tumor and neuroblastoma. Knudson did not attempt to specify the nature of the first hit. The events of his system are stochastic, occurring randomly at a fixed rate. It might be inferred from this that a universal, steady rain of mutagens occurs in nature, accounting for these hits. It is doubtful that Knudson meant to imply this; the model was based in fact, on a mathematical assumption. The concept that only two hits are involved also reflects a mathematical simplification. In reality, many hits are probably required in nature.

At first Knudson did not state whether the first hit might be expressed morphologically. It became clear to him and others that a prenatal first hit, occurring prezygotically or postzygotically, might be expressed as a congenital malformation, a hamartoid hyperplasia of cells, and/or a chromosomal abnormality.[15-19] A summation of how his model has been applied to human carcinogenesis is found in Table 4.

III. CANCER IN EARLY LIFE

Malignancy in newborn and young infants is very rare.[20] It has been estimated that malignant neoplasms occur at a rate of $183.4/10^6$ in infants under 1 year of age, and at a rate of $36.5/10^6$ live births per year in newborns under 1 month. This amounts to 130 neonates with cancer each year. Half are found at birth and two thirds during the first weeks of life. The most common tumors found at this time are neuroblastoma, leukemia, and renal tumors.[9] Neuroblastoma is prevalent, occurring at an annual rate of $62.7/10^6$ infants under 1 year of age and $19.7/10^6$ infants under 1 month of age. It is followed by congenital or infantile leukemia, which occurs at an annual rate of $31.8/10^6$ infants under 1 year of age and at $4.7/10^6$ newborns. Kidney tumors occur at an annual rate $19.7/10^6$ under 1 year of age, and $4.7/10^6$ newborn infants.

It is remarkable to observe that in infants under 1 year of age, the incidence of cancer is three times greater than its mortality. This ratio of incidence to mortality is 10:1 for neuroblastoma in the first year, 5.4:1 for kidney tumors, but only 1.5:1 for leukemia.

The disparity between incidence and mortality may, in part, reflect improved therapy, particularly of kidney tumors. More likely it reflects the essential benignity of the neoplasms or the tendency of regression, and/or cytodifferentiation to mature and benign forms.

Table 4
KNUDSON'S TWO HIT MODEL OF CARCINOGENESIS[18]

First hit effect	Second hit effect
Prezygotic first hit	
Hereditary harmartoses (autosomal dominant)	
Familial polyposis coli	
Colonic polyps	Colonic carcinoma
Neurofibromatosis	
Neurofibromas, Schwannmas	Neurogenic sarcoma, leukemia
Adrenal medullary hyperplasia	Pheochromocytoma
Multiple mucosal neuroma syndrome	
C-cell hyperplasia of thyroid	Medullary carcinoma of thyroid
Basal cell nevus syndrome	Basal cell carcinoma of skin
Childhood cancers	
Treated retinoblastoma	Osteogenic sarcoma
Neuroblastoma *in situ*	Adrenal neuroblastoma
Nodular renal blastema	Bilateral Wilms' tumor
Neuroblastoma (stage IV-S)	
Cytogenetic defects with teratologic syndrome	
Trisomy 21 (Down's)	Leukemia, retinoblastoma
Trisomy 18	
Nodular renal blastema	Wilms' tumor
Sporadic aniridia 11p-13q — deletion syndrome	Bilateral Wilms' tumor
	Retinoblastoma
Sex chromosome abnormalities	
Dysgenetic gonads	Seminoma-dysgerminoma
Autosomal recessive disorders	
Chromosomal fragility	
Ataxia telangiectasia	Lymphoma, leukemia
Bloom's syndrome	Leukemia, gastrointestinal carcinoma
Fanconi's anemia	Leukemia, hepatoma
	Gastrointestinal carcinoma
Xeroderma pigmentosum	Ultraviolet-induced skin cancers
Postzygotic first hit (prenatally induced anomalies)	
Hemihypertrophy (?)[a]	Wilms' tumor
Beckwith-Wiedemann syndrome (?)[a]	
Nodular renal blastema	Wilms' tumor
Fetal adrenal cytomegaly	Adrenocortical carcinoma
Poland syndrome	Leukemia
Genitourinary tract malformations and nephron disorder	Wilms' tumor
Diethylstilbestrol-induced vaginal adenosis	Vaginal carcinoma

[a] There is conflicting evidence whether hemihypertrophy and the Beckwith-Wiedmann syndrome are hereditable.

In infancy, tumors generally originate *in utero* from fetal or embryonal cells, or from vestiges of these tissues persisting after birth. Spontaneous regression may be common. There is, in fact, a period of time, commencing *in utero* and terminating within the first year of life, which we have referred to as the *oncogenic grace period,*[9,21] since tumors emerging at this time tend towards benignity, in spite of the aggressiveness implied by their anaplastic and primitive cytomorphology. Their regression may be manifested by selective necrosis of cancer cells, leaving fibrocalcific residua or no trace whatsoever. The most impressive form of regression is cytodifferentiation into a benign tumor. The best example

Table 5
INFANTILE CONGENERS OF WILMS' TUMOR

Congenital mesoblastic nephroma	Usually a benign fibromyomatoid tumor; the most common tumor in children under 6 months of age; often congenital
Well-differentiated epithelial nephroblastoma	Closely packed, well-differentiated tubules; usually benign; mean age of patients <1 year
Polycystic nephroblastoma or multilocular cystic nephroma	Macrocysts lined by flattened epithelium and fibrous septa; usually benign; mean age of patients <1 year
Fetal rhabdomyomatous nephroblastoma	Predominantly in skeletal muscle; usually benign; one third bilateral; mean age of patients >1 year
Nodular renal blastema-nephroblastomatosis complex	Bilateral, nodular, or confluent subcortical masses of hamaratoid hyperplastic epithelium; precursive of Wilms' tumor, particularly bilateral, hereditary type; may regress to cystic kidneys; associated with teratologic syndromes (sporadic aniridia $11p^-$, Beckwith-Wiedemann syndrome, trisomies 18 and 13)

Table 6
TUMORS OF EARLY LIFE SHOWING BENIGN, REGRESSIVE, AND CYTODIFFERENTIATIVE TENDENCIES

- Infantile congeners of Wilms' tumor
- Neuroblastoma
  - Neuroblastoma *in situ*
  - Congenital neuroblastoma (stage IV-S)
  - Neuroblastoma under 1 year of age
  - Thoracic neuroblastoma
- Hereditary retinoblastoma
- Sacrococcygeal teratoma under 4 months of age
- Congenital and infantile fibromatosis
- Yolk sac carcinoma under 2 years of age
- Hepatoblastoma under 1 year of age

is congenital neuroblastoma which accounts for about 50% of all neonatal malignancies. Here spontaneous regression and cytodifferentiation to ganglioneuroma occur in about 90% of the cases.[22]

Another example is to be found in renal neoplasia occurring in the first year of life.[23-27] Renal tumors in early life were once all diagnosed as Wilms' tumor and treated in an aggressive manner befitting a rapidly growing and potentially lethal malignancy. It is now appreciated that congenital Wilms' tumor is an exceedingly rare event and that the bulk of tumors of the kidney occurring within the first year of life are highly differentiated and, in most instances, benign. We refer to these as the infantile congeners of Wilms' tumor. True Wilms' tumor with its typical morphology and aggressive behavior increases in incidence thereafter reaching its peak between 2 and 3 years of age (Table 5). These renal tumors are related, as they all evolve into their various forms, by the neoplastic transformation of the metanephric blastema. The time of the initiating events may determine the pathobiologic nature of the tumor and its clinical appearance. Table 5 shows how Wilms' tumor may arise from nodular renal blastema, particularly bilateral Wilms' tumor, which is ultimately derived from an autosomal dominant gene.

Examples of the other tumors displaying regression and benign tendencies are listed in Table 6. In most of the conditions cited, these benign tendencies continue for some time

Table 7
ECOGENETIC INTERACTIONS IN HUMAN MALIGNANCY[28,29]

Environmental agent	Genetic trait	Tumor/outcome
Ionizing radiation	Ataxia-telangiectasia with lymphoma	Radiation toxicity
	Retinoblastoma	Sarcoma
	Nevoid basal cell carcinoma syndrome	Basal cell carcinoma
Ultraviolet radiation	Xeroderma pigmentosum	Skin cancer, melanoma
	Cutaneous albinism	Skin cancer
	Dysplastic nevus syndrome	Melanoma
Stilbestrol	XO Turner syndrome	Adenosquamous endometrial carcinoma
Androgen	Fanconi pancytopenia	Hepatic adenomas
Diet(?)	Polyposes coli	Colonic carcinoma
	Lewis antigen (a-b-) (fucosyltransferase activity)	Alimentary tract carcinoma
Iron	Hemochromatosis	Hepatocellular carcinoma
Tyrosine	Tyrosinemia	Hepatocellular carcinoma
Epstein-Barr virus	X-linked lymphoproliferative syndrome	Burkitt and other lymphomas
	HLA-A2, Bw46	Nasopharyngeal carcinoma
Papillomavirus type 5	Epidermodysplasia verruciformis	Skin cancer
N-substituted aryl compounds	*N*-acetyltransferase activity	Urinary bladder cancer

after birth. These oncorepressive influences seem to lose their efficacy within the first year of life, generally before 6 months of age.

IV. ETIOPATHOGENESIS OF CHILDHOOD CANCER

A. Heredito-Familial Aspects

In adults it is widely held that 80% of cancers are due to the environment. In childhood cancer, accounting for 1 to 2% of all cancers, genetic, chromosomal, and familial factors play a far greater role, by rendering individuals unusually susceptible to environmental carcinogens. This has been elegantly crystallized by Mulvihill[28,29] under the rubric ''Ecogenetics of Cancer in the Young''. He points out that of the 2300 single gene traits recorded in McKusick's[30] *Mendelian Inheritance in Man,* 200 of these conditions have neoplastic tendencies, either as a sole feature, a frequent concomitant, or a rare complication. This study is of great importance as it explores the interrelationships between genetic and environmental factors in the pathogenesis of cancer. We have reproduced his analysis of ecogenetic interactions in human malignancy (Table 7).

We shall consider several tumors where the proximate event in carcinogenesis is an inherited mutant gene. This is most striking in retinoblastoma as discussed earlier, where some 40% of cases are hereditary and transmitted as an autosomal dominant trait.

In Wilms' tumor, only 2% of cases are familial; but estimates of the presence of an autosomal dominant gene with incomplete penetrance run as high as 25% of cases. In particular, those cases arising from the matrix of the bilateral nodular renal blastema-nephroblastomatosis complex have been implicated. These precursive hamartoid lesions occur in the Beckwith-Wiedemann syndrome, and hemihypertrophy.[17,19] Often they are interpreted or misdiagnosed as bilateral Wilms' tumor.

There are 23 reported familial aggregations of sporadic neuroblastoma, amounting to 55 cases.[31] The median age at diagnosis is 2.5 years. Before 1 year, 25% are diagnosed. In familial cases the median age of diagnosis is 9 months and 60% are diagnosed before 1 year of age. Of 55 familial cases, 10 presented in newborns. Multiple primaries are characteristic (stage IV-S). It is difficult to determine the incidence and penetrance of the inherited susceptibility to develop neuroblastoma; it may be more prevalent than is now appreciated.

Chances of neuroblastoma developing in siblings or the offspring of an affected individual are about 6%. This figure may be low, in that many potential cases of overt neuroblastomas are obscured by spontaneous regression or transformation into neurofibromatoid forms mimicking von Recklinghausen's disease.[32,33]

B. The Fetal Milieu and Oncogenesis

It would appear from our discussion that the fetal or embryonal milieu is inimical to the development of the oncogenic process. A limited, but important body of experiments has been addressed to the proposition that the embryo restricts and attenuates incipient oncogenesis, causing the cancer cells to differentiate. Brinster[34] showed that, after the injection into mouse blastocysts, followed by blastocyst transfer to pseudopregnant foster mothers, these blastocysts developed into completely normal mice with normal tissues containing markers for the teratocarcinoma cells as well as normal tissues. The cancer cells differentiated completely and were integrated into the organism, now a chimera of normal and differentiated cancer cells. The microenvironment of the blastocyst is apparently able to convert the neoplastic potential of a carcinoma cell into a normal pathway of differentiation.[35] Later experiments by Pierce[36] showed that this was accomplished by cell-to-cell contact of the embryonal carcinoma cells with either trophectoderm or the inner cell mass. Blastocyst regulation with other transplanted experimental tumors such as mouse neuroblastoma has not been so successful.

A fetal cancer-suppressive effect is further illustrated in a recent experiment with Rous sarcoma virus in chick embryos.[37] Injection of the Rous sarcoma virus into newly hatched chicks results in tumors within 1 week of inoculation. Injection into embryos *in ovo* does not produce tumors or malformation. The virus replicates *in ovo* and also expresses the oncogene protein-kinase $pp60^{SRC}$. If the infected embryonal cells are disrupted and placed in culture, they become capable of expression the malignant phenotype within 24 h. It appears that there is a powerful restriction of the expression of the malignant phenotype by the intact embryo.

C. Oncogenes and Antioncogenes

In recent years, brilliant technologic advances in cellular and molecular genetics have quickly brought us to the understanding that the oncogenic process, whether initiated by chemical carcinogens, oncogenic viruses, irradiation, inherited mutant genes, or congenital or acquired cytogenetic defects, is culminated by the activation of cellular oncogenes. The products of these oncogenes are often powerful mitogens which are largely held responsible for the uncontrolled cellular proliferation of the cancer cell phenotype. As these oncogenes are present in the normal genome, it is likely that they strongly influence proliferation in normal development. They, in turn, may be controlled by suppressor genes or regulators, whose major role may be cytodifferentiation. The hostility of the fetal milieu to the full expression of oncogenes may result from the maximal activity of suppressor or cytodifferentiative genes during early development. In 1957, Waddington[38] proposed that developmental equilibrium is maintained following genetic or environmental disturbances in the embryo by a genomic buffering system that restores cell proliferation and differentiation to normal channels following genomic disruption. This he termed ''homeorhesis'', signifying a tendency towards developmental homeostasis. Imperfections in the homeorhesis system would ultimately result in neoplasia or malformation or both.

Matsunaga[39-41] has reasserted this homeorhesis concept through his studies of heritable tumors. He proposed that the penetrance and expressivity of certain oncogenes are determined by a natural host resistance mediated by suppressor genes. No matter if the cancer process is initiated by virus, chemicals, radiation, or mutant genes, cancer develops because of a failure of this host resistance system to control cytodifferentiation. A proximate event in carcinogenesis could then be the loss or inactivation of such regulatory genes. This may occur by deletion of one of an allele pair, bearing the regulator gene(s) which controls the oncogenic activity.

Knudson[42] has described a class of genes he called *antioncogenes* (suppressor genes), which are capable of causing cancer only in a recessive mode. These may be pivotal in the development of retinoblastoma, Wilms' tumors, and possibly neuroblastoma, having a heritable basis. In most other cancers, abnormally activated or mutant oncogenes produce cancer in the heterozygous mode, the mutant allele being dominant. But where the mutant allele is recessive, the normal allele will suppress the oncogenic activity of its abnormal fellow. To develop cancer in the recessive mode, a second event must take place accordingly, which leads to the loss of the normal allele — a submicroscopic loss of chromosomal material, a deletion, or whole chromosomal loss. This would produce a condition of homozygosity or hemizygosity of antioncogenes in the tumor, thus allowing uncontrolled expression of the oncogenes on other chromosomes.

Recent studies of retinoblastomas, neuroblastomas, and Wilms' tumor have supported the antioncogene concept.[43-51] It has been shown in retinoblastoma that tumor development is associated with activation and amplification of the n-*myc* oncogene located on chromosome 2. Cytogenetically, it has been shown that chromosome 13 is lost in whole or in part, creating, respectively, a condition of hemizygosity or homozygosity; this allows expression of the recessive deletion of the long arm of the remaining chromosome 13 (13q14). The recessive 13q14 mutation is probably hereditary. The loss of all or part of the normal chromosome 13 is construed as a second hit effect, which probably causes derepression of n-*myc* and cancer development. Implied in the loss of the chromosomal material is the loss of indigenous suppressor genic activity.

Neuroblastomas are known to be associated with n-*myc* activation and, in advanced stages of the disease, n-*myc* amplification. Chromosomal analyses of the tumor tissue have revealed a deletion of the short arm of chromosome 1 ($1p^-$) in a large proportion of cases. While hemizygosity has not been identified, it is possible that homozygosity at this locus may exist as a result of minute deletions on the normal allele.

The development of Wilms' tumors in aniridia is associated with a deletion of the short arm of chromosome 11 ($11p^-$). In sporadic cases of Wilms' tumor there have been some instances of a deletion of the 11p13 band and restriction length polymorphisms in this region which is adjacent to the H-ras oncogene; there may be homozygous deletion.

These tumors may then be formed by a primary loss of normal antioncogenes, leading to the enhanced activity of an oncogene. It is apparent that enhanced activity of suppressor genes or antioncogenes may be very important in the regression of cancer.

D. Cancer Susceptibility Genomes

It is clear that chromosomal rearrangement predisposes to both carcinogenesis and teratogenesis (Table 1). There has been a dramatic increase in finding chromosomal abnormalities in human cancers. These findings coupled with genetic probing techniques are showing how these derangements predispose to specific oncogene activities.

Attention is now being directed towards other cancer predisposition genomes, notably the Aniridia-Wilms' tumor (Miller's) syndrome and the Beckwith-Wiedemann syndrome. The association of Wilms' tumor with sporadic aniridia was first shown by Miller et al.[52] in 1964. In 1978, Riccardi[53] showed that the complete teratologic syndrome consisted of iris abnormalities, genitourinary anomalies, and mental/motor retardation (AGR triad) and was cytogenetically characterized by an interstitial deletion of chromosome 11 (11p13). Subsequent studies have shown this deletion to be almost invariably present. Not all AGR patients develop the tumor. It has been estimated that 33 to 52% of patients develop Wilms' tumor. Gonadoblastoma has also been reported with deletion 11p11-13. In some cases, the deletion may be passed through generations by unaffected individuals due to the abnormality being carried in a balanced form. Direct analysis of the DNA from the short arm of chromosome 11 has revealed polymorphism for DNA sequences known to be on the short arm of chromosome 11, which also contain genes for globin, H-*ras* oncogene, insulin, and parathormone.[54]

The Beckwith-Weidemann syndrome consists of omphalocele, macrosomia often hemipertrophy, and visceromegaly. There is nodular renal blastema, fetal adrenal cytomegaly, and hyperplasia of the islets of Langarhans. It has been viewed as an ''overgrowth'' syndrome. About 10% develop neoplasms in early life, mostly Wilms' tumor. There have been a few familial cases, but it is mostly sporadic. A variety of abnormalities have again been found in chromosome 11, usually on the short limb.

Further studies of such syndromes for various chromosomal abnormalities and actual oncogene activation will be of great importance in determining if and how the cancers actually arise.

It seems reasonable to assert that a genomic injury may take place in early development, prezygotically or postzygotically. It may or may not be manifested by chromosomal anomaly. This sets the stage for later activation of oncogene, and is accompanied by deletional loss of genes which may be required for cytodifferentiation.

Much less is known about how normal embryogenesis is deranged to cause malformation. The teratogenic process has only begun to be studied in terms of molecular genetics. It remains likely that the greatest proportion of malformations are initiated postzygotically by transplacental or metabolic influences *in utero* in the first trimester of pregnancy. But many of these may produce only a subtle alteration in the genome. This genomic alteration may cause a malformation at one point in development and a cancer later on.

The broader challenge is to detect the individual with a cancer-susceptible genome in very early life, even in those not announced by the presence of a congenital malformation. A beginning has been made by Cavenee and co-workers.[55] Using genetic probes to recognize restriction-fragment-length polymorphisms and isozymic alleles on chromosome 13 in retinoblastoma families, he was able to predict prenatally which offspring were likely to develop retinoblastoma. These findings have implications beyond retinoblastoma.[56] This approach in tumors in which the chromosomal site of an oncogene has been determined — notably Wilms' tumors, multiple endocrine neoplasia type 2, familial renal cell carcinomas, and probably neuroblastoma would be of value. In particular this would be important in teratologic-oncologic syndromes predisposing to cancer.

REFERENCES

1. **Bolande, R. P.,** Models and concepts derived from human teratogenesis and oncogenesis in early life, *J. Histochem. Cytochem.*, 32, 878, 1984.
2. **Kalter, H. and Warkany, J.,** Congenital malformations: etiologic factors and their role in prevention, *N. Engl. J. Med.*, 308, 424, 1983.
3. **Hickey, R. C. and Taylor, J. M.,** Sacrococcygeal teratoma, *Cancer,* 7, 1031, 1954.
4. **Berry, C. L., Keeling, J., and Hilton, C.,** Coincidence of congenital malformations and embryonic tumors of childhood, *Arch. Dis. Child.*, 45, 229, 1970.
5. **Fraumeni, J. F., Jr., Li, F. P., and Dalager, N.,** Teratomas in children. epidemological features, *J. Natl. Cancer Inst.*, 15, 1425, 1973.
6. **Kobayashi, N., Furukawa, T., and Takatsu, T.,** Congenital anomalies in children with malignancy, *Paediatrician,* 16, 31, 1968.
7. **Miller, R. W.,** Relation between cancer and congenital affects in man, *N. Engl. J. Med.*, 275, 87, 1966.
8. **Cohnheim, J. and Mass, H.,** Zur Theorie der Geschwustsmetastasen, *Virchows Arch.*, 70, 161, 1877.
9. **Bolande, R. P.,** Developmental pathology, *Am. J. Pathol.*, 94, 627, 1979.

10. **DiPaolo, J. and Kotin, P.,** Teratogenesis-oncogenesis: a study of possible relationships, *Arch. Pathol.*, 81, 3, 1978.
11. **Rice, J. M.,** An overview of transplacental chemical carcinogenesis, *Teratology*, 8, 113, 1973.
12. **Warkany, J.,** Congenital Malformations, Year Book Medical Publishing, Chicago, 1971.
13. **Herbst, A. L., Poskanzer, D. O., Robboy, S. J., Friedlander, L., and Scully, R. L.,** Prenatal exposure to stilbesterol: a prospective comparison of exposed female offspring with unexposed controls, *N. Engl. J. Med.*, 292, 334, 1975.
14. **Knudson, A. G.,** Mutation and cancer: a statistical study of retinoblastoma, *Proc. Natl. Acad. Sci., U.S.A.*, 60, 820, 1971.
15. **Knudson, A. G. and Strong, L. C.,** The model for Wilms' tumor of the kidney, *J. Natl. Cancer Inst.*, 38, 313, 1972.
16. **Knudson, A. G. and Meadows, A. T.,** Developmental genetics of neuroblastoma, *J. Natl. Cancer Inst.*, 57, 675, 1972.
17. **Bolande, R. P.,** *Childhood Tumors and Their Relationship to Birth Defect in Genetics of Human Cancer*, Mulvihill, J. J., Miller, R. W., and Fraumeni, J. F., Jr., Eds., Raven Press, New York, 1977, 43.
18. **Bolande, R. P. and Vekemans, M.,** Genetic models of carcinogenesis, *Hum. Pathol.*, 8, 658, 1983.
19. **Strong, L. C.,** Genetic and teratogenic aspects of Wilms' tumor, in *Wilms' Tumor*, Pochedly, C., Miller, D., and Finkelstein, J. Z., Eds., John Wiley & Sons, New York, 1976.
20. **Bader, J. L. and Miller, R. W.,** U.S. cancer incidence and mortality in the first year of life, *Am. J. Dis. Child.*, 133, 157, 1979.
21. **Bolande, R. P.,** Benignity of neonatal tumors and the concept of cancer regression in early life, *Am. J. Dis. Child.*, 122, 12, 1971.
22. **Evans, A. E., Gerson, J., and Schnaufer, L.,** Spontaneous regression of neuroblastoma, *Natl. Cancer Inst. Monogr.*, 44, 49, 1976.
23. **Bolande, R. P.,** Spontaneous regression and cytodifferentiation of cancer in early life: the oncogenic grace period, *Sur. Synth. Path. Res.*, 4, 296, 1985.
24. **Bolande, R. P.,** Congenital mesoblastic nephroma, *Perspect. Pediatr. Pathol.*, 1, 222, 1967.
25. **Bolande, R. P.,** Congenital and infantile neoplasms of the kidney, *Lancet*, ii, 1497, 1974.
26. **Gonzalez-Crussi, F.,** *Wilms' Tumor and Related Neoplasms of Childhood*, CRC Press, Boca Raton, Fl., 1984.
27. **Dehner, L. P.,** *Neoplasms of the Fetus and Neonate in Kaufman Perinatal Diseases*, Naeye, R., Kissane, J., and Kaufman, N., Eds., Williams & Wilkins, Baltimore, 1981, 286.
28. **Mulvihill, J. J.,** Ecogenetic origins of cancer in the young: environmental and genetic determinants, in *Cancer in the Young*, Levine, A. S., Ed., Masson, New York, 1982, 13.
29. **Mulvihill, J. J.,** *Clinical Ecogenetics of Human Cancer Genes and Cancer*, Bishop, J. M., Rowley, J. D., and Greaner, M., Eds., Alan R. Liss, New York, 1984.
30. **McKusick, V. A.,** *Mendelian Inheritance in Man*, 4th ed., Johns Hopkins University Press, Baltimore, 1978.
31. **Kushner, B. H., Gilbert, F., and Nelson, L.,** Familial neuroblastoma, *Cancer*, 57, 1887, 1986.
32. **Bolande, R. P. and Towler, W. F.,** A possible relationship of neuroblastoma and von Recklinghausen's disease, *Cancer*, 26, 162, 1970.
33. **Griffin, M. and Bolande, R. P.,** Familial neuroblastoma with regression and maturation to ganglioneuroma, *Pediatrics*, 43, 377, 1969.
34. **Brinster, R. L.,** The effect of cells transferred into the mouse blastocyst by subsequent development, *J. Exp. Med.*, 140, 1049, 1974.
35. **Illmensee, K. and Mintz, B.,** Totipotency and normal differentiation of simple teratocarcinoma cells cloned by injection into blastocysts, *Proc. Natl. Acad. Sci. U.S.A.*, 73, 549, 1976.
36. **Pierce, G. B.,** The cancer cell and its control by the embryo, *Am. J. Pathol.*, 123, 117, 1983.
37. **Dolberg, D. S. and Bissell, M. J.,** Inability of Rous sarcoma virus to cause sarcomas in the avian embryo, *Nature*, 309, 552, 1984.
38. **Waddington, C. H.,** *The Strategy of Genes*, Allen & Unwin, London, 1957.
39. **Matsunaga, E.,** Genetics of Wilms' tumor, *Hum. Genet.*, 57, 231, 1981.
40. **Matsunaga, E.,** Hereditary retinoblastomas — host resistance and age of onset, *Natl. Cancer Inst. Monogr.*, 63, 933, 1979.
41. **Matsunaga, E.,** Retinoblastoma: host resistance and $13q^-$ deletion, *Human Genet.*, 56, 53, 1980.
42. **Knudson, A. G.,** Hereditary cancer, oncogenes and antioncogenes, *Cancer Res.*, 45, 1437, 1985.
43. **Cavenee, W. K., Dryja, T. P., Phillips, R. A., Benedict, W. F., Godbout, R., Gallie, B. L., Murphree, A. L., Strong, L. C., and White, R. L.,** Expression of recessive alleles by chromosomal mechanisms in retinoblastoma, *Nature*, 305, 779, 1983.
44. **Dryja, T. P., Cavenee, W. K., White, R., Rapaport, J. M., Petersen, R., Albert, D. M., and Bruns, G. A.,** Homozygosity of chromosome 13 in retinoblastoma, *N. Engl. J. Med.*, 310, 550, 1984.
45. **Kohl, N. E., Gee, C. E., and Atl, F. W.,** Activated expression of N-*myc* gene in human neuroblastomas and related tumors, *Science*, 226, 1335, 1984.

46. **Brodeur, G. M., Seeger, R. C., Schwab, M., Varnus, H. E., and Bishop, J. M.,** Amplification of N-*myc* in untreated human neuroblastomas correlates with advanced disease stage, *Science,* 224, 1121, 1984.
47. **Gilbert, F., Balaban, G., Moorhead, P., Bianchi, D., and Schlesinger, H.,** Abnormalities of chromosome 1p in human neuroblastoma tumors and cell lines, *Cancer Genet. Cytogenet.,* 7, 33, 1982.
48. **Koufos, A., Hansen, M. F., Lampkin, B. C., Workman, M. L., Copeland, N. G., Jenkins, N. A., and Cavenee, W. K.,** Loss of alleles at loci on human chromsome 11 during genesis of Wilms' tumor, *Nature,* 309, 170, 1984.
49. **Orkin, S. H., Goldman, D. S., and Sallan, S. E.,** Development of homozygosity for chromosome 11p markers in Wilms' tumor, *Nature,* 309, 172, 1984.
50. **Reese, A. E., Housiaux, P. J., Gardner, R. J. M., Chessings, W. E., Grindley, R. M., and Millow, L. J.,** Loss of a Harvey *ras* allele in sporadic Wilms' tumor, *Nature,* 309, 174, 1984.
51. **Fearon, E. R., Vogelstein, B., and Feinberg, A. P.,** Somatic deletion and duplication of genes on chromosome 11 in Wilms' tumor, *Nature,* 130, 176, 1984.
52. **Miller, R. W., Fraumeni, J. R., and Manning, M. D.,** Association of Wilms' tumour with aniridia, hemihypertrophy, and other congenital, *N. Engl. J. Med.,* 27, 922, 1964.
53. **Riccardi, V. M., Sujansky, E., Smith, A. E., and Franke, U.,** Chromosome imbalance in the aniridia — Wilms' tumour association 11p interstitial deletion, *Pediatrics,* 61, 604, 1978.
54. **Cowell, J. K.,** Tracking the cancer genes in paediatric predisposition syndromes, *Cancer Surv.,* 3, 573, 1984.
55. **Cavenee, W. K., Murphree, A. L., Shull, M. M., Benedict, W. F., Sparkes, R. S., Kock, E., and Nordesnkjold, M.,** Prediction of familial predisposition to retinoblastoma, *N. Engl. J. Med.,* 314, 1202, 1986.
56. **Gilbert, F.,** Retinoblastoma and cancer genetics, editorial, *N. Engl. J. Med.,* 314, 1248, 198.

Chapter 5

GENETIC EPIDEMIOLOGY OF CANCER

Takeshi Hirayama

TABLE OF CONTENTS

I. INTRODUCTION

There are selected factors which determine our chances of getting cancer. We usually call such factors "risk modifying factors" or simply "risk factors". There are also factors which affect the prognosis of cancer. Such factors are called "prognosis modifying factors" or simply "prognostic factors". Further, we know there are factors which shorten or prolong the latency period of cancer. We propose that such factors be called latency modifying factors (LMF) or simply latency factors. Both genetics and environment are important components of each of these factors. One should consider the role of genetics in each case.

Both risk factors and prognostic factors must be considered when epidemiological studies are based on mortality. When studies are based on incidence instead of mortality, we are mainly dealing with risk factors, but even in that case, consideration of LMFs is of importance (e.g., cancer of the prostate).

Identification of genetically predisposed individuals was clarified through the observation of cancers for which incidence was 1000 or more times higher in such persons (e.g., retinoblastoma, colon cancer in familial polyposis, and skin cancer in xeroderma pigmentosum). At one time, the main reason for the wide geographical variations which were observed in cancer incidence and/or mortality was believed to be mostly determined by differences in genetic or racial susceptibility. Support for such a view was obtained by studying cancer in migrants. For instance, the Japanese are known to carry an extremely high risk of stomach cancer. If genetic susceptibility were the main reason for such a high risk of this disease, then those Japanese who migrate to other countries such as the U.S. should also show a high incidence of stomach cancer. Such speculation was confirmed by actually comparing the stomach cancer incidence in Hawaii and California. Japanese migrants consistently showed the highest incidence of stomach cancer when compared to other ethnic groups.

Ironically, however, the same observation provided evidence of the rather limited role of genetic factors in determining cancer risk. The fact that the incidence of stomach cancer in Japanese migrants was observed to be significantly lower than for the Japanese living in the motherland, although much higher than other racial groups in the migrated area, strongly suggested the importance of environmental factors to which migrants were exposed after migration. This view was, however, altered to a certain extent by the observation that a similar low incidence of stomach cancer existed in Japanese living in Okinawa, from where the first migrants to Hawaii originated.[1] Further, the stomach cancer incidence steadily decreased first in Japanese who migrated to the U.S. and then, in later years, in Japanese living in the motherland. Such can only be explained by the influence of changes in environmental factors, especially of diet and nutrition. Thus, as more epidemiological studies were conducted, genetic factors appeared to be of lesser importance. Currently, over 90% of cancer of all sites is attributed to environmental factors and the proportion attributed to genetic factors is considered to be quite small and of minor importance.

However, one must be careful in accepting such a simplistic view. Although there is no question that environmental exposure to carcinogens and/or their inhibitors is the key determinant of cancer occurrence, genetic factors do play an important role by acting in combination with such environmental factors. The issue of genetic/environmental interaction should therefore be one of the priority themes of current and future studies of cancer epidemiology.

The best example of the existence of genetic/environmental interaction can be seen in skin cancer in xeroderma pigmentosum patients. Exposure to UV is known to be the key element causing skin cancer in such genetically predisposed patients. Therefore, prevention of skin cancer is possible and is actually being carried out by keeping patients out of UV exposure. Genetic/environmental interaction should also be considered in similar fashion for

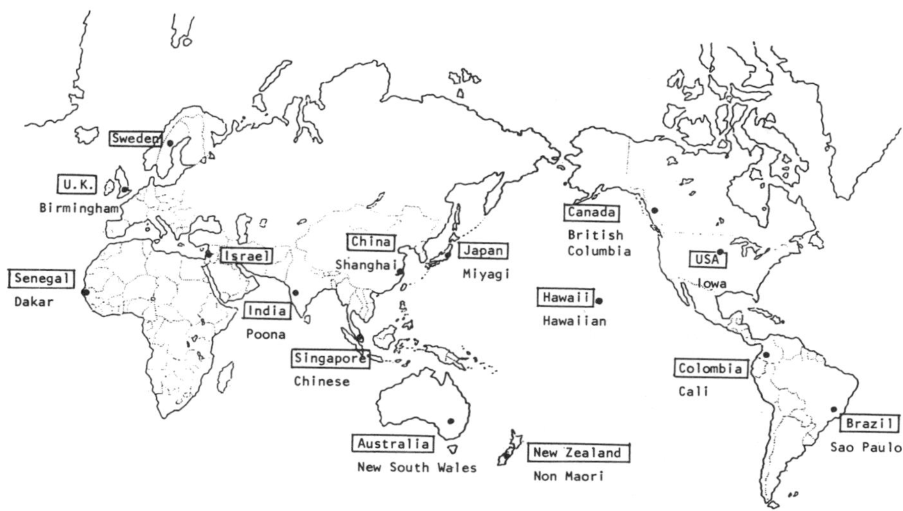

FIGURE 1. Cancer pattern in the world (based on cancer registry data). (From Waterhouse, J., Muir, C., Powell, J., et al., *Cancer Incidents in Five Continents,* Vol. 4, International Agency for Research on Cancer, Lyon, 1982. With permission.)

most other cancers which are commonly encountered. Knudson's[2] two-mutation hypothesis and related reports thereafter must provide theoretical background for such considerations.

In this text, patterns of cancer incidence in the world will be reviewed by each site, taking the influence of genetic factors and their interaction with environmental factors into consideration, using the International Agency for Research on Cancer (IARC) monograph on *Cancer Incidence in Five Continents*[13] as materials.

II. MATERIALS AND METHODS

Figures for cancer incidence in the world have been assembled by means of the establishment and spread of population-based cancer registries in key areas.

Currently, there are more than 80 population-based cancer registries in the world. The results of these cancer registries were compiled by international organizations such as IARC and IACR, and cancer incidence rates adjusted to the world population by each site were calculated and listed in the IARC Monograph on *Cancer Incidence in Five Continents.*[3] Using such materials, cancer patterns in the world were illustrated. For practical purposes of visible comparisons, figures for 15 representative cancer registries were plotted on the world map (Figure 1).

III. RESULTS

When age-standardized incidence rates for cancer of each site in these countries were compared to each other, striking similarities in males and females in the geographical distribution were observed for most cancers, while dissimilarities in the pattern of cancer occurrences in different countries were quite impressive.

A. Cancer of All Sites

Compared to the pattern of cancers of each site, the magnitude of geographical variation

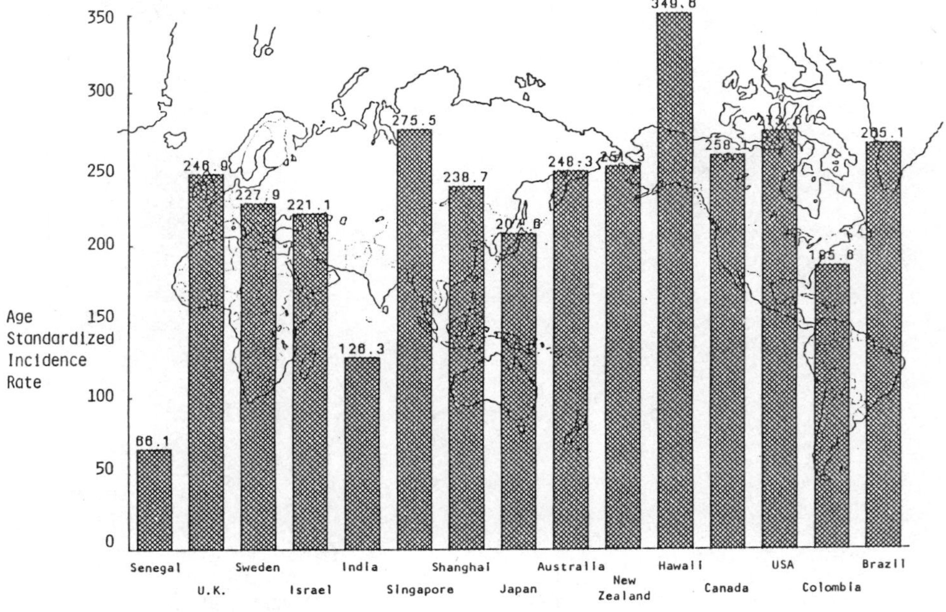

A

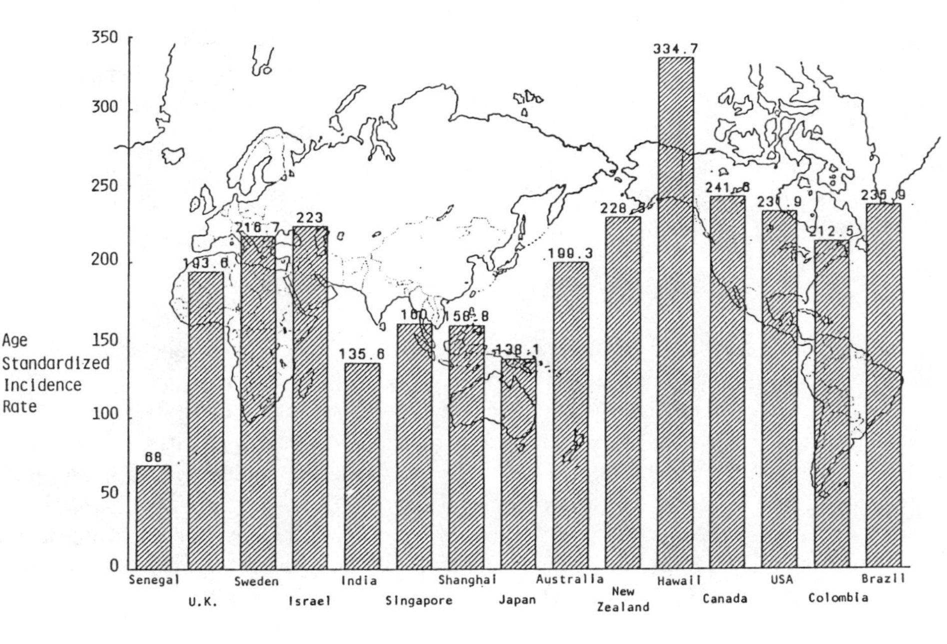

B

FIGURE 2. Cancer of all sites in (A) males and (B) females. (From Waterhouse, J., Muir, C., Powell, J., et al., *Cancer Incidents in Five Continents,* Vol. 4, International Agency for Research on Cancer, Lyon, 1982. With permission.)

in incidence is much smaller in the case of cancer of all sites (Figure 2). The exceptional lower incidence observed in Senegal must be a reflection of the lack of medical care and diagnosis in the community rather than a real difference in risk factors. Similarity in the pattern as well as in the level of incidence between males and females is impressive. The role of genetic factors in the epidemiology of cancer of all sites is not completely known.

Most of the literature on cancer genetics discussed cancer of selected sites except reports on Cancer Family Syndrome or inheritance of a general cancer diathesis. But even in such cases of cancer clustered in families, these are more or less confined to selected sites. Therefore, regarding existence of genetic susceptibility which elevates risks for all types of cancer, more studies are needed.

Registration, mapping, and documentation of cancer families should be included whenever possible in the function of population-based cancer registries.

B. Cancer of the Mouth

The disease is unusually common in India, both in males and females (Figure 3). Undoubtedly, this is due to the habit of chewing betel quids which include areca nut, lime, and tobacco leaves.[4] Cancer of the mouth was observed to be uniformly common in Indians living in different places of the world, such as Bombay, Poona, Singapore, and Natal (Figure 4).

Major known causative factors for cancer of the mouth are tobacco chewing and smoking, plus nutritional deficiencies. There is little information regarding genetic factors except reports on carcinoma of the oral cavity in the X-linked dyskeratosis congenita syndrome, carcinoma of the tongue in sclerotylosis, ectodermal dysplasia, and epidermolysis bullosa dystrophica.

C. Cancer of the Salivary Glands

Berg et al.[5] reported the occurrence of cancer of the salivary gland in association with breast cancer in the same pedigree. Blood group A also appeared to be associated with a higher risk.

D. Cancer of the Esophagus

The standardized incidence rates for cancer of the esophagus are shown in Figure 5. A strikingly wide variation was observed in the rates. The incidence rates of cancer of the esophagus were high in Shanghai and Singapore for males. In females, India showed quite a high incidence of esophageal cancer. Except in India, rates were much higher in males than in females, suggesting the influence of predominantly male lifestyles such as alcohol drinking and cigarette smoking as determinants of risk. Although not shown on the map, there are places of unusually high incidence of esophageal cancer in certain parts of South Africa, northern Iran, and northern China. The incidence ratio is nearly 10.0 or even higher in females in such areas.

The genetic risk for developing esophageal cancer has been studied mainly in relation to tylosis, which is a hyperkeratosis of the palms and soles. Esophageal cancer was also described in celiac disease, scleroderma, and Fanconi's myelopathy, all involving immune system abnormalities.

E. Cancer of the Stomach

Incidence of cancer of the stomach is quite high in Japan in both males and females (Figure 6). Geographical and/or racial distribution is similar in both sexes. As shown in Figure 7, Japanese migrants to Hawaii, San Francisco, and Los Angeles show uniformly elevated incidence of stomach cancer compared to other ethnic groups. This is in favor of a genetic hypothesis. However, the rates are almost half of those for Japanese living in Japan. Environmental factors, especially westernization of diet, are also of importance.

The role of genetic factors has been discussed in relation to consistently elevated risk of stomach cancer in persons belonging to blood group A.[6] Higher risk was also almost uniformly observed for those with a family history of stomach cancer. Age tended to be somewhat younger in such cases. Genetic factors must play an important role in such a

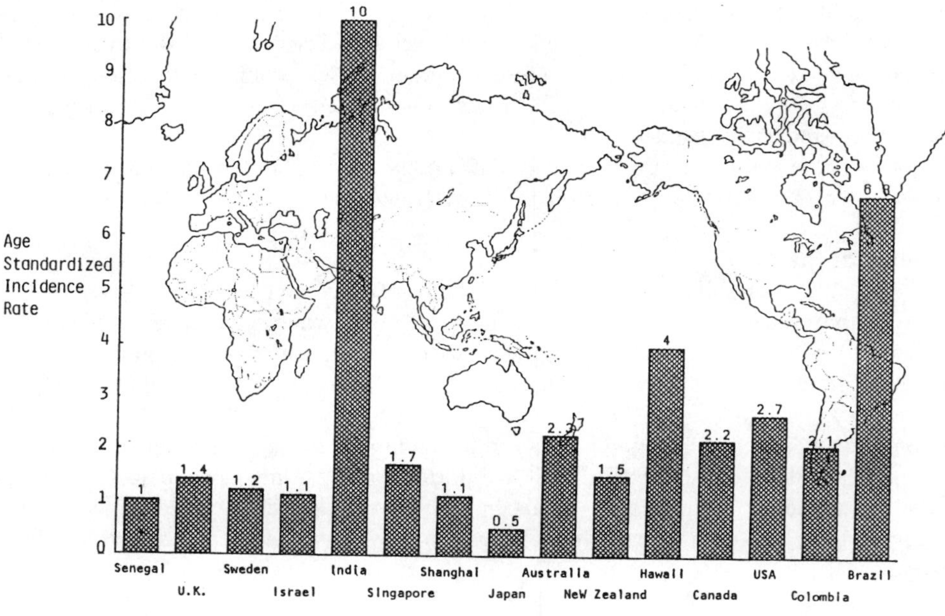

A

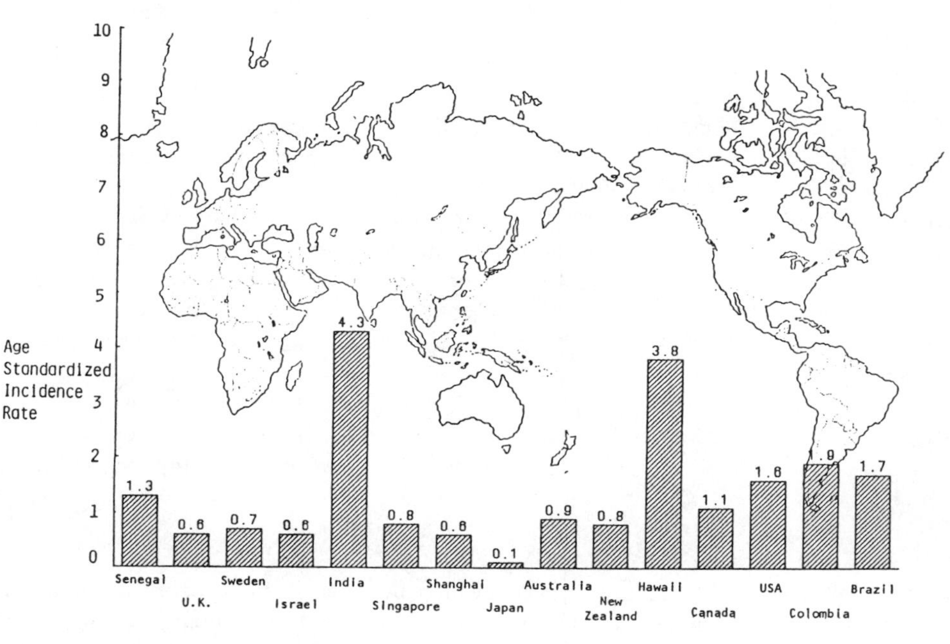

B

FIGURE 3. Cancer of the mouth in (A) males and (B) females. (From Waterhouse, J., Muir, C., Powell, J., et al., *Cancer Incidents in Five Continents,* Vol. 4, International Agency for Research on Cancer, Lyon, 1982. With permission.)

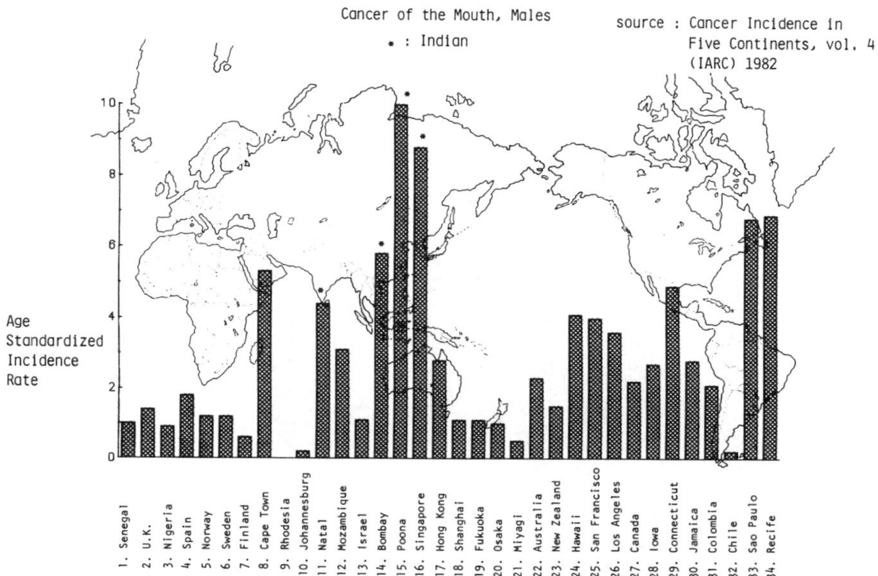

FIGURE 4. Cancer of the mouth in Indian males. (From Waterhouse, J., Muir, C., Powell, J., et al., *Cancer Incidents in Five Continents,* Vol. 4, International Agency for Research on Cancer, Lyon, 1982. With permission.)

clustering of disease in families, although common dietary patterns tend to exist in the same family.

Siurala and Seppala[7] suggested a relationship between gastric carcinoma and atrophic gastritis which may involve a polygenetic factor — pernicious anemia. Bonney et al.[8] reported that the genetic (segregation) analysis showed Mendelian transmission of a recessive autosomal gene with penetrance dependent on age and the mother's chronic atrophic gastritis status.

F. Cancer of the Intestine

The disease is quite common in Australia, New Zealand, Canada, and the U.S. (Figure 8). The incidence rate is similar in males and females as well as in its geographical pattern.

Certain types of colon cancer are known to be closely related to genetic predisposition. The lifetime incidence rate of colon cancer in familial polyposis and Gardner's syndrome (polyposis with soft and hard tissue tumors) reaches nearly 100%. Turcot's syndrome, Cancer Family Syndrome, Peutz-Jegher's syndrome, and juvenile polyposis are also known to be closely associated with colon cancer. Common susceptibility to endometrial, ovarian, or breast cancer in concert with colon cancer has also been described.

Cancer of the duodenum and ampulla of Vater may occur with Gardner's syndrome. Intestinal carcinoid tumors occur in multiple endocrine neoplasia, type I.

G. Cancer of the Pancreas

Cancer of the pancreas is slightly but uniformly higher in males than in females probably due to association with smoking. Similarity with respect to both sexes in its geographical patterns of incidence is impressive (Figure 9). Diabetes is one of the predisposing morbid conditions in pancreatic cancer which is known to be under the influence of genetics. However, information regarding the direct association of genetic factors to cancer of the pancreas remains elusive. There have been reports of the disease in four sibs each in two families.[9,10] Hereditary pancreatitis also poses an increased risk of cancer of the pancreas.

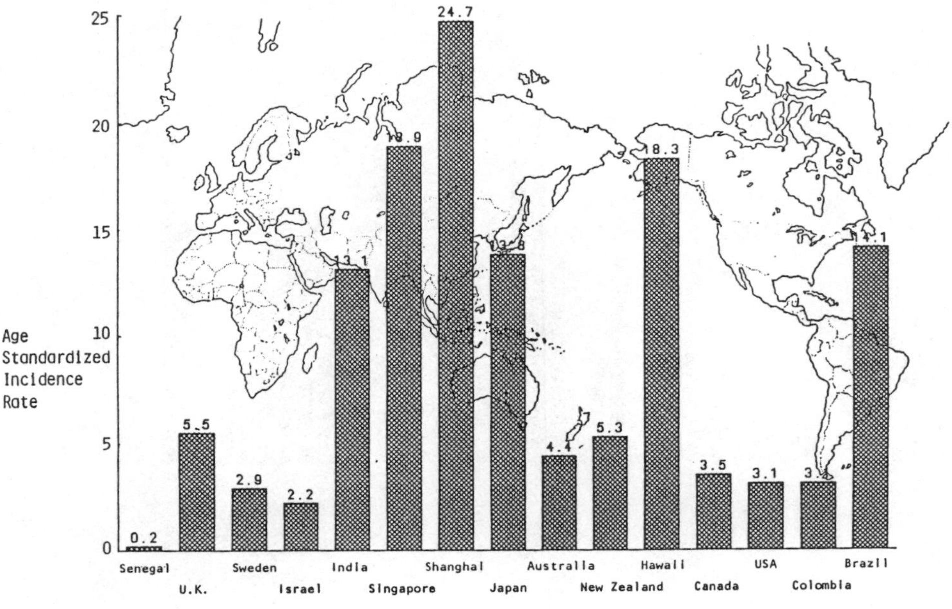

A

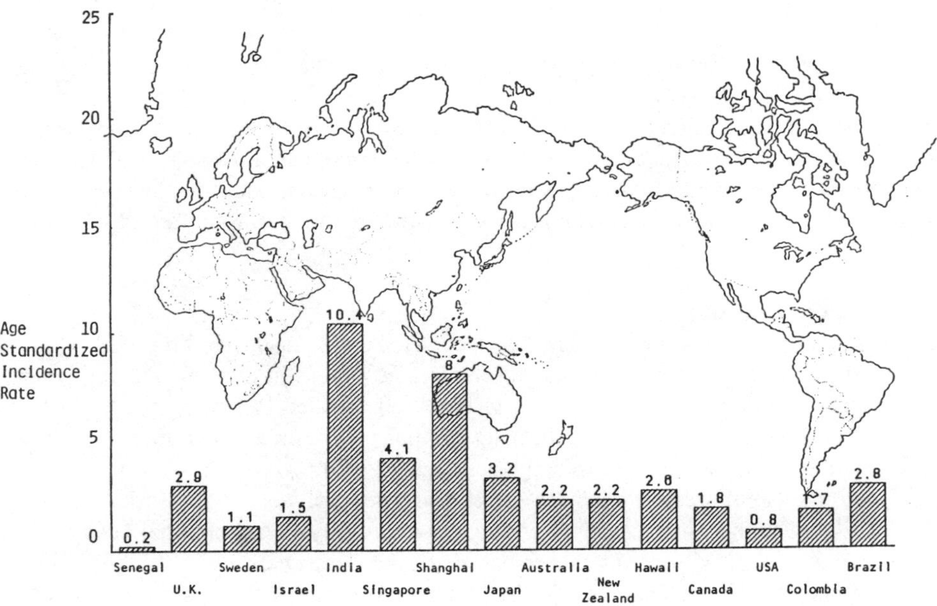

B

FIGURE 5. Cancer of the esophagus in (A) males and (B) females. (From Waterhouse, J., Muir, C., Powell, J., et al., *Cancer Incidents in Five Continents,* Vol. 4, International Agency for Research on Cancer, Lyon, 1982. With permission.)

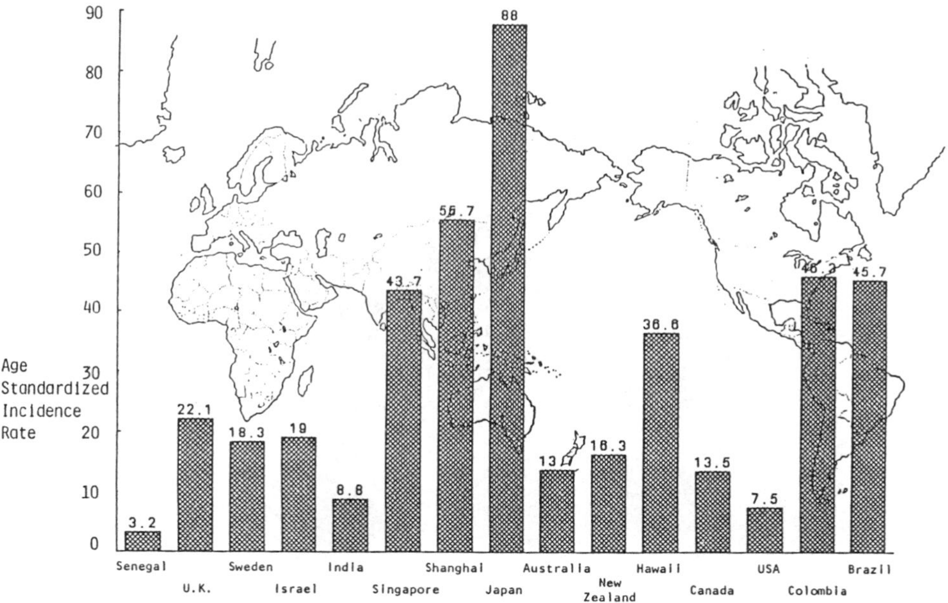

A

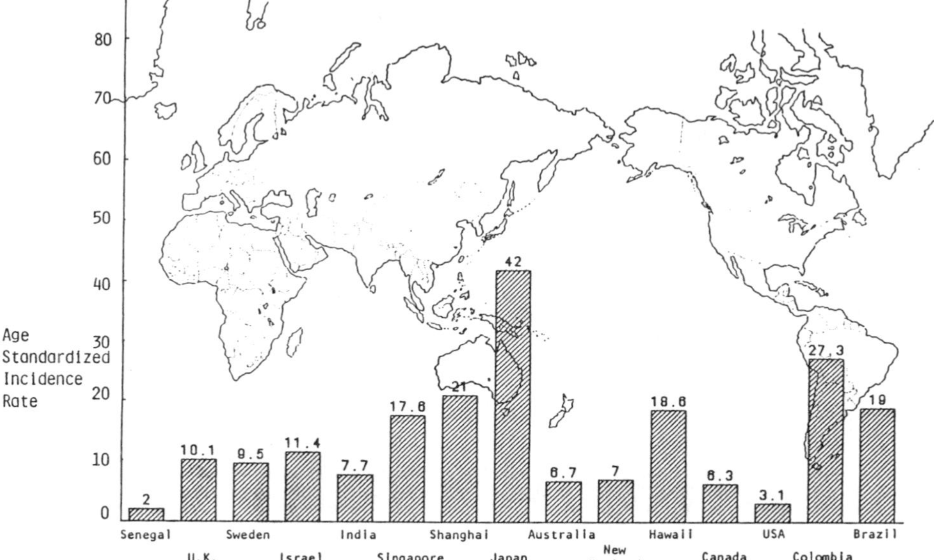

B

FIGURE 6. Cancer of the stomach: (A) males and (B) females. (From Waterhouse, J., Muir, C., Powell, J., et al., *Cancer Incidents in Five Continents,* Vol. 4, International Agency for Research on Cancer, Lyon, 1982. With permission.)

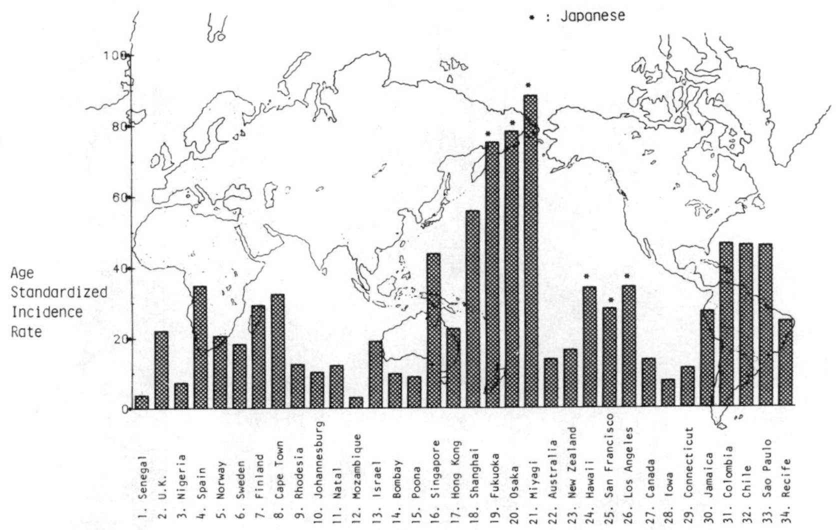

FIGURE 7. Cancer of the stomach in Japanese males. (From Waterhouse, J., Muir, C., Powell, J., et al., *Cancer Incidents in Five Continents,* Vol. 4, International Agency for Research on Cancer, Lyon, 1982. With permission.)

H. Cancer of the Liver

The disease is quite common in Africa and China, both in males and females (Figure 10). This is known to be closely related to high levels of exposure to aflatoxin contamination and also to high levels of hepatitis B virus carriers. Familial patterns of occurrence are mostly the "mother to baby" route due to epigenetic or newborn infection. With regard to genetic predisposition, an increased risk of liver cell carcinoma has been suggested in patients with α-1-antitrypsin deficiency. Familial juvenile cirrhosis associated with hepatoma was also reported.[11]

I. Cancer of the Nasopharynx

The disease incidence in the Chinese is uniquely high in both males and females (Figure 11). Chinese people living in any area of the world, such as Singapore, Hong Kong, Shanghai, Hawaii, San Francisco, and Los Angeles, commonly show a higher incidence of this disease (Figure 12).

This supports the evidence for genetically determined racial susceptibility to the disease. However, the influence of environmental factors (e.g., EB virus infection, consumption of salted fish[12] and croton-oil containg herb drugs[13]) should also be considered.

Clustering in families is frequently reported, particularly for cases of younger age. Nine cases of nasopharyngeal cancer affecting three successive generations were reported by Ho.[14,15] Clustering of Burkitt's lymphoma in the same family was also reported in Canada.[16] A close relationship with certain HLA types was observed in Singapore.[17]

J. Cancer of the Nose and Sinuses

The incidence of this disease is higher in Asia and South America. In most countries, the incidence rates are higher in males than in females (Figure 13).

Chronic exposure to wood dust is suspected as a risk factor. A large scale cohort study in Japan showed a high frequency of nasal sinus cancer in nonsmoking wives who had husbands who smoked, suggesting the risk-enhancing effect of passive smoking which may

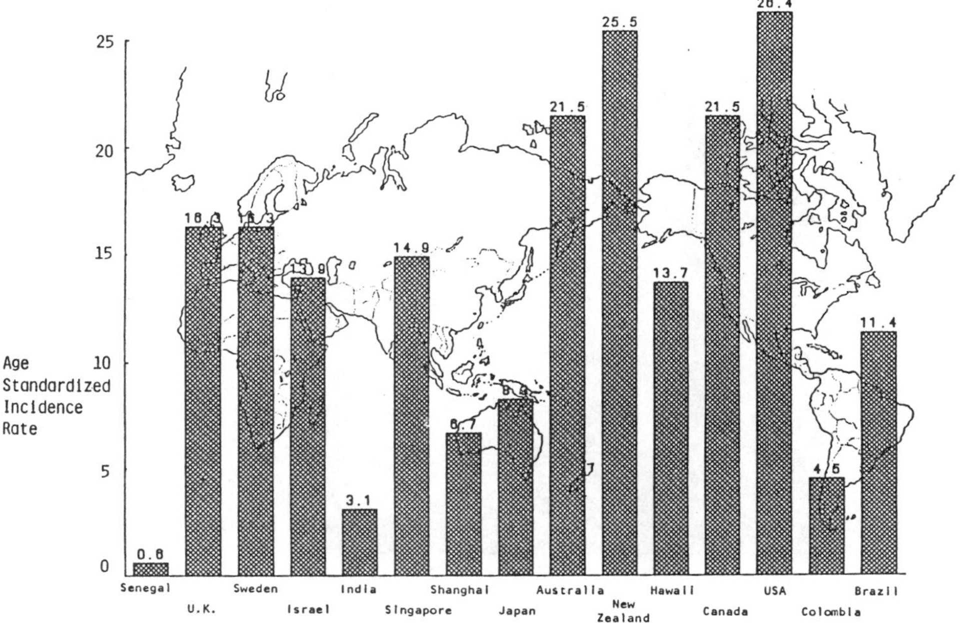

A

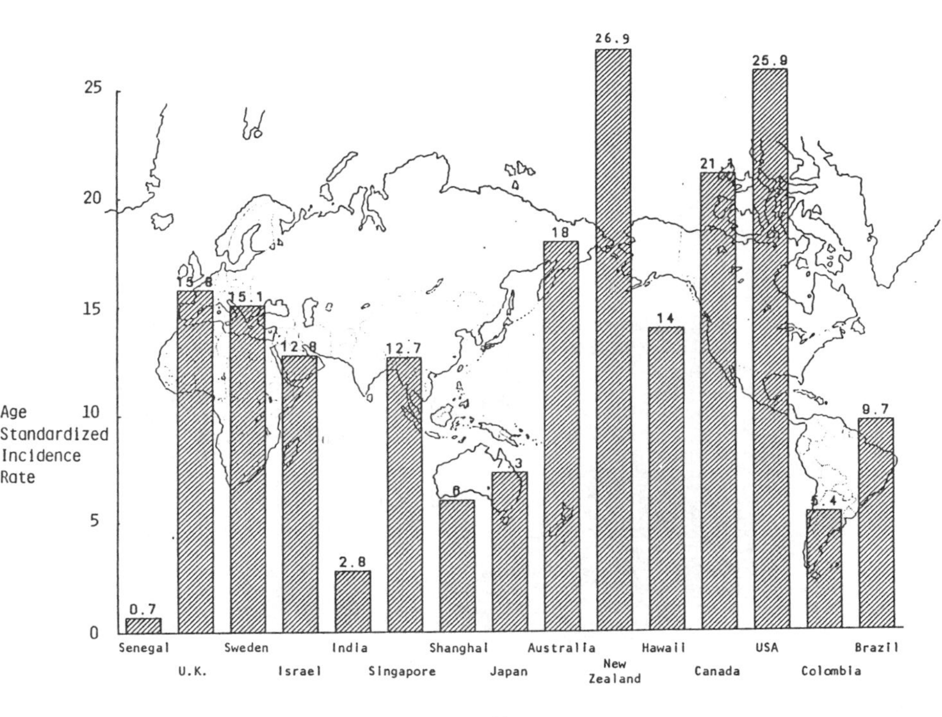

B

FIGURE 8. Cancer of the colon in (A) males and (B) females. (From Waterhouse, J., Muir, C., Powell, J., et al., *Cancer Incidents in Five Continents,* Vol. 4, International Agency for Research on Cancer, Lyon, 1982. With permission.)

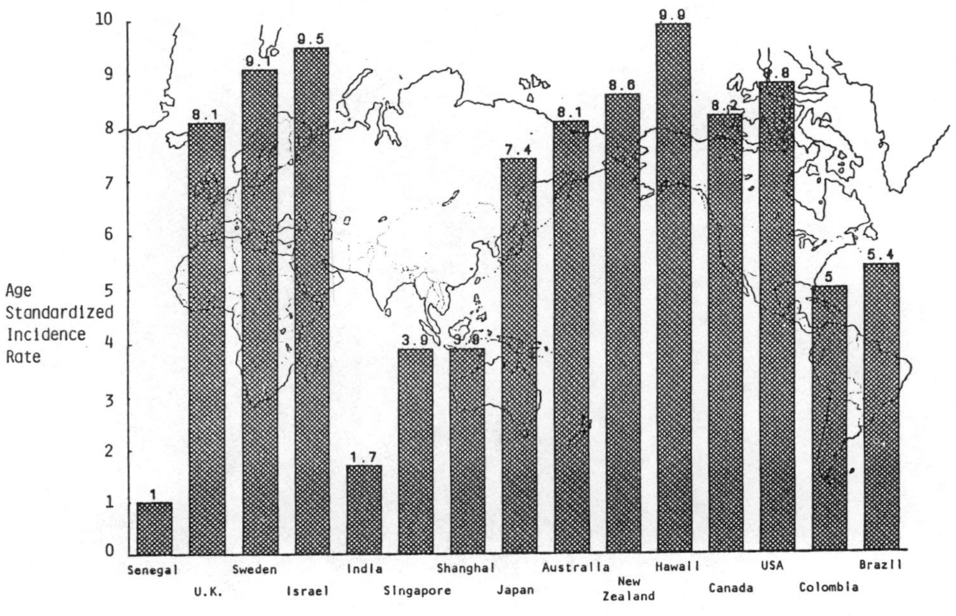

A

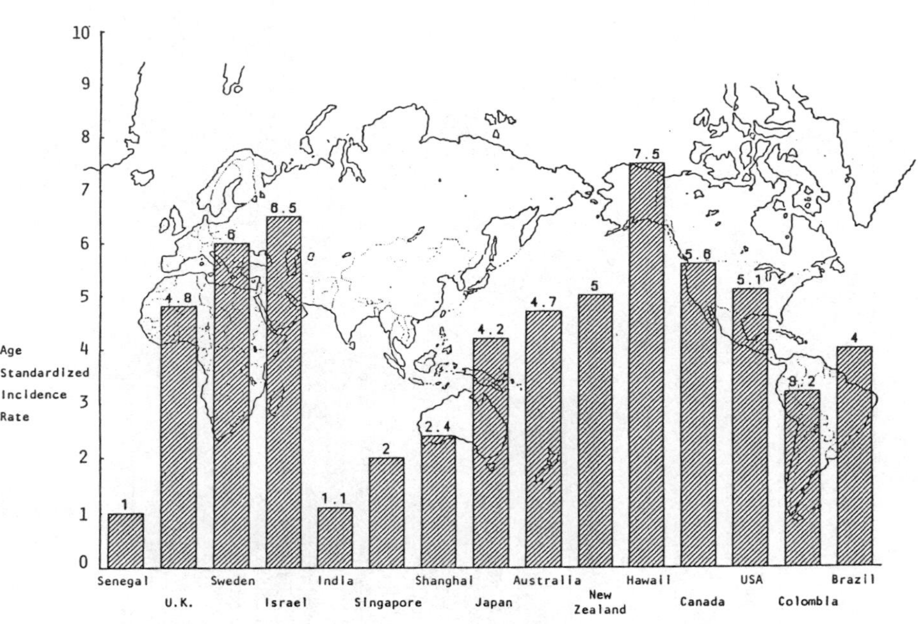

B

FIGURE 9. Cancer of the pancreas in (A) males and (B) females. (From Waterhouse, J., Muir, C., Powell, J., et al., *Cancer Incidents in Five Continents,* Vol. 4, International Agency for Research on Cancer, Lyon, 1982. With permission.)

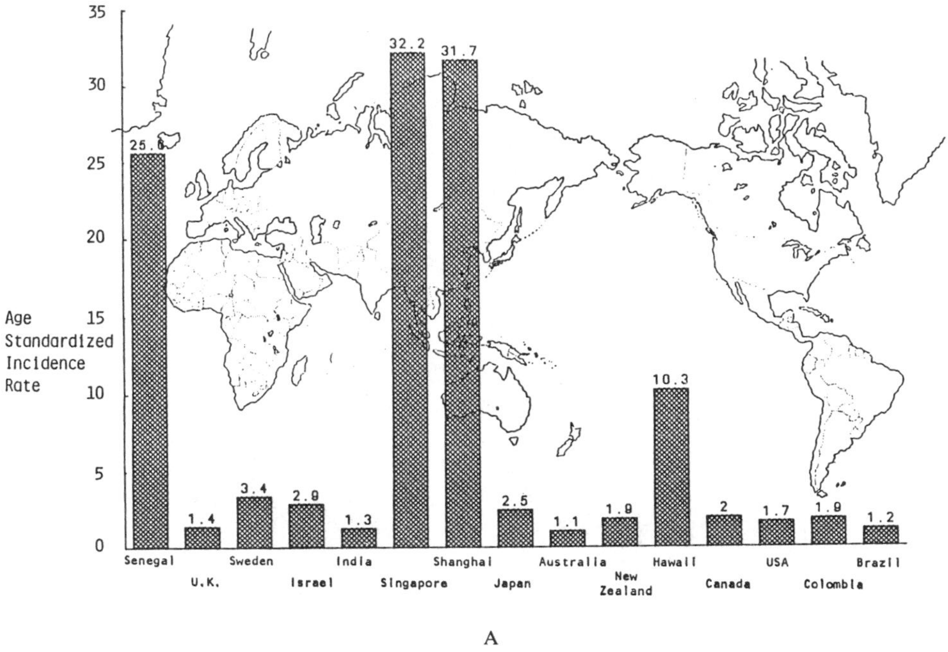

A

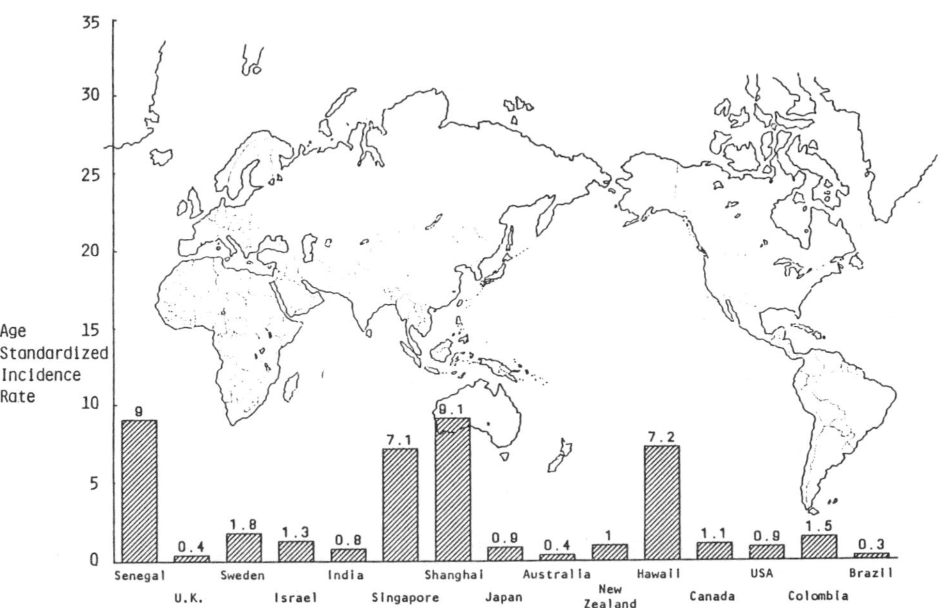

B

FIGURE 10. Cancer of the liver in (A) males and (B) females. (From Waterhouse, J., Muir, C., Powell, J., et al., *Cancer Incidents in Five Continents,* Vol. 4, International Agency for Research on Cancer, Lyon, 1982. With permission.)

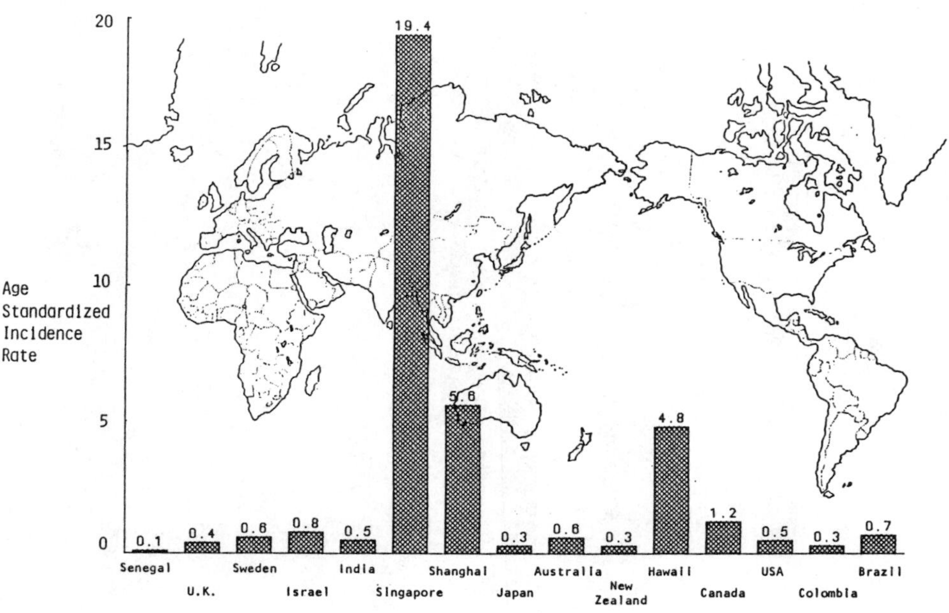

A

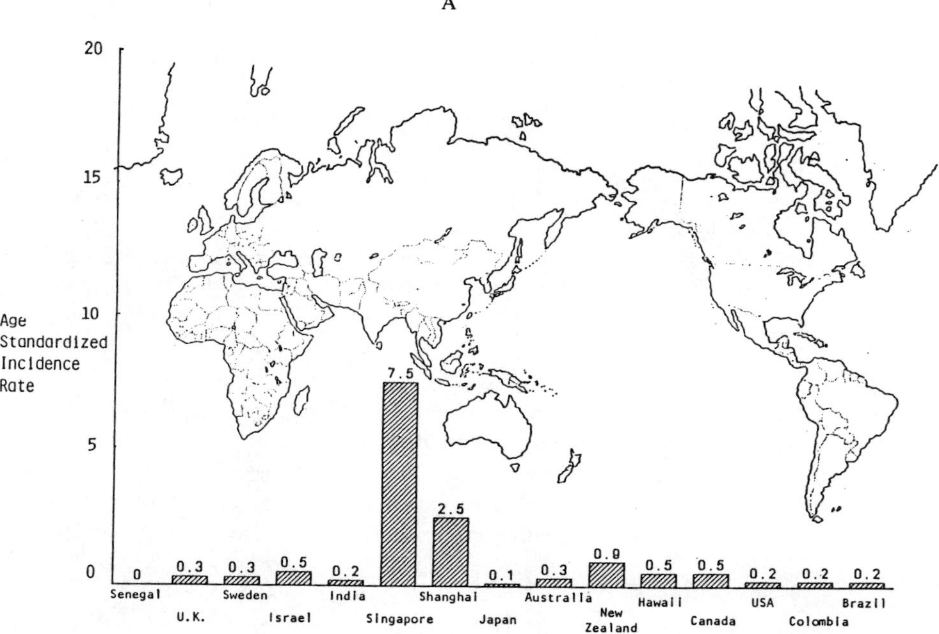

B

FIGURE 11. Cancer of the nasopharynx in (A) males and (B) females. (From Waterhouse, J., Muir, C., Powell, J., et al., *Cancer Incidents in Five Continents,* Vol. 4, International Agency for Research on Cancer, Lyon, 1982. With permission.)

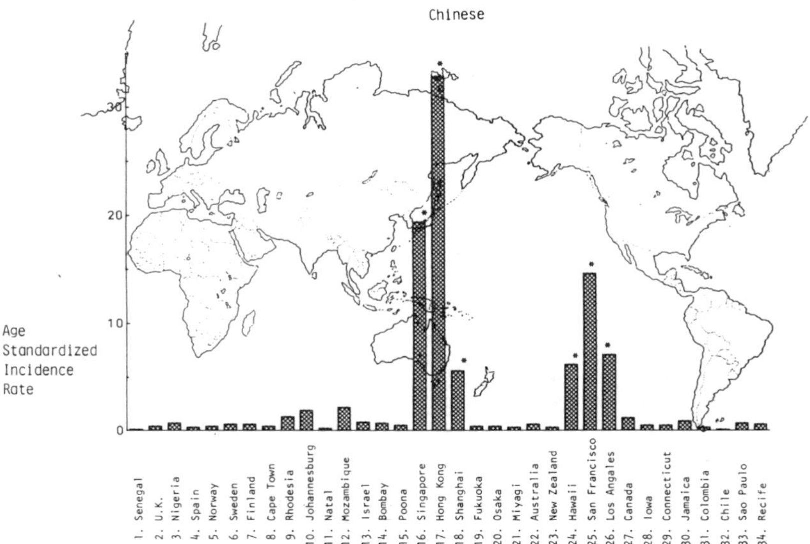

FIGURE 12. Cancer of the nasopharynx in Chinese males. (From Waterhouse, J., Muir, C., Powell, J., et al., *Cancer Incidents in Five Continents,* Vol. 4, International Agency for Research on Cancer, Lyon, 1982. With permission.)

influence the familial aggregation of this disease.[18] Genetic predisposition of the disease is unknown.

K. Cancer of the Larynx

The incidence rates are exceedingly higher in males than in females in most countries of the world (Figure 14). Higher incidence is observed in India and Brazil, reflecting the strong etiological influence of cigarette smoking.

There is insufficient information available with regard to a genetic predisposition. In a study by Trell et al.,[19] a majority of the 65 patients with laryngeal carcinoma carried high levels of inducible aryl hydrocarbon hydroxylase (AHH) enzyme in their lymphocytes.

L. Cancer of the Lung

The disease is far more common in males than in females in most countries, reflecting the causative effect of cigarette smoking (Figure 15). Lung cancer has a tendency to aggregate in families and a synergistic effect of genetic predisposition with cigarette smoking is observed.[20] However, some familial aggregations may be influenced by the possible effect of passive smoking.[18,21] As a genetic marker, inducibility of AHH was postulated.[22]

M. Cancer of the Breast

The disease is quite common in western countries when compared to Asia and Africa. The pattern of geographical variation resembles that of cancer of the prostate, suggesting the existence of certain common backgrounds (e.g., lifestyles) (Figure 16). In view of a report on 24 cases of cancer of the prostate against an expectation of 3.43 in breast cancer families, this particular observation of geographical correlation must be of etiological importance. The incidence was observed to go up in second and later generations of Japanese migrants to Hawaii and California, and in Polish immigrants to the U.S. and Australia. This strongly suggests the influence of diet and nutrition. The increased frequency of breast cancer

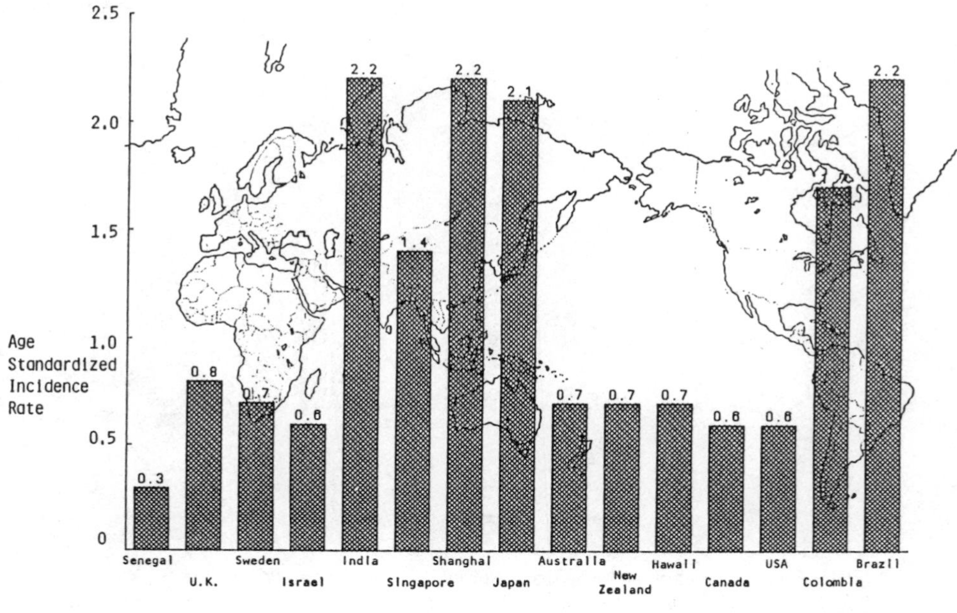

A

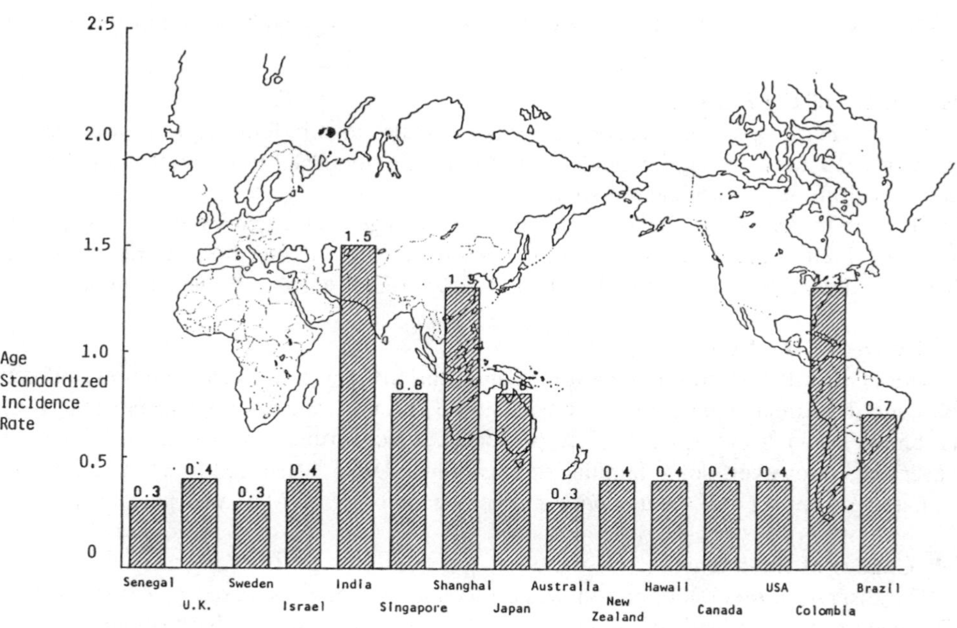

B

FIGURE 13. Cancer of the nose and nasal sinus in (A) males and (B) females. (From Waterhouse, J., Muir, C., Powell, J., et al., *Cancer Incidents in Five Continents,* Vol. 4, International Agency for Research on Cancer, Lyon, 1982. With permission.)

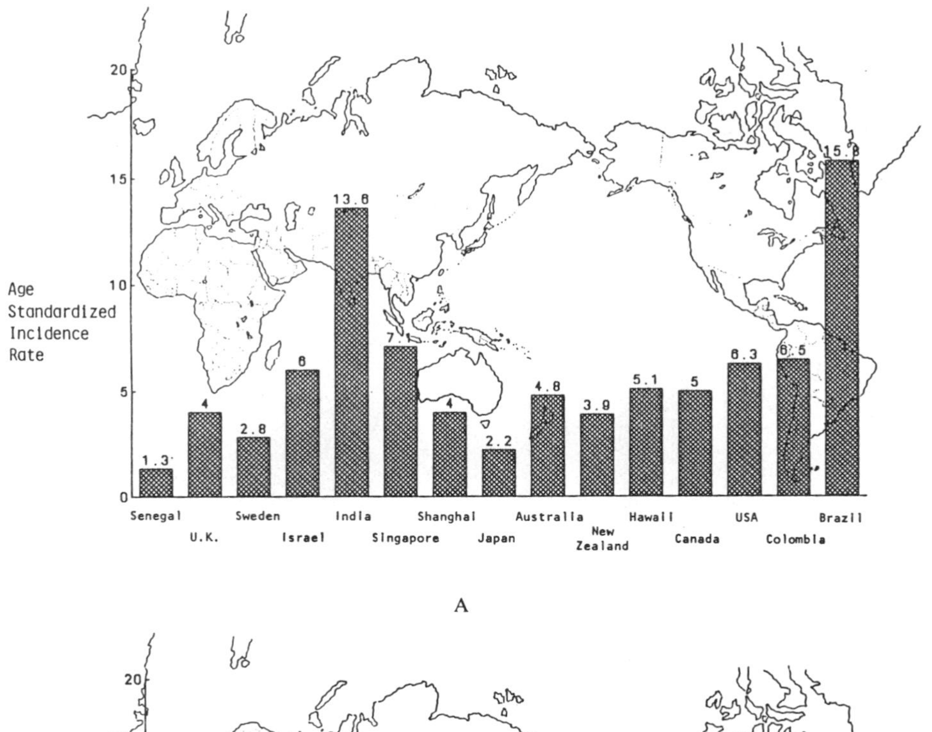

A

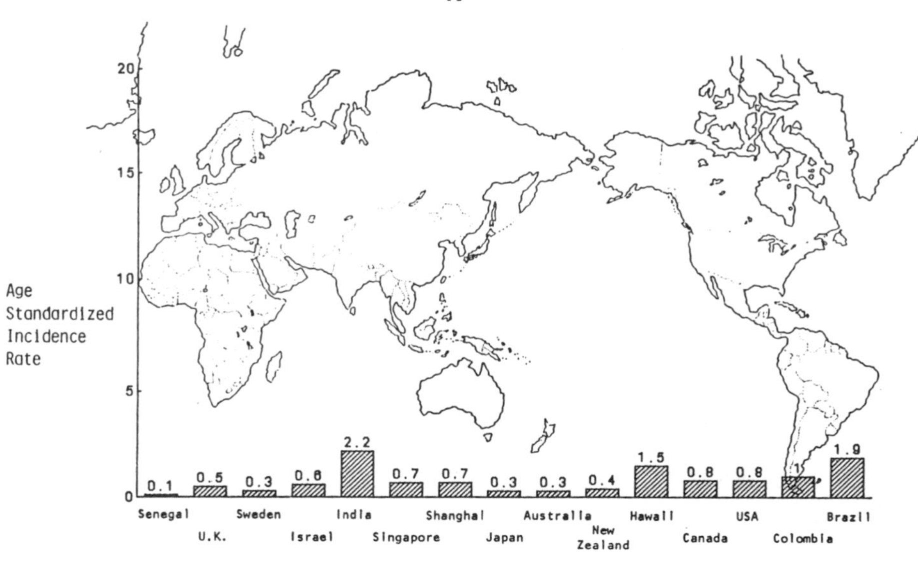

B

FIGURE 14. Cancer of the larynx in (A) males and (B) females. (From Waterhouse, J., Muir, C., Powell, J., et al., *Cancer Incidents in Five Continents,* Vol. 4, International Agency for Research on Cancer, Lyon, 1982. With permission.)

in a family was observed as early as 100 A.D. The incidence is known to increase in women with mothers and/or sisters having breast cancer. The breast cancer-affected women tended to be younger in such cases.

Risk rises twofold if her mother or sister have had it, and sixfold if both had it. If occurring bilaterally, there is about a 30-fold increase. Increased incidence was also reported in phenotypic males with Klinefelter's syndrome. Some high risk families have cancers of multiple sites, including ovary, large bowel, and soft tissue sarcomas. Multiple primary

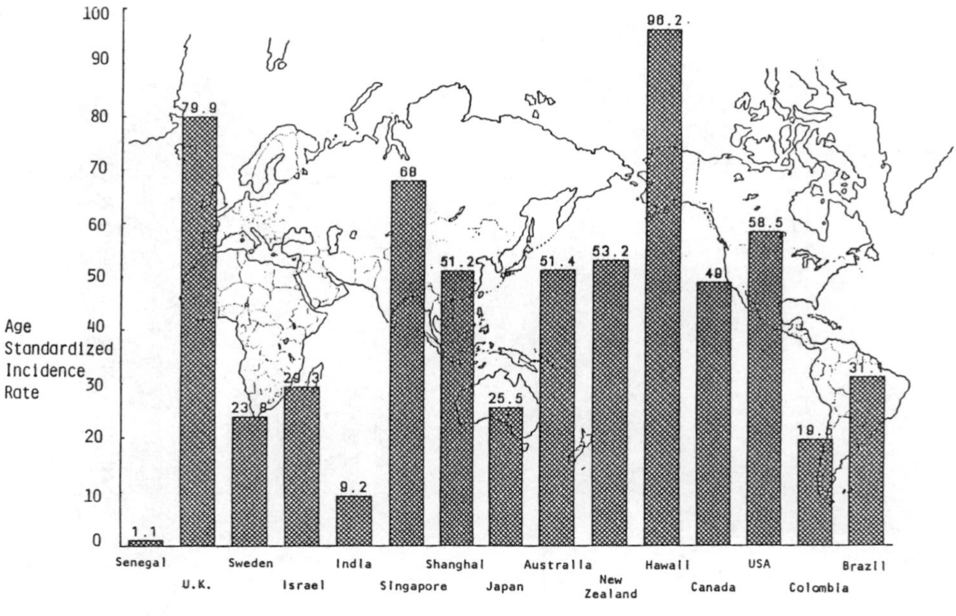

A

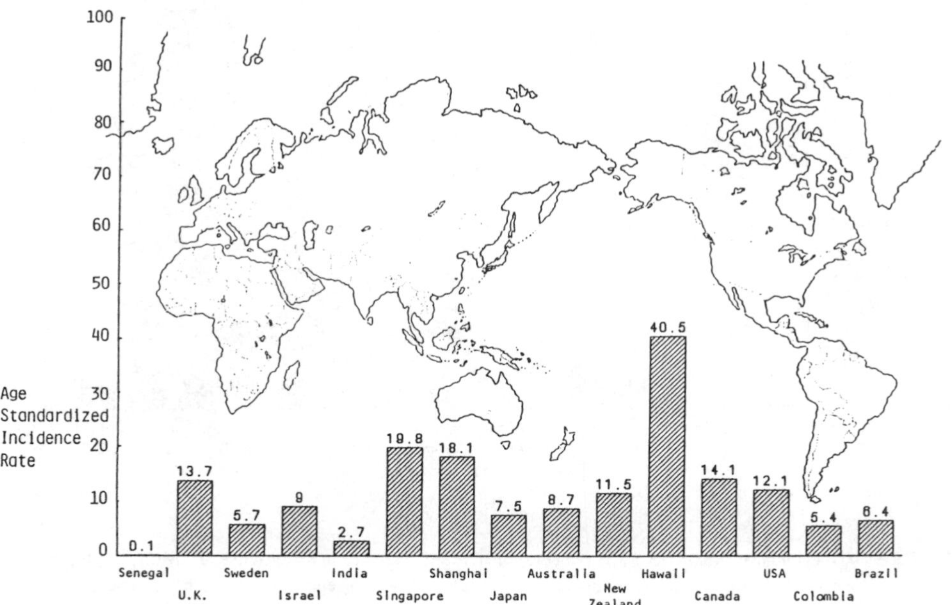

B

FIGURE 15. Cancer of the lung in (A) males and (B) females. (From Waterhouse, J., Muir, C., Powell, J., et al., *Cancer Incidents in Five Continents,* Vol. 4, International Agency for Research on Cancer, Lyon, 1982. With permission.)

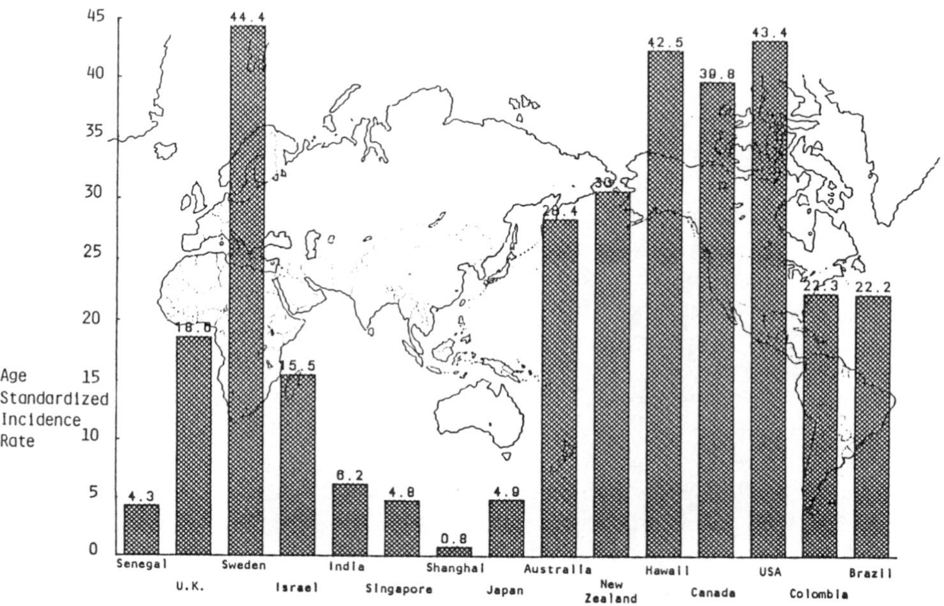

A

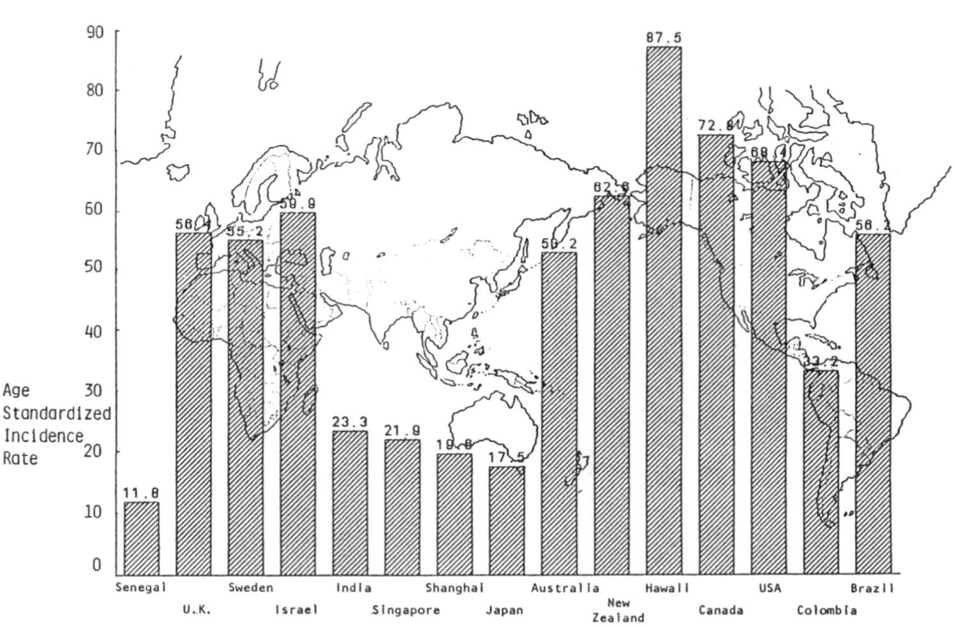

B

FIGURE 16. Cancer of the (A) prostate and (B) breast. (From Waterhouse, J., Muir, C., Powell, J., et al., *Cancer Incidents in Five Continents,* Vol. 4, International Agency for Research on Cancer, Lyon, 1982. With permission.)

neoplasms are mainly endometrial and ovarian cancer. An association exists with colon cancer and salivary gland neoplasms.

N. Cancer of the Cervix

The disease is almost universally common. However, there are countries showing exceedingly high incidence rates such as India and countries in South America. It is of utmost importance to note the geographic correlation with cancer of the penis (Figure 17). The observation strongly suggests common etiology. The hypothesis is being confirmed by identifying the human papilloma virus type 16 and 18 in patients with these two cancers. No specific genetic patterns have been observed.

O. Cancer of the Penis

The incidence of the disease is high in Asia, Africa, and Central and South America (Figure 17). Regions for high incidence often correspond to the variation in ethnic composition (e.g., incidence is low in Java and Indonesia, where mostly circumcised Muslims live, but is also quite high in Bali where the majority are Hindus). In Uganda, the Gisu, the only tribe which practices circumcision, has a low rate for penile cancer.[23] The incidence is known to become lower when penile hygiene is improved (e.g., Indian migrants in Fiji).

P. Cancer of the Prostate

The disease is quite common in western countries and a striking geographical variation exists in the incidence of the disease (Figure 16). The incidence is exceedingly high in blacks in the U.S. Much less variation in rates was observed in occult prostate carcinoma.

The disease was known to become quite common among migrants who came from low-risk countries. This phenomenon is attributed primarily to the differences in diet and nutrition which varies from country to country. A large-scale cohort study in Japan showed a significantly lower mortality rate for prostatic cancer in daily consumers of green/yellow vegetables up to age 74 but not in age 75 or older. This suggests the operation of an LMF of nutritional elements in green/yellow vegetables.

With regard to genetic predisposition, Woolfe[24] and Krain[25] noted that the disease has a tendency to aggregate in families (see Section M).

Q. Cancer of the Testis

The disease is relatively common in western countries. The pattern of geographical distribution is similar to that seen in cancer of the ovary (Figure 18), suggesting the existence of certain common etiologic factors, including genetic susceptibility. Genetic predisposition of seminomas was reported in monozygotic twins.

Genetic abnormalities such as Klinefelter's syndrome and hemaphroditism are predisposing conditions.

R. Cancer of the Ovary

The disease is common in western countries. The pattern of geographical variation is similar to that of cancer of the testis (Figure 18). With regard to genetic predisposition, many high-risk families were reported with cystadenocarcinoma frequently associated with breast cancer. An increased incidence of multiple primary neoplasms, primarily of the breast and corpus uteri, were reported.

S. Cancer of the Kidney

Renal cell carcinoma (hypernephroma) was reported to aggregate in a pedigree, ten cases in three generations of a family, all five living cases having a translocation between chromosomes 3 and 8, with three of the five deceased being obligate carriers of the translocation. The disease was not present in nine adults in the family with normal karyotype.[26]

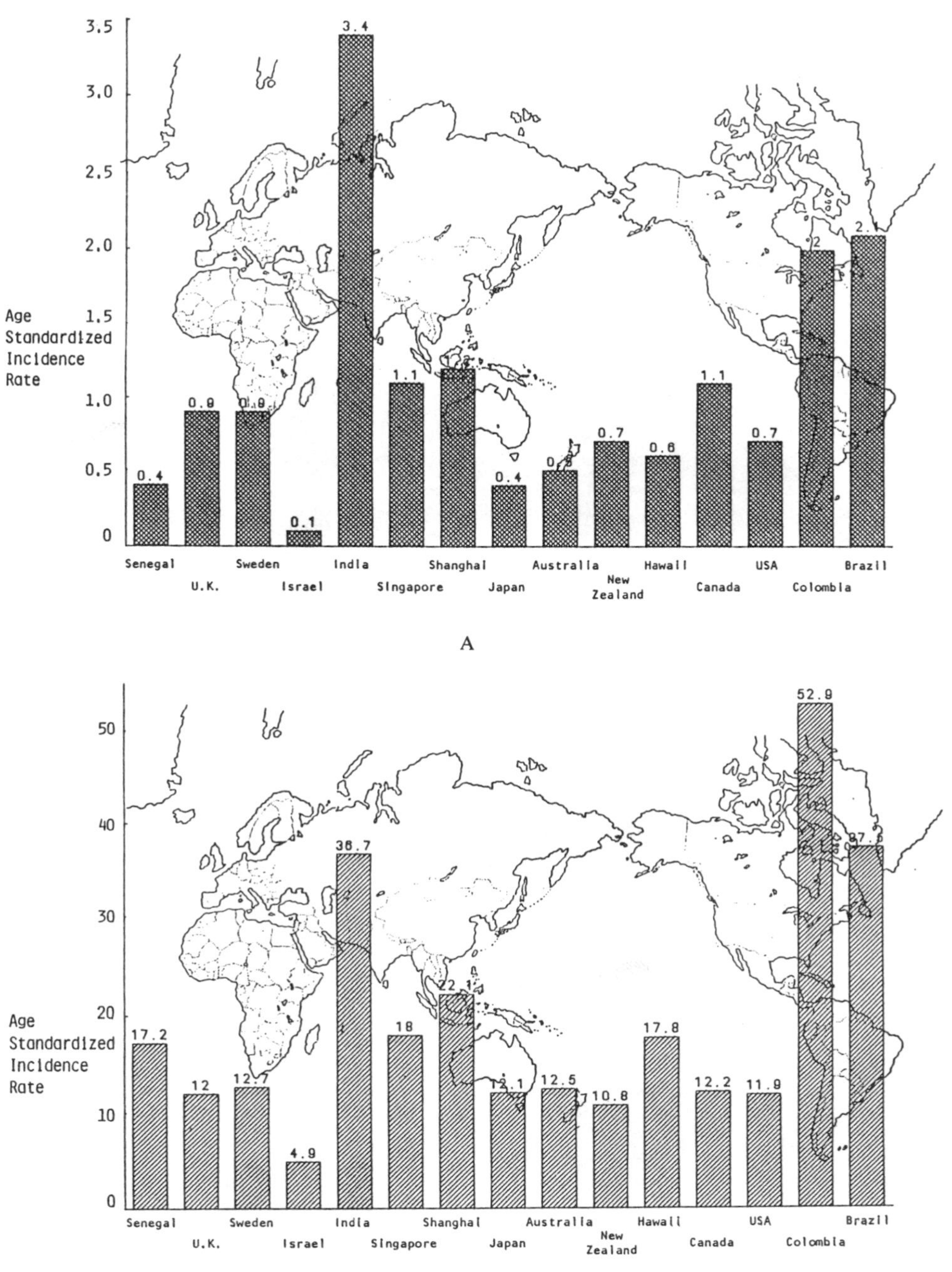

FIGURE 17. Cancer of the (A) penis and (B) cervix. (From Waterhouse, J., Muir, C., Powell, J., et al., *Cancer Incidents in Five Continents,* Vol. 4, International Agency for Research on Cancer, Lyon, 1982. With permission.)

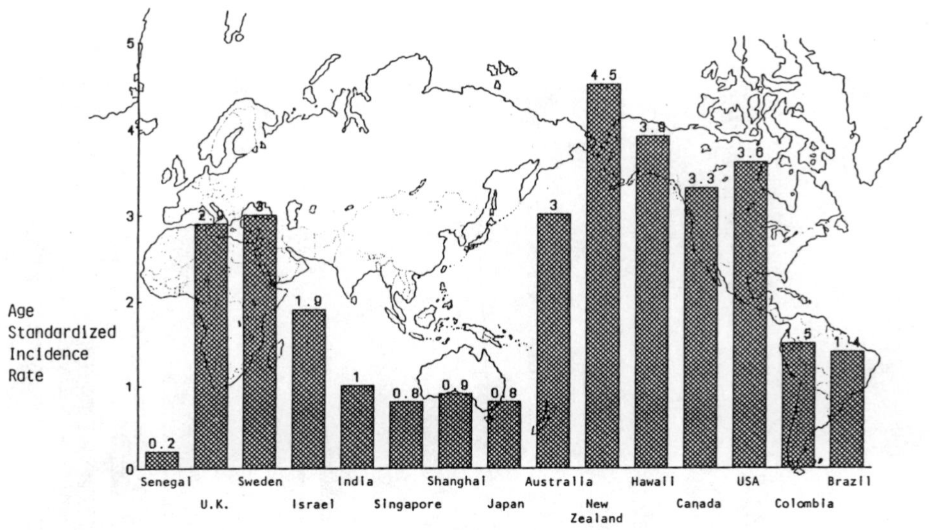

A

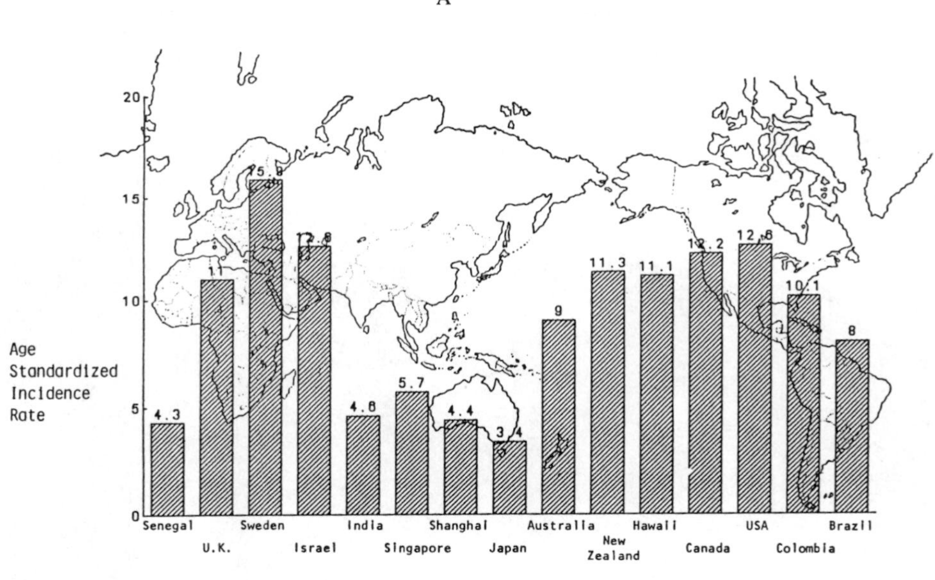

B

FIGURE 18. Cancer of the (A) testis and (B) ovary. (From Waterhouse, J., Muir, C., Powell, J., et al., *Cancer Incidents in Five Continents,* Vol. 4, International Agency for Research on Cancer, Lyon, 1982. With permission.)

T. Cancer of the Urinary Bladder

Transitional cell carcinoma is quite common in western countries while squamous cell carcinoma predominates in Egypt and other African countries (associated with infection with Schistosomiasis haematobium). The disease is much more common in males than in females, reflecting prevalence of smoking habits (Figure 19).

Genetic predisposition reports include possible familial association with tryptophane metabolism. The predominent associated neoplasm is lung cancer, reflecting the association with cigarette smoking as a common etiology.

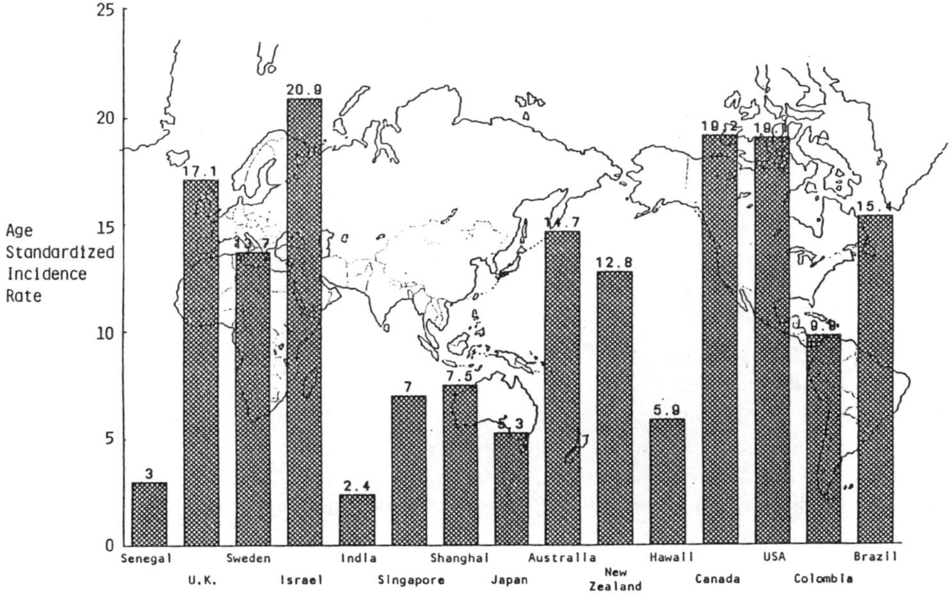

A

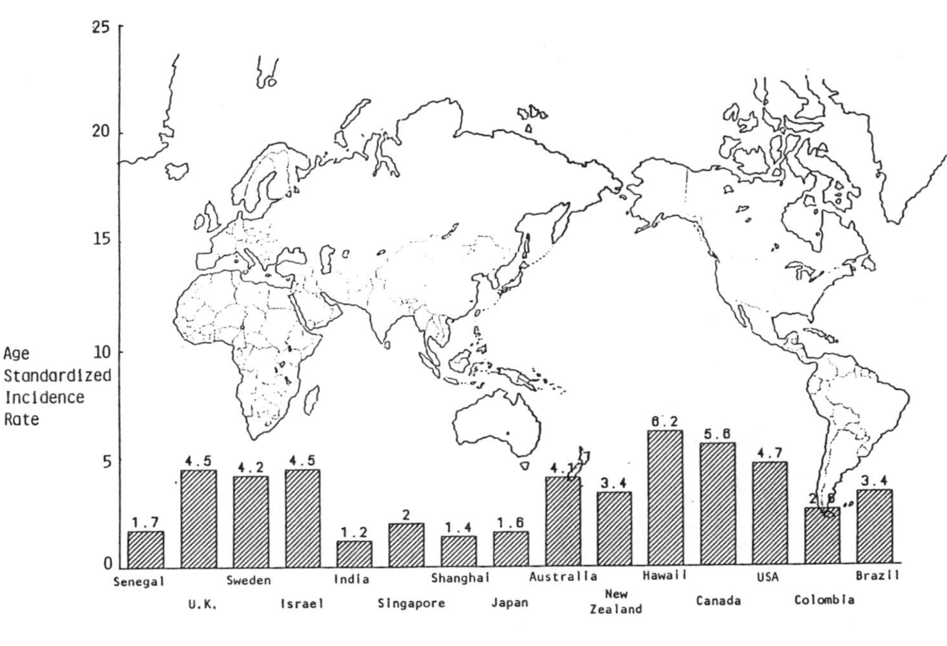

B

FIGURE 19. Cancer of the urinary bladder in (A) males and (B) females. (From Waterhouse, J., Muir, C., Powell, J., et al., *Cancer Incidents in Five Continents,* Vol. 4, International Agency for Research on Cancer, Lyon, 1982. With permission.)

U. Malignant Melanoma

The disease is common in fair-skinned races living in high UV areas such as Australia and New Zealand. The pattern of geographical distribution as well as incidence itself is quite similar in both sexes (Figure 20). However, the distribution by primary site is markedly different for the two sexes. Melanoma of the head, neck, and trunk is higher in males, and in females, the lower extremities are more often affected, which probably reflects differences in dress habits.

Familial susceptibility exists, suggesting the possibility of dominant inheritance. The incidence is also quite high in patients affected by xeroderma pigmentosum. Racial susceptibility is negatively associated with skin pigmentation.

V. Cancer of the Thyroid

The disease is more prevalent in females than in males. However, a high similarity exists in the patterns of geographical variation in both sexes (Figure 21). The disease is quite common in Hawaii in most ethnic groups, suggesting the influence of certain environmental factors specific to the area (e.g., fish consumption).

Genetic predisposition is morphology type dependent. Medullary cancer may be associated with Sipple syndrome (multiple adenomatosis II) which occurs in combination with pheochromocytoma and parathyroid adenoma.

W. Hodgkin's Disease

The disease is more common in western countries (Figure 22). In developed countries, the age distribution is featured by bimodality, one peak being at adolescence and one peak at older ages. Risk was directly related to socioeconomic status and level of education, and was inversely related to family size. Reports on genetic predisposition are controversial. Recent familial studies show a sevenfold higher relative risk among siblings and an association with HLA antigens is suggested.

Premorbid conditions, namely, associations with infectious mononucleosis and immunological disorders (ataxia telangiectasia) have been reported. Prior history of tonsillectomy was also suspected.

X. Non-Hodgkin's Lymphoma

The disease is consistently more frequent in males than in females in any place in the world (Figure 23). Types of lymphoma vary by areas, e.g., follicular lymphoma in U.S. whites, Mediterranean lymphoma (intestinal B-cell lymphoma), Burkitt's tumor in malaria-endemic areas in Africa, adult T-cell lymphoma in southern Kyushu, Japan, parts of the Carribean, Africa, and the southeastern U.S. In each case, virus involvement was proved or strongly suspected. Increased risk was observed in families with immunological defects.[27]

Y. Leukemia

International variation in incidence has more to do with ethnic factors than with geography. The disease is rare in black Africans. Risks are slightly higher in males (Figures 24 and 25). Incidence of chronic lymphocytic leukemia (CLL) is low in Japan. Acute myelocytic leukemia (AML) or acute myelomonocytic leukemia (AMML) with chloroma is found in Ankara, Turkey. The disease occasionally aggregates in families. The elevation is striking in patients who were exposed to maternal antenatal radiation, suggesting genetic/environmental interaction.[28] Risks are generally high in children with a heavy birth weight.[28] Congenital anomalies with chromosome abnormalities are known to be closely related to childhood leukemia (e.g., ALL in Down's syndrome, AMML in Fanconi's aplastic anemia, and non-lymphocytic leukemia in Bloom's syndrome). Ataxia telangiectasia predisposes to ALL. Some CML cases show typical chromosome patterns (Philadelphia chromosome).

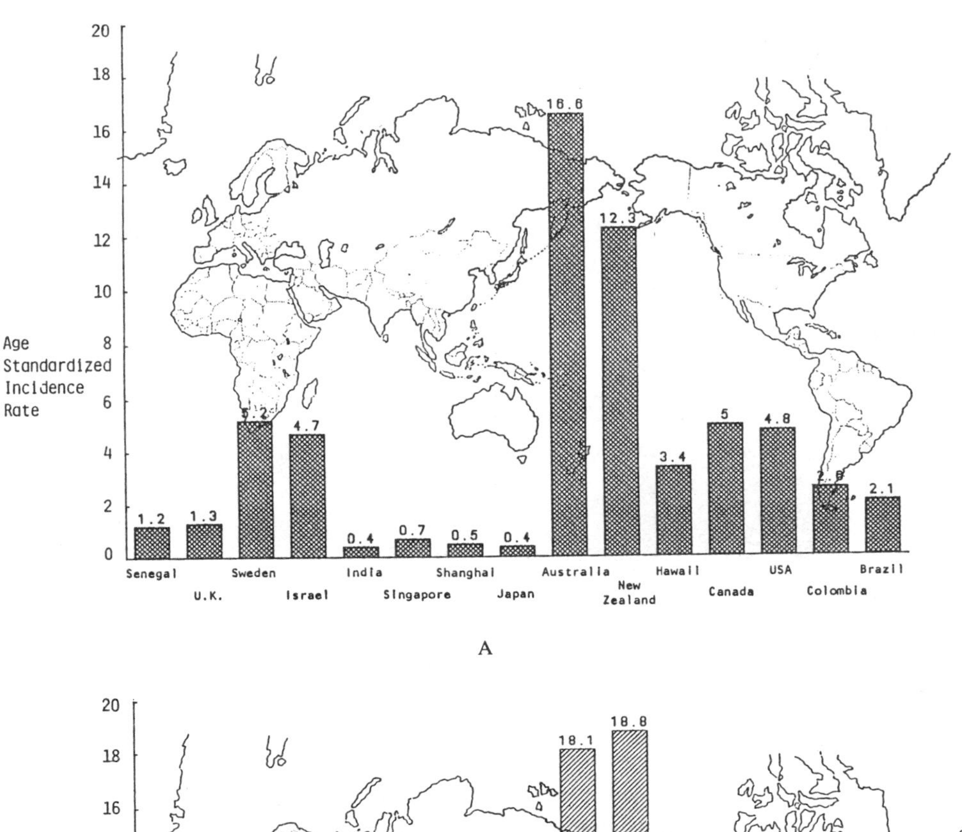

A

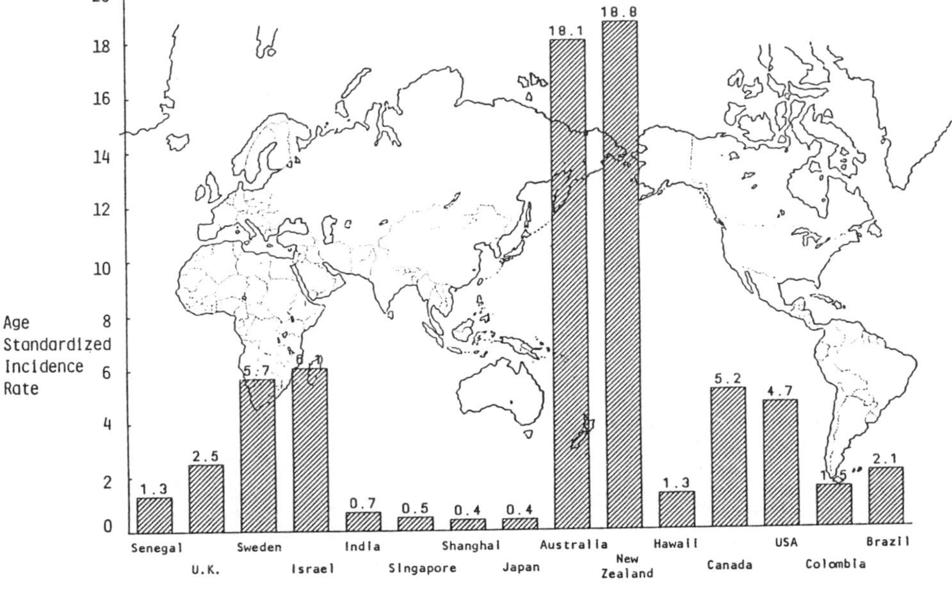

B

FIGURE 20. Melanoma in (A) males and (B) females. (From Waterhouse, J., Muir, C., Powell, J., et al., *Cancer Incidents in Five Continents*, Vol. 4, International Agency for Research on Cancer, Lyon, 1982. With permission.)

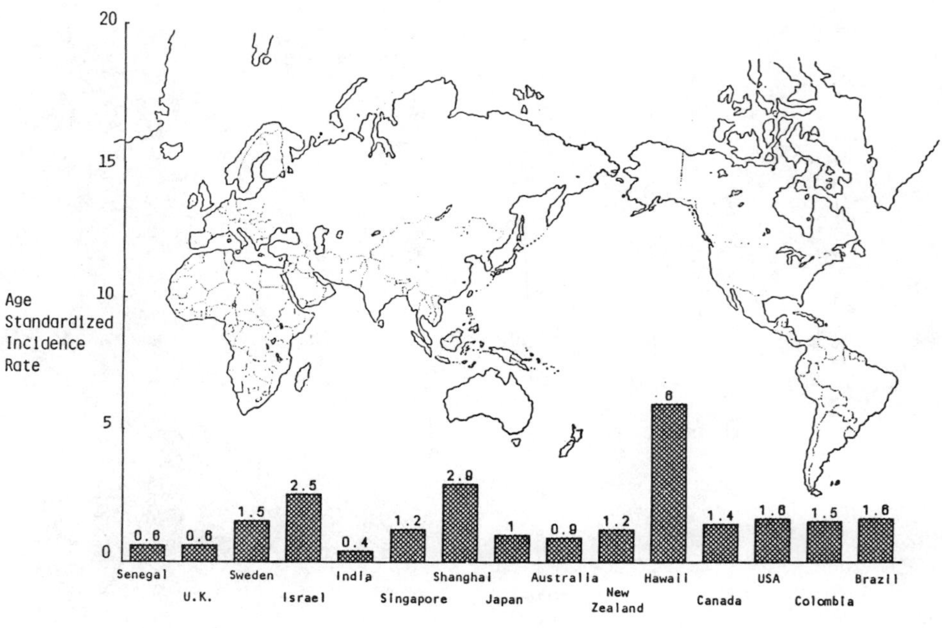

A

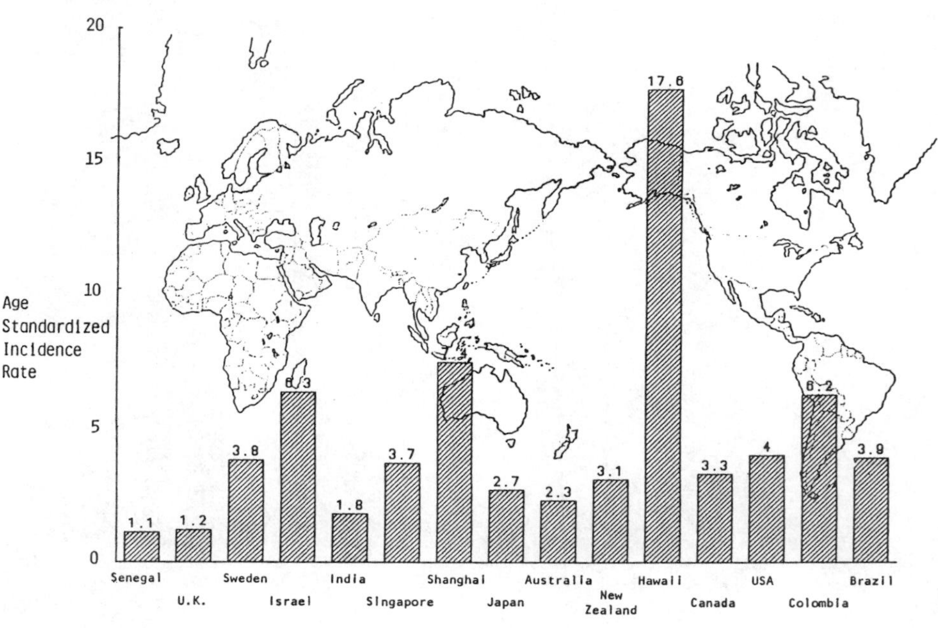

B

FIGURE 21. Cancer of the thyroid in (A) males and (B) females. (From Waterhouse, J., Muir, C., Powell, J., et al., *Cancer Incidents in Five Continents,* Vol. 4, International Agency for Research on Cancer, Lyon, 1982. With permission.)

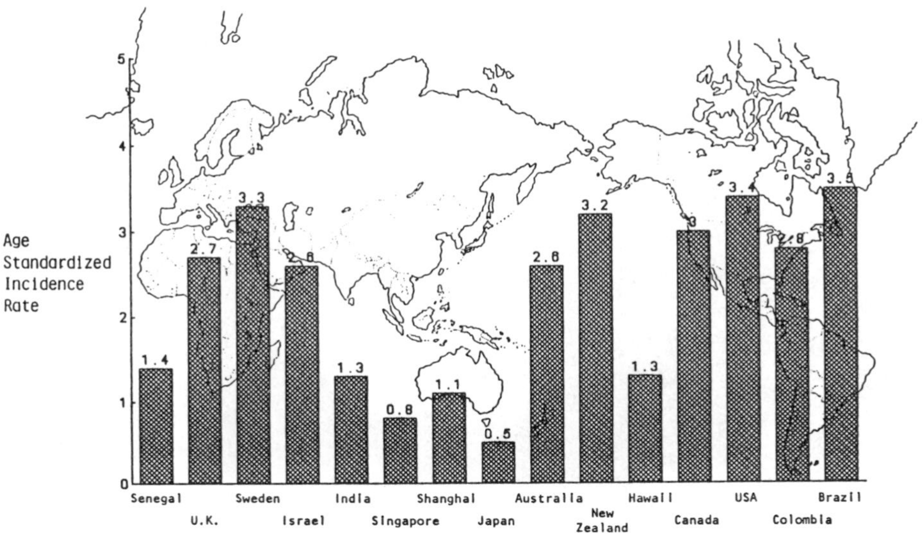

A

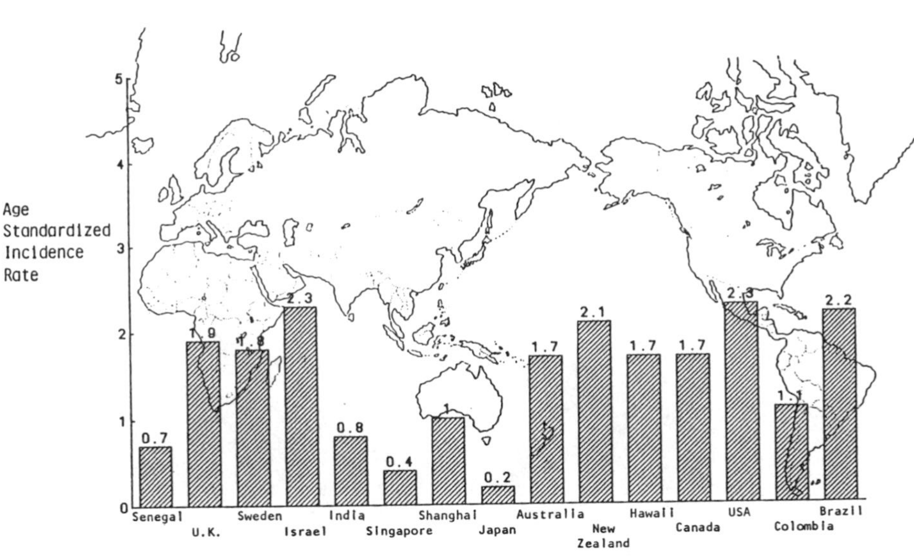

B

FIGURE 22. Hodgkin's disease in (A) males and (B) females. (From Waterhouse, J., Muir, C., Powell, J., et al., *Cancer Incidents in Five Continents,* Vol. 4, International Agency for Research on Cancer, Lyon, 1982. With permission.)

Z. Childhood Malignancies

There is little geographical variation in the incidence of childhood malignancies (Figure 26). The slight variation observed may reflect different levels of expertise in medical diagnosis in these countries since the pattern is similar in males and females.

AA. Wilms' Tumor

The geographic distribution of Wilms' tumor or nephroblastoma is nearly uniform around the world. The disease aggregates in families.[29] Multifocal familial cases have a prezygotic

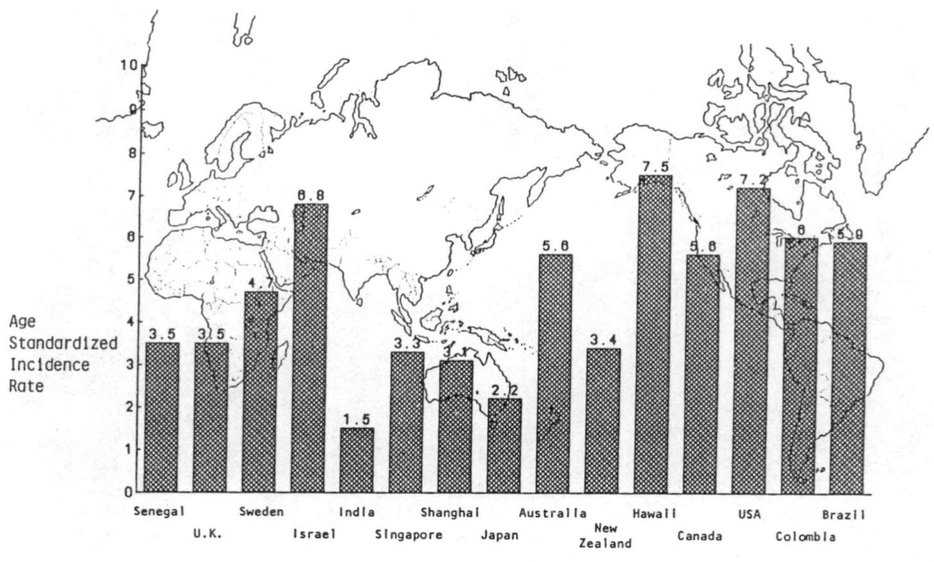

A

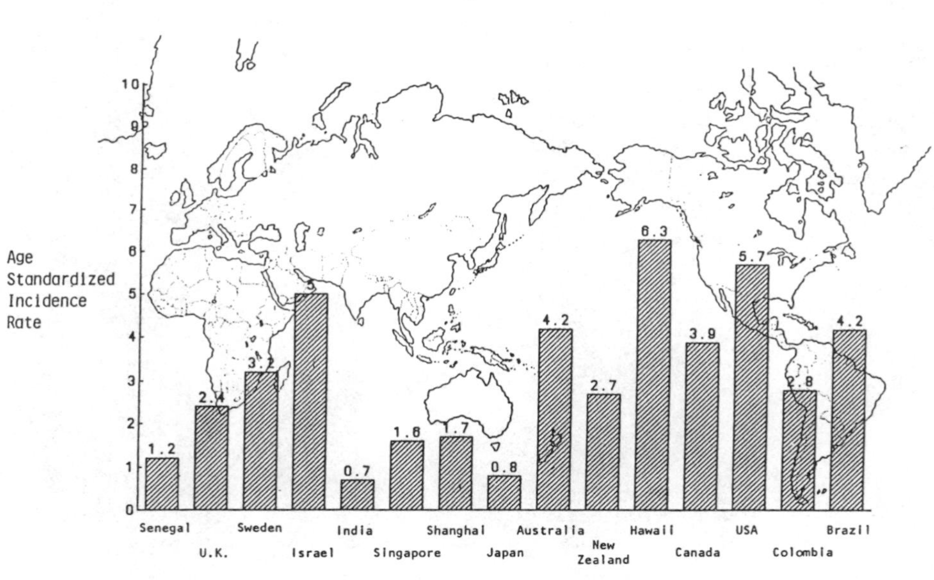

B

FIGURE 23. Lymphosarcoma in (A) males and (B) females. (From Waterhouse, J., Muir, C., Powell, J., et al., *Cancer Incidents in Five Continents,* Vol. 4, International Agency for Research on Cancer, Lyon, 1982. With permission.)

first step and postzygotic malignant transforming step. Bilateral Wilms' tumor shows renal dysplasia in nonmalignant subcapsular renal tissue. Generally, any disorder with genitourinary anomalies may have renal dysplasia that predisposes to Wilms' tumor (e.g., hemihypertrophy, aniridia, horseshoe kidney, or male pseudohemaphroditism). A chromosome abnormality (11p-) is observed in patients with aniridia and Wilms' tumor.[30]

BB. Retinoblastoma

There is little international variation in the incidence of the disease. The incidence is

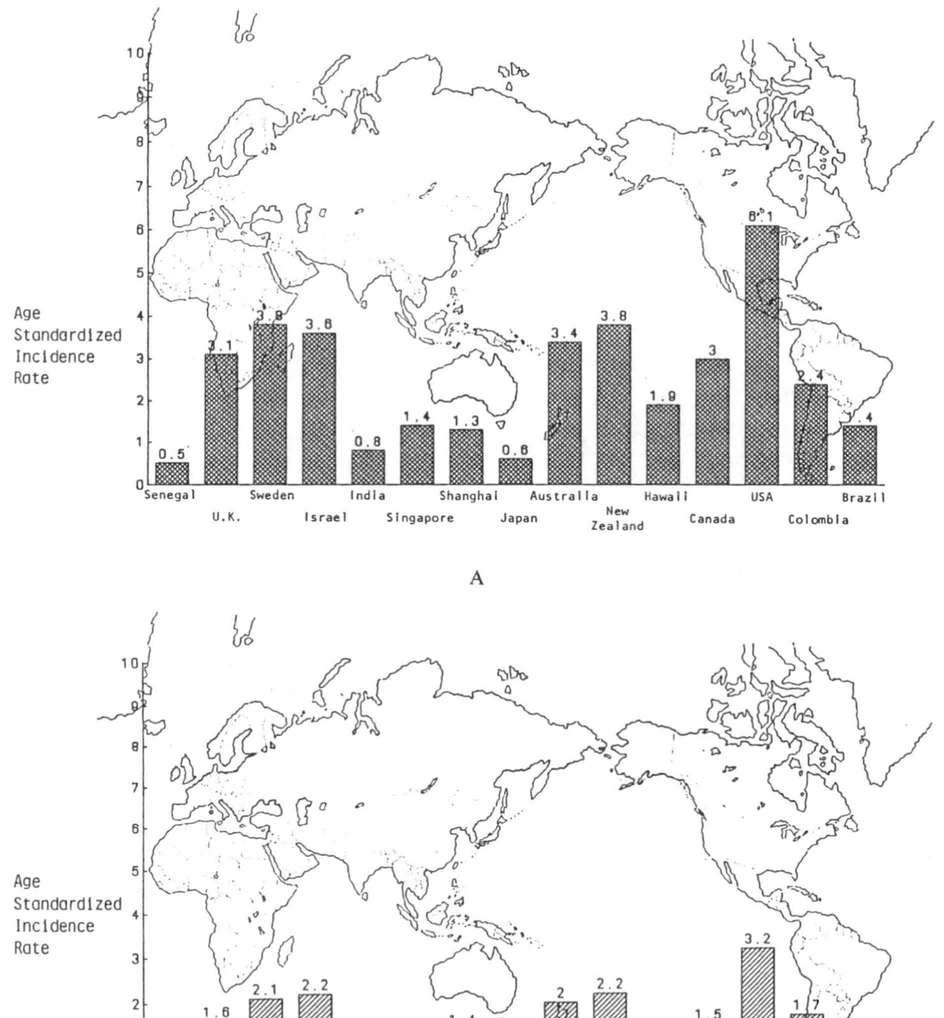

FIGURE 24. Lymphatic leukemia in (A) males and (B) females. (From Waterhouse, J., Muir, C., Powell, J., et al., *Cancer Incidents in Five Continents,* Vol. 4, International Agency for Research on Cancer, Lyon, 1982. With permission.)

slightly higher in males. Approximately 40% of retinoblastoma cases have a genetic basis (autosomal dominant inheritance).[31] These generally have an earlier age of onset and the majority are bilateral.[2] Multiple primary neoplasms include osteosarcoma, fibrosarcoma, adenocarcinoma, and pinealblastoma in the irradiated site in bilateral cases.[32,33] Wilson observed an abnormality in chromosome 13-q (34).

CC. Cancer of the Bone

Osteosarcoma is a common primary tumor of bone. Other malignancies include chon-

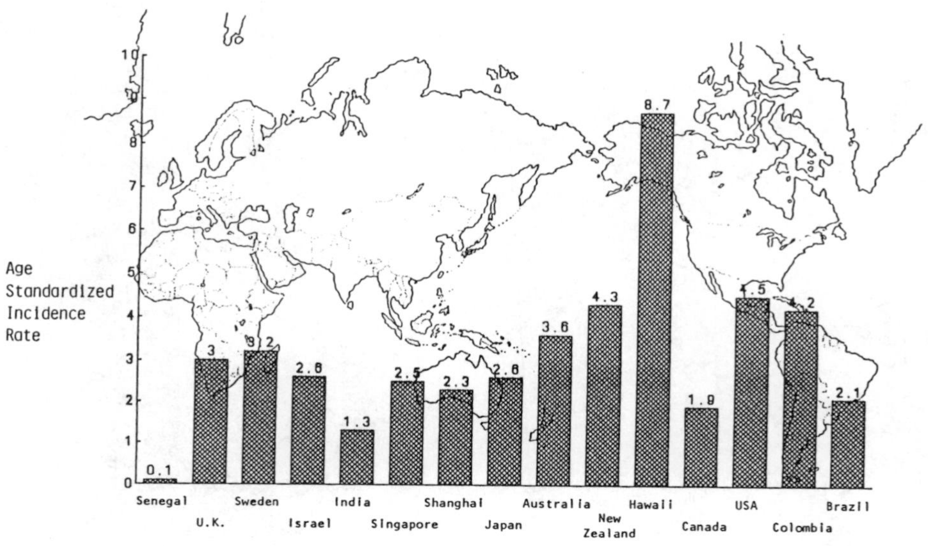

A

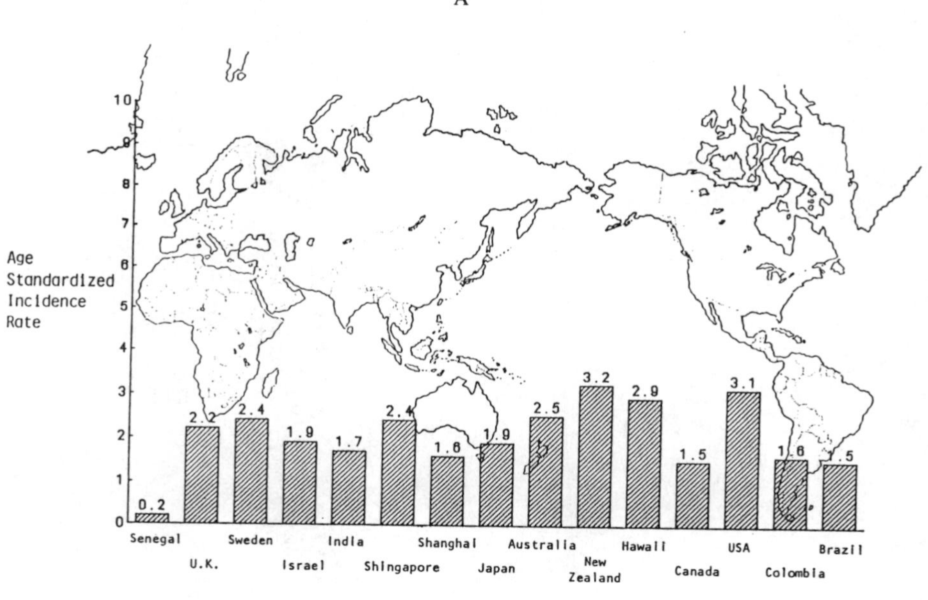

B

FIGURE 25. Myeloid leukemia in (A) males and (B) females. (From Waterhouse, J., Muir, C., Powell, J., et al., *Cancer Incidents in Five Continents,* Vol. 4, International Agency for Research on Cancer, Lyon, 1982. With permission.)

drosarcoma and Ewing's sarcoma. In osteogenic sarcoma, the geographical variation is related to the prevalence of Paget's disease. International variations in the incidence of Ewing's sarcoma have been considered to be closely related to racial factors.[35] Blacks in all geographical areas appear to have a resistance to Ewing's sarcoma. This is apparent in both African and American blacks, suggesting a racially determined resistance to the tumor. Multiple exostoses, an autosomal dominant disorder, produces osteochondromas and a 5 to 11% risk of chondrosarcoma, which often occurs at an early age.

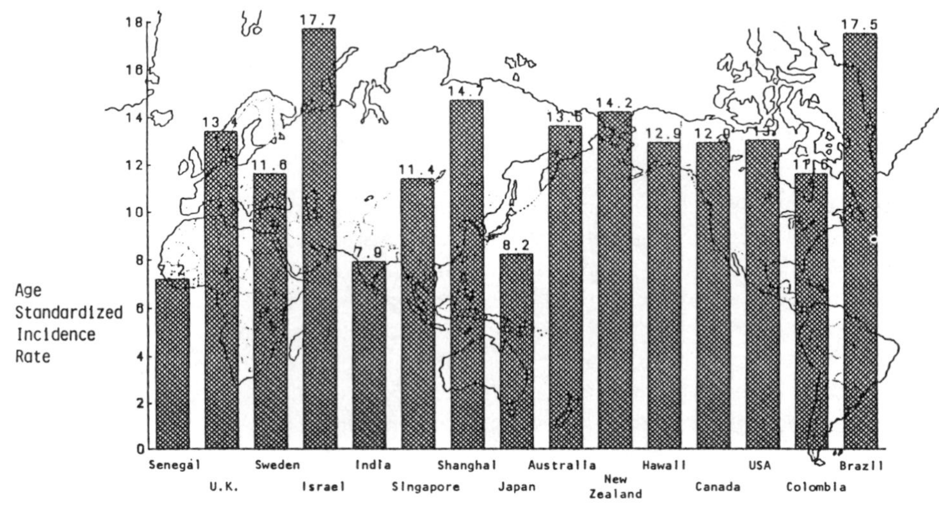

A

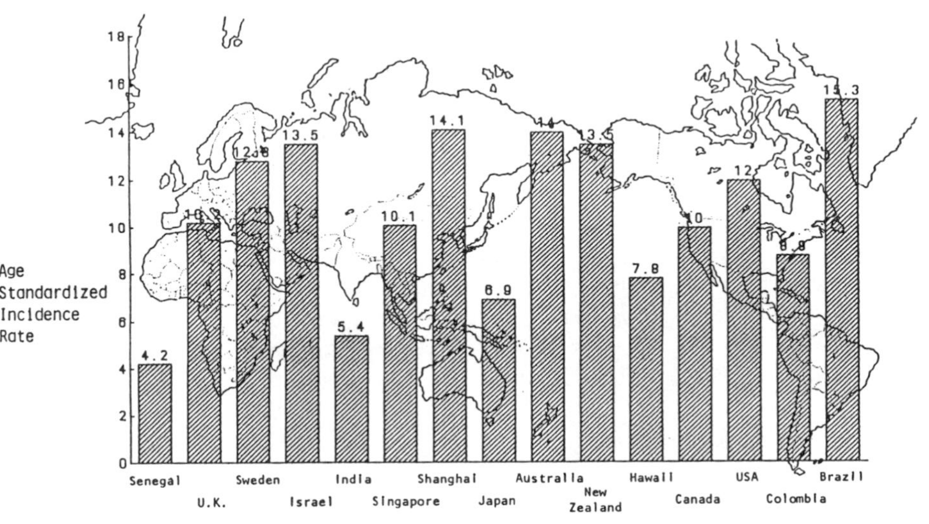

B

FIGURE 26. Childhood malignancy in (A) males and (B) females. (From Waterhouse, J., Muir, C., Powell, J., et al., *Cancer Incidents in Five Continents,* Vol. 4, International Agency for Research on Cancer, Lyon, 1982. With permission.)

Hereditary retinoblastoma, an autosomal dominant disorder, is associated with an increased risk for radiation-induced and spontaneous osteogenic sarcomas.

DD. Brain Tumors

Tumors of the pineal gland occur six to nine times more frequently in Japan when compared with other brain tumors. Within Japan, regional variations are striking, with the highest incidence being in Aomori prefecture.[28] Gliomas are more often observed in whites, while meningiomas occur more often in blacks. Glioblastoma multiforme and medulloblastoma are seen more frequently in males, while astrocytoma, neurinoma, and meningiomas are more common in females.

Risks of brain tumor are reported to be higher when epilepsy is present in siblings.[36] Brain tumors are also reported to be significantly higher in those exposed to passive smoking.[18] The effect of nitrosamine in sidestream smoke has been suspected.[37]

IV. DISCUSSION

Geographical distribution of cancer incidence was observed by each cancer site and interpreted in relation to racial and genetic characteristics. In most cases, it is evident that observed unique geographical patterns are similar in males and females, strongly suggesting that factors affecting such geographical differences operate in similar fashion in both sexes.

Further, an interesting similarity was observed in certain pairs of cancers of sex-specific sites (e.g., cancer of the prostate and breast, cancer of the testis and ovary, and cancer of the penis and cervix). In such cases, special risk factors including genetic predisposition may be commonly operating in cancer of different sites in different sexes.

Whether or not such factors are genetic, environmental, both, or artificial (e.g., different levels of expertise in diagnosis) must be a subject of future epidemiologic study. Possibilities of genetic/environmental interacton must always be considered. Further careful observation of cancer patterns in migrants may clarify such issues. Racial characteristics usually remain as such in migrants, strongly suggesting the existence of genetic factors in determining levels of cancer incidence, although rates in migrants are in general lower than those in their motherland. In this context, comparison of the incidence in migrants and those in the motherland are of crucial importance (e.g., stomach cancer incidence in Japanese in Okinawa and Japanese in Hawaii).

When details of site distribution of the leading cause of cancer in males and females in selected countries were compared, dissimilarities in the pattern of cancer occurrence in different countries were impressive. There seemed to be regional similarities, and groups of neighboring countries tended to show rather similar patterns (e.g., oral cancer in India and Sri Lanka, cervical cancer in most of Latin America, stomach cancer in China, Japan, and Korea, liver cancer in most countries in Africa and Asia, malignant lymphoma in the Middle East, gallbladder cancer in Bolivia and New Mexico). Environmental conditions as well as genetic factors must be considered in interpreting such phenomena. Such regional cancer patterns also suggest the desirability of a regional approach in global cancer control programs.

REFERENCES

1. **Hirayama, T.,** Epidemiology of stomach cancer in Japan with special reference to the strategy for the primary prevention, *Jpn. J. Clin. Oncol.*, 14, 159, 1984.
2. **Knudson, A. G.,** Mutation and cancer: statistical study of retinoblastoma, *Proc. Natl. Acad. Sci., U.S.A.*, 68, 820, 1971.
3. **Waterhouse, J., Muir, C., Powell, J., et al.,** *Cancer Incidence in Five Continents,* Vol. 4, IARC Sci. Publ. No. 42, International Agency for Research on Cancer, Lyon, 1982.
4. **Hirayama, T.,** An epidemiological study of oral and pharyngeal cancer in Central and Southeast Asia, *Bull. WHO,* 34, 41, 1966.
5. **Berg, J. W., Hutter, R. V. P., and Foote, F. W., Jr.,** The unique association between salivary gland cancer and breast cancer, *JAMA,* 204, 771, 1968.
6. **Aird, I. and Bentall, H. H.,** A relationship between cancer of the stomach and the ABO blood groups, *Br. Med. J.*, 17, 799, 1951.
7. **Siurala, M. and Seppala, K.,** Atrophic gastritis as a possible precursor of gastric carcinoma and pernicious anemia — results of followup exam, *Acta Med. Scand.*, 166, 455, 1960.
8. **Bonney, G. E., Elston, R. C., Correa, P., et al.,** Genetic etiology of gastric carcinoma. I. Chronic atrophic gastritis, *Genet. Epidemiol.*, 3, 213, 1986.

9. **Friedman, J. M. and Fialkow, P. J.,** Familial carcinoma of the pancreas, *Clin. Genet.*, 9, 463, 1976.
10. **Macdermot, R. P. and Kramer, P.,** Adenocarcinoma of the pancreas in four siblings, *Gastroenterology*, 65, 137, 1973.
11. **Miller, M. C.,** Familial cirrhosis with hepatoma, *Am. J. Dig. Dis.*, 12, 633, 1967.
12. **Armstrong, R. W., Armstrong, M. J., Yu, M. C., and Henderson, B. E.,** Salted fish and inhalants as risk factors for nasopharyngeal carcinoma in Malaysian Chinese, *Cancer Res.*, 43, 2967, 1983.
13. **Hirayama, T. and Ito, Y.,** A new view of the etiology of nasopharyngeal carcinoma, *Prev. Med.* 10, 614, 1981.
14. **Ho, H. C.,** Genetic and environmental factors in nasopharngeal carcinoma, in *Recent Advances in Human Tumor Virology and Immunology*, Nakahara, W., Nishioka, K., and Hirayama, T., et al., Eds., University of Tokyo Press, Tokyo, 1971, 275.
15. **Ho, H. C.,** Current knowledge of the epidemiology of nasopharnygeal carcinoma — a review, *Oncogenesis and Herpesviruses*, Biggs, P. M., de-The, G., and Payne, L. N., Eds., IARC Sci. Publ. No. 2, International Agency for Research on Cancer, Lyon, 1972, 357.
16. **Joncas, J. H., Rioux, E., Robitaille, R., and Wastiaux, J. P.,** Multiple cases of lymphoepithelioma and Burkitt's lymphoma in a Canadian family, *Bibl. Haematol.*, 224, 1975.
17. **Simons, M. J., Wee, G. B., Goh, E. H., Chan, S. H., Shanmugaratnam, K., Day, N. E., and de-The, G.,** Immunogenetic aspects of nasopharyngeal carcinoma. IV. Increased risk in Chinese of nasopharyngeal carcinoma associated with a Chinese-related HLA profile, *J. Natl. Cancer Inst.*, 57, 977, 1976.
18. **Hirayama, T.,** Cancer mortality in nonsmoking women with smoking husbands based on a large-scale cohort study in Japan, *Prev. Med.*, 13, 680, 1984.
19. **Trell, E., Korsgaard, R., Hood, B., Kitzing, P., Norden, G., and Simonsson, B. G.,** Aryl hydrocarbon hydroxylase inducibility and laryngeal carcinomas, *Lancet*, ii, 140, 1976.
20. **Tokuhata, G. K. and Lilienfeld, A. M.,** Familial aggregation of lung cancer in humans, *J. Natl. Cancer Inst.*, 30, 289, 1963.
21. **Hirayama, T.,** Non-smoking wives of heavy smokers have a high risk of lung cancer; a study from Japan, *Br. Med. J.*, 282, 183, 1981.
22. **Kellerman, G., Shaw, C. R., and Luyten-Kellemann, M.,** Aryl hydrocarbon hydroxylase inducibility and bronchogenic carcinoma, *N. Engl. J. Med.*, 289, 934, 1973.
23. **Schmauz, R. and Jain, D. K.,** Geographical variation of carcinoma of the penis in Uganda, *Br. J. Cancer*, 25, 25, 1971.
24. **Woolf, A. M.,** An investigation of the familial aspects of carcinoma of the prostate, *Cancer*, 13, 739, 1960.
25. **Krain, L. S.,** Some epidemiologic variables in prostate carcinoma in California, *Prev. Med.*, 3, 154, 1974.
26. **Li, F. P., Marchetto, D. J., and Cohen, A. J.,** Familial renal cell carcinoma associated with a constitutional chromosomal translocation: biological and clinical implications, *Proc. AACR*, 19, 384, 1978.
27. **Purtilo, D. T.,** Opportunistic non-Hodgkin's lymphoma in X-linked recessive immunodeficiency and lymphoproliferative syndromes, *Semin. Oncol.*, 4, 335, 1977.
28. **Hirayama, T.,** Descriptive and analytical epidemiology of childhood malignancy in Japan, in *Recent Advances in Management of Children with Cancer*, Proc. Int. Symp. Children's Cancer, 1979, Tokyo, 1980, 27.
29. **Knudson, A. G., Jr. and Strong, L.,** Mutation and cancer: a model for Wilms' tumor of the kidney, *J. Natl. Cancer Inst.*, 48, 313, 1972.
30. **Riccardi, V. M., Sujansky, E., Smith, A. C., et al.,** Chromosomal imbalance in the aniridia-Wilms' tumor association: 11p interstitial deletion, *Pediatrics*, 61, 604, 1971.
31. **Knudson, A. G., Jr.,** Retinoblastoma: a prototypic hereditary neoplasm, *Semin. Oncol.*, 5, 57, 1978.
32. **Jensen, R. D. and Miller, R. W.,** Retinoblastoma: epidemiologic characteristics, *N. Engl. J. Med.*, 285, 307, 1971.
33. **Tucker, M. A., Meadows, A. T., Boice, J. D., Jr., Hoover, R. N., and Fraumeni, J. F., Jr.,** Cancer risk following treatment of childhood cancer, in *Radiation Carcinogenesis, Epidemiology and Biological Significance*, Boice, J. D. and Fraunmeni, J. F., Jr., Eds., Raven Press, New York, 1984, 211.
34. **Wilson, M. G., Ebin, A. J., Towner, J. W., et al.,** Chromosomal anomalies in patients with retinoblastoma, *Clin. Genet.*, 12, 1, 1977.
35. **Polednak, A. P.,** Primary bone cancer incidence in black and white residents of New York state, *Cancer*, 55, 2883, 1985.
36. **Gold, E., Gordia, L., Tonascia, J., and Szklo, M.,** Risk factors for brain tumors in children, *Am. J. Epidemiol.*, 109, 309, 1979.
37. **Presto-Martin, S. and Henderson, B. E.,** N-nitroso compounds and human intracranial tumours, IARC Sci. Publ. NO. 57, International Agency for Research on Cancer, Lyon, 1984, 887.

Chapter 6

CANCER OCCURRENCE IN PERSONS WITH INBORN ERRORS OF METABOLISM

Robert E. Grier and R. Rodney Howell

TABLE OF CONTENTS

I. INTRODUCTION

Since Garrod[1] made the correlation between the occurrence of alkaptonuria and a defective enzyme reaction, human inborn errors of metabolism have been increasingly informative. Many steps and even entire pathways of intermediary metabolism have been elucidated due to investigation of these rare inherited enzyme defects. The direct health effects of the enzyme defect may range from unimportant and incidential to life threatening and from acute to chronic. Onset of symptoms may be at birth or may occur well into adulthood.

In addition to the immediate clinical problems of patients with inborn errors, we now recognize that several metabolic defects carry a distinctly increased risk of malignancy.[2] This chapter will review several inborn errors of metabolism which have a clear association with cancer.

II. GENETIC DEFECTS WITH ASSOCIATED MALIGNANCY

A. Glucose-6-Phosphatase Deficiency

Glucose-6-phosphatase (G-6-Pase) deficiency produces a defect of glycogen metabolism (glycogen storage disease, GSD, type I, or von Gierke's disease) inherited as an autosomal recessive trait.[3] Two variants of G-6-Pase deficiency have been delineated and designated type Ia and type Ib, respectively.[4] Type Ia involves an abnormality of the enzyme glucose-6-phosphatase per se. Type Ib is due to a deficiency of the transport of glucose-6-phosphate formed in the cytosol of the cell, across the microsomal membrane. The clinical results of these deficiencies are quite similar.

All patients with type Ia G-6-Pase deficiency develop hepatic adenomas which appear about puberty or later in life.[5] These are usually multiple lesions which are most likely prehepatoma lesions.[6] Hepatic cirrhosis does not occur in patients with G-6-Pase deficiency and adenomas have been reported to regress with dietary therapy.[7] This later suggestion is not yet proven.

Several hypotheses have been put forward to explain the etiology of these hepatomas. These hepatic adenomata have been observed in older patients over many years and have maintained a benign histologic appearance. Although unproven, we have felt these adenomata could arise from the continual hormonal stimulation (by glucagon) of the liver in the futile effort of the body to maintain euglycemia.

On rare occasions, highly malignant tumors arise in areas of the liver which, at least in some instances, had been previously biopsied and shown to be histologically benign.

The malignancy is thought to be an indirect manifestation of the metabolic defect, not a direct pleiotophic effect of the gene mutation.[2] The possibility of an abnormal metabolite(s) acting as a carcinogen is certainly a plausible theory but no compound from these individuals has been identified which is known to be carcinogenic.[8] The liver could, of course, be responding to the physical problem of glycogen and fat-laden cells which may not function normally.[5] An attractive hypothesis is the theory that the chronic state of hyperglucagonemia and suppressed insulin levels may induce malignancy.[9] A hormonal influence on tumor formation is documented. The development of hepatocellular carcinoma in adolescents is exceedingly rare. The fact that GSD type Ia affected patients develop hepatoma without cirrhosis occuring would point to a malignant propensity with this genetic metabolic defect.[9]

A case was reported recently of a patient with type Ib G-6-Pase deficiency who developed myelogenous leukemia.[10] Type Ib patients are known to have abnormalities of the granulocytes. The occurence of myelogenous leukemia in a type Ib patient is suggestive of a malignancy predisposing metabolic condition caused by G-6-Pase deficiency. This, however, could be only a chance occurrence.

The reports of several patients with hepatic carcinoma in the very rare glucose-6-phosphatase glycogen storage disease clearly indicates an increased incidence of hepatic carcinoma in this situation.

B. β-Glucocerebrosidase Deficiency

β-Glucocerebrosidase deficiency, also known as Gaucher's disease, is inherited as an autosomal recessive trait.[11] The abnormal storage of glucocerebroside(s) is primarily within the recticuloendothelial system. The enzymatic deficiency results in a clinical picture of hepatosplenomegaly, hypersplenism, and osteoportic erosion of the long bones, hip joints, and vertebrae. Several clinical presentations of the disorder have been delineated. Type 1 is the chronic adult nonneuronopathic form. Type 2 is the acute neuronopathic or infantile form. Type 3 is the subacute neuronopathic or juvenile form. All three types have subnormal β-glucocerebrosidase activity.

Several patients with Type 1 β-glucocerebrosidase deficiency have developed malignancy.[12,13] The lymphatic system is the location of most of these reported malignancies, diagnosed as chronic lymphocytic leukemia or Hodgkin's disease. The cells are seen to store large amounts of β-glucocerebroside in the lysosome which results in physical crowding by the engorged cells which could restrict blood flow.[11]

Gery et al.[14] have found that macrophages respond to the intake of toxic compounds by increased release of lysosomal hydrolases, fibroblast-stimulating factors, cytolytic factors, and lymphocyte-activating factors. Bradfield and Souhami[15] noted that blockage of macrophage function by stored materials leads to hepatocyte damage, cirrhosis, and therefore increased levels of circulating toxins to be handled by the macrophage. This chronic stimulation of the immune system by internal glucocerebroside accumulation and external stimulation by toxins, hydrolases, and factors may lead to macrophage proliferation. The same phenomenon is occuring with B-cell storage, which could result in B-cell proliferation or the interruption of B-cell development and maturation.[16,17] These mechanisms, individually or in concert, could be causing the malignant transformation.

A tumor of the right tibia has been reported in a Japanese patient with Gaucher's disease.[18] The bone marrow was found to be replaced by Gaucher's cells which lead progressively to atrophy and ischemic necrosis. The insult of β-glucocerebroside accumulation could possibly be seen to cause a malignant response, directly or indirectly.

C. Galactosemia

Galactosemia due to galactose-1-phosphate uridyl transferase deficiency is inherited as an autosomal recessive trait.[19] Hepatosplenomegaly, liver disease, malnutrition, mental retardation, and cataracts are the clinical features seen early in an affected child. Treatment by the removal of milk and milk products from the diet results in significant clinical improvement and usually normal development. This autosomal recessive trait has an incidence of approximately 1:60,000 in the general U.S. population.

Much research has been carried out to identify the compound which is toxic in galactosemia patients.[20] Increased intracellular levels of galactose (and particularly galactose phosphate) contribute largely to the galactose toxicity. Even on a galactose-free diet, the body synthesizes necessary galactose. This could produce a continuous "self-intoxication" of the tissues with the toxic metabolite.[21] Cirrhosis is found even in some patients diagnosed and treated early. One case of hepatic adenoma has been reported.[22] The patient's liver was cirrhotic and contained numerous small nodules. The malignancy seen here could well be the type recognized frequently in the livers of patients with cirrhosis from any cause.

D. α-1-Antitrypsin Deficiency

α-1-Antritrypsin deficiency is an abnormality of a serum regulatory protein ordinarily secreted from the hepatocyte.[23] α-1-Antitrypsin is an inhibitor of several serine proteases and is thereby protective of lung, liver, and skeletal joint tissues. The predominant allele for this single polypeptide chain protein is designated M. Individuals who are homozygous or heterozygous are phenotypically normal. Rare individuals who have approximately 50% of normal serum α-1-antitrypsin levels, or less, may experience clinical symptoms of α-1-antitrypsin deficiency. The abnormal genotypes include SS, SZ, and ZZ, with the ZZ individual having approximately 12% of normal serum α-1-antitrypsin. A very rare null allele has been recognized which produces no product.

Complications of α-1-antitrypsin deficiency include destructive lung disease, joint disease, and hemorrhagic episodes. In addition to PAS-positive granules being formed in the hepatocyte, several hepatic complications usually appear in affected individuals, including cholestasis, bile duct proliferation, and fibrosis of the portal system, resulting in cirrhosis in approximately 10% of affected individuals.

This genetic disease is manifested in Z homozygous individuals, but clinical disease is sometimes seen in heterozygotes.[23] A study in 1979 found primary hepatic carcinoma in association with α-1-antitrypsin positive intracellular globules in 18% of a series of patients.[24] This was in comparison to an unselected series of autopsies where the incidence of PAS-positive globules was 6%. Cirrhosis is not always correlated with hepatic carcinoma in α-1-antitrypsin-deficient individuals. Schleissner and Cohen[25] report such a case and suggest that α-1-antitrypsin deficiency may be causative of hepatic carcinoma by a mechanism not related to cirrhotic damage of the liver.[25]

A study of α-1-antitrypsin-deficient patients from Sweden found an extraordinary 23% to have hepatic carcinoma; 75% of individuals with α-1-antitrypsin deficiency and who also had cirrhosis, had malignancy of the liver.[26] These authors feel that cirrhosis in association with α-1-antitrypsin deficiency should be considered a precancerous condition. These investigators hypothesize that the accumulation of PAS-positive bodies within the hepatocytes predispose them to injury by continuous hypoxia or constant exposure to other (toxic) factors which the hepatocytes are unable to overcome.

E. Hereditary Tyrosinemia

Hereditary tyrosinemia is an autosomal recessive trait which presents with failure to thrive, fever, edema, vomiting and diarrhea, and hepatomegaly. If untreated with dietary restriction of tyrosine, death usually occurs by 6 to 8 months of age.[27] Fumarylacetoacetate hydrolase is the enzyme most likely deficient in affected individuals, although this is not clear and other enzymes have been found to have low activity in patients.

If affected children survive to age 2 years, they then face a 30 to 40% risk of developing hepatic malignancy.[28] Virtually all patients are found to have cirrhosis of the liver. Of affected patients, 30 to 40% develop hepatocarcinoma, an uncommon tumor in children. Hepatocarcinoma, much more common in adults, has an incidence of only 4% in adults who die with cirrhosis. This clearly suggests that cirrhosis is certainly not the sole causative factor inducing malignancy in children affected with tyrosinemia.[29] One could hypothesize about a toxic compound(s) not being properly metabolized by these children, which could first produce cirrhosis and then hepatocarcinoma. This sequence could be considered a vicious cycle leading to malignancy.

F. Xeroderma Pigmentosum

Xeroderma pigmentosum (XP) is a recessively inherited disease which involves the DNA of the cell directly.[30] UV light overlaps the absorption spectra of nucleic acids and proteins. The absorption of the UV energy by these molecules results in their alteration. Most UV damage is repaired by normal tissue whereas XP patients are unable to repair specific damage to their DNA due to a genetic defect in a repair enzyme. Affected individuals experience severe photosensitivity with a high incidence of skin cancer. These malignancies include basal cell carcinoma, squamous cell carcinoma, and malignant melanoma.[31]

Adjacent thymine bases may form dimers when excited by UV energy. Normal repair involves the excision of the dimer and replacement of the excised bases. Xeroderma patients are unable to carry out this multistep process.[32] Patients can be divided into at least seven complementation groups based upon the ability to repair DNA containing thymine dimers subsequent to cell fusion of patient cells from different familial groups.[32]

Several hypotheses have been proffered to explain the etiology of malignancy in XP. Unexcised thymine dimers may be directly involved in carcinogenesis but more likely they play an indirect role.[33,34] Robbins et al. noticed an increase in the number of sister chromatid exchanges in XP cell lines, secondary to thymine dimer production.[35] Sister chromatid exchanges are known to be an indication of chromosome stability and their increased frequency has been implicated as a risk factor for malignancy. Another secondary effect is the damage to the immunologic system from UV irradiation.[33] This damage, in conjunction with or in addition to thymine dimer formation, could lead to a protracted ability of the body to recognize and eliminate newly transformed cells.

G. α-L-Iduronidase Deficiency

An animal model of α-L-iduronidase deficiency (mucopolysaccharidosis type I, also Hurler Syndrome or Hurler-Scheie Syndrome) in cats is informative for the human condition. The clinical presentation in the cat is very similar to that in man. Haskins and McGrath[36] have reported on the necropsy of seven young cats with α-L-iduronidase deficiency. Four were found to have meningiomas while the leptomeninges appeared abnormal and included nodules in the remaining three cats. The physical location of the lesions was very similar in all four animals. The investigators could not report a clear relationship between α-L-iduronidase deficiency and meningiomas. They did find interesting the occurrence of meningiomas in young cats with α-L-iduronidase deficiency and wondered about a common etiology or predisposition for malignancy with this enzyme deficiency.

Malignancies have not been reported in humans with α-L-iduronidase deficiency at this time. The long-term survivors should be carefully watched.

III. SUMMARY

The basic mechanisms leading to malignancy in the genetic metabolic defects discussed in this chapter are for the most part not known. The idea that physical cell damage, such as cell engorgement with stored material, subsequent cell crowding, hypoxia, and cell damage, as a cause of malignancy, is probably simplistic. The altered repair process(es) (such as in XP) may be a more logical area of investigation, based upon our knowledge that cancer is an altered condition of cell growth. This would also apply to organ damage, i.e., liver cirrhosis.

The concept that a toxic compound(s) which is formed, stored, released, or not properly metabolized may cause malignancy is an attractive one. The recognized serious aberrations in hormonal balance in the glycogen storage diseases are certainly causes of abnormal cellular proliferation. External environmental compounds are known to cause cell transformation. Therefore, internally synthesized molecules which are harmful could also lead to malignancy by a variety of mechanisms, including disruption of metabolic pathways, interference with the genome, and altered cell repair.

The complexity of the immune system has recently become apparent. Recognition of self and not-self is vital to survival of the organism. Perturbation of the immune system could lead to altered growth of a cell clone which was not recognized as abnormal. Transformation could occur and not be recognized. The underlying process of cell growth and differentiation (the cell cycle) is susceptible to alteration. The immune system is a vital component of homeostasis in the organism and is correctly receiving intensive scrutiny as to its normal and abnormal functioning.

Direct changing of cell function by altering the genome is not fully appreciated. What are the pathways for maintenance and repair of the DNA? How does the genome check the validity of itself? It is easy to see how change at the DNA level can lead to cell metabolism changes which could lead to cell transformation.

Advances have been recently made by Tsuji et al.[37] in the cloning and analysis of the defective gene believed to be etiologic for Gaucher's disease. Beaudet[38] has discussed therapies for Gaucher's disease. This primarily involves enzyme replacement. The important problems which are associated with these particular therapeutic approaches were discussed.

Lev and Sundaram[39] discuss the use of a specific inhibitor of cerebroside synthesis for Gaucher's disease. This therapy is a logical approach in that cerebrosides and glucocerebrosides accumulate in the brain, spleen, liver, and bone marrow in patients with Gaucher's disease. The anatomic site of accumulation is dependent upon the particular type of Gaucher's disease.[11] Thus, given this background, it is clear that genetically induced metabolic changes occur in this disorder which are steadily being elucidated through molecular analyses. Treatment and prevention are dependent upon these laboratory epidemiology and molecular biology technologies. The ultimate achievement one day may involve gene replacement.

Children with inherited metabolic defects have often died early of acute illness. A growing number of these children are living longer with the medical care of today. The illustrations in this chapter would indicate that at least some genetic metabolic defects predispose or precipitate malignancy. Therefore, the longer these children survive, the greater their risk of developing cancer. Do other genetic metabolic defects carry this same type of risk for cancer development? Further investigation and time will tell.

From another point of view, what percentage of childhood-young adult malignancy is the result of a genetic defect(s)? The percentage could certainly be higher than that recognized today. Children who develop malignancy may be carrying an unrecognized metabolic defect. This is perhaps an unexplored area for genetic research.

REFERENCES

1. **Garrod, A. E.,** Inborn errors of metabolism (Croonian Lectures), *Lancet,* 2, 214, 1908.
2. **Stevenson, R. E., Ben-Menachem, Y., Dudrick, S., and Howell, R. R.,** Hepatocellular carcinoma in Type I glycogen storage disease, *Proc. Greenwood Genet. Cent.,* 3, 39, 1984.
3. **Cori, G. T. and Cori, C. F.,** Glucose-6-phosphatase of the liver in glycogen storage disease, *J. Biol. Chem.,* 199, 661, 1952.
4. **Narisawa, K., Igarashi, Y., Otomo, H., and Tada, K.,** A new variant of glycogen storage disease type 1 probably due to a defect in the glucose-6-phosphatase transport system, *Biochem. Biophys. Res. Commun.,* 83, 1360, 1978.
5. **Howell, R. R., Stevenson, R. E., Ben-Menachem, Y., Philiky, R. L., and Berry, D. H.,** Hepatic adenomata with type 1 glycogen storage disease, *JAMA,* 236, 1481, 1976.
6. **Miller, J. H., Gates, G. F., Landing, B. H., Kogut, M. D., and Roe, T. F.,** Scintigraphic abnormalities in glycogen storage disease, *J. Nucl. Med.,* 19, 354, 1978.
7. **Parker, P., Burr, I., Slonim, A., Ghishan, F. K., and Greene, H.,** Regression of hepatic adenomas in Type Ia glycogen storage disease with dietary therapy, *Gastroenterology,* 81, 534, 1981.
8. **Zangeneh, F., Limbeck, G. A., Brown, B. I., Emch, J. R., Arcasoy, M. M., Goldenberg, V. E., and Kelley, V. C.,** Hepatorenal glycogenosis (Type I glycogenosis) and carcinoma of the liver, *J. Pediatr.,* 74, 73, 1969.
9. **Fink, A. S., Appelman, H. D., and Thompson, N. W.,** Hemorrhage into a hepatic adenoma and Type Ia glycogen storage disease: a case report and review of the literature, *Surgery,* 91, 117, 1985.
10. **Simmons, P. S., Smithson, W. A., Gronert, G. A., and Haymond, M. W.,** Acute myelogenous leukemia and malignant hyperthermia in a patient with Type Ib glycogen storage disease, *J. Pediatr.,* 105, 428, 1984.

11. **Brady, R. O. and Barranger, J. A.,** Glucosylceramide lipidoses: Gaucher's disease, in *The Metabolic Basis of Inherited Disease,* 5th ed., Stanbury, J. B., Wyngaarden, J. B., Fredrickson, D. S., Goldstein, J. L., and Brown, M. S., Eds., McGraw-Hill, New York, 1983, 842.
12. **Bruckstein, A. H., Karanas, A., and Dire, J. J.,** Gaucher's disease associated with Hodgkin's disease, *Am. J. Med.,* 68, 610, 1980.
13. **Krause, J. R., Bures, C., and Lee, R. E.,** Acute leukaemia and Gaucher's disease, *Scand. J. Haematol.,* 23, 115, 1979.
14. **Gery, I., Zigler, J. S., Jr., Brady, R. O., and Barranger, J. A.,** Selective effects of glucocerebroside (Gaucher's storage material) on macrophage cultures, *J. Clin. Invest.,* 68, 1182, 1981.
15. **Bradfield, J. W. B. and Souhami, R. L.,** Hepatocyte damage secondary to Kupffer cell phagocytosis, in *The Reticuloendothelial System and the Pathogenesis of Liver Disease,* Liehr, H. and Grun, M., Eds., Elsevier, New York, 1980, 165.
16. **Fox, H., McCarthy, P., Andre-Schwartz, J., Shoenfeld, Y., and Miller, K. B.,** Gaucher's disease and chronic lymphocytic leukemia, *Cancer,* 54, 312, 1984.
17. **Schoenfeld, Y., Gallant, L. A., Shaklai, M., Livni, E., Djaldetti, M., and Pinkhas, J.,** Gaucher's disease: a disease with chronic stimulation of the immune system, *Arch. Pathol. Lab. Med.,* 106, 338, 1982.
18. **Wantanabe, M., Yanagisawa, M., Sonobe, S., Matsumoto, J., and Miura, H.,** An adult form of Gaucher's disease with a huge tumour formation of the right tibia, *Int. Orthopaed.,* 8, 195, 1984.
19. **Segal, S.,** Disorders of galactose metabolism, in *The Metabolic Basis of Inherited Disease,* 5th ed., Stanbury, J. B., Wyngaarden, J. B., Fredrickson, D. S., Goldstein, J. L., and Brown, M. S., Eds., McGraw-Hill, New York, 1983, 167.
20. **Gitzelmann, R. and Hansen, R. G.,** Galactose metabolism, hereditary defects and their clinical significance, in *Inherited Disorders of Carbohydrate Metabolism,* Burman, D., Holton, J. B., and Pennock, C. A., Eds., MTP Press, Lancaster, England, 1980, 61.
21. **Smetana, H. F. and Olen, E.,** Hereditary galactose disease, *Am. J. Clin. Pathol.,* 38, 3, 1962.
22. **Edmonds, A. M., Hennigar, G. R., and Crooks, R.,** Galactosemia: report of case with autopsy, *Pediatrics,* 10, 40, 1952.
23. **Gadek, J. E. and Crystal, R. G.,** Alpha-1-antitrypsin deficiency, in *The Metabolic Basis of Inherited Disease,* 5th ed., Stanbury, J. B., Wyngaarden, J. B., Fredrickson, D. S., Goldstein, J. L., and Brown, M. S., Eds., McGraw-Hill, New York, 1983, 1450.
24. **Reintoft, I. and Hagerstrand, I. E.,** Does the Z gene variant of alpha-1-antitrypsin predispose to hepatic carcinoma?, *Hum. Pathol.,* 10, 419, 1979.
25. **Schleissner, L. A. and Cohen, A. H.,** Alpha-1-antitrypsin deficiency and hepatic carcinoma, *Am. Rev. Respir. Dis.,* 111, 863, 1975.
26. **Eriksson, S. and Hagerstrand, I.,** Cirrhosis and malignant hepatoma in α-1-antitrypsin deficiency, *Acta Med. Scand.,* 195, 451, 1974.
27. **Goldsmith, L. A.,** Tyrosinemia and related disorders, in *The Metabolic Basis of Inherited Disease,* 5th ed., Stanbury, J. B., Wyngaarden, J. B., Fredrickson, D. S., Goldstein, J. L., and Brown, M. S., Eds., McGraw-Hill, New York, 1983, 287.
28. **Weinberg, A. G., Mize, C. E., and Worthen, H. G.,** The occurrence of hepatoma in the chronic form of hereditary tyrosinemia, *J. Pediatr.,* 88, 434, 1976.
29. **Fisch, R. O., McCabe, E. R. B., Doeden, D., Koep, L. J., Kohlhoff, J. G., Silverman, A., and Starzl, T. E.,** Homotransplantation of the liver in a patient with hepatoma and hereditary tyrosinemia, *J. Pediatr.,* 93, 592, 1978.
30. **Cleaver, J. E.,** Xeroderma pigmentosum, in *The Metabolic Basis of Inherited Disease,* 5th ed., Stanbury, J. B., Wyngaarden, J. B., Fredrickson, D. S., Goldstein, J. L., and Brown, M. S., Eds., McGraw-Hill, New York, 1983, 1227.
31. **Robbins, J. H., Kraemer, K. H., Lutzner, M. A., Festoff, B. W., and Coon, H. G.,** Xeroderma pigmentosum: an inherited disease with sun sensitivity, multiple cutaneous neoplasms, and abnormal DNA repair, *Ann. Intern. Med.,* 80, 221, 1974.
32. **Kripke, M., Urback, F., and Witkop, C.,** Ultraviolet radiation carcinogenesis, in *Biology of Skin Cancer,* Laerum, O. D. and Iversen, O. H., Eds., International Union Against Cancer, Geneva, 1981, chap. 6.
33. **Epstein, W. L., Fukuyama, K., and Epstein, J. H.,** UV light, DNA repair and skin carcinogenesis in man, *Fed. Proc. Fed. Am. Soc. Exp. Biol.,* 30, 1766, 1971.
34. **Zajdela, F. and Latarjet, R.,** Inhibition of skin carcinogenesis *in vivo* by caffeine and other agents, *Natl. Cancer Inst. Monogr.,* 50, 133, 1978.
35. **Robbins, J. H.,** Significance of repair of human DNA: evidence from studies of xeroderma pigmentosium, *J. Natl. Cancer Inst.,* 61, 645, 1978.
36. **Haskins, M. E. and McGrath, J. T.,** Meningiomas in young cats with Mucopolysaccharidosis. I, *J. Neuropathol. Exp. Neurol.,* 42, 664, 1983.

37. **Tsuji, S., Choudary, P. V., Martin, B. M., et al.,** A mutation in the human glucocerebrosidase gene in neutropathic Gaucher's disease, *N. Engl. J. Med.*, 316, 570, 1987.
38. **Beaudet, A. L.,** Gaucher's disease, *N. Engl. J. Med.*, 316, 619, 1987.
39. **Lev, M. and Sundaram, K. S.,** Gaucher's disease, *N. Engl. J. Med.*, 317, 572, 1987.

Chapter 7

FAMILY HISTORY IN CHILDHOOD MALIGNANCIES WITH SPECIAL REFERENCE TO GENETIC-ENVIRONMENTAL INERACTION

Takeshi Hirayama

TABLE OF CONTENTS

I. INTRODUCTION

Certain types of childhood malignancies such as retinoblastoma are known to be etiologically linked to primary genetic factors. In order to determine whether or not such a relationship could be observed for each type of childhood cancer, a comprehensive check of familial history was attempted using records of the National Childhood Malignancies Registry in Japan.

II. MATERIALS AND METHODS

During the period of 1966 to 1982 in Japan, 16,555 cases of childhood malignancies were registered. This is the largest registry of the disease in the world involving practically all major hospitals, medical institutes, and clinics in the country. Standardized registry cards were used which included information regarding key risk factors such as family history, prenatal and postnatal exposure to radiation, maternal age, weight at birth, congenital anomalies, and medical history.[1]

Major focus of attention was given to the collection of family history of cancer through second-degree relatives (grandparents, aunts, uncles). Out of 16,555 cases of childhood malignancies registered, 2926 cases or 17.7% showed a family history of cancer of any site. Expected frequency was calculated from the proportion with a family history of cancer of each site in the 2926 cases of all types of childhood malignancies with cancer family histories. Details by anatomic site are presented in Section III.

III. RESULTS

A. Leukemia

Of the cases who had leukemia, a family history of cancer was observed in 1355 cases. Cases with a family history of leukemia were significantly higher than expected (121 vs. 80.6, $X^2 = 20.25$). Histories of no other malignancies were found in excess (Table 1).

B. Malignant Lymphoma

Out of 286 cases with positive cancer family histories, the following 2 types of cancer were observed in excess: cancer of the esophagus — observed 17 vs. expected 9.0, $X^2 = 7.11$ and malignant lymphoma — observed 7 vs. expected 3.1, $X^2 = 4.91$) (Table 1).

C. Brain Tumors

Out of 168 positive cancer family histories, only the history of brain tumor was in excess (observed 8 vs. expected 3.6, $X^2 = 5.38$) (Table 1).

D. Neuroblastoma

Out of 271 cases with positive cancer family history, histories of the following two types of cancer were in excess: cancer of the larynx — observed 11 vs. expected 3.2, $X^2 = 19.01$ and neuroblastoma — observed 3 vs. expected 0.06, $X^2 = 9.60$) (Table 1).

E. Retinoblastoma

Out of 260 cases with positive cancer family history, only history of retinoblastoma showed an excess (observed 68 vs. expected 6.3, $X^2 = 604.27$) (Table 1).

F. Wilms' Tumor

Out of 142 cases with positive cancer family history, only history of rectal cancer was observed in excess (observed 11 vs. expected 5.1, $X^2 = 6.83$) (Table 1).

Table 1
CANCER FAMILY HISTORY AND CHILDHOOD MALIGNANCIES

Type	Leukemia		Malignant		Brain		Neuro-		Retino-		Wilms		Others		Total
Cancer			lymphoma		tumor		blastoma		blastoma		tumor				
family history of	O	E	O	E	O	E	O	E	O	E	O	E	O	E	O
Oral, pharynx	4	5.6	4	1.2	2	0.7		1.1		1.1	1	0.6	1	1.8	12
Tongue	5	4.2	2	0.9		0.5		0.8		0.8		0.4	2	1.4	9
Esophagus	31	42.6	17	9.0	9	5.3	7	8.5	7	8.2	6	4.5	15	14.0	92
Stomach	489	462.2	91	97.5	68	57.3	84	92.4	76	88.7	40	48.4	150	151.4	998
Intestine	22	24.1	7	5.1	3	3.0	6	4.8	5	4.7	3	2.5	6	7.9	52
Rectum	45	49.1	9	10.4	3	6.1	12	9.8	6	9.4	11	5.1	20	16.1	106
Bile duct	6	8.8	1	1.9	3	1.1	1	1.8	3	1.7	1	0.9	4	2.9	19
Liver	82	79.7	18	16.8	12	9.9	17	15.9	10	15.3	9	8.3	24	26.1	172
Pancreas	31	30.6	8	6.5	6	3.8	5	6.1	3	5.9	3	3.2	10	10.0	66
Peritoneum	2	3.7		0.8	1	0.5	2	0.7	1	0.7	1	0.4	1	1.2	8
Nose		0.5		0.1		0.1	1	0.1		0.1		0.0		0.2	1
Parotic gland	1	0.5		0.1		0.1		0.1		0.1		0.0		0.2	1
Larynx	11	16.2	4	3.4	1	2.0	11	3.2	1	3.1	2	1.7	5	5.3	35
Maxilla	12	6.9	2	1.5		0.9		1.4		1.3		0.7	1	2.3	15
Axilla	2	0.9		0.2		0.1		0.2		0.2		0.1		0.3	2
Lung	95	92.6	16	19.5	15	11.5	14	18.5	12	17.8	10	9.7	38	30.3	200
Pleura		0.5		0.1		0.1		0.1		0.1		0.0	1	0.2	1
Breast	52	61.6	19	13.0	7	7.6	14	12.3	13	11.6	5	6.5	23	20.2	133
Uterus	104	100.5	18	21.2	9	12.5	24	20.1	15	19.3	9	10.5	38	32.9	217
Ovary	18	19.4	6	4.1	3	2.4	2	3.9	3	3.7	1	2.0	9	6.4	42
Prostate	6	4.2		0.9		0.5	1	0.8		0.8		0.4	2	1.4	9
Testis	1	2.3	1	0.5		0.3	2	0.5		0.4		0.2	1	0.8	5
Kidney	6	7.4	3	1.6	1	0.9	1	1.5	1	1.4	2	0.8	2	2.4	16
Bladder	9	12.0	6	2.5	1	1.5	3	2.4	2	2.3	2	1.3	3	3.9	26
Skin	6	5.1	1	1.1		0.6	1	1.0		1.0	3	0.5		1.7	11
Thyroid	7	9.3	4	2.0		1.1	5	1.9		1.8	3	1.0	1	3.0	20
Retinoblastoma	2	32.9		6.9		4.1	1	6.6	68	6.3		3.4		10.8	71
Brain	27	29.2	8	5.2	8	3.6	7	5.8	4	5.6	4	3.1	5	9.6	63
Bone	15	10.2		2.2	2	1.3	2	2.0	2	2.0		1.1	1	3.3	22
Lymphoma	15	14.8	7	3.1		1.8	1	3.0		2.8	2	1.6	7	4.9	32
Neuroblastoma	1	3.2		0.7		0.4	3	0.6		0.6		0.3	3	1.1	7
Hodgkin's	1	1.4		0.3		0.2		0.3		0.3		0.1	2	0.5	3
Reticulo. sarcoma	9	13.0	2	2.7	3	1.6	4	2.6	4	2.5		1.4	6	4.2	28
Fibroma	4	1.9		0.4		0.2		0.4		0.4		0.2		0.6	4
Endothelioma	2	1.4		0.3		0.2	1	0.3		0.3		0.1		0.5	3
Leukemia	121	80.6	16	17.0	4	1.0	9	16.1	8	15.5	4	8.4	12	26.4	174
Others	111	116.2	16	24.5	7	14.4	30	23.2	16	22.3	20	12.2	51	38.1	251
Total	1,355		286		168		271		260		142		444		2,926

Note: O = observed; E = expected.

Material derived from the National Childhood Malignancy Registry, 1969 to 1982.

G. Other Childhood Malignancies

With regard to family history of cancer of any type, no significant association was observed for other childhood malignancies (Table 1).

In summary, family history of malignancies of the same site or same type was observed in excess of leukemia, malignant lymphoma, brain tumor, neuroblastoma, and retinoblastoma. It is also of importance to note the family history of esophageal cancer was found in excess of the cases of malignant lymphoma and family history of rectal cancer was observed in excess of the cases of Wilms' tumor.

Table 2
CANCER FAMILY HISTORY AND CHILDHOOD LEUKEMIA BY CELL TYPE

	Acute Myeloid Leukemia		Acute Lymphatic Leukemia		Others		Total
	O	E	O	E	O	E	
Oral, pharynx	2	1.5	2	3.0		1.0	4
Tongue		1.1	3	2.3	2	0.8	5
Esophagus	15	11.6	8	23.3	8	7.8	31
Stomach	135	125.5	254	252.4	100	84.2	489
Intestine	6	6.6	13	13.2	3	4.4	22
Rectum	11	13.3	24	26.8	10	8.9	45
Bile duct	1	2.4	4	4.8	1	1.6	6
Liver	21	21.6	47	43.5	14	14.5	82
Pancreas	3	8.3	24	16.7	4	5.6	31
Peritoneum	1	1.0	1	2.0		0.7	2
Nose		0.1		0.3		0.1	
Parotic gland		0.1	1	0.3		0.1	1
Larynx	4	4.4	5	8.9	2	3.0	11
Maxilla		1.9	8	3.8	4	1.3	12
Axilla	1	0.3	1	0.5		0.2	2
Lung	24	25.2	52	50.6	19	16.9	95
Pleura		0.1		0.3		0.1	
Breast	14	16.7	30	33.6	8	11.2	52
Uterus	25	27.3	65	54.9	14	18.3	104
Ovary	2	5.3	13	10.6	3	3.5	18
Prostate		1.1	6	2.3		0.8	6
Testis		0.6		1.3	1	0.4	1
Kidney		2.0	5	4.0	1	1.4	6
Bladder	8	3.3		6.6	1	2.2	9
Skin	1	1.4	2	2.8	3	0.9	6
Thyroid	1	2.5	6	5.1		1.7	7
Retinoblastoma		8.9	1	18.0	1	6.0	2
Brain	8	7.9	15	15.9	4	5.3	27
Bone	7	2.8	7	5.6	1	1.9	15
Lymphoma	5	4.0	9	8.1	1	2.7	15
Neuroblastoma		0.9	1	1.8		0.6	1
Hodgkin's		0.4	1	0.8		0.3	1
Reticulo. sarcoma	2	3.5	6	7.1	1	2.4	9
Fibroma	1	0.5	3	1.0		0.3	4
Endothelioma		0.4	2	0.8		0.3	2
Leukemia	45	21.9	57	44.0	19	14.7	121
Others	25	31.6	64	63.5	22	21.2	111
Total	368		740		247		1,355

Note: O = observed; E = expected.

Material derived from the National Childhood Malignancy Registry, 1969 to 1982.

H. Cancer Family History in Leukemia by Cell Types

In acute lymphatic leukemia, out of 740 cases with positive cancer family histories, the family history of leukemia was observed in 57 cases when only 44 cases were expected, observed/expected (OE) ratio being 1.30 ($X^2 = 3.84$) (Table 2). In acute myeloid leukemia, out of 368 cases with cancer family history, leukemia family history was noted in 45 cases when only 21.9 cases were expected, OE ratio being 2.05 ($X^2 = 24.37$) (Table 2).

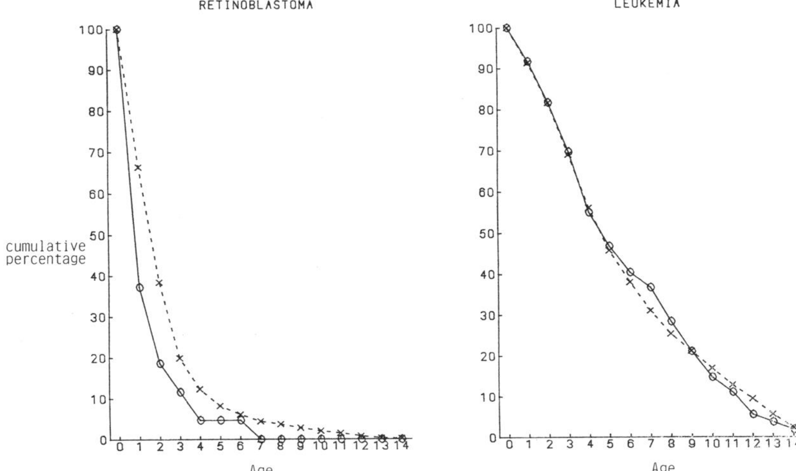

FIGURE 1. Cumulative age distribution for retinoblastoma and leukemia. Solid line = cases with family history of the same disease and dotted line = total cases.

In other childhood leukemias, out of 247 cases with cancer family history, leukemia family history was observed in 19 cases when 14.7 cases were expected, OE ratio being 1.29 (X^2 = 1.26, not significant) (Table 2). In short, association with family history of leukemia was most striking in acute myeloid leukemia.

I. Age at First Diagnosis and Cancer Family History

As shown in Figure 1, earlier age at first diagnosis was observed in cases with family history of the same site for retinoblastoma, median age being 11 months earlier (8 months of age for cases with family history vs. 1 year and 7 months for total cases). No difference in age at first diagnosis was observed for leukemia cases with positive leukemia family history and for total cases, median age for both being 4 years and 7 months (Figure 1). Similar relationships were observed for cases of malignant lymphoma — 8 years, 3 months for those with a positive family history vs. 8 years, 5 months for total cases. Age at first diagnosis of brain tumors for cases of brain tumors was 8 years of age for cases with positive family histories vs. 6 years and 9 months for total cases.

J. Genetic-Environmental Interaction in Childhood Leukemia

Family history of leukemia and history of exposure to prenatal radiation were compared between childhood leukemia cases (male 4233, female 3268) and controls (other childhood malignancies — male 4607, female 4447). Compared to children with neither factor, the relative risk for those with a history of prenatal radiation exposure was only 1.50 (1.38 to 1.63) and that for those with leukemia family history was only 2.87 (2.16 to 3.82). When both factors exist, the relative risk was 4.69 (2.19 to 10.03) (see Figure 2). Mantel-Haenszel X^2 values were 77.74, 37.11, and 11.14 respectively, all being significant at the 0.1% level.

The mode of interaction of leukemia family history and history of exposure to prenatal radiation appears to be multiplicative rather than additive (observed relative risk = 4.69. Expected by additive model — 0.50 + 1.87 = 3.37; expected by multiplicative model — 1.50 × 2.87 = 4.31).

IV. DISCUSSION

It was impressive that only family history of malignancy of the same type was observed with statistical significance in the National Childhood Malignancy Registry in Japan (1969

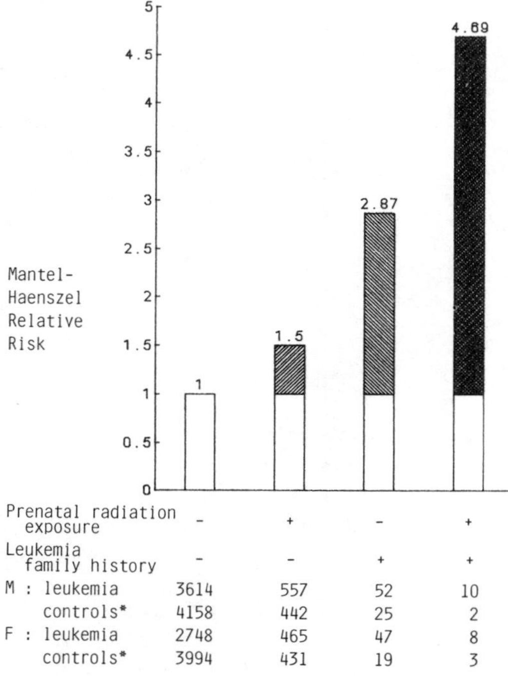

FIGURE 2. Relative risk of childhood leukemia by presence or absence of prenatal radiation exposure and by presence or absence of leukemia family history. From the National Childhood Malignancy Registry, 1969 to 1982.

to 1982). This clearly indicates that genetic predisposition is cell type specific, which is in accord with many of the reports in the literature.[2]

Among 209 patients with leukemia, 17 or 8.1% were found to have at least one leukemia relative.[3] In the current study among 1355 patients with leukemia, 121 or 8.9% were found with a positive leukemia family history. Regarding cell type, the likelihood of having a genetic origin was considered to be stronger for cases of CLL than for cases of other variants.[4] However, in the current study association with leukemia, a positive family history was most striking in AML.

Regarding retinoblastoma, there are numerous reports on its familial aggregation and, based on such observation, Knudson[5] formulated the two mutation hypothesis. The average interval of age at onset among cases with or without a positive family history in the literature is 11 months, which also corresponds to the median age observed in the current study. Knudson's hypothesis was extended to Wilms' tumor[6] and neuroblastoma.[7] In the current study, a significant familial aggregation was also observed for neuroblastoma. However, no such familial aggregation was observed for Wilms' tumor.

With regard to brain tumors, a ninefold increase over expected was reported in the incidence of CNS tumors in sibs.[8] A significant, more than twofold increase over expected was noted in the current study.

Both malignant lymphoma and cancer of the esophagus are known to occur with high frequency in cases with immunological disorders. In the current study, an excess incidence of esophageal cancer was observed in the family members of malignant lymphoma affected in addition to the excess of malignant lymphoma family history.

Regarding interaction of leukemia family history and prenatal radiation exposure, reports are limited in the literature. The mode of interaction was observed to be multiplicative rather than additive. This must be of importance in considering the mechanisms underlying the possible genetic-environmental interaction.

It was also of interest to note that the relative risk of leukemia in cases with a history of prenatal radiation exposure is similar to the relative risk reported in the literature.[9]

V. SUMMARY

Association with family history of cancer of each site was examined for each type of childhood malignancy using data from the National Childhood Malignancy Registry in Japan (n = 16,555). There were 2926 cases identified with positive cancer family history. Family history of same type malignancy was found significantly in excess for leukemia, malignant lymphoma, brain tumor, neuroblastoma, and retinoblastoma. When observed by cell type, association with family history of leukemia was most striking in acute myeloid leukemia. Median age at first diagnosis of retinoblastoma was 11 months earlier when family history of retinoblastoma existed.

Family history of leukemia and history of exposure to prenatal radiation exposure were found to enhance relative risk for childhood leukemia when combined, suggesting the existence of genetic-environmental interaction. Mode of interaction was interpreted as multiplicative.

These observations must be of importance, both for etiological studies and for consideration of strategies, for prevention of childhood malignancies.

REFERENCES

1. **Hirayama, T.,** Descriptive and analytical epidemiology of childhood malignancy in Japan, in *Recent Advances in Management of Children with Cancer,* Proc. Int. Symp. Children's Cancer, Tokyo, 1979, The Children's Cancer Association of Japan, Tokyo, 1980, 27.
2. **Stewart, A. and Barber, R.,** The epidemiological importance of childhood cancers, *Br. Med. Bull.,* 27, 64, 1971.
3. **Videbaek, A.,** Familial leukemia: a preliminary report, *Acta Med. Scand.,* 127, 26, 1947.
4. **Heath, C. W.,** Hereditary factors in leukemia and lymphoma, in *Cancer Genetics,* Lynch, H. T., Ed., Charles C Thomas, Springfield, IL, 1976, 233.
5. **Knudson, A. G.,** Mutation and cancer: statistical study of retinoblastoma, *Proc. Natl. Acad. Sci. U.S.A.,* 68, 820, 1971.
6. **Knudson, A. G. and Strong, L. C.,** Mutation and cancer: a model for Wilms' tumor of the kidney, *J. Natl. Cancer Inst.,* 48, 313, 1972.
7. **Knudson, A. G. and Strong, L. C.,** Mutation and cancer: neuroblastoma and pheochromocytoma, *Am. J. Hum. Genet.,* 24, 514, 1972.
8. **Miller, R. W.,** Deaths from childhood cancer in sibs, *N. Engl. J. Med.,* 279, 122, 1968.
9. **Graham, S., Levin, M. L., Lilienfeld, A. M., et al.,** Preconception, intrauterine, and postnatal irradiation as related to leukemia, *Natl. Cancer Inst. Monogr.,* 19, 347, 1966.

Chapter 8

GENETIC EPIDEMIOLOGY OF RETINOBLASTOMA

E. Matsunaga

TABLE OF CONTENTS

I. INTRODUCTION

Since Falls and Neel[1] first attempted to apply both genetic and epidemiologic approaches to an analysis of nonrandom distribution of retinoblastoma in human populations, our knowledge about genetics and genesis of this tumor has increased tremendously. First, follow-up studies of survivors of the tumor revealed that all bilateral, whether familial or sporadic (isolated), and about 10% of sporadic unilateral cases are heritable in an autosomal dominant fashion, whereas 90% of sporadic unilateral cases are nonheritable.[2] Second, the development of human cytogenetics, especially with the aid of banding technique, showed that a minority of cases is associated with a constitutional deletion of chromosome band 13q14,[3] which usually results in 50% of esterase D activity in normal cells of the patients.[4] Third, the attractive two-mutation hypothesis advocated by Knudson[5] stimulated both cytogeneticists and molecular biologists and led them to discover that the *Rb* gene is located on 13q14,[6] and that homozygosity for the mutant allele is a prerequisite for the genesis of retinoblastoma, irrespective of the heritable or nonheritable form,[7-11] although additional nonrandom chromosomal changes may be necessary for its development.[12] The term homozygosity here used means the effective loss of activity of both normal alleles at a locus; it can be brought about by several somatic chromosomal mechanisms, including nondisjunctional loss of the homologue carrying the wild-type allele, reduplication of the mutant chromosome, and mitotic recombination between the two homologues. Thus, retinoblastoma is a recessive cancer at the cellular level. We may anticipate that cloning of the *Rb* gene will soon lead to the understanding of the molecular nature of mutation at this locus.

In the meantime, however, few epidemiologic studies have been conducted to investigate possible environmental factors associated with germinal or somatic mutation leading to heritable or nonheritable retinoblastoma. Obviously, the rarity of this disease makes it difficult to collect a sufficiently large number of sporadic bilateral or unilateral cases to give an epidemiologically sound conclusion. On the other hand, taking advantage of reduced penetrance and variable expressivity of the *Rb* gene, data from familial cases have been utilized to analyze possible host factors that can modify the process of tumor development when the primary genetic change is already present in all the target cells. Moreover, studies of clinical epidemiology have provided much information about increased risk of other cancers in patients with retinoblastoma and their relatives. This chapter reviews these and other studies, with special reference to their epidemiologic aspects.

II. VARIATION IN INCIDENCE

In contrast to most adult cancers, the incidence of retinoblastoma is fairly uniform worldwide. According to Vogel[2] who reviewed relevant data from 16 different populations published up to 1977, the most reliable estimates for the incidence range between about 1:28,000 and 1:15,000, and there is a tendency for studies covering more recent periods to give higher values. This tendency may be attributed largely to more complete ascertainment in the more recent studies but partly to increasing number of cases inherited from survivors of the disease.

Table 1 shows additional data on the incidence from seven series that were not covered by Vogel.[2] Most of the recent data give estimates higher than 1:20,000 newborns. It is striking that the Navajo Indians show an exceptionally high value. Berkow and Fleshman[19] speculate on the possibility that silent expression of the *Rb* gene occurs more frequently among the Navajo population compared with other populations. However, if this was the case, one could have observed more familial cases having unaffected parents, but actually none of the 11 affected children observed were found within the same family. Possible increase in germinal mutation associated with uranium-mining activities, an important source of income for the Navajo Indians, cannot be supported because the children included only

Table 1
INCIDENCE OF RETINOBLASTOMA

Population	Time covered	Number of cases	Incidence	Remarks	Ref.
Ireland	1955—1970	36	1:26,595	Population-based; 4 familial and 32 sporadic (10 bilateral, 22 unilateral) cases	13
U.S.					
Whites	1969—1971	52	1:19,600	Population-based, indirect estimate	14
Blacks		7	1:22,000		
Japanese	1975	121	1:16,400	Hospital-based, nationwide; 6 familial and 115 sporadic (31 bilateral, 84 unilateral) cases	15
U.S.					
Whites	1974—1976	49	1:21,800	Population-based, indirect estimate	16
Blacks		9	1:16,700		
Other nonwhites		12	1:8,260		
New Zealand	1948—1977	100	1:17,500	5 familial and 95 sporadic (25 bilateral, 70 unilateral) cases	17
Greater Delaware Valley					
Whites	1970—1979	63	1:17,300	Population-based, indirect estimate	18
Nonwhites		19	1:12,650		
Navajo Indians	1966—1981	11	1: 6,550	All sporadic (2 bilateral, 9 unilateral)	19

two bilateral cases. Further ophthalmologic surveillance of children, together with epidemiologic investigation on possible maternal exposure during pregnancy, should be made in that population. In this connection, Pendergrass[16] noted that, although no difference in incidence of retinoblastoma was found for U.S. whites and blacks, other nonwhites had much higher incidence. However, the number of other nonwhite patients in his series was only 12 including 1 American Indian, which is too small to draw any conclusion. While the figure for the Japanese[15] is comparable to those for European populations, population-based data from other areas in the world, particularly Asia and Africa, are necessary to answer the problem of possible ethnic difference in incidence of this tumor.

III. DISTRIBUTION OF SPORADIC VS. FAMILIAL CASES BY LATERALITY

Because of the etiological heterogeneity, it is important for epidemiologic studies to classify retinoblastoma cases by laterality and sporadic or familial occurrence. While the diagnosis of bilateral involvement is definite, that of unilateral disease is tentative. However, in more than 90% of bilateral cases, the interval between diagnosis in first and second eye lies within 1 year,[20] so that misclassification of bilateral cases as unilaterally affected could be minimized if ophthalmologic surveillance of the patients is made for at least 1 year.

Table 2 gives relevant data from two surveys in Japan; one[21] was a population-based survey aiming at complete ascertainment of retinoblastoma cases that occurred during 1945 to 1957 in Hokkaido, and the other[22] was a nationwide registry made by ophthalmologists in 1975 to 1976. While the fraction of familial cases has been increased from 1.4 to 4.7% during the last 20 years, sporadic cases represent the overwhelming majority, for which the ratio of unilateral to bilateral cases remains to be approximately 2:1. The pattern of this distribution is comparable to that in most other populations so far investigated.

A word may be said about the changing picture of familial cases with improved medical care services. Prior to the advent of modern surgery, the disease was almost always fatal,

Table 2
DISTRIBUTION OF RETINOBLASTOMA IN JAPAN BY LATERALITY AND SPORADIC VS. FAMILIAL OCCURRENCE

Laterality	Sporadic	Familial	Total	Ref.
Unilateral	46	0	46	21
Bilateral	22	1	23	21
Total	68	1 (1.4%)	69	21
Unilateral	392	11	403	22
Bilateral	179	17	196	22
Total	571	28 (4.7%)	599	22

and the original pattern of familial cases was characterized by two or more siblings or collateral relatives affected without expression in parents (Figure 1). While this pattern of inheritance still persists and will persist, cases inherited from the survivors are gradually increasing in number (Table 3).

IV. AGE-SPECIFIC INCIDENCE

Onset of retinoblastoma tends to be much earlier in bilateral cases than in unilateral cases, and age-specific incidence data have been analyzed for testing fitness with various mathematical models.[5,23-25] However, there is a certain interval, which can be varied appreciably by socioeconomic factors, between the time when parents first notice something wrong with the eye in the child and the time when the diagnosis is made by a physician. In Japan, for example, the mean age at diagnosis of unilateral cases has been lowered from 31.5 to 23.6 months, and that of bilateral cases from 17.1 to 10.4 months during the last 20 years.[24] This change may be ascribed to increased availability of medical care services and medical awareness by the public as well as to increased parental care resulting from small families that have been prevalent since 1950 in this country. Therefore, comparison of age-specific incidence data between different populations should be made cautiously, taking into account sociocultural backgrounds.

Table 4 gives recent Japanese data for the distribution of ages at diagnosis of 244 bilateral, 31 familial unilateral, and 435 sporadic unilateral cases. Of the bilateral cases, 191 were sporadic and 53 were familial, and their respective distributions were essentially the same;[24] this is consistent with the notion that all bilateral cases are due to germinal mutation, irrespective of sporadic or familial occurrence. While about half of the familial bilateral and unilateral cases were taken from the literature compiled by Matsunaga,[26] all the sporadic cases were ascertained by a nationwide registration since 1975.

It is clear from the table that, although the range of age at diagnosis extends up to 7 years or over, i.e., long after embryonic retinal cells have ceased cell division, a significant proportion of the bilateral as well as unilateral cases were diagnosed shortly after birth, implying that tumors can be induced during the later fetal period involving the minimal number of carcinogenic steps. On the other hand, of the 435 sporadic unilateral cases, a great majority of which can be regarded as nonheritable, 20 were diagnosed after the age of 5 years, whereas there were only 3 such cases among the 275 heritable cases. The earlier onset of heritable than nonheritable cases is consistent with the Knudson's[5] theory that only one hit of somatic mutation is required for the development of a heritable tumor, whereas two such events are needed to occur for a nonheritable tumor. However, both mean and variance of ages at diagnosis of the familial unilateral cases were considerably greater than those of the bilateral cases. Since age at diagnosis of patients with heritable cases can be regarded as latency period, this finding may suggest that patients with familial unilateral

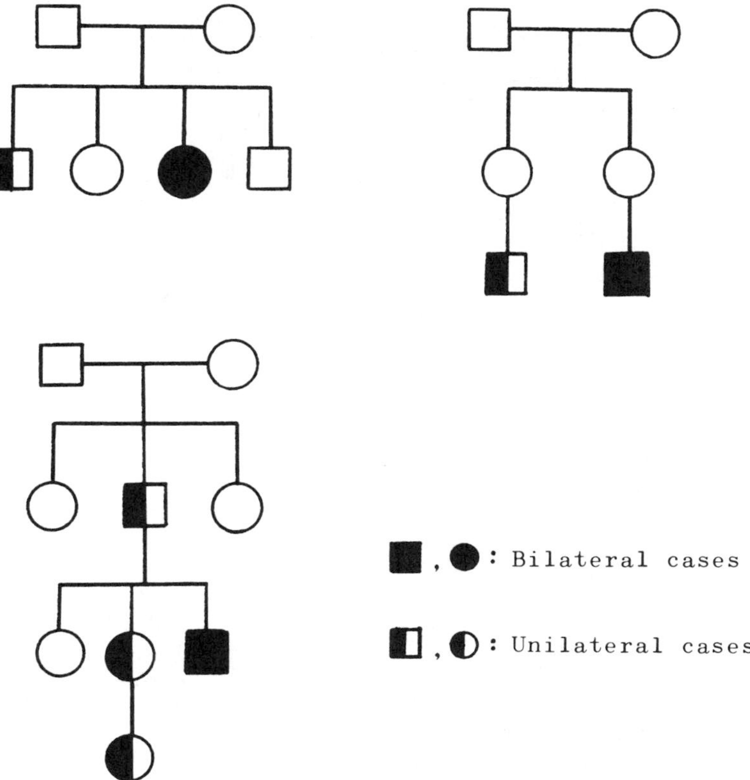

FIGURE 1. Pattern of familial cases of retinoblastoma in representative pedigrees. The above two represent the prototype, while the below is emerging with prevalence of medical care service.

Table 3
NUMBER OF KINDREDS WITH FAMILIAL RETINOBLASTOMA BY YEAR OF PUBLICATION IN JAPAN

Year of publication	Both parents normal	One parent affected		Total
		Unilateral	Bilateral	
1925—1955	5	0	0	5
1956—1965	3	2	1	6
1966—1976	6	16	10	32
Total	14	18	11	43

Table 4
AGES OF PATIENTS AT DIAGNOSIS OF BILATERAL AND UNILATERAL RETINOBLASTOMA

Age at diagnosis (months)	Number of cases		
	Bilateral	Familial unilateral	Sporadic unilateral
0—4	81	6	57
5—9	64	3	48
10—14	34	5	50
15—19	27	1	50
20—29	26	5	112
30—39	7	7	54
40—49	3	2	27
50—59	1	0	17
60—69	1	1	7
70—79	0	1	6
≥80	0	0	7
Total	244	31	435
Mean age	10.5	21.9	23.6
Variance	100.6	328.0	395.2

cases represent a more resistant group than those who present bilateral involvement.[24] This point will be discussed later in more detail.

V. SEARCH FOR ENVIRONMENTAL RISK FACTORS

The somatic mutation in nonheritable retinoblastoma may be caused by maternal exposure during pregnancy to ionizing radiation, certain oncogenic virus, or chemical mutagens. However, Japanese children who were *in utero* at the time of the atomic bombings do not have an increased cancer risk.[27] Although epidemiologic studies have shown that a low-dose prenatal X-ray irradiation may increase the risk of childhood cancer,[28-30] the increased risk appears to refer to cancer in general, an observation that conflicts markedly with well-established knowledge of radiation carcinogenesis in adults. Thus, the problem of possible causal relationship between fetal irradiation and childhood cancers including retinoblastoma remains to be answered.[31]

Recently a case-control study in Sweden of childhood cancer, not including retinoblastoma, disclosed a dose-response relationship between maternal smoking during pregnancy and cancer risk in the offspring.[32] The risk was doubled for non-Hodgkin lymphoma, acute lymphoblastic leukemia, and Wilms' tumor. Similar epidemiologic studies including cases of retinoblastoma should be done to confirm the result.

Possible viral etiology has been suggested from time to time, not only for nonheritable retinoblastoma but also for the appearance of what has been called delayed mutation.[2,33] In experiments with rodents and baboons, retinoblastoma-like tumors can be produced by intraocular injection of human adenovirus 12[34] and *in vitro* experiments; the viral DNA can induce malignant transformation of human embryonic retinal cells.[35] However, the viral hypothesis has never been tested by epidemiologic studies or by an examination of patients for antiviral antibodies.

Seasonal variation in births of patients with sporadic unilateral retinoblastoma could suggest that the disease is influenced by certain environmental agents such as viral infection. Earlier reports[1,17,36,37] failed to show clustering in a specific season. But this would be expected, because they were based on a rather small number of patients. We were able to

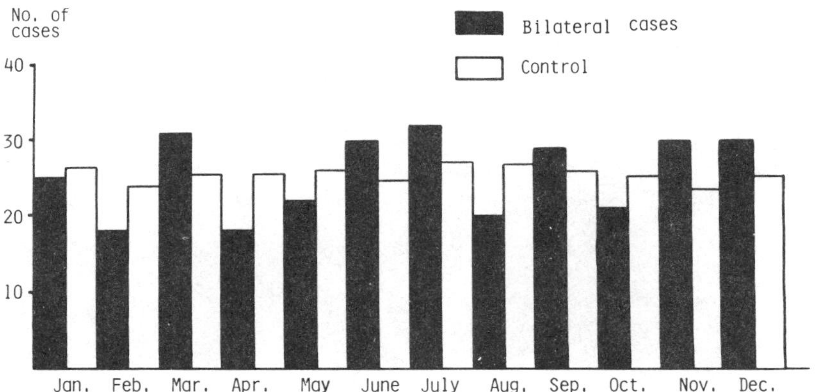

FIGURE 2. Distribution by month of births of 306 sporadic cases of bilateral retinoblastoma born in 1965 to 1981.

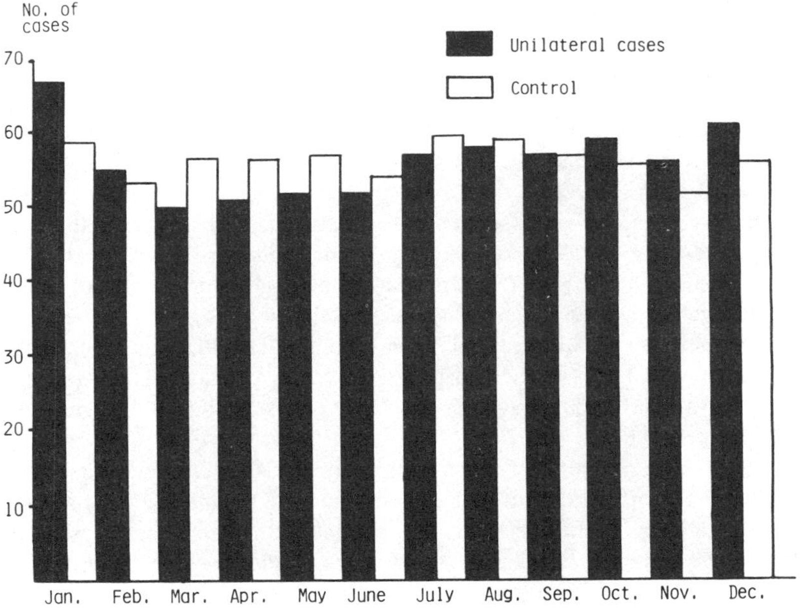

FIGURE 3. Distribution by month of births of 675 sporadic cases of unilateral retinoblastoma born in 1965 to 1981.

analyze distributions of the months of births of 981 sporadic cases of retinoblastoma (675 unilateral and 306 bilateral) ascertained by the nationwide registration.[38] These children were born during the period from 1965 to 1981, and the control was constructed on the basis of the vital statistics data in all Japan, adjusted by the year of births of the patients. As shown in Figure 2, the frequency of the bilateral cases fluctuates to some extent by month of births, but there was no statistically significant deviation from the control. In the unilateral cases (Figure 3), there appears to be a slight excess of births of the patients beginning from October through February, whereas a slight deficit is seen from March through August, although the differences from the controls were not significant. In general, the distribution of the unilateral cases was closer to the control than that of the bilateral cases, probably because of the larger number of cases. We may conclude that the occurrence of nonheritable retinoblastoma is not likely to be associated with those viruses whose activity varies markedly with season.

Table 5
MEAN AGES OF THE PARENTS OF CHILDREN WITH SPORADIC RETINOBLASTOMA

Bilateral cases			Unilateral cases			Controls		
Number of cases	Father	Mother	Number of cases	Father	Mother	Father	Mother	Ref.
21	34.4	28.9	45	33.0	28.9	32.0[a]	28.4[b]	40
17	33.5	31.7	51	32.5	27.7	31.5	28.4	41
155	32.3	28.2	289	30.9	27.7	31.1[c]	27.6[c]	42
225	30.2	27.3	408	30.2	27.2	30.1[b]	27.3[b]	42a

[a] Vital statistics for 1952.
[b] Vital statistics, adjusted by the year of births of the patients.
[c] Vital statistics for 1956.

It is well known that paternal age has a profound effect on the production of mutations leading to certain dominant bone anomalies such as achondroplasia, acrocephalosyndactyly, and Marfan's syndrome. With respect to sporadic retinoblastoma, Vogel and Rathenberg[39] reviewed the literature and concluded that there seems to be a paternal age effect in the bilateral but not in the unilateral cases, although the extent of the effect is much smaller than in the dominant bone anomalies. This problem is interesting because, in contrast to the case in female gametogenesis, the spermatogonia are continuously dividing and therefore defects due to a failure to copy the DNA correctly at cell division should increase with advancing paternal age. However, epidemiologic evidence for the paternal age effect is not strong. First, previous studies were based on a small number of cases, with the exception of Pellié et al.[42] Second, it is generally difficult to obtain appropriate control data for paternal age; data for paternal age distribution are seldom available in vital statistics. Pellié et al.[42] compared paternal ages of 444 sporadic cases of retinoblastoma with French vital statistics for 1956. The year of births of these patients, however, extended over more than 10 years including 1951 to 1960,[43] during which paternal age distribution in the general population must have changed gradually.

We analyzed parental ages of 633 patients with sporadic retinoblastoma (408 unilateral and 225 bilateral) born in 1965 to 1968 and 1975 to 1982. Japanese vital statistics provide distributions of all legitimate live births by paternal and maternal ages for these years and the controls were adjusted by year of births of the patients. The results were somewhat unexpected: there was no difference at all in the mean paternal or maternal age between bilateral and unilateral cases, and they were respectively virtually the same as the controls (Table 5). The negative finding may be due, in part, to diminishing variance in parental ages during the last 30 years in this country, resulting from increasing concentration of childbearing at around 30 and 27 years of paternal and maternal ages, respectively. Therefore, our results do not necessarily exclude the possibility of a slight paternal age effect, but they do suggest that paternal exposure to ionizing radiation or chemical mutagens, which should have an accumulated effect with advancing age, does not play a major role in the production of germinal mutation for retinoblastoma.

VI. HOST FACTORS

Examination of families with two or more affected members clearly indicates that there are three phenotypes of individuals carrying the *Rb* gene: unaffected, unilaterally affected, and bilaterally affected (Figure 1). Variable expressivity means that the primary genetic change alone is not always sufficient to develop retinoblastoma. Two lines of evidence show

Table 6
SEGREGATION RATIO OF FAMILIAL CASES OF RETINOBLASTOMA AND PROPORTION OF BILATERALITY AMONG AFFECTED

Phenotype of carrier parents	Porportion of children affected	Proportion of bilaterality among affected
Unaffected	0.31 ± 0.03	133/246 = 0.541
Unilateral	0.42 ± 0.05	96/126 = 0.762
Bilateral	0.49 ± 0.05	79/88 = 0.898

From Matsunaga, E., *Am. J. Hum. Genet.*, 30, 406, 1978. With permission.

Table 7
MEAN AGE OF PATIENTS AT DIAGNOSIS OF INHERITED CASES OF RETINOBLASTOMA ACCORDING TO PHENOTYPE OF CARRIER PARENTS

	Affected children					
	Bilateral			Unilateral		
Phenotype of carrier parents	Number	Mean age (months)	SD	Number	Mean age (months)	SD
Unaffected	17	13.9	15.41	16	21.5	14.53
Unilateral	20	9.4	8.46	6	15.7	13.49
Bilateral	12	9.3	11.42	1	1	—

From Matsunaga, E., *J. Natl. Cancer Inst.*, 63, 933, 1979. With permission.

that both environmental and genetic factors can modify the process of tumor development in the carriers. The participation of some unknown environmental factors is suggested by occasional case reports about discordant pairs of identical twins, in whom one twin was bilaterally affected while the other was totally unaffected.[44] Regarding genetic factors, analysis of family data for inherited cases of retinoblastoma showed that not only the segregation ratio of affected children but also the degree of expressivity as measured by the proportion of bilaterally affected and age at diagnosis of the children varied consistently with expressivity in carrier parents (Tables 6 and 7).[24,45]

Formally, such a correlation can be ascribed to a variety of mechanisms, including multiple alleles, modifier genes, chromosomal mechanisms, maternal effect, delayed mutation,[46] and mutational mosaicism.[47] The existence of multiple alleles with different expressivity can be ruled out because all the three phenotypes occur frequently within the same family.[48] Maternal effect was also excluded because the proportion of bilateral involvement in the affected children did not change with the sex of the carrier parents.[49] Strong et al.[50] reported a large kindred with familial cases of 13q14 deletion, in which the deletion in the patients was transmitted from a balanced insertional translocation carried by an unaffected parent. Therefore, apparent nonexpression in carriers in certain families may be due to chromosome rearrangement in a balanced state. However, the same mechanism cannot account for the appearance of unaffected carriers in offspring of unilaterally or bilaterally affected parents. Delayed mutation has been referred to for interpreting some unusual pedigrees in which multiple cases of retinoblastoma appeared among distant collateral relatives.[51,52] However, analysis of comprehensive data suggested that, although the possibility of delayed mutation could not be excluded, there was no need to postulate it if one accepts modifier genes.[45,51] Moreover, there was some circumstantial evidence against the model of mutational mosaicism.[53]

We therefore proposed that host resistance or modifier genes at other loci play an important role in the development of heritable retinoblastoma. In other words, unaffected carriers are inherently resistant to tumor formation, whereas persons with bilateral cases are the most susceptible, hereditary unilateral cases being the intermediate. Since most unaffected carriers show no abnormality in the retinae by ophthalmoscopic examination, the modifier genes appear to be concerned mainly with the process of malignant transformation of the embryonic retinal cells, a process now known to be shifting by various somatic chromosomal mechanisms from heterozygosity to homozygosity for the mutant allele on 13q14, although progression phase may also be modified by genetic factors, as suggested by infrequent spontaneous regression of bilateral retinoblastoma.[54,55] The number of the modifier genes seems to be small.

So far, few studies have been carried out to search for possible association of genetic markers with susceptibility to develop retinoblastoma. Bertrams et al.[56] claimed an association with Bw35 and B12 antigens of the HLA system, but Gallie et al.[57] failed to find any such association. These authors found that in families with multiple cases of retinoblastoma, HLA type did not segregate with the disease, and that HLA type apparently had no effect on the rate of spontaneous regression. We investigated ABO blood groups of patients with bilateral and sporadic unilateral cases separately and found that the blood group distribution in those with early onset, who may be regarded as most susceptible, was essentially the same as in the general population.[58] In order to study the nature of the presumptive host resistance genes, a large kindred in which all the three phenotypes of the *Rb* gene carriers occurred over generations should be examined using a variety of polymorphic DNA markers (RFLPs). Such studies could identify a specific DNA segment correlated with host resistance in the gene carriers.

VII. RISK OF OTHER CANCERS IN PATIENTS WITH HERITABLE RETINOBLASTOMA AND THEIR RELATIVES

It is well established that survivors of heritable retinoblastoma, but not survivors of nonheritable tumor, are prone to develop a second primary neoplasm, mainly osteosarcoma, not only in the area of irradiation but also outside this zone.[59,60] From this, Kitchin and Ellsworth[61] argued that the increased risk of second primary tumors is a pleiotropic effect of the *Rb* gene. In fact, nonradiogenic osteosarcoma can occur not infrequently even in the gene carriers who did not develop retinoblastoma.[20] We collected from the literature 26 cases of nonradiogenic osteosarcoma that developed in patients with retinoblastoma and in their close relatives, and on the basis of their distribution we argued that in the gene carriers resistance to osteosarcoma is also genetically determined and it is not correlated with the resistance to retinoblastoma. In other words, the presumed host resistance genes are tissue specific.[62]

According to Abramson et al.[63] incidence of second tumors, including radiogenic ones, in patients with heritable retinoblastoma increases with time after the diagnosis of a primary ocular tumor: at 30 years, the incidence was 90%, and that of nonradiogenic tumors was 68%. However, their figures were based on a retrospective analysis of patients treated in one hospital and therefore probably overestimated due to biased ascertainment. A systematic follow-up investigation of the patients should be done to provide more reliable incidence figures. It is interesting that these authors found no relationship between incidence of tumors and dose of therapeutic radiation, although Sagerman et al.[59] demonstrated a positive result.

We do not know about the molecular basis for the inherent tendency of patients with heritable retinoblastoma to develop second primary tumors after irradiation. Weichselbaum et al.[64] and Nove et al.[65] reported that, *in vitro* experiments, fibroblast strains from patients with heritable retinoblastoma, and some strains from patients with 13q deletion were abnormally radiosensitive, but their results could not be confirmed by Ejima et al.[66] On the other hand, recent molecular genetic studies have demonstrated that homozygosity at chromosome 13q is involved in the genesis of nonradiogenic osteosarcoma in patients with heritable retinoblastoma as well as in individuals who had no previous retinoblastoma or family history of retinoblastoma.[67,68]

Recently, Bader et al.[69] reported 11 patients with bilateral retinoblastoma who developed pinealoblastoma and called this condition ''trilateral retinoblastoma''. Since the pineal contains vestigial photoreceptor tissue, the pineal tumor represents an additional focus of multicentric retinoblastoma rather than a true second primary neoplasm in the gene carriers. However, pinealoblastoma is rarely observed in patients with bilateral retinoblastoma. Johnson et al.,[70] who described three additional cases of this condition, pointed out that, in contrast to bilateral retinoblastomas alone, the ocular tumors in trilateral retinoblastoma develop before the age of 6 months, and they argued that low host resistance of trilateral retinoblastoma is evident by the early age of presentation and the multicentric occurrence of the tumor.

We have seen that the *Rb* gene has a pleiotropic effect, and tissue-specific resistance genes at other loci are presumably involved in the manifestation of that gene. It is therefore anticipated that relatives of patients with heritable retinoblastoma are, inasmuch as they are carriers of the *Rb* gene, prone to develop certain other neoplasms, notably osteosarcoma. We do not know, however, whether the relatives are at increased risk of common cancers such as stomach and breast cancers.

Fedrick and Baldwin[71] observed an overall excess in cancer incidence in relatives of 11 patients with retinoblastoma. However, the data were small and most of the probands appeared to be sporadic unilateral cases. Bonaïti-Pellié and Briard-Guillemot[72] also reported excess of cancer deaths in grandparents of 308 children with retinoblastoma, regardless of unilateral or bilateral, sporadic or familial occurrence. However, this excess, which was found in all types of common cancers and not in a specific type, seemed to affect only deaths over age 50 years, a finding that conflicts with well-established knowledge of earlier onset of genetically determined cancers.

Recently, Strong et al.[73] presented most comprehensive data obtained by a retrospective survey. Their data suggested that, compared with death rates for the general population, there was a slight excess in cancer deaths among relatives of patients with bilateral and/or familial retinoblastoma, but not among relatives of patients with sporadic unilateral cases. The excess was most marked for relatives at young ages, for fathers, and for obligate gene transmitters. Specific tumor types in excess included early-onset lung cancer and melanoma, tumors also observed in survivors of heritable retinoblastoma. There was no excess of osteosarcoma, but this may be due to selection of relatives who have survived the adolescent age. The authors speculated that the excess might be attributable to an unexpressed *Rb* gene or some kind of ''premutation'' in particular kindreds. However, most striking in their data was a marked deficit of deaths from noncancer causes among relatives of the patients. Follow-up studies of close relatives of these patients with appropriate controls are desirable to confirm the above findings.

VIII. SUMMARY

Recent studies of genetic epidemiology of retinoblastoma are reviewed, and major conclusions drawn are as follows:

1. Retinoblastoma occurs in heritable or nonheritable form. The primary genetic change in the heritable form is a point mutation or deletion at a locus on 13q14. For the genesis of a tumor in either form, the loss or inactivation of both alleles at this locus is a prerequisite, although additional events may be needed for its development.
2. Information about environmental risk factors for the occurrence of heritable or nonheritable retinoblastoma is still meager. Although viral etiology for nonheritable tumor cannot be excluded, an extensive epidemiologic study revealed no seasonal variation in births of patients with sporadic unilateral cases, a great majority of which may be regarded as due to somatic mutation. Moreover, there was no paternal age effect at all on the occurrence of sporadic bilateral cases arising from germinal mutations. Paternal exposure to ionizing radiation or chemical mutagens, which should have an accumulated effect with advancing age, does not seem to play a major role in the production of germinal mutation at the *Rb* locus.
3. Family studies show that host resistance genes at other loci can modify the process of tumor development when the primary genetic change is already present in all the target cells. Unaffected gene carriers may be regarded as inherently resistant to tumor formation, whereas persons who present early onset of bilateral tumors are the most susceptible. In certain families, however, nonexpression in the carriers may be due to chromosomal rearrangement in a balanced state. The resistance genes seem to be tissue specific.
4. The *Rb* gene has a pleiotropic effect of developing not only ocular and ectopic retinoblastomas but also osteosarcoma and possibly other neoplasms. These tumors seem to develop in the most susceptible subgroup of the gene carriers.
5. There seems to be a modest overall cancer excess in relatives of patients with heritable retinoblastoma. Whether the excess is attributable to a pleiotropic effect of the *Rb* gene remains to be answered.

REFERENCES

1. **Falls, H. F. and Neel, J. V.,** Genetics of retinoblastoma, *Arch. Ophthalmol.*, 46, 367, 1951.
2. **Vogel, F.,** Genetics of retinoblastoma, *Hum. Genet.*, 52, 1, 1979.
3. **Yunis, J. J. and Ramsay, N.,** Retinoblastoma and subband deletion of chromosome 13, *Am. J. Dis. Child.*, 132, 161, 1978.
4. **Sparkes, R. S., Sparkes, M. C., Wilson, M. G., Towner, J. W., Benedict, W., Murphree, A. L., and Yunis, J. J.,** Regional assignment of genes for human esterase D and retinoblastoma to chromosome band 13q14, *Science*, 208, 1042, 1980.
5. **Knudson, A. G., Jr.,** Mutation and cancer: statistical study of retinoblastoma, *Proc. Natl. Acad. Sci. U.S.A.*, 68, 820, 1971.
6. **Sparkes, R. S., Murphree, A. L., Lingua, R. W., Sparkes, M. C., Field, L. L., Funderburk, S. J., and Benedict, W. F.,** Gene for hereditary retinoblastoma assigned to human chromosome 13 by linkage to esterase D, *Science*, 219, 971, 1983.
7. **Benedict, W. F., Murphree, A. L., Banerjee, A., Spina, C. A., Sparkes, M. C., and Sparkes, R. S.,** Patient with 13 chromosome deletion: evidence that the retinoblastoma gene is a recessive cancer gene, *Science*, 219, 973, 1983.
8. **Godbout, R., Dryja, T. P., Squire, J., Gallie, B. L., and Phillips, R. A.,** Somatic inactivation of genes on chromosome 13 is a common event in retinoblastoma, *Nature*, 304, 451, 1983.
9. **Cavenee, W. K., Dryja, T. P., Phillips, R. A., Benedict, W. F., Godbout, R., Gallie, B. L., Murphree, A. L., Strong, L. C., and White, R. L.,** Expression of recessive alleles by chromosomal mechanisms in retinoblastoma, *Nature*, 305, 779, 1983.
10. **Dryja, T. P., Cavenee, W., White, R., Rapaport, J. M., Petersen, R., Albert, D. M., and Bruns, G. A. P.,** Homozygosity of chromosome 13 in retinoblastoma, *N. Engl. J. Med.*, 310, 550, 1984.
11. **Cavenee, W. K., Hansen, M. F., Nordenskjold, M., Kock, E., Maumenee, I., Squire, J. A., Phillips, R. A., and Gallie, B. L.,** Genetic origin of mutations predisposing to retinoblastoma, *Science*, 228, 501, 1985.

12. **Murphree, A. L. and Benedict, W. F.,** Retinoblastoma: clues to human oncogenesis, *Science,* 223, 1928, 1984.
13. **Barry, G. and Mullaney, J.,** Retinoblastoma in the Republic of Ireland, *Trans. Ophthalmol. Soc. U.K.,* 91, 839, 1971.
14. **Young, J. L., Jr. and Miller, R. W.,** Incidence of malignant tumors in U.S. children, *J. Pediatr.,* 86, 254, 1975.
15. **Minoda, K.,** National registration of retinoblastoma in 1975, *Acta Soc. Ophthalmol. Jpn.,* 80, 1648, 1976.
16. **Pendergrass, T. W.,** Incidence of retinoblastoma in the United States, *Arch. Ophthalmol.,* 98, 1204, 1980.
17. **Suckling, R. D., Fitzgerald, P. H., Stewart, J., and Wells, E.,** The incidence and epidemiology of retinoblastoma in New Zealand: a 30-year survey, *Br. J. Cancer,* 46, 729, 1982.
18. **Kramer, S., Meadows, A. T., Jarrett, P., and Evans, A. E.,** Incidence of childhood cancer: experience of a decade in a population-based registry, *J. Natl. Cancer Inst.,* 70, 49, 1983.
19. **Berkow, R. L. and Fleshman, J. K.,** Retinoblastoma in Navajo Indian children, *Am. J. Dis. Child.,* 137, 137, 1983.
20. **Gordon, H.,** Family studies in retinoblastoma, *Birth Defects: Orig. Artic. Ser.,* 10(10), 185, 1974.
21. **Matsunaga, E. and Ogyu, H.,** Genetic study of retinoblastoma in a Japanese population, *Jpn. J. Hum. Genet.,* 4, 156, 1959.
22. **Minoda, K.,** The International Symposium on Retinoblastoma, Kyoto, May 20-21, 1978, *Jpn. J. Ophthalmol.,* 22, 299, 1978.
23. **Bonaiti-Pellié, C., Briard-Guillemot, M. L., Feingold, J., and Frézal, J.,** Mutation theory of carcinogenesis in retinoblastoma, *J. Natl. Cancer Inst.,* 57, 269, 1976.
24. **Matsunaga, E.,** Hereditary retinoblastoma: host resistance and age at onset, *J. Natl. Cancer Inst.,* 63, 933, 1979.
25. **Hirayama, T.,** Descriptive and analytical epidemiology of childhood malignancy in Japan, in *Recent Advances in Managements of Children with Cancer,* Kobayashi, N., Ed., The Children's Cancer Association of Japan, Tokyo, 1980, 27.
26. **Matsunaga, E.,** Hereditary retinoblastoma: penetrance, expressivity and age of onset, *Hum. Genet.,* 33, 1, 1976.
27. **Jablon, S. and Kato, H.,** Childhood cancer in relation to prenatal exposure to atomic-bomb radiation, *Lancet,* 2, 1000, 1970.
28. **Stewart, A., Webb, J., and Hewitt, D.,** A survey of childhood malignancies, *Br. Med. J.,* 1, 1495, 1958.
29. **MacMahon, B.,** Prenatal X-ray exposure and childhood cancer, *J. Natl. Cancer Inst.,* 28, 1173, 1962.
30. **Harvey, E. B., Boice, J. D., Honeyman, M., and Flannery, J. T.,** Prenatal X-ray exposure and childhood cancer in twins, *N. Engl. J. Med.,* 312, 541, 1985.
31. **MacMahon, B.,** Prenatal X-ray exposure and twins, *N. Engl. J. Med.,* 312, 576, 1985.
32. **Stjernfeldt, M., Berglund, K., Lindsten, J., and Ludvigsson, J.,** Maternal smoking during pregnancy and risk of childhood cancer, *Lancet,* 1, 1350, 1986.
33. **Zimmerman, L. E.,** Changing concepts concerning the pathogenesis of infectious diseases, *Am. J. Ophthalmol.,* 69, 947, 1970.
34. **Mukai, N., Kalter, S. S., Cummins, L. B., and Matthews, V. A.,** Retinal tumor induced in the baboon by human adenovirus 12, *Science,* 210, 1023, 1980.
35. **Byrd, P., Brown, K. W., and Gallimore, P. H.,** Malignant transformation of human embryonic retinoblasts by cloned adenovirus 12 DNA, *Nature,* 298, 69, 1982.
36. **Vogel, F.,** Über Genetik und Mutationsrate des Retinoblastoms (Glioma retinae). Nebst einigen allgemeinen Bemerkungen über die Methoden zur Mutationsratenschätzung beim Menschen, *Z. Menschl. Vererb. u. Konstitutionslehre,* 32, 308, 1954.
37. **Ogyu, H.,** Genetico-epidemiological study on the occurrence of retinoblastoma in a Japanese population, *Acta Soc. Ophthalmol. Jpn.,* 63, 2702, 1959.
38. **Matsunaga, E. and Minoda, K.,** Examination of seasonal variation in the births of patients with sporadic retinoblastoma, *Jpn. J. Hum. Genet.,* 29, 237, 1984.
39. **Vogel, F. and Rathenberg, R.,** Spontaneous mutation in man, *Adv. Hum. Genet.,* 5, 223, 1975.
40. **Matsunaga, E.,** Parental age and sporadic retinoblastoma, *Annu. Rep. Natl. Inst. Genet.,* 16, 121, 1965.
41. **Tünte, W.,** Human mutations and paternal age, *Humangenetik,* 16, 77, 1972.
42. **Pellié, C., Briard, M. L., Feingold, J., and Frézal, J.,** Parental age in retinoblastoma, *Humangenetik,* 20, 59, 1973.
42a. **Matsunaga, E. and Minoda, K.,** unpublished results.
43. **Briard-Guillemot, M. L., Bonalti-Pellié, C., Feingold, J., and Frézal, J.,** Étude génétique du rétinoblastome, *Humangenetik,* 24, 271, 1974.
44. **Kanter, Y. C. and Harris, J. E.,** Retinoblastoma occurring in one of a pair of identical twins, *Arch. Ophthalmol.,* 72, 783, 1964.
45. **Matsunaga, E.,** Hereditary retinoblastoma: delayed mutation or host resistance?, *Am. J. Hum. Genet.,* 30, 406, 1978.

46. **Herrmann, J.,** Delayed mutation as a cause of retinoblastoma: application to genetic counseling, *Birth Defects: Orig. Artic. Ser.*, 12(1), 79, 1976.
47. **Carlson, E. A. and Desnick, R. J.,** Mutational mosaicism and genetic counseling in retinoblastoma, *Am. J. Med. Genet.*, 4, 365, 1979.
48. **Macklin, M. T.,** A study of retinoblastoma in Ohio, *Am. J. Hum. Genet.*, 12, 1, 1960.
49. **Matsunaga, E.,** Hereditary retinoblastoma: lack of maternal effect, *Hum. Genet.*, 62, 124, 1982.
50. **Strong, L. C., Riccardi, V. M., Ferrel, R. E., and Sparkes, R. S.,** Familial retinoblastoma and chromosome 13 deletion transmitted *via* an insertional translocation, *Science*, 213, 1501, 1981.
51. **Bundey, S. and Morten, J. E. N.,** An unusual pedigree with retinoblastoma. Does it shed light on the delayed mutation and host resistance theories?, *Hum. Genet.*, 59, 434, 1981.
52. **Connolly, M. J., Payne, R. H., Johnson, G., Gallie, B. L., Allderdice, P. W., Marshall, W. H., and Lawton, R. D.,** Familial, *EsD*-linked, retinoblastoma with reduced penetrance and variable expressivity, *Hum. Genet.*, 65, 122, 1983.
53. **Matsunaga, E.,** Retinoblastoma: mutational mosaicism or host resistance?, *Am. J. Med. Genet.*, 8, 375, 1981.
54. **Boniuk, M. and Girard, L. J.,** Spontaneous regression of bilateral retinoblastoma, *Trans. Am. Acad. Ophthalmol. Otolaryngol.*, 73, 194, 1969.
55. **Morris, W. E. and Lapiana, F. G.,** Spontaneous regression of bilateral multifocal retinoblastoma with preservation of normal visual acuity, *Ann. Ophthalmol.*, 6, 1192, 1974.
56. **Bertrams, J., Schildberg, P., Höpping, W., Böhme, U., and Albert, E.,** HLA antigens in retinoblastoma, *Tissue Antigens*, 3, 78, 1973.
57. **Gallie, B. L., Dupont, B., Whitsett, C., Kitchin, F. D., Ellsworth, R. M., and Good, R. A.,** Histocompatibility typing in spontaneous regression of retinoblastoma, in *HLA and Malignancy*, Murphy, G. P., Cohen, E., Fitzpatrick, J. E., and Pressman, D., Eds., Alan R. Liss, New York, 1977, 229.
58. **Matsunaga, E. and Minoda, K.,** Retinoblastoma and ABO blood groups, *Hum. Genet.*, 63, 87, 1983.
59. **Sagerman, R. H., Cassady, J. R., Tretter, P., and Ellsworth, R. M.,** Radiation induced neoplasia following external beam therapy for children with retinoblastoma, *Am. J. Roentgenol.*, 105, 529, 1969.
60. **Jensen, R. D. and Miller, R. W.,** Retinoblastoma: epidemiologic characteristics, *N. Engl. J. Med.*, 285, 307, 1971.
61. **Kitchin, F. D. and Ellsworth, R. M.,** Pleiotropic effects of the gene for retinoblastoma, *J. Med. Genet.*, 11, 244, 1974.
62. **Matsunaga, E.,** Hereditary retinoblastoma: host resistance and second primary tumors, *J. Natl. Cancer Inst.*, 65, 47, 1980.
63. **Abramson, D. H., Ellsworth, R. M., Kitchin, F. D., and Tung, G.,** Second nonocular tumors in retinoblastoma survivors. Are they radiation-induced?, *Ophthalmology*, 91, 1351, 1984.
64. **Weichselbaum, R. R., Nove, J., and Little, J. B.,** X-ray sensitivity of diploid fibroblasts from patients with hereditary or sporadic retinoblastoma, *Proc. Natl. Acad. Sci. U.S.A.*, 75, 3962, 1978.
65. **Nove, J., Little, J. B., Weichselbaum, R. R., Nichols, W. W., and Hoffman, E.,** Retinoblastoma, chromosome 13, and in vitro cellular radiosensitivity, *Cytogenet. Cell Genet.*, 24, 176, 1980.
66. **Ejima, Y., Sasaki, M. S., Utsumi, H., Kaneko, A., and Tanooka, H.,** Radiosensitivity of fibroblasts from patients with retinoblastoma and chromosome-13 anomalies, *Mutat. Res.*, 103, 177, 1982.
67. **Hansen, M. F., Koufos, A., Gallie, B. L., Phillips, R. A., Fodstad, Ø., Brøgger, A., Gedde-Dahl, T., and Cavenee, W. K.,** Osteosarcoma: a shared chromosomal mechanism revealing recessive predisposition, *Proc. Natl. Acad. Sci. U.S.A.*, 82, 6216, 1985.
68. **Dryja, T. P., Rapaport, J. M., Epstein, J., Goorin, A. M., Weichselbaum, R., Koufos, A., and Cavenee, W. K.,** Chromosome 13 homozygosity in osteosarcoma without retinoblastoma, *Am. J. Hum. Genet.*, 38, 59, 1986.
69. **Bader, J. L., Meadows, A. T., Zimmerman, L. E., Rorke, L. B., Voute, P. A., Champion, L. A. A., and Miller, R. W.,** Bilateral retinoblastoma with ectopic intracranial retinoblastoma: trilateral retinoblastoma, *Cancer Genet. Cytogenet.*, 5, 203, 1982.
70. **Johnson, D. L., Chandra, R., Fisher, W. S., Hammock, M. K., and McKeown, C. A.,** Trilateral retinoblastoma: ocular and pineal retinoblastoma, *J. Neurosurg.*, 63, 367, 1985.
71. **Fedrick, J. and Baldwin, J. A.,** Incidence of cancer in relatives of children with retinoblastoma, *Br. Med. J.*, 1, 83, 1978.
72. **Bonaïti-Pellié, C. and Briard,-Guillemot, M. L.,** Excess of cancer deaths in grandparents of patients with retinoblastoma, *J. Med. Genet.*, 17, 95, 1980.
73. **Strong, L. C., Herson, J., Haas, C., Elder, K., Chakraborty, R., Weiss, K. M., and Majumder, P.,** Cancer mortality in relatives of retinoblastoma patients, *J. Natl. Cancer Inst.*, 73, 303, 1984.

Chapter 9

XERODERMA PIGMENTOSUM: GENETIC EPIDEMIOLOGY OF A CANCER-PRONE DISEASE

Hiraku Takebe, Chikako Nishigori, and Yoshiaki Satoh

TABLE OF CONTENTS

I. INTRODUCTION

Xeroderma pigmentosum (XP) is an autosomal recessive hereditary disease associated with a high incidence of skin cancer. Hypersensitivity of the skin of the patients to sunlight was attributed to UV light which had been regarded as the cause of cancer. In 1968, Cleaver[1] discovered that cultured fibroblast cells originating from XP patients were defective in DNA repair of UV damage. XP and other cancer-prone hereditary diseases may represent mutations in human cells which enhance the susceptibility to cancer, and investigation on these diseases may lead to an understanding of not only the genetics of the diseases but also the mechanisms by which they associate with the cause of cancer in general.

A joint research group on XP in Japan (H. Takebe, chief investigator) was started in 1975 and an extensive survey of the patients both in clinical and DNA repair characteristics has been carried out. The joint research has been assisted by the participation of many dermatologists throughout Japan and several cell biologists interested in DNA repair studies.

International cooperative studies on XP have also been carried out by exchanging information about the patients as well as the cells originating from these patients. XP is one of the very few diseases in which both clinical and cellular characteristics have been extensively investigated, and may serve as a good example of experimental genetic epidemiology.

This article intends to summarize our studies on XP patients and their cells, and to compare our results with those from other countries. Aspects of the mechanisms of disease with emphasis on skin cancer will be discussed.

II. CLINICAL AND DNA REPAIR CHARACTERISTICS OF XERODERMA PIGMENTOSUM IN JAPAN

Table 1 gives the age distribution of XP patients in Japan with clinical and DNA repair characteristics. Ages of the patients are recorded at the time of the first visit to the clinics and may not reflect the age of onset of the symptoms. Skin cancer consists of basal cell carcinoma (BCC), squamous cell carcinoma (SCC), and malignant melanoma (MM). In our previous reports[2-5] some keratoacanthomas were included in the survey as skin cancer, but they are excluded in the present survey as noted in Table 1.

Neurological abnormalities of unknown etiology occur in XP patients. In our survey, they are mainly represented by mental retardation. Hearing difficulty and gait disturbances are also often observed. Detailed description of the neurological abnormalities are given by Robbins et al.[6] and the early detection in some of our patients was reported by Mimaki et al.[7] Patients were listed as unknown either because of lack of information or because they were too young to be diagnosed neurologically.

DNA repair characteristics are represented by the relative amounts of unscheduled DNA synthesis (UDS) after UV irradiation in the cells cultured from the patient. Normal human skin fibroblast cells are taken as the standard. XP patients without UDS data are not included in the table and will not be discussed in this article unless otherwise specified.

Major characteristics of XP patients in Japan are presented in Table 1 as follows. Nearly 40% of the patients were under 10 years old and the majority of them showed neurological abnormalities. Cells of the patients in the 0 to 9 age group had extremely low UDS levels with a small number of exceptions. In patients 30 years of age and over, few had neurological abnormalities and essentially no cell strains from this group had extremely low UDS levels. When we started the survey, we assumed that patients with low DNA repair capacity might develop the capacity later, but follow-up studies denied such possibility. Consequently, absence of patients in very low (less than 5% of normal level) UDS at ages 30 and over suggest that the patients might have died by age 30 years. Patients whose cells have relatively high (more than 60%) UDS levels are older than other patients, and some have not developed

Table 1
AGE DISTRIBUTION, CLINICAL SYMPTOMS, AND DNA REPAIR OF XERODERMA PIGMENTOSUM PATIENTS IN JAPAN

Age	Number of patients	Neurological abnormalities			UDS (% of normal)			
		Yes	No	Unknown	<5	5—30	31—60	>60
0—9	102(21)	56	15	31	81(18)	15(3)	4(0)	2(0)
10—19	51(28)	24	17	10	27(20)	7(5)	3(1)	14(2)
20—29	28(19)	3	20	5	4(3)	4(4)	3(1)	17(11)
30—39	31(19)	2	15	14	0	2(1)	7(7)	22(11)
40—49	24(15)	2	15	7	0	6(3)	2(2)	16(10)
50≦	26(12)	0	14	12	1(0)	5(4)	2(1)	18(7)
Total	262(114)	87	96	79	113(41)	39(20)	21(12)	89(41)

Note: (n): patients with skin cancer. Keratoacantoma: 35 patients, 13 without other skin cancer. Primary non-skin cancer: 4 patients.

cancer at 50 or more years of age. Relatively few patients had intermediate (5 to 60%) UDS values. It appears that these intermediate groups constitute the majority of XP patients in Europe and the U.S., but no reliable statistics from this viewpoint have been reported so far. In general, correlation may exist between DNA repair deficiency as represented in relative UDS and development of clinical symptoms. Although cutaneous pathology other than cancer is not shown in Table 1, the development of skin lesions is generally much faster and more severe in the patients with low UDS levels than those with high UDS levels. Such a correlation was also shown in the development of skin cancer in the patients and will be discussed later.

III. GENETICS OF DNA REPAIR DEFICIENCY

A. Genetic Analysis

Genetic analysis of families of XP patients in our survey supported the autosomal recessive inheritance of the disease. Sex ratio of the patients is 1:1. As expected, none of the parents of the patients are affected with XP. Appearance of the patients in the same sibships was noted. Frequency of consanguinous marriage in parents was high. First cousin marriages were approximately 30%, whereas that in the general population in Japan has been 1% or less in recent years. Due to the accelerated population movement from rural areas to large cities in Japan after World War II, the frequency of first cousin marriages changed extensively from 6% in 1947 to less than 1% in 1972.[8] This makes the estimate of the gene frequency based on the coefficient of inbreeding rather difficult. If we take 2% as the frequency of first cousin marriages as the average estimate in the general population during the period corresponding to the marriages of parents of XP patients in Table 1, the frequency of the XP gene in Japanese is approximately 1/300 and the frequency of the XP patients in the newborn babies is 1/100,000.

B. Complementation Groups and Their Distribution in the World

Genetic complementation test by cell fusion revealed the presence of different complementation in XP cells.[9] When cells from different patients, both having low UDS levels, are fused, the resulting heterodikaryon may have normal UDS level by genetic complementation, i.e., exchange of genetic information without recombination of genes. The number of complementation groups identified in XP has increased from an original five in 1975[10]

Table 2
GENETIC GROUP OF XP PATIENTS

Area	Complementation groups									Variant
	A	B	C	D	E	F	G	H	I	
Japan	30	0	5	4	2	11	1	0	0	21
U.S.	3	1	5	5	0	0	0	1	0	2
Europe	10	0	14	8	5	1	2	0	2	5
Egypt	7	0	12	0	0	0	0	0	0	5

Note: Compiled at the 16th International Congress of Dermatology, Tokyo, 1982, with additional reports thereafter. A group F patient in Europe is by personal communication from F. Giannelli.

to nine, and were labeled A to I[11-14] in 1985. Among them, group F was first found in Japan.[11] In addition to nine complementation groups, there are variants whose cells show normal levels of UDS although clinically the patients have XP.[6] Cells from variant patients were reported to have reduced postreplication repair[15] while cells from nine complementation groups had reduced ability to repair UV damage by the excision-resynthesis mechanism. Detailed description of DNA repair deficiency in XP cells has been given in several review articles.[3,6,16-18] Table 2 shows the distribution of genetic complementation groups and variants in different areas of the world.[5,19-25] Patients in Japan are dominated by group A and variants, while group C is the most frequent group in other countries obtained. Patients belonging to group F are still mainly found in Japan. The distribution of these groups in Japan may account for the clinical and DNA repair characteristics of XP patients in Japan as shown in Table 1. All XP patients belonging to complementation group A in Table 2 except one showed neurological abnormalities and extremely low UDS levels in their cells. In Table 1, they correspond to the patients with neurological abnormalities and with UDS levels of less than 5% of normal level; they are the most frequently found XP patients in Japan. Also, the high frequency of patients with UDS levels over 60% are mainly represented by the variant groups.

Cells originating from complementation group F showed rather unique characteristics. Although their UDS levels are relatively low, most of the patients belonging to group F showed mild symptoms. Arase et al.[11] and Hayakawa et al.[26] found that group F cells have considerably higher DNA repair capacity than expected from the UDS levels, presumably because of long-lasting excision repair. The standard UDS measurement in our study depends on the first 3 h after UV irradiation and does not represent the slow repair process in group F cells. Most of the relatively old patients with low UDS (Table 1) have been identified as belonging to group F.

IV. SKIN CANCER

Ages of XP patients depending on genetic groups and ages of onset of skin cancer are given in Table 3. Patients listed in Tables 3, 4, and 5 are the same patients as listed in Table 1. Age distribution of the patients for both time of the first visit and the onset of skin cancer may be segregated into two groups: (1) those less than 10 years old consisting of groups A (and less than 5% UDS) and C, and (2) those over 10 years old in the remaining groups. This again appears to be related to the levels of DNA repair deficiency. The lower the repair capacity, the earlier the symptom and skin cancer develop. Since the number of patients belonging to groups C to G are small, precise correlation between genetic groups and clinical characteristics, if it exists, is not clear. Essentially no differences were noted in the ages of onset of three histopathologically different types of skin cancers. Although

Table 3
AGE DISTRIBUTION AND AGE OF ONSET OF SKIN CANCERS IN XP PATIENTS

Groups	Number of patients[b]	Average age (years)	Age of onset (Years)		
			BCC	SCC	MM
A and less than 5%[a]	115(41)	7.9	9.3	8.2	7.5
C	3(3)	8.3	9.7	8.3	11
D	3(1)	20.3	—	41	—
E	2(0)	11.5			
F	11(3)	28.3	45.5	64	—
G	1(1)	32	32		
Other intermediate UDS	38(24)	28.6	45.4	41.5	14.0
Variant and over 60%	89(41)	38.1	40.8	42.0	46.8

[a] UDS as in Table 1.
[b] (n): with skin cancer.

Table 4
SKIN CANCER OF XP PATIENTS IN JAPAN

Group	Number of patients		Patients with skin cancer		BCC		SCC		MM	
A and less than 5% UDS	115		41		35		20		5	
C	3	} 20	3	} 8	3	} 6	3	} 5	2	} 2
D	3		1		0		1		0	
E	2		0		0		0		0	
F	11		3		2		1		0	
G	1		1		1		0		0	
Other intermediate UDS	38		24		11		10		2	
Variants and over 60% UDS	89		41		30		14		9	
Total	262		114		82		49		18	

no comparable data are available for skin cancer in general in Japanese, onset of BCC could be much later than that of SCC in skin cancer patients in Japan. This is based on comparison between two surveys on skin cancer in Japanese carried out 15 years apart, 1956 to 1960[27] and 1971 to 1975.[28] The later survey reported a nearly fourfold increase in BCC compared with the earlier report and the increase was mainly in the older population, presumably reflecting longer exposure to sunlight due to increased longevity in Japan. This may imply that DNA repair deficiency may have a greater effect in solar induction of BCC than of SCC.

Such possibility is supported by the relative incidence of different histopathologic types of skin cancer as shown in Table 4. The number of patients having BCC is much higher than those having SCC. In skin cancer patients in general, BCC and SCC were found at almost equal frequency by Tada and Miki[28] in their 1971 to 1975 survey. The frequency of MM in skin cancer patients in Japan in their survey was 12.6%, which is about equal to the frequency of MM in skin cancer of XP patients. MM appeared in 15.8% of XP patients having skin cancer and in 12.1% when multiple skin cancers are counted separately depending on the histopathologic types. The site of MM is quite different in ordinary MM patients and XP patients. The latter patients have their MM limited to sun-exposed areas while XP patients have their MM anywhere on the cutaneous surface. The relative incidence of different histopathological types does not correlate to the capacity of DNA repair in the cells.

Table 5
MULTIPLE SKIN CANCERS OF DIFFERENT HISTOPATHOLOGICAL TYPES IN XP PATIENTS

DNA repair levels	Number of patients	BCC + SCC	BCC + MM	SCC + MM	BCC + SCC + MM	Total
Less than 5% of normal UDS	113(41)	8	2	1	1	12
Intermeidate UDS	60(32)	6	0	0	3	9
Over 60% of normal UDS	89(41)	6	0	1	3	10
Total	262(114)	20	2	2	7	31

Note: (n): patients having skin cancers.

Table 6
XP PATIENTS IN KOREA IN COMPARISON WITH PATIENTS IN OSAKA, JAPAN

	Kwangju and Pusan (Korea)	Osaka (Japan)
Number of patients	23	36
Average age	13.6	13.8
Patients with neurological abnormalities	0	21
Consanguinity per number of families	0/17	12/34
Neurological abnormalities in patients in families with consanguinity	—	6/11
Neurological abnormalities in patients in families without consanguinity	—	13/22

Table 5 lists the occurrence of multiple skin cancers of different histopathological types. Essentially no skin cancer patients other than those with XP have multiple skin cancer in Japan, and the XP patients in Table 5 may represent almost all recorded cases of multiple skin cancer consisting of different histopathological types. Also, nearly half of the XP patients with skin cancer have multiple skin cancer of the same histopathological type. These results suggest the involvement of DNA repair deficiency in the etiology of skin cancer in XP patients.

V. XERODERMA PIGMENTOSUM IN KOREA AND CHINA

In collaboration with colleagues in Korean and China, surveys of XP patients in these countries are in progress. Although cellular studies are still at the planning stage, genetic epidemiological studies in comparison to Japanese patients have been carried out. Table 6 compares XP patients in two southern cities in Korea — Kwangju[29] and Pusan — and those in Osaka, Japan. Thses cities are at almost identical latitudes and weather conditions so that the effects of solar UV light are expected to be similar. Striking difference was noted in the frequency of patients with neurological abnormalities, despite almost similar average age of the patients. Another major difference is that no consanguinous marriage in parents of the patients were recorded in Korea, while 35% of Osaka families were consanguinous. This is probably due to the law and tradition in Korea to avoid consanguinous marriage. As shown in Table 6, incidence of neurological abnormalities is not related to consanguinity. Possible reason for the absence of the patients with neurological abnormalities could be due to the different distribution of genetic complementation groups in Korea and Japan. For example, if complementation group C is predominant in Korea, XP patients in Korea could develop symptoms as early as group A patients but essentially no neurological abnormalities would develop. One XP patient in Korea has been identified as belonging to complementation group C[30] and two others with low UDS levels were found not belonging to group A (Takebe, unpublished) suggesting this possibility. Further DNA repair tests are planned. In China, 44 patients were recorded and 7 had neurological abnormalities. Consanguinous marriages were involved in approximately half of the patients, and the age distribution of the patients appears to be similar to that in Japanese, but data are still too few to draw conclusions.[31]

VI. DNA REPAIR DEFICIENCY AND CANCER

A. Cancer-Prone Hereditary Diseases with Possible DNA Repair Defects

Among the several cancer-prone hereditary diseases which are suggested to involve DNA repair deficiency, XP is the only disease with solid evidence of the defect in repair of DNA damage. Also, the exact cause of skin cancer in XP is clearly solar UV light. Other diseases such as ataxia telangiectasia, Bloom's syndrome, and Fanconi's anemia may be associated with DNA repair deficiency, but no dependable experimental data exists to explain the mechanism of disease or the cause of cancer in these patients. Another difference between XP and other cancer-prone diseases is that XP cells behave normally unless they are subjected to some agents such as UV or UV-mimetic chemicals, while ataxia telangiectasia, Bloom's syndrome, and Fanconi's anemia have "built-in" defects which cause chromosome instability without any treatment by external agents. Consequently, discussions relating to DNA repair deficiency and the mechanism of carcinogenesis should be confined to XP.

B. Mutation in Xeroderma Pigmentosum Cells

One of the most attractive hypotheses for the mechanism of carcinogenesis is the somatic mutation theory. Ample evidence supporting the hypothesis that mutation is the initiating event for cancer has been presented. Recent progress in the studies on oncogenes supplies further support. Induction of mutation in XP cells by UV and some carcinogenic chemicals clearly showed that the XP cells are hypermutable against the agents which give higher cytotoxicity to XP cells than to normal cells.[32,33]

In microorganisms, the mechanism of UV mutagenesis has been extensively investigated and the SOS response has been implicated with solid supporting evidence. In human cells, no mutant cell lines corresponding to the key prokaryote mutants in investigating the SOS responses, such as *recA*, *lexA*, and *umuC*, have been isolated, nor found in cells originating from hereditary diseases. Attempts to demonstrate the presence of an SOS-type inducible error-prone repair in human cells have not yielded reliable evidence despite the pioneering work by Sarasin.[34] Consequently, even in XP cells, the somatic mutation theory of cancer still remains as a hypothesis.

In other cancer-prone hereditary diseases of autosomal recessive inheritance (ataxia telangiectasia, Bloom's syndrome, and Fanconi's anemia), little data has been presented to show the relationship between mutation and cancer.[35] In these diseases, the chromosome instability could be more responsible than the processing of DNA damages through repair or replication, although no experimental evidence has been presented.

As already mentioned, association of neurological abnormalities in some of the patients has not been explained. Neurological abnormalities are found in most XP patients belonging to complementation groups A and D, group A patients being much more severe than group D in general. Possible damage in neuron cells due to the reduced repair capacity during early stage of development was suggested[36] but the absence of similar damage in group C patients whose repair capacities are also considerably reduced is not clearly explained.

C. DNA Repair Genes and Mechanisms

Despite enzymatic studies of DNA repair process in human cells, our understanding of the mechanism of DNA repair deficiency is far from complete. The presence of nine complementation groups may imply that the enzyme, presumably UV-DNA endonuclease, may consist of nine subunits if analogy with *Escherichia coli* is taken. No experimental data concerning the mechanism of complementation have been presented. A gene compensating the defect in group A XP cells was mapped on human chromosome #1, provisionally. Attempts to clone the genes responsible for human DNA repair have not been successful except for a gene compensating DNA repair defect in Chinese hamster cells, ERCC1.[37]

Successful restoration of repair capacity in XP group A cells by transfecting normal human DNA was reported[38] but has not been reproducible in many laboratories.

D. Non-Skin Cancers in Xeroderma Pigmentosum Patients

Although correlation between DNA repair defect and skin cancer is well established in XP, a question was raised whether XP patients develop more cancers of internal organs than normal subjects.[39] Kraemer et al.[40] surveyed more than 700 published records of XP patients and found that the age-adjusted frequency of non-skin cancer in XP patients 0 to 19 years of age was approximately 12 times higher than in the normal control population. Only four non-skin cancers were found in XP patients listed in Table 1, and no conclusion may be drawn from this survey. A high incidence of skin cancer in parents of XP patients was reported and the enhanced cancer susceptibility in heterozygotes of XP genes was proposed[41] as in heterozygotes of the ataxia telangiectasia gene.[42] In our survey, none of the parents of XP patients developed skin cancer, presumably reflecting the very low susceptibility of Japanese to skin cancer. Whether XP heterozygotes are more susceptible to cancer of organs other than skin remains to be answered.

ACKNOWLEDGMENTS

The authors wish to thank the Japanese Cancer Association for permission to reproduce data in the tables, and Drs. Takehito Kozuka, Kenji Sato, Masao Inoue, Masao S. Sasaki, Kiyoji Tanaka, Mituo Ikenaga, and Yoshisada Fujiwara for their continuous cooperation throughout the survey. Cooperation by Drs. Y. P. Kim and Z. -S. Jiang in obtaining data from Korea and China, respectively, is greatly appreciated. This work was supported by Grant-in-Aid for Cancer Research from the Ministry of Education, Science, and Culture, the Japan Society for Promotion of Sciences, and by Nissan Science Foundation.

REFERENCES

1. **Cleaver, J. E.,** Defective repair replication of DNA in xeroderma pigmentosum, *Nature,* 218, 652, 1968.
2. **Takebe, H., Miki, Y., Kozuka, T., Furuyama, J., Tanaka, K., Sasaki, M. S., Fujiwara, Y., and Akiba, H.,** DNA repair characteristics and skin cancers of xeroderma pigmentosum in Japan, DNA repair characteristics and skin cancers of xeroderma pigmentosum in Japan, *Cancer Res.,* 37, 490, 1977.
3. **Takebe, H.,** Xeroderma pigmentosum: DNA repair defects and skin cancer, in *Progress in Cancer Biochemistry* (Gann Monograph on Cancer Research, 24), Sugimura, T., Endo, H., Ono T., and Sugano, H., Eds., Japan Scientific Society Press, Tokyo, 1979, 103.
4. **Takebe, H., Yagi, T., and Satoh, Y.,** Cancer-prone hereditary diseases in relation to DNA repair, in *Biology of Cancer,* Vol 1, (13th Int. Cancer Congress, Part B), Mirand, E. A., Hutchinson, W. B., and Mihichi, E., Eds., Alan R. Liss, New York, 1983, 267.
5. **Takebe, H., Tatsumi, K., and Satoh, Y.,** DNA repair and its possible involvment in the origin of multiple cancer, *Jpn. J. Clin. Oncol.,* 15(Suppl. 1), 299, 1985.
6. **Robbins, J. H., Kraemer, K. H., Lutzner, M. A., Festoff, B. W., and Coon, H. G.,** Xeroderma pigmentosum. An inherited disease with sun sensitivity, multiple cutaneous neoplasmas, and abnormal DNA repair, *Ann. Intern. Med.,* 80, 221, 1974.
7. **Mimaki, T., Itoh, N., Abe, J., Tagawa, T., Sato, K., Yabuuchi, H., and Takebe, H.,** Neurological manifestations in xeroderma pigmentosum, *Ann. Neurol.,* 20, 70, 1986.
8. **Imaizumi, Y., Shinozaki, N., and Aoki, H.,** Inbreeding in Japan: results of a nation-wide study, *Jpn. J. Hum. Genet.,* 20, 91, 1975.
9. **de Weerd-Kastelein, E. A., Keijzer, W., and Bootsma, D.,** Genetic heterogeneity of xeroderma pigmentosum demonstrated by somatic cell hybridization, *Nature, New Biol.,* 238, 80, 1972.
10. **Kraemer, K. H., de Weerd-Kastelein, E. A., Robbins, J. H., Keijzer, W., Barrentt, S. F., Petinga, R. A., and Bootsma, D.,** Five complementation groups of xeroderma pigmentosum, *Mutat. Res.,* 33, 327, 1979.

11. **Arase, S., Kozuka, T., Tanaka, K., Ikenaga, M., and Takebe, H.,** A sixth complementation group of xeroderma pigmentosum, *Mutat. Res.,* 59, 143, 1979.
12. **Keijzer, W., Jaspers, N. G. J., Abrahams, P. J., Taylor, A. M. R., Arlett, C. F., Zelle, B., Takebe, H., Kinmont, P. D. S., and Bootsma, D.,** A seventh complementation group in excision deficient xeroderma pigmentosum, *Mutat. Res.,* 62, 183, 1979.
13. **Moshell, A. N., Ganges, M. B., Lutzner, M. A., Coon, H. G., Barrett, S. F., Dupuy, J. M., and Robbins, J. H.,** A new patient with both xeroderma pigmentosum and Cockayne syndrome establishes a new xeroderma pigmentosum complementation group H, in *Cellular Responses to DNA Damage,* Friedberg, E. C. and Bridges, B. A., Eds., Alan R. Liss, New York, 1983, 209.
14. **Fischer, E., Keijzer, W., Thielman, H. W., Popanda, O., Bohnert, E., Edler, L., Lung, E. G., and Bootsma, D.,** A ninth complementation group in xeroderma pigmentosum, XP. I, *Mutat. Res.,* 145, 217, 1985.
15. **Lehmann, A. R., Kirk-Bell, S., Arlett, C. F., Paterson, M. C., Lohman, P. H., de Weerd-Kastelein, E. A., and Bootsma, D.,** Xeroderma pigmentosum cells with normal levels of excision repair have a defect in DNA synthesis after UV irradiation, *Proc. Natl. Acad. Sci. U.S.A.,* 72, 219, 1975.
16. **Cleaver, J. E. and Bootsma, D.,** Xeroderma pigmentosum. Biochemical and genetic characteristics, *Annu. Rev. Genet.,* 9, 18, 1975.
17. **Kraemer, K. H.,** Heritable diseases with increased sensitivity to cellular injury, in *Update: Dermatology in General Medicine,* Fizpatrick, T. B., Eisen, A. Z., Wolff, K., Freedberg, I. M., and Austin, K. F., Eds., McGraw-Hill, New York, 1983, 113.
18. **Freidberg, E. C.,** *DNA Repair,* W. H. Freeman, New York, 1984, chap. 9.
19. **Fujiwara, Y. and Satoh, Y.,** Assignment of two Japanese xeroderma pigmentosum patients to complementation group D and their characteristics, *Jpn. J. Cancer Res. (Gann),* 76, 162, 1985.
20. **Fujiwara, Y., Uehara, Y., Ichihashi, M., and Nishioka, K.,** Xeroderma pigmentosum complementation group F: more assignments and repair characteristics, *Photochem. Photobiol.,* 41, 629, 1985.
21. **Fujiwara, Y., Uehara, Y., Ichihashi, M., Yamamoto, Y., and Nishioka, K.,** Assignment of two patients with xeroderma pigmentosum to complementation group E, *Mutat. Res.,* 135, 51, 1985.
22. **Ichihashi, M., Fujiwara, Y., Uehara, Y., and Matsumoto, A.,** A mild form of xeroderma pigmentosum assigned to complementation group G and its repair heterogeneity, *J. Invest. Dermatol.,* 85, 284, 1985.
23. **Fujiwara, Y., Ichihashi, M., Uehara, Y., Matsumoto, A., Yamamoto, Y., Kano, Y., and Tanakura, Y.,** Xeroderma pigmentosum groups C and F: additional assignments and a review of the subjects in Japan, *J. Radiat. Res.,* 26, 443, 1985.
24. **Ichihashi, M. and Fujiwara, Y.,** Clinical and photobiological characteristics of Japanese xeroderma pigmentosum variant, *Br. J. Dermatol.,* 105, 1, 1981.
25. **Fischer, E., Schnyder, U. W., and Jung, E. G.,** Report of three sisters with XP-E, a rare xeroderma pigmentosum complementation group, *Photodermatology,* 1, 242, 1984.
26. **Hayakawa, H., Ishizaki, K., Inoue, M., Yagi, T., Sekiguchi, M., and Takebe, H.,** Repair of ultraviolet radiation damage in xeroderma pigmentosum cells belonging to complementation group F, *Mutat. Res.,* 80, 381, 1981.
27. **Miyaji, T.,** Skin cancers in Japan: a nationwide 5-year survey, 1956—1960, *Natl. Cancer Inst. Monogr.,* 10, 55, 1962.
28. **Tada, M. and Miki, Y.,** Malignant skin tumors among dermatology patient in university hospitals of Japan. A statistical survey 1971—1975, *J. Dermatol.,* 11, 313, 1984.
29. **Hwang, S. W., Yoo, Y. E., and Kim, Y. P.,** The genetics and clinical studies of xeroderma pigmentosum, *Korean J. Dermatol.,* 20, 879, 1982.
30. **Park, S. D. and Chung, H. Y.,** Characterization of a Korean xeroderma pigmentosum cell strain, XP1SE, by somatic cell hybridization and complementation studies, *Korean J. Genet.,* 4, 69, 1982.
31. **Jiang, Z., Hu, Y., Chen, Q., and Yang, L.,** Study of DNA repair enzyme system. I. Ultraviolet-induced ^{3}H-TdR unscheduled incorporation in xeroderma pigmentosum lymphocytes, *Acta Genet. Sinica,* 8, 310, 1981.
32. **McCormick, J. J. and Maher, V. M.,** Mammalian cell mutagenesis as a biological consequence of DNA damage, in *DNA Repair Mechanisms,* Hanawalt, P. C., Friedberg, E. C., and Fox, C. F., Eds., Academic Press, New York, 1979, 739.
33. **Tatsumi, K., Toyoda, M., Hashimoto, T., Furuyama, J., Kurihara, T., Inoue, M., and Takebe, H.,** Differential hypersensitivity of xeroderma pigmentosum cell lines to ultraviolet light mutagenesis, *Carcinogenesis,* in press.
34. **Sarasin, A.,** The use of DNA viruses as probe for studying DNA repair pathways in eucaryotic cells, in *Radiation Research* Proc. 6th Int. Cong. Radiation Research, Okada, S., Imamura, M., Terashima, T., and Yamaguchi, H., Eds., Maruzen, Tokyo, 1979, 462.
35. **Takebe, H. and Tatsumi, K.,** Genetically high-risk population for cancer and mutation by environmental mutagens, in *Genetic Toxicology of Environmental Chemicals, Part B: Genetic Effects and Applied Mutagenesis,* Proc. 4th Int. Conf. Environ. Mutagens, Ramel, C., Lambert, B., and Magnusson, J., Eds., Alan R. Liss, New York, 1986, 213.

36. **Andrews, A. D., Barrett, S. A., and Robbins, J. H.,** Xeroderma pigmentosum neurological abnormalities correlate with colony-forming ability after ultraviolet radiation, *Proc. Natl. Acad. Sci. U.S.A.*, 75, 1984, 1978.
37. **Westerveld, A., Hoeijmakers, J. H. J., van Duin, M., de Wit, J., Odijk, H., Pastink, A., Wood, R. D., and Bootsma, D.,** Molecular cloning of a human DNA repair gene, *Nature,* 310, 425, 1984.
38. **Takano, T., Noda, M., and Tamura, T.,** Transfection of cells from a xeroderma pigmentosum patient with normal human DNA confers UV resistance, *Nature,* 296, 269, 1982.
39. **Cairns, J.,** The origin of human cancers, *Nature,* 289, 353, 1981.
40. **Kraemer, K. H., Lee, M. M., and Scotto, J.,** DNA repair protects against cutaneous and internal neoplasia: evidence from xeroderma pigmentosum, *Carcinogenesis,* 5, 511, 1984.
41. **Swift, M. and Chase, C.,** Cancer in families with xeroderma pigmentosum, *J. Natl. Cancer Inst.*, 62, 1415, 1979.
42. **Swift, M., Shlomon, L., Perry, M., and Chase, C.,** Malignant noeplasms in the families of patients with ataxia telangiectasia, *Cancer Res.*, 36, 209, 1976.

Chapter 10

ATAXIA TELANGIECTASIA AND OTHER α-FETOPROTEIN-ASSOCIATED DISORDERS

John A. Johnson

TABLE OF CONTENTS

I. INTRODUCTION

Ataxia telangiectasia (AT) has been exhaustively described, discussed, and investigated for several decades. Various aspects of the disorder have been analyzed by experts, and will be briefly discussed as appropriate. Instead of extensive coverage of thoroughly discussed subjects, I propose to present a biochemist's view of a topic that is often mentioned in association with AT, but rarely discussed in detail: elevated serum α-fetoprotein (AFP). Since AFP is the subject of about 400 reports per year,[1] its possible relationship to AT merits close attention. Two other hereditary disorders, tyrosinemia type I and adenosine deaminase deficiency, are also characterized by elevated AFP. These disorders will be discussed to provide insight concerning elevated AFP and metabolic disease, but only AT will receive the full treatment of an epidemiologic discussion.

II. OCCURRENCE AND PROGNOSIS

AT is an autosomal recessive disorder characterized by the occurrence of cerebellar ataxia at an early age, followed by oculocutaneous telangiectasia and symptoms of immundeficiency.[2,3] Consistent with immunologic flaws, patients often have an undeveloped thymus or lack it completely. This feature, and consistently elevated serum AFP, suggest a defect in tissue differentiation or maturation. Reduced levels of immunoglobulin A, the component imparting immunity to mucosal surfaces,[4] renders patients susceptible to recurrent sinopulmonary infections. These persons also exhibit clinical and experimental hypersensitivity to X-rays and other forms of γ-radiation.

The prevalence of AT in California has been estimated at 1 in 40,000 persons.[2] On the other hand, Swift et al.[5] estimated the incidence of AT in the U.S. in the years 1965 to 1969 was 3 per 1 million live births. As noted by Boder,[2] the disease is relentlessly progressive. Because of the great variety of symptoms, treatment is highly individualized and designed to slow progression of the disorder. Carefully planned physical therapy may keep patients ambulatory until young adulthood. Because of the high risk for pulmonary disease and cancer, many patients have not survived to adulthood. However, in a current case-finding study, Swift[6] reported that about 50% of white probands live to age 20. Malignancy occurs in patients at a rate of 10%[7] to 20%.[8] Of the 52 cancers reported by Morrell et al.,[8] the overwhelming majority were lymphomas (60%) and leukemias (27%). Spector et al.[9] noted that about one third of the cases collected in the Immunodeficiency Cancer Registry are AT patients. A list of malignancies in 108 patients from 22 countries included lymphomas (55%) and leukemias (24%). Kraemer et al.[3] pointed out that cancer types in AT patients are those encountered in immunodeficiency disease rather than those induced by γ-radiation. Not surprisingly, cancer is a major cause of death in AT. Boder[2] noted that in 57 published cases and 44 of her patients, about 20% died of malignancy, 50% of pulmonary disease, and 30% of both. Some investigators[10] are not convinced that pulmonary disease is a major risk factor. This circumstance may reflect greater current awareness of AT, resulting in diagnosis of less severe cases, and rigorous application of prophylactic measures. Because reduction of pulmonary infections will allow patients to live longer, malignancy may become the dominant lethal factor in AT. Consequently, the need for future epidemiologic studies is even more pressing than it has been in the past.

III. EXPERIMENTAL INVESTIGATIONS

A. Biochemical Studies

Extensive studies have been conducted with skin fibroblasts and lymphoblastoid cell lines to examine their responses to γ-radiation and chemical agents. This topic has been discussed in detail by McKinnon.[11] The major type of DNA damage consists of single- and double-strand breaks. This damage appears to be repaired in normal fashion; however, a high resolution technique[12] revealed that more unrepaired breaks occurred in AT cells than in controls. Furthermore, Cox et al.[13] addressed a topic that is often overlooked: fidelity of DNA repair. They reported that the rate of misrepair of double-strand breaks in AT cells was much higher than normal.

Although the nature of the defect in DNA repair is unresolved, AT cells exhibit two characteristic responses to γ-radiation: (1) hypersensitivity as reflected by reduced survival and (2) radioresistance, in that DNA replication is not inhibited as it is in control cells. These characteristics are separable, as demonstrated by Lehmann et al.[14] They isolated a clone from cultured AT cells that had acquired normal radiosensitivity but retained radioresistant DNA synthesis. Also, Mohamed and Lavin[15] reported that extracts of AT lymphoblastoid cells conferred radioresistant DNA synthesis on control cells. Alternatively, Fiorilli et al.[16] described two patients with late onset of symptoms whose irradiated lymphoblastoid cells exhibited normal inhibition of DNA synthesis.

B. Cytogenetic Studies

A consistent finding with AT patients is the high level of spontaneous and radiation-induced chromosomal abnormalities in lymphocytes and cultured fibroblasts. Experimental studies have been discussed in a current review[11] and will not be detailed here. The *in vivo* development of lymphocyte clones in association with leukemia and lymphoma merits comment.

Al Saadi et al.[17] monitored four patients for several years, and followed the development of clones with 14;14 translocations. They proposed that chromosomes of AT cells undergo numerous alterations, most of which do not permit cell survival. Cells with rearranged chromosome 14 were stable and underwent clonal selection. The authors cited examples in support of the premise that rearrangement, t(14q12;14q32), and loss of the small centric portion of the broken 14 may precede development of cancer. Kaiser-McCaw and Hecht[18] described three cases where T-cell leukemia clones emerged with t(14q12;14q32) and loss of the 14q-chromosome. Thus, it appears that AT lymphocytes have 14q12 break points that confer selective advantage before development of malignancy. On the other hand, a fourth patient had some cells with the 14;14 translocation, but the malignant clone developed from cells with normal chromosomes.

In keeping with the numerous observations of chromosomal abnormalities, a clastogenic factor has been detected in plasma of AT patients and in the medium of cultured fibroblasts.[19] The presence of such a factor in amniotic fluid has been employed for prenatal diagnosis of AT.[20,21]

IV. PHENOTYPIC EXPRESSION OF THE ATAXIA TELANGIECTASIA GENE

A. Heterogeneity of the Disorder

Because of the wide variety of symptoms and the variable age of onset of specific defects, it was long suspected that AT is a heterogeneous disorder. Hecht and Kaiser-McCaw[22] tentatively defined several classes, mainly by clinical criteria. Chen et al.[23] conducted complementation studies by fusing lymphoblastoid cell lines from four normals, five heterozygotes and seven homozygotes. They classified the AT cell lines into four complementation groups, and demonstrated a gene dosage effect of increasing radiosensitivity with increasing number of AT alleles in heterokaryons. Jaspers et al.[24] reviewed 4 different studies (including the above-mentioned one) of patients from 17 unrelated families, and concluded there were at least 4 and possibly 9 complementation groups. Thus, both clinical and genetic heterogeneity are well established.

B. Cancer Risk of Heterozygotes

A convenient test for carriers of the AT gene is long overdue. Recent studies have been conducted on the basis of cellular hypersensitivity to chronic γ-radiation,[25] radiation-induced chromosomal abnormalities,[26] postirradiation cumulative labeling index,[27] and G2 chromosomal radiosensitivity.[28] Many procedures are cumbersome because they require cultured skin fibroblasts; some[26] employ lymphoblastoid cell lines. Rosin and Ochs[29] developed a procedure based on oral-cavity swabs and urine samples. This noninvasive exfoliated cell micronucleus test detected the seven AT heterozygotes tested, but it is not clear how specific the test is for the AT gene.

Although Reed et al.[30] noted the increased frequency of cancer in relatives of AT patients, lack of a definitive test for heterozygosity impeded statistical validation. Despite this lack, Swift and colleagues have amassed increasingly convincing evidence of elevated cancer risk in blood relatives. Swift et al.[31] studied 110 newly identified white AT families. Relatives had a considerable excess of breast cancer, as well as excess numbers of bladder, endometrial, prostate, and skin cancers. There was also an excess of hematologic and lymphoid malignancies, including lymphomas and leukemias. The pattern of cancer types in relatives resembles that of homozygous patients, with elevated occurrence of late-onset malignancy such as breast cancer. Swift and colleagues have established a registry for AT in the U.S., with two primary goals (Swift, personal communication): (1) identification of new probands and families, and prospective follow-up of known families and (2) establishment of lymphoblastoid cell lines from patients and their relatives. A portion of each cell line is deposited in the Human Genetic Cell Depository (Institute for Medical Research, Camden, NJ) for use by interested investigators; the remainder is stored for linkage studies and in anticipation of development of a test for heterozygosity. (Such future testing would constitute the ultimate "blind" study.)

Since AT carriers are at increased risk for cancer, it is important to know the frequency of the AT gene. Estimates based on disease incidence must be adjusted for the existence of complementation groups by a factor of approximately the square root of the number of groups. This conclusion is based on the assumption that gene carriers from different complementation groups cannot have affected offspring. However, it must be noted that the existence of complementation groups has not been established to the degree that has been documented for xeroderma pigmentosum patients. Also, it is not certain that the endpoints of the various AT complementation assays truly represent phenotypic expression of the disease. Swift et al.,[5] on the basis of four complementation groups, estimated a gene frequency range of 0.68 to 7.7%, with a best estimate of 2.8%. Currently[31] they employed an estimate of 1.4% to calculate that 8.8% of all persons with breast cancer are heterozygous for AT.

C. α-Fetoprotein

One of the most intriguing aspects of AT is the occurrence of elevated plasma AFP in most but not all patients (Berkel, discussion after Dugaiczyk et al., Reference 32 and References 33 to 37). Unfortunately, heterozygous relatives do not have intermediate levels; they may be normal[35] or even have very high AFP.[33] There are many tantalizing clues linking AFP with a variety of metabolic disorders. Consequently, the topic will be discussed in detail in hopes of providing new insight into the relationship of AFP to AT. Since human AFP differs from that of other species in several important aspects, remarks will refer to the human protein unless otherwise noted.

1. Instances of Elevated α-Fetoprotein

Because plasma AFP is elevated in pregnancy, much attention has been directed to its immunosuppressive actions. Keller et al.[38] discussed the possible relationship of AFP to the immunodeficiency symptoms of AT. Although there appeared to be no direct connection, it was suggested that lack of cell-surface AFP receptors may be one aspect of tissue immaturity in AT. Plasma AFP is elevated in a variety of dissimilar circumstances: impaired liver function,[39] carcinoma,[40,41] tyrosinemia type I,[42] and in patients with severe combined immunodeficiency disease (SCID), with and without adenosine deaminase (ADA) deficiency.[43] In addition, elevated AFP has been reported in systemic lupus erythematosus[44] and instances of benign hereditary elevated AFP have been reported.[45]

2. Glycosylation Variants of α-Fetoprotein and Their Diagnostic Value

Usual sources of AFP are fetal liver, yolk sac and gastrointestinal tract,[46,47] and germ-cell[46] and hepatic carcinomas.[40] The elevated AFP in AT patients is thought to arise from immature liver cells; and indeed, Ohama and Ikuta[48] demonstrated AFP in hepatocytes of autopsy specimens. Likewise, although liver symptoms are absent or mild, about 45% of AT patients have abnormal function tests.[40] Several glycosylation forms of AFP are known[49] and their distribution pattern is characteristic of the tissue source. Therefore, AFP has been studied not only as a tumor marker[50-52] but also a diagnostic aid for tumor type.[53,54] The AFP levels in AT patients range from normal to very high, vary widely between siblings and even in the same patient, and are not correlated with liver function (see Reference 32). Therefore, it seems advisable to determine the variant pattern(s) of plasma AFP in AT patients. This was suggested by Berkel (discussion after Dugaiczyk et al.,[32]) but appears not to have been reported yet.

3. Control of the α-Fetoprotein Gene

What, then, might be the relationship, if any, of AFP to the clinical expression of AT? Perhaps consideration of control of the AFP gene will be helpful.

a. Developmental Expression

Embryonic production of AFP begins in the yolk sac and later switches to the liver. In this later stage, all fetal liver cells except the hematopoietic ones produce AFP.[46] As development proceeds, AFP production tapers off; synthesis of a homologous protein, albumin, becomes increasingly important. Although AFP production and albumin synthesis are coordinated in reciprocal fashion, the processes are independent. Thus, in analbuminemic rats, AFP synthesis decreased almost normally after birth.[55]

b. Hypomethylation and Gene Expression

Much attention is being directed to the topic of gene expression and methylation of DNA. Holliday[56] described control of gene expression by postsynthetic methylation of cytosine. This activity is catalyzed by a maintenance transmethylase which acts on hemimethylated DNA after replication. Since hypomethylation is associated with gene expression, hereditary defects in methylation could lead to inappropriate expression of, or failure to turn off, fetal genes. The controversy concerning methylation and gene expression has been discussed in detail by Sell et al.[57] Some contradictions may be explained on the basis that undermethylation may be a necessary but not sufficient condition for transcription, as observed by Ott et al.[58] for albumin production by cultured rat hepatoma cells. A similar rationale was presented by Locker et al.[59] They observed that liver tumors arising in rats on a choline-deficient diet had a methylation pattern similar to that of the active AFP gene of fetal liver, but did not produce increased amounts of AFP messenger RNA. Other anomalies may be resolved by the model proposed by Weiss et al.[60] for the albumin gene: expression seems to retard its methylation, whereas inactivity permits slow methylation to occur. Once methylation occurs, the probability of gene expression is low, but it can occur in an unstable fashion.

Whatever the ultimate relationship between methylation and gene expression, it is tempting to propose that elevated AFP in AT is due to defective methylation. The compulsion is strengthened by the suggestion[61] that hypomethylation may cause carcinogenic chromosomal rearrangement, a process that occurs in AT patients (see Section III.B).

4. Hereditary Tysosinemia Type I, Elevated α-Fetoprotein, and Hepatocarcinoma

This rare autosomal recessive disorder is characterized by high plasma tyrosine, methionine and AFP,[42] and vitamin D-resistant rickets.[62] The latter symptom may be significant in view of the homology between AFP and vitamin D binding protein.[63] Some patients excrete high levels of δ-aminolevulinic acid (ALA) and exhibit symptoms of acute intermittent porphyria (AIP).[64] Those children born with severe hepatorenal disturbance have a poor prognosis because of progressive cirrhosis and early development of hepatomas. Early initiation of a diet low in tyrosine and phenylalanine is helpful. The diet may also resolve methioninemia[65] but methionine restriction (at least initially) is required for some patients.[66-68] Neonates with severe involvement may not benefit from dietary restriction.[69] Most reports relate to persons with severe hepatorenal disease, but some patients survive to young adulthood.

Low levels of several hepatic enzymes involved in tyrosine degradation have been reported. The key deficiency appears to be lack of fumarylacetoacetate hydrolase (FAH),[64] perhaps accompanied by low levels of *p*-hydroxyphenylpyruvic acid (*p*-HPPA) oxidase.[70,71] Since only liver and kidney contain *p*-HPPA oxidase, the enzyme catalyzing the first irreversible step in tyrosine catabolism, these tissues are most susceptible to damage by tyrosine metabolites. Activity of FAH may provide a test for heterozygosity, since parents of tyrosinemia patients have intermediate levels in their erythrocytes[72] and lymphocytes.[73] Deficient hepatic FAH activity results in accumulation of fumarylacetoacetate and two unusual derivatives, succinylacetoacetate (SAA) and succinylacetone (SA). The fact that SA strongly inhibits ALA dehydratase[74] explains the elevated ALA levels and occurrence of symptoms of AIP. It has also been reported that SA strongly inhibits DNA methylase in rat liver.[75]

Several observations suggest an association between reduced methionine utilization (i.e., decreased methylation capacity) and persistance of AFP production in tyrosinemia patients. Thus, hepatic methionine adenosyltransferase (MAT) is low[76] and ATP (MAT cosubstrate) is greatly reduced.[75] Belanger et al.[42] observed that in patients who responded to administration of pyridoxine and ATP to improve methionine metabolism, serum AFP decreased in concert with methionine. These observations are consistent with the premise that reduced methylation capacity delays methylation of the AFP gene, allowing AFP production to persist. Hancock[77] employed a similar rationale to link tyrosinemia, AFP, and hepatocarcinoma.

The foregoing considerations imply that defective tyrosine catabolism accounts for the major biochemical aberrations of tyrosinemia type I. However, the relationship is not absolute for methionine, as evidenced by the need (mentioned earlier) to restrict methionine intake of patients. With regard to AFP, I have encountered no reports of long-term monitoring of AFP levels during dietary restriction. Elevated AFP is only partially resolved by dietary restriction of tyrosine[71] or tyrosine, phenylalanine, and methionine.[66,78] Failure of dietary restriction to reduce AFP levels to normal is consistent with the concept that the tyrosinemia patient's liver is locked in a fetal state of differentiation.[42] This premise is supported by the observations of Liau et al.[79] on three tyrosinemia patients who died of massive cirrhosis; liver specimens displayed a fetal isozyme pattern for MAT. Likewise, fetal-type pyruvate kinase and aldolase were present in livers of five patients.[80]

Patients with severe hepatorenal involvement are at high risk for hepatocellular carcinoma. Weinberg et al.[81] reported a 37% incidence in 43 patients, with median age at time of death from tumor of 5 years. All liver cancer patients had preceding hepatorenal dysfunction, not a surprising circumstance considering the rapid onset of tumors. Although a diet low in phenylalanine and tyrosine prolongs life, patients are still at risk for hepatomas. Therefore, it has been proposed that early liver transplantation, under semi-elective conditions, be considered.[71,82] It has also been pointed out that renal failure may occur if a patient lives long enough, and could be a late manifestation after liver transplantation.[83] Significantly, the three patients mentioned by Kvittingen et al.[83] were young adults (20, 22, and 23 years old).

Tyrosinemia type I has been discussed in detail, in hopes of discovering clues to the significance of elevated AFP in AT. Attempts to relate AFP to tyrosinemia were frustrated by conflicting reports of enzyme deficiencies and biochemical abnormalities, and by clinical heterogeneity of the disorder. Restriction of dietary tyrosine and phenylalanine seems to reduce massive AFP levels to moderately high ones, perhaps as a consequence of improved liver function. Subsequent accumulation of excessive AFP may be due to development of hepatomas[82] or hepatic fibrosis.[78,83] Resolution of the present confusion requires precise definition of tyrosinemia type I. Grenier et al.[84] pointed out that initiation of blood AFP determination as an adjunct to screening for blood tyrosine reduced the frequency of false positive results from 1 to 0.4%. Addition of a test for urinary SAA + SA virtually eliminates false positives. Inherent in this rationale is the assumption that tyrosinemia type I is defined by elevated plasma tyrosine and AFP, *and* FAH deficiency (as revealed by assay of liver tissue or presence of urinary SAA + SA). However, it is not clear at present that all patients with severe hepatorenal disturbance and high risk for liver cancer have FAH deficiency. The most consistent data available are from liver transplant patients. All three patients of Tuchman et al.[78] had urinary SAA and SA. Two patients had reduced urinary levels post-operatively, indicating FAH deficiency in extrahepatic tissue(s) as well. The patient of Kvittingen et al.[83] also excreted reduced amounts of SA after liver transplantation. Van Thiel et al.[71] had two patients with markedly decreased or absent hepatic FAH, and a third with reduced FAH who excreted SA. A fourth patient had reduced FAH (20% of normal) and nearly absent *p*-HPPA oxidase (4% of normal), yet excreted SA. Thus all eight patients with liver damage severe enough to justify transplantation had deficient hepatic FAH activity.

5. Hereditary Adenosine Deaminase Deficiency and Elevated α-Fetoprotein

As noted earlier (Section IV.C.1), some patients with SCID have elevated AFP.[43] This relationship was observed in 6 of 21 SCID patients with normal ADA activity, and appeared in 6 of 6 patients with ADA deficiency. Hereditary ADA deficiency is a rare autosomal recessive disorder occurring in about 20% of all SCID cases.[85] Most patients have moderate to severe leukopenia, impaired T-cell and B-cell function,[86] and virtual absence of T cells.[87] Approximately 90% of obligate heterozygotes have intermediate erythrocyte ADA levels that are characteristic for the carrier state.[85] Patients lacking ADA have high levels of the substrates adenosine and deoxyadenosine. The latter causes irreversible inactivation of *S*-adenosylhomocysteine hydrolase, thus interfering with methionine metabolism and with methylation reactions requiring the amino acid. Deoxy ATP also accumulates, and is cytotoxic to T cells. This action, coupled with reduced methylation capacity, strongly interferes with T-cell proliferation. These observations have been applied therapeutically with the use of deoxycoformycin, an ADA inhibitor, for treatment of T-cell leukemias.[86] The compromised methylation capacity of ADA-deficient persons provides a rationale for persistence of AFP production. However, although it must be recalled that some ADA-competent SCID patients also have elevated AFP,[43] it remains to be determined if all ADA-deficient persons tested will exhibit elevated AFP.

Severe ADA deficiency, if untreated, is fatal within the first 2 years of life.[87] Enzyme replacement by erythrocyte transfusion is effective for a few patients[87] but must be considered a stopgap measure. Currently, Hershfield et al.[88] reported success with intramuscular injection of ADA modified to increase its plasma half-life. This new procedure, of course, requires long-term evaluation. Transfusion of allogeneic histocompatible bone marrow from an unaffected sibling affords a permanent care, but the small size of many families limits the availability of compatible bone marrow.[87] Transplantation of haplocompatible parental bone marrow has been successful in many cases, but requires further validation.[87] The ultimate cure for ADA deficiency may be gene therapy, i.e., insertion of a normal ADA gene into the patient's bone marrow cell.[87]

Despite short life spans, SCID patients have an increased incidence of cancer.[89] However, little information is available for ADA-deficient persons. Of such persons identified in the Immunodeficiency Cancer Registry from the fall of 1975 to the spring of 1977, 18 did not have cancer.[90] Heterozygosity does not impart risk, since cancer incidence was not elevated in nine families of ADA-deficient SCID patients.[91] Because bone marrow transplantation is affording long-term survival of ADA-deficient patients, elevated incidence of specific cancer types may become apparent in the future.

Since ADA deficiency appears to be associated with elevated AFP levels as well as impaired methylation capacity, it is of interest to know the ADA status of AT patients. In conversations with several investigators, I gained the impression that extensive screening programs for impaired purine metabolism have been conducted for various immunodeficiency disorders, probably including AT. However, normal enzyme and metabolite levels were obtained and were not published. Frazelle et al.[92] reported that fibroblasts from patients with Fanconi anemia were hypersensitive to purine analogues, whereas AT cells exhibited normal survival. Although it appears the purine metabolism in AT patients is normal, I have encountered no direct evidence that ADA activity in AT erythrocytes has been examined. It is noteworthy that there are cases with little or no erythrocyte ADA, but with substantial activity in lymphoid cells.[93] These children are immunocompetent at 1 to 2 years of age, but there is reason to believe that their partial ADA deficiency may lead to a spectrum of immunodeficiency disorders as they become older.[85] The important point for consideration is that ADA can be absent in erythrocytes, while enzyme production in other blood cells affords partial or total compensation. If this condition existed in AT patients, then carriers might have intermediate erythrocyte values, and the long-awaited test for heterozygosity would be at hand. Development of such a test is so important that, no matter how low the chance of success, erythrocyte ADA in AT patients should be surveyed. If the study has been done and enzyme levels found to be normal, it merits publication.

6. *Significance of Elevated α-Fetoprotein in Ataxia Telangiectasia*

As revealed in Section II, AT patients are at high risk for lymphomas and leukemias, as is the case for SCID patients. At first glance, it appears that AT patients have little in common with tyrosinemia patients, since the latter have an overwhelming risk of hepatocellular carcinoma. However, this cancer is not unknown in AT; at least six cases have been reported since discussion of the first one in 1979.[9,94-97] Significantly, hepatic carcinoma developed in AT siblings[97] and in at least one instance, the cancer was discovered at autopsy.[95] The latter observation suggests that clinically silent hepatomas may have been overlooked in the past. It is also noteworthy that the four cases whose ages were specified were 13, 15, 22, and 24 years old. As improved therapy increases the life spans of AT patients, more of them may survive to develop late-onset symptoms such as hepatocellular carcinoma. Since plasma AFP is often a marker for hepatic tumors, it should be monitored in all AT patients. Special attention should be devoted to liver function of those who exhibit consistently high AFP levels.

V. ENVIRONMENTAL FACTORS AND ATAXIA TELANGIECTASIA

A. Etiology

Understanding the influence of environment on disease is facilitated by knowing the etiology of the disorder. However, development of a unifying concept for the multiple symptoms of AT is a formidable task. This model must reconcile such phenomena as neurologic disfunction, cutaneous abnormalities, immunodeficiencies, failure of tissue differentiation or maturation, and increased cancer risk in patients and their relatives. Waldman et al.[3] pointed out that radiosensitivity and potential defects in repair or synthesis of DNA may cause the degenerative changes of AT, whereas abnormal tissue differentiation could account for failure of tissue maturation and for immunodeficiency. Since these proposals are not mutually exclusive, a unifying principle may be involved. It was suggested that DNA repair enzymes could serve other cellular functions. Consequently, deficiencies causing aberrant DNA repair could also affect cellular recombination events and organ maturation.

An alternate unifying approach is consideration of defective cytoskeletal structure.[11] Although these aberrations are not conducive to normal embryonic development, McKinnon[11] suggested that defects such as actin anomalies might be expressed only at certain developmental stages. These aberrant expressions could affect tissue differentiation and maturation, as well as DNA repair processes.

Chromosome changes and leukemia were discussed in Section III.B. In a current report, Hecht and Kaiser-McCaw[98] pointed out that the frequent chromosome rearrangements of AT lymphocytes are simply a magnification of the normal condition. They also noted that the six preferred breakpoints in AT all involve genes of the immune system. This observation, plus the association of 14;14 translocations with leukemia (Section II.B), connect the immune system to lymphoid cancer.

B. Environmental Factors

1. Sunlight

The oculocutaneous telangiectasias of AT are of mainly venous origin,[2] and tend to be localized in sun-exposed areas.[2,30] Cohen et al.[96] reported telangiectasias not confined to sun-exposed areas, but their patients exhibited various degrees of photophobia. The excessive skin changes in AT patients after extensive sun exposure[30] and occurrence of multiple basal cell carcinomas and actinic keratoses in two patients in their twenties[2] suggests that sunlight is an etiologic factor in the cutaneous aspects of AT.

2. Cancer Therapy

In 1967, Gotoff et al.[99] reported for the first time that radiation treatment of AT patients has serious sequelae. Although the patient's lymphosarcoma was eliminated by a moderate tumor dose of 300 rad over 3 weeks, he died several months later as a result of severe radiation damage. In the interval since this classic report, oncologists have struggled with the problem of treating radiosensitive tumors in AT patients. Pritchard et al.[100] described a patient with Hodgkin's disease who succumbed to the effects of therapy several months after receiving 3000 rad of Cobalt radiation over 26 d. Radiation tests with cultured fibroblasts established the diagnosis of AT, but unfortunately the results were not available until after the therapy had been completed. The authors suggested that, if malignant cells of AT patients are also hypersensitive to radiation, smaller therapeutic doses may be effective. Abadir and Hakami[101] employed a similar rationale for treatment of lymphoma in an AT patient. Chemotherapy for 6 weeks, followed by 1600 rad of Cobalt radiation in 11 d, resolved the tumor. The patient was alive, without evidence of cancer, 5 years after initiation of treatment. Toledano and Lange[102] reviewed 20 known cases of AT and acute lymphoblastic leukemia. They reported 3-years remission in their patient after chemotherapy, and noted a few other prolonged remissions from the literature.

REFERENCES

1. **Bergstrand, C. G.,** Alphafetoprotein in paediatrics, *Acta Paediatr. Scand.*, 75, 1, 1986.
2. **Boder, E.,** Ataxia-telangiectasia: an overview, in *Ataxia-Telangiectasia: Genetics, Neuropathology, and Immunology of a Degenerative Disease of Childhood,* Gatti, R. A. and Swift, M., Eds., Alan R. Liss, New York, 1985, 1.
3. **Waldmann, T. A., Misiti, J., Nelson, D. L., and Kraemer, K. H.,** Ataxia-telangiectasia: a multisystem hereditary disease with immunodeficiency, impaired organ maturation, X-Ray hypersensitivity, and a high incidence of neoplasia, *Ann. Intern. Med.*, 99, 367, 1983.
4. **Berman, B. A. and Ross, R. N.,** Ataxia telangiectasia and immotile cilia syndrome: what do these disorders have in common?, *Cutis,* 29, 428, 1982.
5. **Swift, M., Morrell, D., Cromartie, E., Chamberlin, A. R., Skolnick, M. H., and Bishop, D. T.,** The incidence and gene frequency of ataxia-telangiectasia in the United States, *Am. J. Hum. Genet.*, 39, 573, 1986.
6. **Swift, M.,** Genetics and epidemiology of ataxia-telangiectasia, in *Ataxia-Telangiectasia: Genetics, Neuropathology, and Immunology of a Degenerative Disease of Childhood,* Gatti, R. A. and Swift, M., Eds., Alan R. Liss, New York, 1985, 133.
7. **Gelfand, E.,** General discussion, in *Ataxia-Telangiectasia: Genetics, Neuropathology, and Immunology of a Degenerative Disease of Childhood,* Gatti, R. A. and Swift, M., Eds., Alan R. Liss, New York, 1985, 353.
8. **Morrell, D., Cromartie, E., and Swift, M.,** Mortality and cancer incidence in 263 patients with ataxia-telangiectasia, *J. Natl. Cancer Inst.*, 77, 89, 1986.
9. **Spector, B. D., Filipovich, A. H., Perry, G. S., III, and Kersey, J. H.,** Epidemiology of cancer in ataxia-telangiectasia, in *Ataxia-Telangiectasia: A Cellular and Molecular Link Between Cancer, Neuropathology, and Immune Deficiency,* Bridges, B. A. and Harnden, D. G., Eds., John Wiley & Sons, New York, 1982, 103.
10. **Jason, J. M. and Gelfand, E. W.,** Diagnostic considerations in ataxia-telangiectasia, *Arch. Dis. Child.*, 54, 682, 1979.
11. **McKinnon, P. J.,** Ataxia-telangiectasia: an inherited disorder of ionizing-radiation sensitivity in man, *Hum. Genet.*, 75, 197, 1987.
12. **Cornforth, M. N. and Bedford, J. S.,** On the nature of a defect in cells from individuals with ataxia-telangiectasia, *Science,* 227, 1589, 1985.
13. **Cox, R., Debenham, P. G., Masson, W. K., and Webb, M. B. T.,** Ataxia-telangiectasia: a human mutation giving high-frequency misrepair of DNA double-stranded scissions, *Mol. Biol. Med.*, 3, 229, 1986.
14. **Lehmann, A. R., Arlett, C. F., Burke, J. F., Green, M. H. L., James, M. R., and Lowe, J. E.,** A derivative of an ataxia-telangiectasia (A-T) cell line with normal radiosensitivity but A-T like inhibition of DNA synthesis, *Int. J. Radiat. Biol.*, 49, 639, 1986.
15. **Mohamed, R. and Lavin, M. F.,** Ataxia-telangiectasia cell extracts confer radioresistant DNA synthesis on control cells, *Exp. Cell. Res.*, 163, 337, 1986.
16. **Fiorilli, M., Antonelli, A., Russo, G., Crescenzi, M., Carbonari, M., and Petrinelli, P.,** Variant of ataxia-telangiectasia with low-level radiosensitivity, *Hum. Genet.*, 70, 274, 1985.
17. **Al Saadi, A., Palutke, M., and Kumar, G. K.,** Evolution of chromosomal abnormalities in sequential cytogenetic studies of ataxia telangiectasia, *Hum. Genet.*, 55, 23, 1980.
18. **Kaiser-McCaw, B. and Hecht, F.,** Ataxia-telangiectasia; chromosomes and cancer, in *Ataxia-Telangiectasia: A Cellular and Molecular Link Between Cancer, Neuropathology, and Immune Deficiency,* Bridges, B. A. and Harnden, D. G., Eds., John Wiley & Sons, New York, 1982, 243.
19. **Shaham, M., Becker, Y., and Cohen, M. M.,** A diffusable clastogenic factor in ataxia telangiectasia, *Cytogenet. Cell. Genet.*, 27, 155, 1980.
20. **Becker, Y.,** Cancer in ataxia-telangiectasia patients: analysis of factors leading to radiation-induced and spontaneous tumors, *Anticancer Res.*, 6, 1031, 1986.
21. **Tsukahara, M., Masuda, M., Ohshiro, K., Kobayashi, K., Kajii, T., Ejima, Y., and Saskai, M. S.,** Ataxia telangiectasia with generalized skin pigmentation and early death, *Eur. J. Pediatr.*, 145, 121, 1986.
22. **Hecht, F. and Kaiser-McCaw, B.,** Ataxia-telangiectasia: genetics and heterogeneity, in *Ataxia-Telangiectasia: A Cellular and Molecular Link Between Cancer, Neuropathology, and Immune Deficiency,* Bridges, B. A. and Harnden, D. G., Eds., John Wiley & Sons, New York, 1982, 197.
23. **Chen, P., Imray, F. P., and Kidson, C.,** Gene dosage and complementation analysis of ataxia telangiectasia lymphoblastoid cell lines assayed by induced chromosome aberrations, *Mutat. Res.*, 129, 165, 1984.
24. **Jaspers, N. G. J., Painter, R. B., Paterson, M. C., Kidson, C., and Inoue, T.,** Complementation analysis of ataxia-telangiectasia, in *Ataxia-Telangiectasia: Genetics, Neuropathology, and Immunology of a Degenerative Disease of Childhood,* Gatti, R. A. and Swift, M., Eds., Alan R. Liss, New York, 1985, 147.

25. **Paterson, M. C., MacFarlane, S. J., Gentner, N. E., and Smith, B. P.,** Cellular hypersensitivity to chronic γ-radiation in cultured fibroblasts from ataxia-telangiectasia heterozygotes, in *Ataxia-Telangiectasia: Genetics, Neuropathology, and Immunology of a Degenerative Disease of Childhood,* Gatti, R. A. and Swift, M., Eds., Alan R. Liss, New York, 1985, 73.
26. **Kidson, C., Chen, P., and Imray, P.,** Ataxia-telangiectasia heterozygotes: dominant expression of ionizing radiation sensitive mutants, in *Ataxia-Telangiectasia: A Cellular and Molecular Link Between Cancer, Neuropathology, and Immune Deficiency,* Bridges, B. A. and Harnden, D. G., Eds., John Wiley & Sons, New York, 1982, 363.
27. **Nagasawa, H., Kramer, K. H., Shiloh, Y., and Little, J. F.,** Detection of ataxia telangiectasia heterozygous cell lines by postirradiation cumulative labeling index: measurements with coded samples, *Cancer Res.,* 47, 398, 1987.
28. **Shiloh, Y., Parshad, R., Sanford, K. K., and Jones, G. M.,** Carrier detection in ataxia-telangiectasia, *Lancet,* 1, 689, 1986.
29. **Rosin, M. P. and Ochs, H. D.,** In vivo chromosomal instability in ataxia-telangiectasia homozygotes and heterozygotes, *Hum. Genet.,* 74, 335, 1986.
30. **Reed, W. B., Epstein, W. L, Boder, E., and Sedgwick, R.,** Cutaneous manifestations of ataxia-telangiectasia, *JAMA,* 195, 746, 1966.
31. **Swift, M., Reitnauer, P. J., Morrell, D., and Chase, C. L.,** Breast and other cancers in families with ataxia-telangiectasia, *N. Engl. J. Med.,* 316, 1289, 1987.
32. **Dugaiczyk, A., Harper, M. E., and Minghetti, P. P.,** Chromosomal localization, structure, and expression of the human α-fetoprotein gene, in *Ataxia-Telangiectasia: Genetics, Neuropathology, and Immunology of a Degenerative Disease of Childhood,* Gatti, R. A. and Swift, M., Eds., Alan R. Liss, New York, 1985, 181.
33. **Gatti, R. A, Bick, M., Tam, C. F., Medici, M. A., Oxelius, V. A., Holland, M., Goldstein, A. L., and Border, E.,** Ataxia-telangiectasia: a multiparameter analysis of eight families, *Clin. Immunol. Immunopathol.,* 23, 501, 1982.
34. **Richkind, K. A., Boder, E., and Teplitz, R. L.,** Fetal proteins in ataxia-telangiectasia, *JAMA,* 248, 1346, 1982.
35. **Simons, M. J. and Hosking, C. S.,** A.F.P. and ataxia-telangiectasia, *Lancet,* 1, 1234, 1974.
36. **Sugimoto, R., Sawada, R., Tozawa, M., Kidowaki, T., Kusunoki, T., and Yamaguchi, N.,** Plasma levels of carcinoembryonic antigen in patients with ataxia-telangiectasia, *J. Pediatr.,* 92, 436, 1978.
37. **Waldman, T. A. and McIntire, K. R.,** Serum-alpha-fetoprotein levels in patients with ataxia-telangiectasia, *Lancet,* 2, 1112, 1972.
38. **Keller, R. J., Atwater, J. A., Martin, R. A., and Tomasi, T. B.,** Ataxia telangiectasia, immunodeficiency, and AFP: is there a relationship?, *UCLA Forum Med. Sci.,* 20, 27, 1978.
39. **Alpert, E. and Feller, E. R.,** α-Fetoprotein (AFP) in benign liver disease: evidence that normal liver regeneration does not induce AFP synthesis, *Gastroenterology,* 74, 856, 1978.
40. **Crandall, B. F.,** Alpha-fetoprotein: a review, *Crit. Rev. Clin. Lab. Sci.,* 15, 127, 1981.
41. **Klavins, J. V.,** Advances in biological markers for cancer, *Ann. Clin. Lab. Sci.,* 13, 275, 1983.
42. **Belanger, L., Baril, P., Guertin, M., Gingras, M. C., Gourdeau, H., Anderson, A., Hamel, D., and Boucher, J. M.,** Oncodevelopmental and hormonal regulation of α-fetoprotein gene expression, *Adv. Enz. Regul.,* 21, 73, 1983.
43. **Ammann, A. R., Cowan, M., Wara, D., Heyman, M., Thaler, M. M., Buckley, R., Lawton, A., and Hirschhorn, R.,** Alpha-fetoprotein levels in immunodeficiency, *N. Engl. J. Med.,* 314, 717, 1986.
44. **Wollina, U.,** Alpha1-fetoprotein-relation to impaired macrophage function in systemic lupus erythematosus?, *Dermatol. Monatsschr.,* 170, 703, 1984.
45. **Staples, J.,** Alphafetoprotein, cancer, and benign conditions, *Lanct,* 2, 1277, 1986.
46. **Abelev, G. I.,** Cellular aspects of alpha-fetoprotein synthesis, *Onco-Developmental Gene Expression,* Fishman, W. H. and Sell, S., Eds., Academic Press, New York, 1976, 191.
47. **Toran-Allerand, C. D.,** On the genesis of sexual differentiation of the central nervous system: morphogenetic consequences of steroidal exposure and possible role of α-fetoprotein, *Progr. Brain Res.,* 61, 63, 1984.
48. **Ohama, E. and Ikuta, F.,** Ataxia-telangiectasia: immunocytochemical demonstration of α-fetoprotein and hepatitis B surface antigen in the liver, *Acta Neuropathol.,* 56, 13, 1982.
49. **Ishiguro, T., Sakaguchi, H., Fukui, M., and Sugitachi, I.,** Alpha-fetoprotein subfractions in amniotic fluid identified by a modification of the method of concanavalin A, lentil lectin or phytohemagglutinin-E affinity crossed-line immunoelectrophoresis, *Tumour Biol.,* 6, 195, 1985.
50. **Aoyaki, Y., Suzuki, M., Isemura, M., Soga, K., Ozaki, T., Ichida, T., Inoue, K., Sasaki, H., and Ichida, F.,** Differential reactivity of α-fetoprotein with lectins and evaluation of its usefulness in the diagnosis of hepatocellular carcinoma, *Gann,* 75, 809, 1984.
51. **Buamah, P. K., Harris, R., James, O. F. W., and Skillen, A. W.,** Lentil-lectin-reactive alpha-fetoprotein in the differential diagnosis of benign and malignant liver disease, *Clin. Chem.,* 32, 2083, 1986.

52. **Neville, A. M.,** Some immunobiochemical approaches for the detection of metastases, *Invasion Metas.*, 2, 2, 1982.
53. **Kitagawa, H., Ohkouchi, E., Hata, J., Tsuchida, Y., Fukuda, A., and Tada, T.,** Monoclonal antibodies with fine specificities distinguishing alpha-fetoproteins of hepatoma and yolk sac tumor origin, *Jpn. J. Cancer Res.*, 77, 1012, 1986.
54. **Tsuchida, Y., Kaneko, M., Saito, S., and Endo, Y.,** Differences in the structure of alpha-fetoprotein and its clinical use in pediatric surgery, *J. Pediatr. Surg.*, 20, 260, 1985.
55. **Makino, R., Esumi, H., Takahashi, Y., Sato, S., and Sugimura, T.,** Molecular mechanism of change in serum α-fetoprotein concentration during neonatal development of analbuminemic rats, *Ann. N.Y. Acad. Sci.*, 417, 31, 1983.
56. **Holliday, R.,** Testing molecular theories of cellular aging, in *Dimensions in Aging, the 1986 Sandoz Lectures in Gerontology,* Bergener, M., Ermini, M., and Stahelin, H. B., Eds., Academic Press, New York, 1986, 21.
57. **Sell, S., Longley, M. A., and Boulter, J.,** Lack of correlation of methylation and alphafetoprotein and albumin gene expression during liver growth, in hepatocellular carcinomas, and during hepatocarcinogenesis, *Tumour Biol.*, 6, 133, 1985.
58. **Ott, M. O., Sperling, L., Cassio, D., Levilliers, J., Sala-Trepat, J., and Weiss, M. C.,** Undermethylation at the 5′ end of the albumin gene is necessary but not sufficient for albumin production by rat hepatoma cells in culture, *Cell,* 30, 825, 1982.
59. **Locker, J., Hutt, S., and Lombardi, B.,** α-Fetoprotein gene methylation and hepatocarcinogenesis in rats fed a choline-devoid diet, *Carcinogenesis,* 8, 241, 1987.
60. **Weiss, M. C., Sellem, C. H., Ott, M. O., Levilliers, J., Cassio, D., and Sperling, L.,** Relationship between expression of the albumin gene and its state of methylation, in *Biochemistry and Biology of DNA Methylation,* Cantoni, G. L. and Razin, A., Eds., Alan R. Liss, New York, 1985, 177.
61. **Feinberg, A. P.,** The molecular biology of human cancer, in *Biochemistry and Biology of DNA Methylation,* Cantoni, G. L. and Razin, A., Eds., Alan A. Liss, New York, 1985, 279.
62. **Belanger, L., LaRochelle, J., Belanger, M., and Prive, L.,** Tyrosinosis: hereditary persistence of alpha-1-fetoprotein, in *Onco-Developmental Gene Expression,* Fishman, W. H. and Sell, S., Eds., Academic Press, New York, 1976, 155.
63. **Peters, T., Jr.,** Intracellular precursor forms of plasma proteins: their functions and possible occurrence in plasma, *Clin. Chem.*, 33, 1317, 1987.
64. **Linblad, B., Lindstedt, S., and Steen, G.,** On the enzymatic defects in hereditary tyrosinemia, *Proc. Natl. Acad. Sci. U.S.A.*, 74, 4641, 1977.
65. **Scriver, C. R., LaRochelle, J., and Silverberg, M.,** Hereditary tyrosinemia and tyrosyluria in a French Canadian geographic isolate, *Am. J. Dis. Child.*, 113, 41, 1967.
66. **Ameen, V. A., Powell, G. K., and Rassin, D. K.,** Cholestasis and hypermethioninemia during dietary management of hereditary tyrosinemia type 1, *J. Pediatr.*, 108, 949, 1986.
67. **Gaull, G. E., Rassin, D. K., Solomon, G. E., Harris, R. C., and Sturman, J. A.,** Biochemical observations on so-called hereditary tyrosinemia, *Pediat. Res.*, 4, 337, 1970.
68. **Michals, K., Matalon, R., and Song, P. W. K.,** Dietary treatment of tyrosinemia type I, *J. Am. Diet. Assoc.*, 73, 507, 1978.
69. **Gray, R. G. F., Patrick, A. D., Preston, F. E., and Whitfield, M. F.,** Acute hereditary tyrosinemia type I: clinical, biochemical, and haematological studies in twins, *J. Inher. Metab. Dis.*, 4, 37, 1981.
70. **Furukawa, N., Kinugasa, A., Seo, T., Ishii, T., Ota, T., Machida, Y., Inoue, F., Imashuku, S., Kusunoki, T., and Takamatsu, T.,** Enzyme defect in a case of tyrosinemia type I, acute form, *Pediatr. Res.*, 18, 463, 1984.
71. **Van Thiel, D. H., Gartner, L. M., Thorp, F. K., Newman, S. L., Lindahl, J. A., Sonter, E., New, M. I., and Starzl, T. E.,** Resolution of the clinical features of tyrosinemia following orthotopic liver transplantation for hepatoma, *J. Hepatol.*, 3, 42, 1986.
72. **Holme, E., Linblad, B., and Lindstedt, S.,** Possibilities for treatment and for early prenatal diagnosis of hereditary tyrosinaemia, *Lancet,* 1, 527, 1985.
73. **Kvittingen, E. A., Halvorsen, S., and Jellum, E.,** Deficient fumarylacetoacetate fumarylhydrolase activity in lymphocytes and fibroblasts from patients with hereditary tyrosinemia, *Pediat. Res.*, 17, 541, 1983.
74. **Berger, R., van Faassen, H., and Smith, G. P. A.,** Biochemical studies on the enzymatic deficiencies in hereditary tyrosinemia, *Clin. Chim. Acta,* 134, 129, 1983.
75. **Gourdeau, H., LaRochelle, J., Belanger, M., and Belanger, L.,** Nouvelles observations sur la cirrhose hepatique foetale associee a la tyrosinemie hereditaire, *Union Med. Can.*, 114, 762, 1985.
76. **Gauil, G. E., Rassin, D. K., and Sturman, J. A.,** Significance of hypermethionaemia in acute tyrosinosis, *Lancet,* 1, 1318, 1968.
77. **Hancock, R. L.,** Theoretical mechanisms for synthesis of carcinogen-induced embryonic proteins. XIII. Mutational and non-mutational mechanisms as subsets of a more general mechanism, Part B: Hereditary tyrosinemia, *Med. Hypoth.*, 16, 183, 1985.

78. **Tuchman, M., Freese, D. K., Sharp, H. L., Ramnaraine, M. L. R., Ascher, N., and Bloomer, J. R.,** Contribution of extrahepatic tissues to biochemical abnormalities in hereditary tyrosinemia type I: study of three patients after liver transplantation, *J. Peditar.*, 110, 399, 1987.
79. **Liau, M. C., Chang, C. F., Belanger, L., and Grenier, A.,** Correlation of isozyme patterns of *S*-adenosylmethionine synthetase with fetal stages and pathological states of the liver, *Cancer Res.*, 39, 162, 1979.
80. **Guguen-Guillouzo, C., Szajnert, M. F., Schapira, F., Belanger, L., and Grenier, A.,** Liver fetal isozymes in hereditary tyrosinemia, *Eur. J. Cancer,* 15, 1131, 1979.
81. **Weinberg, A. G., Mize, C. E., and Worthen, H. G.,** The occurrence of hepatoma in the chronic form of hereditary tyrosinemia, *J. Pediatr.*, 88, 434, 1976.
82. **Starzl, T. E., Zitelli, B. J., Shaw, B. W., Iwatsuki, S., Gartner, J. C., Gordon, R. D., Malatack, J. J., Fox, I. J., Urbach, A. H., and Van Thiel, D. H.,** Changing concepts: liver replacement for hereditary tyrosinemia and hepatoma, *J. Pediatr.*, 106, 604, 1985.
83. **Kvittingen, E. A., Jellum, E., Stokke, O., Flatmark, A., Bergan, A., Sodal, G., Halvorsen, S., Schrumpf, E., and Gjone, E.,** Liver transplantation in a 23-year-old tyrosinaemia patient: effects on the renal tubular dysfunction, *J. Inher. Metab. Dis.*, 9, 216, 1986.
84. **Grenier, A., Lescault, A., LeBerge, C., Gagne, R., and Mamer, O.,** Detection of succinylacetone and the use of its measurement in mass screening for hereditary tyrosinemia, *Clin. Chim. Acta,* 123, 93, 1982.
85. **Hirschhorn, R.,** Inherited enzyme deficiencies and immunodeficiency: adenosine deaminase (ADA) and purine nucleoside phosphorylase (PNP) deficiencies, *Clin. Immunol. Immunopathol.*, 40, 157, 1986.
86. **Kredich, N. M. and Hershfield, M. S.,** Immunodeficiency diseases caused by adenosine deaminase deficiency and purine nucleoside phosphorylase deficiency, in *The Metabolic Basis of Inherited Disease,* Stanbury, J. B., Wyngaardern, J. B., Fredrickson, D. S., Goldstein, J. L., and Brown, M. S., Eds., McGraw-Hill, New York, 1983, 1157.
87. **Hirschhorn, R.,** Adenosine deaminase deficiency., *Hosp. Pract.*, 22, 149, 1987.
88. **Hershfield, M. S., Buckley, R. H., Greenberg, M. L., Melton, A. L., Schiff, R., Hatem, C., Kurtzberg, J., Markert, M. L., Kobayashi, R. H., Kobayashi, A. L., and Abuchowski, A.,** Treatment of adenosine deaminase deficiency with polyethylene glycol-modified adenosine deaminase, *N. Engl. J. Med.*, 316, 589, 1987.
89. **Filipovich, A. H., Spector, B. D., and Kersey, J.,** Immunodeficiency in humans as a risk factor in the development of malignancy, *Prevent. Med.*, 9, 252, 1980.
90. **Spector, B. D., Perry, G. S., III, and Kersey, J. H.,** Genetically determined immunodeficiency diseases (GDID) and malignancy: report from the Immunodeficiency-Cancer Registry, *Clin. Immunol. Immunopathol.*, 11, 12, 1978.
91. **Morrell, D., Chase, C. L., and Swift, M.,** Cancer in families with severe combined immune deficiency, *J. Natl. Cancer Inst.*, 78, 455, 1987.
92. **Frazelle, J. H., Harris, J. S., and Swift, M.,** Response of Fanconi anemia fibroblasts to adenine and purine analogues, *Mutat. Res.*, 80, 373, 1981.
93. **Hirschhorn, R.,** Genetic deficiencies of adenosine deaminase and purine nucleoside phosphorylase: overview, genetic heterogeneity and therapy, *Birth Defects,* 19, 73, 1983.
94. **Kumar, G. K., Al Saadi, A., Yang, S. S., and McCaughey, R. S.,** Ataxia-telangiectasia and hepatocellular carcinoma, *Am. J. Med. Sci.*, 278, 157, 1979.
95. **Yoshitoma, F., Zaitsu, Y., and Tanaka, K.,** Ataxia-telangiectasia with renal cell carcinoma and hepatoma, *Virchows Arch. Pathol. Anat. Histol.*, 389, 119, 1980.
96. **Cohen, L. E., Tanner, D. J., Schaefer, H. G., and Levis, W. R.,** Common and uncommon cutaneous findings in patients with ataxia-telangiectasia, *J. Am. Acad. Dermatol.*, 10, 431, 1984.
97. **Weinstein, S., Scottolini, A. G., Loo, S. Y. T., Caldwell, P. C., and Bhagavan, N. V.,** Ataxia-telangiectasia with hepatocellular carcinoma in a 15-year-old girl and studies of her kindred, *Arch. Pathol. Lab. Med.*, 109, 1000, 1985.
98. **Hecht, F. and Kaiser-McCaw, B.,** Chromosome changes connect immunodeficiency and cancer in ataxia-telangiectasia, *Am. J. Pediatr. Hematol. Oncol.*, 9, 185, 1987.
99. **Gotoff, S. P., Amirmokri, E., and Liebner, E. J.,** Ataxia telangiectasia. Neoplasia, untoward response to X-irradiation, and tuberous sclerosis, *Am. J. Dis. Child.*, 114, 617, 1967.
100. **Pritchard, J., Sandland, M. R., Breatnach, F. B., Pincott, J. R., Cox, R., and Husband, P.,** The effects of radiation therapy for Hodgkin's disease in a child with ataxia telangiectasia, *Cancer,* 50, 877, 1982.
101. **Abadir, R. and Hakami, N.,** Ataxia telangiectasia with cancer. An indication for reduced radiotherapy and chemotherapy doses, *Br. J. Radiol.*, 56, 343, 1983.
102. **Toledano, S. R. and Lange, B. J.,** Ataxia-telangiectasia and acute lymphoblastic leukemia, *Cancer,* 45, 1675, 1980.

Chapter 11

THE ENVIRONMENT AND CANCER-ASSOCIATED GENODERMATOSES

Ramon M. Fusaro

TABLE OF CONTENTS

I. INTRODUCTION

Our environment has many physical and chemical agents which have been known for centuries to be harmful to man. Historically the literature has noted many examples of agents which have been nonspecifically (occurs in all persons) cytotoxic to skin with an immediate response within a few minutes to hours of inflammation and direct death of tissue. The classic example of universal immediate cytotoxicity is a burn with heat. The sunburn is also a cytotoxic phenomenon which is delayed by 8 h and reaches its peak damage at 24 h. Because of the delayed dermatitis, the patient has no immediate indicator of the damaging action that they are undertaking while sunbathing. There is a more prolonged delayed form of primary cytotoxic damage to the skin which occurs from repetitive daily exposure to minute amounts of chemicals in the environment. The classic example is the hand dermatitis seen in housewives and bartenders. In this situation there is the accumulative nonspecific minute cytotoxic effect of soap on the integument; however, once the dermatitis is established, the effect of exposure to the soap is within hours and days. The delayed dermatitis of allergic contact dermatitis is a different uniquely specialized immunologic response of certain individuals to a highly specific environmental agent which normally is not directly cytotoxic but, under the altered immunologic response of recognized foreignous of nonself, it becomes cytotoxic producing an acute or chronic dermatitis when the specific agent comes into contact with a specific sensitized individual. These are some of the biologic mechanisms through which the environment damages the skin. Superimposed upon these mechanisms is the spectrum of genetic heritage of individuals and their different abilities to respond to the above array of stimuli.

The environment in modern times is being filled with chemicals which are directly and indirectly toxic to man. At the present time we are dumping hundreds of new chemicals into the environment at a rate which is impossible to ascertain the damaging effect on man except in a retrospective manner when it is already a fait accompli. The agents may not be cytotoxic in a manner described above but they can alter in subtle ways the chemical structure of critical portions of the cell and thereby alter the biologic function of the cell. This alteration can in some instances cause an immediate effect but usually the cell function is altered such that there is a delayed expression of function which usually becomes manifest many years later. The classic example of the latter is the cutaneous effect of tar and the resulting skin cancers seen several decades later.

Nature has provided us with a universal environment agent of sunlight which has a bimodal effect in that in adequate amounts it is beneficial but in excessive amounts it is damaging to biologic tissue. The beneficial effect of vitamin D production by sunlight has been known for over a century. The damaging effects of electromagnetic radiation of the common UV wavelengths and X-rays have become apparent only in the last 50 years or so. Within the last 2 decades, we have also realized that we are destroying the protective ozone barrier with chemical pollutants of our modern industrial development. Thus we are changing the quality and quantity of UV light reaching the surface of the earth from the sun. These UV wavelengths also interact with chemical pollutants which come into contact with the skin. These new UV-altered compounds may produce accelerated adverse biologic effects.

UV radiation is part of the electromagnetic spectrum which ranges across a broad band of heat (infrared), visible light (red to blue), UV light and up into the higher energies of X-rays and high energy particles. Man is exposed to significant amounts of high energy particles or X-rays from artificial sources such as diagnostic X-ray machines and therapeutic radiation equipment used in cancer therapy or accidentally in industry. With respect to UV light, our main significant source is sunlight which gives us the UV A (320 to 400 nm), B (290 to 320 nm), and C (200 to 290 nm); the latter is only present in the upper atmosphere and not at the surface of the earth. At the surface of the earth, there are only two UV bands,

UV A and B, with the latter including the sunburn rays at approximately 300 nm. In our modern environment there are potential sources of UV exposure. These include fluorescent lamps, welding arcs, germicidal lamps, mercury vapor lamps, industrial curing/drying UV chambers, lasers, etc., but in our consideration of cancer they are probably insignificant. However, a new significant introduction of UV A in the last decade has been the high output UV A lamps originally designed for the treatment of psoriasis with concomitant use of oral psoralen but their use in suntan parlors as a so-called safe suntanning procedure has become their major use. The safety of these public tanning parlors has been questioned as will be discussed later.

Medicine has long recognized that in some individuals an excessive and normal amount of sunlight can be damaging in that UV causes, in a delayed response curve, skin cancer which may take years to manifest. Albinism was one of the first disorders to be recognized historically as the product of an adverse delayed reaction of the skin to sunlight exposure in a person who lacks the normal protective qualities of melanin pigmentation. Within the last century, we have discovered many disorders which are affected by sunlight exposure. We have also begun to realize that many of these disorders have a genetic basis in their susceptibility to the delayed cytotoxic effects of electromagnetic radiation which alters intracellular chemical structure, especially DNA, both directly and indirectly through the formation of highly reactive short-lived chemical intermediates which attach cytologic and chromosomal structures and thereby create abnormal biologic functions which may be detrimental to the cell and the whole organism as in the case of uncontrolled cancer. The major concern of this chapter is the cancer-associated genodermatoses which have the capacity to produce cancer in response to the environmental factors. The chapter will concentrate mostly on the following disorders: albinism, basal cell nevus syndrome, epidermolysis bullosa, porokeratoses, porphyria, familial atypical multiple mole melanoma syndrome, hemochromotosis, and hereditary cutaneous cancer in Celts. Two cancer associated genodermatoses, xeroderma pigmentosum and ataxia telangiectasia, will be discussed separately in chapters by other authors.

II. CAUCASIANS, CELTS, AND SKIN CANCER

The etiologic role of UV light in the formation of skin cancer has been the subject of many studies during the past 50 or so years.[1-3] These epidemiologic studies have brought to our attention the consequences to the skin of man from large amounts of sunlight exposure, especially during the most intense sunlight at midday with high noon at the center of the 4-h period. In addition, we have begun to realize the importance of total sunlight exposure accumulated not only as an adult but throughout the individual's whole life span starting with infancy.

The most damaging and carcinogenic part of the electromagnetic spectrum of natural sunlight is from 290- to 330-nm range (UV B or short UV light).The intact ozone layer of the upper atomosphere effectively cuts out wavelengths lower than 290 nm. UV wavelengths lower than 290 nm are very carcinogenic and damaging to biolgoic tissue (germicidal lamps used 254 nm as their principal output). There is evidence to suggest that even the so-called safe UV A (330 to 400 nm) which passes through window glass may be somewhat carcinogenic but it certainly promotes the effects of UV B. The safety of so-called tanning parlors which use high intensity UV A booths is under serious question. Diffey[4] reported that questionnaires of patrons using suntan parlors noted that 28% of them experienced itching and 8% developed a rash or nausea after the treatment. Staberg et al.[5] showed that hairless mice exposed to artificial sunlight for 3 months, followed by UV A for up to 6 months (conditions similar to sunlight exposure in summer and UV A sunparlor exposure in winter) had a higher incidence of skin tumors than those receiving artificial sunlight or UV B only for 3 months.

The range of wavelengths in UV B region is effectively removed from sunlight by passage through window glass or reduced through air containing high concentrations of condensed water vapor (clouds). Thus, dry sunny climates are the most dangerous for acquiring the detrimental effects of sunlight exposure. It is important to inform patients that as much as 50 to 65% of these UV rays can reach the skin not in a direct straight line from the sun but as reflection from sand (snow is a 100% reflector) or scattered from the blue sky, especially on a lake where there is an absence of buildings or trees to obstruct exposure to the dome of blue light which emits UV from every part of the sky above the horizon. An individual forgets that as one goes higher in altitude, there is less volume of air to filter out the UV light so that sunlight exposure in the high mountain country is many times worse than at sea level; in fact, it is difficult to get a sunburn on the shores of the Dead Sea in the Middle East of Asia Minor as it is below sea level.[6,7] The importance of latitude and local cloudless days, both natural and artificial from pollutants, are critical to the understanding of the effects of sunlight.

These epidemiologic studies have emphasized our awareness of the role of racial melanin pigmentation and the distribution of clinical cancers on the exposed integument as primafacie evidence implicating sunlight in the pathophysiologic process of skin cancer. Carcinoma of skin of the exposed cutaneous surface in the Caucasian is common but conversely it is very rare in heavily pigmented skin of other racial groups, especially the black clans out of Africa or the darkly pigmented aborigines of Australia. The dramatic protection of melanin pigmentation is exemplified by the prodigious occurrence of skin cancer in the albino of black heritage. Carcinoma of the skin is most prevalent in sunny countries where there are the descendants of the Caucasians who migrated from the relatively sunless environments of Europe. These adopted geographical areas are noted for their intense continuous sunny clear days: southern part of the U.S., South Africa, Australia, parts of Central America, northern South America, and north Africa. In these areas there is intense sun and on occasion wind in certain geographic areas which has given the white, fair-complexioned, blue-eyed, blond or red-head individual the potential for a significant pathologic amount of UV exposure that his ancestors had never experienced. Cutaneous squamous and basal cell cancers are so common in this group of individuals that they themselves often recognize the clinical lesions and seek medical care. Within the U.S., the incidence of skin cancer of the squamous and basal cell types in white people increases as their place of residence moves closer to the equator and is very low in cloudy places such as Seattle.[8] These rates are increasing as shown by surveys in Texas.[9,10] Even in the less sunny and wintry climates as in Minnesota, the rates of skin cancer have doubled in the last 2 decades.[11] With respect to malignant melanoma whose occurrence is also considered related to sunlight exposure, the mortality rates show a progressive increase in number of deaths from the malignancy.[12]

These recent increases in skin cancer may not reflect the changes in our environmental exposure vis-a-vis chemical pollutants and increased UV light from the decreased ozone layer in the atomosphere but may be the result of significant changes in the behavioral patterns of the affluent population of the predominantly Caucasian areas of the world. This evidence is circumstantial but highly suspicious. Within this century, several factors have greatly influenced our outdoor exposure. The ''sign of the tan'' has become a social marker of wide acceptance. It is thus, especially among the youth of this group, an indicator of health, physical attributes, social position, wealth, and sexual vigor. These attitudes have led to the failure of use of present day sunscreens by young white teenagers and adult population. Because of shorter working hours in the work week and inexpensive rapid transportation, the middle class white population of Europe, the U.S., and Australia has embarked on an unprecedented human experience with outdoor sports activities during the daylight hours. This increased outdoor exposure is life long and starts in early infancy, a hitherto unknown behavioral pattern for families. Mass production of sports equipment with the resulting lower unit costs of each sports item and the accompanying scanty attire of clothes, also mass produced, used in these sports, have made outdoor sports activities available and affordable to the majority for the first time in history. Outdoor pleasures no longer are solely possesed by the wealthy. Not only are the working classes and their progeny out in the summer time in excessive UV exposure but in the winter they travel ''en masse'' to high altitudes to ski or to warm sunny climates for one to two or more weeks a year of intense ''fun in the sun'' with very insufficient use of present day sunscreens as they are cumbersome to apply and interrupt the immediate pleasures of the vacation activities. In addition, most young people want to acquire a healthy tan. For the active young person, the occurrence of skin cancer 20 to 30 years down the road of life is a harmful reward too far removed from the immediate pleasurable stimulus of the vacation in order to have any deterrent effect on an occurrence of overexposure to sunlight.

Within this group of suspectible Caucasians, there is a singular ethnic group which seems to have an extraordinary susceptibility to the development of skin cancer. The group of Celts from Ireland and Scotland who have migrated to the U.S. and Australia have a high rate of squamous cell and basal cell carcinoma of the skin.[13,14] Recent studies also indicate an increase in the incidence of malignant melanoma but this may not be just one racial group in the Caucasians and also may be related to the familial atypical multiple mole melanoma (FAMMM) syndrome (see later discussion) which is a separate genetic entity in which the dominant genetic trait is established in contrast to unknown genetic mechanism of the incidence of squamous and basal cell skin cancers in Celts.

III. ALBINISM

In the hereditary disorders of melanin production and metabolism, albinism is that group of cancer-associated genodermatosis in which there is a distinct identifiable environmental factor intricately involved in the pathologic process of cancer. The external factor is sunlight and it is coupled with the absence of the normal melanization process which appears to be crucial in the protection of skin against the UV radiation deleterious effect of neoplasia of the integument. Neoplasia usually consists of squamous cell carcinoma, basal cell epithelioma, and to a far lesser degree malignant melanoma. It is of interest that in vitiligo in which there is a complete absence of melanin along with the melanocyte, there is not a significant increase in incidence of cutaneous neoplasia.[15] That observed phenomenon may be a quantitative effect of the total amount of accumulative UV radiation, rather than a qualitative effect in that vitiligo usually appears later in life; however, even in patients who have had vitiligo most of their lives, there does not appear to be the significant amount of cutaneous neoplasia as expressed in albinism. There is evidence to suggest that there are a variety of molecular mechanisms through which photoactivated intermediates of melanin metabolism may damage crucial cellular components and thereby produce cutaneous cancers.[16] Normally these intermediates of melanin metabolism are not allowed to accumulate in abnormal concentration in the melanocytes and surrounding keratinocytes which absorb the melanin products, but in the array of metabolic defects associated with albinism numerous and selective intermediates probably accumulate depending upon the respective genetic disorder. In any case, the absence of the normal melanization process in this group of disorders is significant in the carcinogenic process.

The basic genetic component in this group of disorders is the control of melanin production by the melanocyte.[17,18] In man it is not known how many genes are involved in the production of melanin; it must be assumed there is more than one from our basic understanding of the process. In mice, there are approximately 130 genes at 50 loci which are known to affect the final color of mice.[19] When we consider albinism, we cannot restrict ourselves to the melanocyte but most consider the whole process of migration of the melanocyte from the neural crest to its final abode in the epidermis. In addition, the melanocyte does not rest in isolation with its fellow partners, the keratinocytes. The latter cells play an active role in the distribution and final disposal of melanin. Their instructions in this process are certainly under some control from another set of gene(s). This epidermal/melanocytic family or unit which consists of the melanocyte and its associated keratinocytes represents a complex genetic process of many steps in the coloration of the skin, hair, and eyes of man. Thus, the array of disorders which can be assigned to the aberrations of this complex process grows with each decade as we develop technologies which help us separate out the nature of the color of man along with its interraction with the UV environment.

The normal color of the skin, as perceived by the eye, is a composite in varying qualitative and quantitative elements of the red (oxyhemoglobin), blue (deoxygenated hemoglobin), yellow (carotene), and brown-black (melanin) which are in a constant state of flux. The constitutive cutaneous color is that genetically controlled color or normal unexposed (under the clothes) skin such as seen on the sun-deprived areas of the buttocks or axillae. These colors represent the various racial characteristics of man. The facultative cutaneous color applies to the tanned skin which also reflects the genetic capacity of the skin to deepen in brown color in response to UV light exposure. It is obvious that the facultative cutaneous color can be constantly changing during the seasons of the year and, depending on our degree of outdoor activity, the constitutive cutaneous color can also be in a state of flux relevant to the disease states in the skin and the general health of the individual.

Within the melanocyte of the integument, two kinds of melanin are produced: (1) eumelanin or brown-black melanin which is found in ellipsoid melanosomes and gives the skin and hair its brown-black color and (2) pheomelanin or yellow-red melanin which is found in spherical melanosomes and imparts the color for yellow-red hair. There is a third black melanin known as neuromelanin which is formed within nerve cells by an enzymic metabolic pathway different from that process responsible for the formation of eumelanin and pheomelanin. It is assumed that the latter is not involved in the cancer-associated genodermatoses known as albinism.

Clinically, albinism is a loose group of disorders in which there is hypomelanosis or amelanosis with eye involvement. We will be discussing that group of albinism designated the oculocutaneous type (OCA). The other large group is the ocular type of albinism in which the process is essentially limited to the eye; this group will not be discussed as cutaneous neoplasia is not a part of its clinical spectrum.

Albinism is an inherited disorder of melanin metabolism which affects the skin, eyes, and hair of the patient.[20] These patients have congenitally white (noncolored) skin, white hair, nystagmus, and photophobia. The inheritance is autosomal recessive in all except the dominant oculocutaneous albinoidism. Within this OCA recessive group there are the following types: tyrosinase-positive (ty-pos), tyrosinase-negative (ty-neg), Chediak-Higashi syndrome (CHS), Hermansky-Pudlak syndrome (HPS), Cross-McKusick-Breen syndrome (CMBS), yellow-mutant OCA (Ym-OCA), brown OCA (B-OCA), rufous OCA (R-OCA), platinum OCA (Pt-OCA), and black locks-albinism-deafness syndrome (BADS). These disorders have decreased or absent melanin in hair, skin, and eyes along with nystagmus, photophobia, and decreased visual acuity. The dominant albinoidism has hypomelanosis but with essentially normal eyes. In all these disorders except BADS and ocular albinism, the malanocytes are distributed normally throughout the skin and eyes but the normal amounts of melanin are not being synthesized.

The reported incidence of albinism is about 1:20,000 births.[21,22] Ty-pos OCA is the most common albinsim in the U.S. and is more common than the ty-neg OCA. This is probably true for the rest of the world. In the U.S., the Mennonites and Amish Caucasians have a particularly higher incidence of the disease.

A. Susceptibility to Skin Neoplasia

Patients with albinism have extreme cutaneous susceptibility to damage from UV light. Though the short UV light (far) 290- to 320-nm range has been implicated for many years as the major UV spectrum which is damaging to DNA, it is now realized that the long UV light (near) 320 to 400 nm is no longer safe but can also be damaging to the epithelium such that cutaneous neoplasia will be enhanced. The following table gives the relative susceptibility to skin neoplasia of the various forms of Albinism discussed with the weakest at 1+ and the most susceptible at 4+.

SUSCEPTIBILITY TO CUTANEOUS NEOPLASIA

Diseases	ty-neg	ty-pos	Ym	HPS	CHS	BADS	CMBS	Pt	R-OCA	B-OCA	Dominant albinoidism
Susceptibility	4+	3+	Unknown	3+	2+	4+	Unknown	4+	Low	Akin to whites in Africa	Unknown

B. Tyrosinase-Positive OCA

This form of albinism was called complete perfect albinism or albinism II. It is by far the most common form in the U.S. and the most common among the Chinese and American Indians who were tested.[23] These individuals form some melanin in skin, hair, and eyes but its occurrence may not be present at birth so that ty-pos and ty-neg albinos appear identical. If the child is of a black racial heritage, the ty-pos child will appear darker in color than a normal fair-skin, blond Caucasian. As these individuals grow older, the fair color becomes yellow, cream colored, light brown, or red. The eye color may change from its light gray to any within the spectrum of brown, hazel, yellow, or blue. The iris is diaphanous and on transillumination shows cartwheeling which indicates pigment accumulation. The red reflex is present in ty-pos Caucasians but in American Indians and blacks racial groups it may be absent or diminished. Any other ocular abnormalities are similar to ty-neg OCA but are less severe.

The pathologic mechanism of ty-pos OCA is at present unknown. The dopa reaction reveals the presence of tyrosinase and there is not any data to indicate any inhibitory factor(s). The hair bulb incubation test is positive. An electron microscopic examination of the melanocytes shows many stage I and II melanosomes, some partially pigmented stage III melanosomes and very rarely fully pigmented stage IV melanosomes. Within this disorder there are two subtypes. Type I has a two- to fourfold increase in tyrosinase activity compared to hair bulb assays of normal hair and type II has values that appear to be normal.[23]

C. Tyrosinase-Negative OCA

This was named in the past as the imperfect albinism or albinism I. These patients have snow-white hair, pink-white skin (in all racial groups), gray to gray-blue irides without cartwheeling, photophobia, macular hypoplasia, markedly decreased visual acuity, and severe nystagmus. The false yellow coloring of the hair may be due to the biochemical changes in the keratin from exposure to UV radiation. The electron microscopic studies of patients' hair bulbs show melanosomes packed into the dendrites of the melanocytes. Most of the melanosomes are in stage I with some unmelanized stage II melanosomes observed. The dopa reaction is negative. There are no serum inhibitory factors present and the ty-neg OCA appears to be allelic with Ym-OCA and Pt-OCA but not with ty-pos OCA.[22,24,25] The incubation of ty-pos OCA hair bulb in ty-pos OCA serum does not inhibit pigment formation. The hair bulb incubation test will detect heterozygotes with the finding of markedly reduced amounts of free tyrosinase in anagen hairs incubated in tritiated tyrosine substrate.[26]

D. Chediak-Higashi Syndrome

CHS is a rare type of OCA which is characterized by pigmentary dilution, recurrent infections in early life, neurologic abnormalities, hematologic aberrations, and early death by the 2nd decade. Characteristically, there are giant melanin organelles within the melanocytes and abnormal inclusions in leukocytes, Schwann cells, and other tissues.[27] By the early 1970s, there had been only 59 cases reported but their distribution in the world includes North and South America, Europe, and Asia but not in black racial groups.[28] Approximately 50% of the reported cases have pigmentary dilution of hair, eyes and skin which varies from a light cream to slate gray but may darken slightly with sun exposure.[29] The hair color is light blond to brunette and can even assume a frosted metallic-gray sheen. The irides are blue-violet to brown. In addition, there may be squint, photophobia, and reduced retinal pigmentation.

On histologic examination, the melanocytic size and number are normal and contain fully melanized stage IV melanosomes. While some melanosomes are normal, others appear abnormally large but are still present in the keratinocytes.[25,30-33] These giant melanosomes may be the result of fusion of single melanosomes of all stages. Similar melanosomes are present in hair follicles, retina, choroid plexus, and pia-arachnoid.[33-36]

CHS leukocytes contain azurophilic staining granules.[37,38] These lysosomaloid organelles are found in the mucosa of the mouth, stomach, and duodenum, as well as the adrenal and pituitary glands, pancreas, liver, kidney, spleen, bone marrow, iris, skin, and hair.[31,39,40] This abnormality may be a fusion of lysosome-like cytoplasmic organelles.[41]

Even though routine childhood inoculations are well tolerated by these patients, they have recurrent staphylococcal and streptococcal infections at an early age. By the middle of the 1st decade, they manifest convulsions and later develop anemia, thrombocytopenia, and neutropenia. In the final stages, they develop hepatosplenomegaly, hilar adenopathy, leukemic-like gingivitis, hilar adenopathy, and pseudomembranous destruction of the buccal mucosa. Early death will result from lymphoreticular malignancy.

E. Hermansky-Pudlak Syndrome

HPS is another rare form of albinism which is ty-pos and has a hemorrhagic diathesis secondary to a storage pool platelet abnormality with accumulation of ceroid-like substance in the reticuloendothelial system, lung, mucosa of the oral cavity and intestine, and urine.[42] With over 200 reported cases, it is most common in Puerto Ricans and natives of Madras in India but it has been seen in Japanese, Jews, and Europeans with an area of southern Holland showing an unusually common prevalence.[20] This recessive trait may be the result of the pleiotrophic effect of a single gene mutation or from two or more closely linked mutations.[43] These individuals have fair skin color and resemble ty-pos OCA with their pigmentary dilution of the hair and irides and in their severity of photophobia, visual acuity, loss of vision, and nystagmus.

Patients with HPS have hemorrhagic episodes with histories of easy bruisability, epistaxis, hemoptysis, gingival bleeding, hemorrhage following tooth extraction, and excessive postpartum bleeding, all of which has on occasion been fatal. Other tissues such as the lung show interstitial pulmonary fibrosis secondary to ceroid-like substance in the alveolar macrophages; restrictive pulmonary disease may become manifest during the 3rd decade.[44] Inclusions in the cardiac muscle and tubular epithelium of the kidney may result in cardiac and renal failure. Ulcerative colitis may occur in up to one third of HPS patients.

At the electron microscopic level, melanocytes show numerous, irregular, atypical pigmented melanosomes which are round and spotted with pigment and thus resemble pheomelanosomes. Melanosomes of the stage I, II, and III types are present but there is on rare occasion a type IV melanosome present. Other structures such as atypical large melanosomes, giant melanin organelles, and vacuolated melanocytes have been reported.[45]

F. Cross-McKusick-Breen Syndrome

This disorder, which is also known as oculocerebral-hypopigmentation syndrome or hypopigmentation with microophthalmia, is a very rare syndrome which was first described in an Amish kindred from Ohio in which there were multiple consanquinous marriages[30,36] (see above). Since that report, families have been reported from Uruguay, Italy, and the U.S. These patients have a skin color of white with blond hair of a yellow-gray metallic sheen character. Their eyes are small with cloudy corneas and they have a jerky nystagmus. The mental and physical development is severely retarded and on oral examination, there is gingival fibromatosis. The afflicted child exhibits a writhing motion of the arms and legs in addition to a weak high-pitched cry.

The basic defect of CMBS is unknown but the dopa reaction of hair bulbs is weakly positive. On electron microscopy, there are a few melanocytes present with small clusters of melanosomes in all stages of development.[22,44]

G. Black Locks, Albinism, Deafness Syndrome

This disorder has only been reported in two kindreds in which there is sensory neural hearing loss in which the patients have the unusual appearance of amelanotic skin and hair with locks of black hair and coin-like brown cutaneous macules. The irides are gray and there is marked nystagmus with poor acuity. The melanocytes are absent in the amelanotic areas. On ophthalmologic examination of the fundus, there are hyperpigmented and hypopigmented regions.[46]

H. Yellow Mutant OCA

Ym-OCA[20] is common in the Amish communities of the U.S. and is on occasion seen in Polish and German Americans. It is also seen in Ceylon and blacks from America and Africa. These individuals have yellow-red or yellow-brown hair with fair, light skin which can tan slightly after sun exposure. If nevi are present, they are pigmented. At birth, they are indistinguishable from ty-neg OCA patients. By midinfancy, the irides become pigmented but by mid-1st decade, transillumination may reveal a cartwheeling effect. On ophthalmologic examination, slight retinal pigmentation may be seen. The amount of nystagmus, reduced visual acuity, and photophobia are less pronounced than in the patients with ty-pos OCA.

Stage I, II, and III melanosomes are seen in the melanocytes by electron microscopy but they have matrices which are unevenly pigmented and resemble red hair pheomelanosomes. Incubation of Ym hair bulb in L-tyrosine results in no increase in pigmentation; however, incubation with L-tyrosine and L-cysteine reveals the formation of round, small, stage III prepheomelanosomes.

I. Brown OCA

This form of OCA has been seen in black individuals in the New Guinea and Nigeria regions. They have a medium brown hair with tan to olive skin. They may have hazel, blue, or brown (apparent only after dark adaptation) irides along with photophobia and moderate nystagmus. Although these individuals are darker than ty-pos OCAs at birth, progressive darkening occurs with aging and marked delayed tanning does not occur in B-OCA. All stages of melanosomes are seen on electron microscoy. The hair bulb incubation test shows mostly stage III melanosomes as seen in normal Caucasian brown hair.[47]

J. Rufous OCA

This rare form of OCA[48] has been described in New Guineans and Afro-American blacks with the feature of mahogany-red-brown skin and hair which is deep mahogany to sandy red in color. The irides are red brown and with slight translucency. There is mild nystagmus and photophobia but visual acuity may be only mildly to moderately affected. The hair bulb incubation test is positive.

K. Platinum OCA

This is a rare disorder in which the skin is pink to red color with no pigmented nevi, the hair is platinum or cream colored and the eye color is gray to blue. There is an absence of fundal pigment and a red reflex is present. The patients are usually legally blind with a marked photophobia and nystagmus. Incubation of hair bulb in tyrosine shows little to no pigmentation. On electron microscopy, the malanocytes show stage I and II melanosomes with a few stage III melanosomes present.

L. Oculocutaneous Albinoidism

This disorder is different from the other OCAs as it is an autosomal dominant hypomelanosis of the skin, eye, and hair in which the other features of the OCA group are rarely found.[49] The skin is white but may tan slightly on exposure to sunlight. The patients have white to yellow or red hair. The irides are blue and the foveal reflex is absent. On transillumination there is a diffuse punctate, hypopigmentation pattern in the retina. The incubation assay of a hair bulb shows pigmentation.

IV. BASAL CELL NEVUS SYNDROME

This is an autosomal dominant cancer-associated genodermatosis with high penetrance and variable expressivity which has many clinical and pathologic manifestations which result from the pleiotropic effects of a single gene. It is also known as Gorlin's syndrome and nevoid basal cell carcinoma syndrome. The syndrome, which affects males and females equally, is uncommon but not rare. The exact frequency of the disorder is not known but its expression can be manifest over a broad age range with the hallmark of the syndrome, multiple basal cell carcinomas, beginning at an early young age, averaging about 15 years at onset. At the present time, there is not any satisfactory explanation which encompasses the large amount of abnormalities that have been recorded in this syndrome (Table 1).[50-56]

There are several neoplastic problems listed in Table 1 but the only one which has any apparent relationship to the environment is the basal cell carcinoma. This is the most common cutaneous abnormality in this disorder. These multiple basal cell epitheliomas are true carcinomas. Although they may occur early in life on cutaneous sites which are shielded from sunlight by clothes, the tumors are more common on the exposed areas of the body and can be very generalized. The number of lesions vary from just a few to many hundreds in a single patient. When these lesions appear, they may not appear as the classic basal cell epitheliomas, but may be brown, red, and flesh-colored small papules and nodules. When they are brown color, they may be mistaken for ordinary nevi with the result that they have been referred to as nevi. These lesions may remain locally dormant for years before they become locally destructive and invasive as any other basal cell epitheliomas if neglected.[57]

As the majority of the basal cell carcinomas tend to appear in greater number on the exposed areas of the body, it has been assumed that UV radiation from sunlight plays a prominent role in initiating these tumors. This concept has been further strengthened by the relatively few basal cell carcinomas that appear in dark pigmented individuals of black heritage who have this syndrome.[58-62] There is a reservation to this concept as it is possible that in black individuals there is a modifying gene which alters the phenotypic expression of the basal cell carcinoma such that sunlight has no effect and thus there is a false impression that the UV protective effect of malanin is real.

Patients with this disorder have had the following internal malignancies or locally destructive tumors reported: ameloblastomas of the oral cavity, ovarian fibromas, fibrosarcoma of the jaw, teratomas, cystadenomas, cerebellar astrocytomas, meningiomas, craniopharyngiomas, and medulloblastomas. In the treatment of the latter neoplasm with radiation therapy, there has been a major complication of the skin with numerous basal cell carcinomas

Table 1
CLINICAL FINDINGS OF BASAL CELL NEVUS SYNDROME

- Cutaneous
  - Multiple basal cell epitheliomas (carcinoma)
  - Keratin "pits" of the palms and soles
  - Benign lesions
    - Lipomas
    - Fibromas
    - Epithelial cysts
    - Milia
    - Cafe au lait
- Central nervous system
  - Seizures
  - Mental retardation
  - Agenesis of corpus callosum
  - Medulloblastoma
  - Cerebellar astrocytoma
  - Meningioma
  - Craniopharyngioma
  - Congenital hydrocephalus
  - Nerve deafness
  - Lamellar calcification of falx and dura
  - Electroencephalographic changes
  - Cortical atrophy
- Ocular
  - Hypertelorism
  - Dystropia canthorum
  - Strabismus, internal
  - Congenital blindness
  - Colobomas
  - Cataracts
  - Glaucoma
  - Corneal opacities
  - Microophthalmia
- Reproductive tract
  - Hypogonadism in males: absent or undescended testes
  - Ovarian and uterine fibromas
- Osseous abnormalities
  - Multiple jaw cysts
  - Bifid, synostoses, splaying, rudimentary ribs
  - Spina bifida occulta
  - Fusion of vertebra
  - Scoliosis
  - Kyphoscoliosis
  - Bridging of sella
  - Frontal, temporoparietal bossing
  - Oligodactyly or syndactyly
  - Pes planus, hallus valgus
  - Defective clavicle
  - Pectus excavatum or carinatum
  - Brachymetacarpalism, fourth
  - Sprengel's deformity of scapula
- Oral/facial
  - Fibrosarcomas of the jaw
  - Mandibular prognathism
  - Cleft palate and lip
  - Defective dentition
  - Ameloblastoma
  - Broad nasal root

Table 1 (continued)
CLINICAL FINDINGS OF BASAL CELL NEVUS SYNDROME

Miscellaneous findings
- Renal abnormalities
- Inguinal hernias
- Lymphatic mesenteric cysts
- Lung cysts

Features of other syndromes
- Marfan's
- Turner's
- Gardner's
- Weil-Marchesani
- Pseudohypoparathyroidism
- Neurofibromatosis

Table 2
CLASSIFICATION OF PORPHYRIAS

Tissue	Name of specific porphyria
Erythropoietic	Erythropoietic porphyria
	Erythropoietic coproporphyria
	Erythropoietic protoporphyria
Hepatic	Acute intermittent porphyria
	Porphyria cutanea tarda
	Variegate porphyria
	Hereditary coproporphyria
Hepatic-erytheopoietic	Hepatoerytheopoietic porphyria

appearing relatively rapidly in the skin which was exposed to the radiotherapy.[63] Thus there appears to be an X-ray hypersensitivity of the cutaneous tissue which allows the patient to develop basal cell carcinomas at a more rapid rate than expected in this syndrome under normal environmental conditions. It may well be that the basal cell epitheliomas seen usually in this syndrome are also the result of the radiation in our environment but, because of the much lower doses in our natural environment, the cancers of the integument are slower to appear.

V. HEREDITARY PORPHYRIA

The porphyrias are a group of disorders (Table 2) which are intimately involved in one of the most important biosynthetic pathways of tissues. This important metabolic sequence has as its final product heme which is the prosthetic group for a number of proteins such as hemoglobin, catalases, peroxidases, myoglobin, and cytochromes. These proteins and enzymes play key roles in our biologic function. This tetrapyrole is the central pin in these most important biochemical processes of our tissues. Porphyrins are ubiquitous and essential biochemical constituents of all living things. In plants, chlorophyll, a magnesium-chelating porphyrin is the essential cornerstone of the crucial oxygen-producing metabolic process of photosynthesis which is an energy-storing system of our planet by which light and carbon dioxide are converted into a chemically stabilized energy storage form through a sequence of oxidation-reduction reactions. These plants with their stored energy in the forms of carbohydrates become the basis for the support of all higher forms of life which consume them. In all higher forms of life, including man, the iron-chelated tetrapyroles are biologically

Table 3
ACTIVITIES OF ENZYMES IN PORPHYRIAS

Enzyme	Tissue	Proposed enzyme defect
δ-Aminolevulinic acid synthase	Liver, kidney fibroblasts, lymphocytes	Increased activity in AIP, HCP, and VP
δ-Aminolevulinic acid dehydrase	Liver, kidney, erythrocytes	Decreased from lead intoxication
Porphobilinogen deaminase	Liver, fibroblasts, amnion cells, erythrocytes, lymphocytes	Decreased in AIP
Uroporphyrinogen-III cosynthase	Erythrocytes, fibroblasts	Decreased in EP
Uroporphyrinogen decarboxylase	Erythrocytes, liver	Decreased in PCT and HEP
Coproporphyrinogen oxidase	Liver, fibroblasts, lymphoctes	Decreased in HCP
Protoporphyrinogen oxidase	Liver, fibroblasts	Decreased in VP
Ferrochelatase	Erythropoietic >80%; nonerythropoietic (including liver <20%)	Decreased in EPP and lead poison, ? in VP

important in their capacity to act as mediators of oxidation reactions which metabolize these carbohydrates and release the stored chemical energy for consumption.

The porphyric disorders result from either an inherited or acquired abnormality in heme synthesis which allows excessive accumulation of intermediates of heme synthesis in various body tissues. Thus, each type of porphyria may be characterized by a specific enzyme deficiency (Table 3).

The porphyric disorders can be found in many animals but those in Table 3 have been identified in man. In only one of these disorders was an *in vivo* double radioactive isotope study ever done. Schwartz et al.[64] clearly established for the first time the dynamics of how the vast majority of excess protoporphyrins were made in the erythropoietic tissue and not in the liver as previosuly suspected.[65] The rest of the nonerythropoietic tissue such as liver, kidney, etc. produced less than 20% of the excess protoporphyrins. The model concepts for analyzing the dynamics of porphyrin metabolism developed by these investigators are applicable to all the porphyrias.

In all porphyrias except AIP, these excess porphyrins produce photosensitivity of the skin when the porphyric patients are exposed to adequate amounts of long UV light particularly at the Soret band at 405 nm. Depending upon the porphyrin, its concentration in the blood and skin, and the amount of long UV light exposure within a period of time, these porphyric patients will develop in their sunlight-exposed skin an inflammatory reaction composed of erythema, hives, papules, vesicles, bullae, and erosions. The cutaneous collagen and capillaries in the papillary region of the dermis are slowly damaged by the photoactivated porphyrins which chemically react with the dermal tissue so that its tissue strength is weakened. This results in blisters and erosions from the slightest trauma to these exposed areas. The long-term result of this damage is a scarred or a sclerodermoid cutaneous appearance. Interestingly, cutaneous neoplasia is not a consequence of this trauma. It is in only two disorders of porphyria, PCT and VP, that there are malignancies which result from the disease process and these malignancies are internal.

Porphyria cutanea tarda (PCT) has two forms. The classic symptomatic PCT is a nonhereditary form which appears to have all the same traits as the hereditary form which is inherited as an autosomal dominant disorder. Symptomatic PCT is assumed to be an acquired abnormality due to the effects of environmentally encountered toxins: ethyl alcohol, hexachlorobenzene, estrogenic hormones, iron, chlorinated phenols, tetrachlorodibenzo-*p*-dioxin, and polychlorinated biphenyls. It may well be that the susceptibility of individuals and family members to these agents may have a genetic basis which as yet has not been elucidated. Many previous cases of symptomatic PCT are now being recognized as genetic.[66] In both the hereditary and symptomatic PCT there is a deficiency of the enzyme uroporphyrinogen decarboxylase. The distribution of symptomatic PCT is worldwide in all races and continents but the hereditary form of PCT has been reported in far fewer countries which may reflect the economic medical status of medicine.

Variegate porphyria (VP) which is also called mixed porphyria was first described in South Africa by Barnes[67] but later clarified by Dean and Barnes.[68] It has been estimated to occur in 1 in 300 whites of South Africa.[69] This autosomal dominant trait has symptoms of PCT and AIP and was thought to be seen only in South African whites and blacks who traced their ancestry back to one of the Dutch immigrants who migrated from Holland. Mustajoki[70] noted the occurrence of VP in the U.K., U.S., South Africa, Finland, and several regions of Europe. Although reported before in the U.S., five new families were just reported in the New England region which means the disorder is probably universal and is not being easily detected.[71] Recent studies have indicated a deficiency of protoporphyrinogen oxidase.[72]

Patients with PCT or VP can develop hepatomas which may be the result of the disease or the porphyric liver being stressed with a liver toxin such as alcohol. In these patients, hepatomas are a long term problem which needs periodic surveillance coupled with environment control in which all chemicals capable of liver toxicity are eliminated or severely restricted. In both the hereditary forms (HPCT and VP) and the nonhereditary form of PCT, malignancies of the liver are of major concern in the long term care of these patients. Hepatomas in these patients may be more prominent than previously realized.[73-75] In routine autopsy reports the incidence of hepatomas is less than 1%. In two series, the incidence of hepatocellular carcinoma in patients with PCT was 47 and 39%. This information strongly suggests that the incidence of hepatomas is many times greater in PCT and VP than in the general population.

VI. POROKERATOSIS

Porokeratosis is a cancer-associated genodermatosis in which there is a faulty keratinization process which is not limited to the orifices of the eccrine pore but involves the whole epidermis. Cutaneous malignancies have been reported in all forms; however, the link to an environmental factor has only been demonstrated in one of the forms, disseminated superficial actinic porokeratosis (DSAP).[76] The environmental factor is sunlight which unequivocally causes increases in cutaneous lesions. It is assumed that, since malignancy develops in the skin of these patients, the malignancy is linked to the environmental factor of UV exposure. It cannot be assumed that UV light plays any role in the production of cutaneous malignancies in the other forms of porokeratosis. There are four basic forms of porokeratosis: (1) porokeratosis of Mibelli, (2) DSAP, (3) porokeratosis palmaris, plantaris et disseminata (PPPD), and (4) linear porokeratosis. A fifth variant, punctate porokeratosis, is associated with either the Mibelli or linear variants. In all the variants, except linear porokeratosis, the mode of inheritance is an autosomal dominant trait.

Porokeratosis of Mibelli is an autosomal dominant disorder which has its onset in early childhood with a M/F ratio of 3:1.[77] This asymptomatic, slowly progressive disorder is usually found on the acral areas of the extremities, the thighs, and the perigenital regions. This localized, invariably unilateral, relatively large eruption has a diagnostic prominent hyperkeratotic and verrucous peripheral furrow which is more than a millimeter in height and contains a linear serpiginous groove. The center of the lesion is atrophic, anhirotic, hypo/hyperpigmented, and hairless.

DSAP is a bilateral, generalized symmetrical eruption mainly on the exposed part of the extremities. The lesions are small, superficial, fairly uniformly distributed, keratotic papules of 1 to 3 mm which are hyperkeratotic and too numerous to count. Their color is varied from a red or pigmented tan to normal flesh tones. Though the center of these lesions may be atrophic with the periphery hyperkeratotic, the characteristic furrow is invariably not seen. The individual lesions are dry and anhidrotic. This is a relatively common autosomal dominant trait with reduced penetrance. It has not been reported in childhood and is always seen by the 3rd and 4th decade of life with an equal sex ratio.[78] Summertime causes a mild aggravation of the clinical findings. Autotransplantation shows recipient site governs the clinical expression.[79] DSAP, which is the most common of these disorders, has not been reported in blacks.

PPPD, which is an autosomal dominantly inherited trait with a 2:1 M/F ratio, has its onset late in the 2nd decade with a small, superficial and generalized eruption which includes both sunlight and nonexposed cutaneous sites. The initial onset is on the soles and palms with extension elsewhere of hundreds of lesions which are hyperkeratotic and on the palms and soles may have a peripheral furrow. There is no exacerbation of PPPD in the summer as in DSAP.[80,81]

The histopathology of these disorders has the cornoid lamella as its characteristic microscopic feature. It is found at the periphery of the lesion and consists of a tightly packed column of parakeratotic cells extending through the entire height of the surrounding orthokeratotic stratum corneum. Whereas the periphery of the lesion is hyperkeratotic, the epidermis in the center of the lesion is atrophic with liquifaction degeneration of the basal cells, flattening of rete ridges, and colloid body formation.[82] These findings are found in all forms of porokeratosis but in DSAP and PPPD the cornoid lamella is less pronounced and therefore less informative histologically. Structures similar to the cornoid lamella are found in other disorders but the correlation of the clinical and histologic findings offer security in diagnosis.

The development of cutaneous cancer on the exposed areas has been observed in each of the hereditary disorders but with varying rates of expression with DSAP showing the most rapid appearance. This phenomenon is probably related to the sunlight exposure factor which is so prominent clinically in DSAP. The cutaneous malignancies reported include Bowen's disease, basal cell epithelioma, and squamous cell carcinoma with none of them ever being reported as metastasizing to internal organs.[83-89]

VII. THE FAMILIAL ATYPICAL MULTIPLE MOLE MELANOMA (FAMMM) SYNDROME

The familial atypical multiple mole melanoma (FAMMM) syndrome is an autosomally dominantly inherited cancer-associated genodermatosis which has extant heterogeneity and variable expressivity. This syndrome is characterized by the patient having a greater than normal occurrence of cutaneous malignant melanoma (CMM) multiple large cutaneous (>4 mm) atypical nevi (AN), and systemic primary cancers of the following organ systems: breast, eye (IOM), respiratory tract, gastrointestinal canal, and lymphatic system.[90-92]

AN are usually characteristic in their clinical expression when they are over 4 mm in diameter. These AN are usually macular but they can be papular. AN are usually found on the trunk and proximal portions of both upper and lower extremities but can be seen anywhere, especially the scalp. They vary in color from red through light tan into the dark brown which can be almost black. The pigment in these lesions is rarely uniform but variegated in distribution such that it may be regularly or irregularly spotted and on occasion such that one side of the mole is darker in color than the other side. The borders of these lesions are not usually regular and are sharply delineated as in normal moles but show an irregular serpiginous pattern which gives the impression that the color of the nevi is leaking from the border of the moles in an indiscriminate fashion. At other times, the borders will only show a diffusion of pigment into the surrounding skin. The clinical spectrum of AN is very broad but the classic AN is easy to recognize when the lesions are greater than 4 mm. When their size decreases to between 1 and 3 mm, none of the above clinical expression can be discerned easily, even with a magnifying 5× hand lens. One must apply the ABCDE rule to consider the possibility of CMM in monitoring of these classic larger AN, i.e.,

1. A — Asymmetry becomes more prominent
2. B — The borders are enlarging in an irregular manner
3. C — The color is variegated
4. D — The diameter of the lesion increases at least in one dimension
5. E — Significant elevation in size occurs

Any of these changes may mean malignant degeneration. If more than one of the above changes, immediate excision is indicated.

The histologic picture is characteristic in the classic clinical lesions and shows cellular atypica, architectural atypia, and a dermal mesenchymal host response. Bergman[93] defines architectural atypia as including

1. Junctional activity [increased melanocytic proliferation either lentiginous or nevoid (nests)]
2. Melanocytic preference for the tips of rete ridges absent
3. Configuration of the rete ridges are elongated, club-shaped, and irregular with considerable variation in size/shape
4. Nests are pleomorphic, i.e., there is wide variation in size and shape
5. Bridging is present between contiguous rete ridges
6. There is impairment of maturation of the dermal nevocellular elements

The features of cellular atypia include

1. Large or pleomorphic melanocytes
2. Nuclear pleomorphism
3. Melanocytic nuclei larger than those of surrounding keratinocytes
4. Melanocytic nucleoli prominent
5. Presence of dusty melanin pigment in the cytoplasm of melanocytes
6. The presence of prominent melanocytic retraction artifacts

The dermal mesenchymal response covers

1. Lymphocytic infiltrates which are perivascular (slight), aggregate-like (moderate), and band-like (severe)
2. Increase collagen fibers surrounding the rete and lamellar fibrosis in the reticular dermis
3. Vascular proliferation in the papillary dermis
4. The presence of melanophages in the dermis

The definition of the standard terms of atypia and dysplasia are under question as they are used differently by different investigators. Ackerman has discussed the range of definitions and also feels very strongly that the majority of malignant melanoma *in situ* are not associated with preexisting malanocytic nevi but seem to arise *de novo*.[94]

The wide spectrum of clinical and histologic variations is such that, as one approaches the minimal criteria for diagnosis, the margins of error will increase dramatically. We often see classic AN which on histologic examination are normal nevi. Conversely, removal of normal nevi from a patient who is a member of a FAMMM pedigree but appears to be clinically normal will on occasion show classic histologic features of FAMMM moles. Thus, a positive histologic picture can establish the diagnosis of a FAMMM phenotype, but a negative histologic finding in a clinically suspicious phenotype indicates the need for further excisions of more AN to confirm the presence of the clinical phenotype.

At present the occurrence of the FAMMM gene in the general population is not known. It has been estimated that between 3 to 9% of the Caucasian population of the U.S. has clinically atypical nevi[95] but it is not known how many of these individuals are hereditary and belong to the FAMMM syndrome. All studies have not made the critical genetic analysis of the first and second degree members of all patients with AN seen in their studies. Such a study would require the verification of all medical records for primary and secondary relatives in these pedigrees. This lack of verification has led to the conflict over the occurrence of primary systemic cancers in this syndrome.[96-97]

The role of the environment in the occurrence of CMM in the FAMMM syndrome is not known. There have been studies involving patients with melanomas and the occurrence of melanomas in different races, in Caucasians with type I through IV skin, and in individuals with different eye color, hair color, ability to tan or sunburn easily, and the number of nevi on the study subjects.[98-103] There have been studies of the occurrence of melanoma in different geographic areas, latitudes, and climatic conditions (sunny vs. cloudy or rainy vs. dry desert regions), but in all these studies there is no clear-cut separation of the hereditary melanoma patients and their relatives from the sporadic cases of CMM.[104-105] In all these studies, the results indicate that certain types of individuals have a greater tendency for CMM and that UV light from sunlight both on a continuous and intermittent basis (the latter appears to be more significant, especially when severe sunburns occur) plays a significant role in inducing the increased rate of CMM being seen today.[106] There is some question even concerning the indoor exposure to UV light through fluorescent lighting but there is a lack of acceptance of this data by dermatologists.[107-110]

Despite the many publications concerning sunlight and the occurrence of malignant melanoma, there has recently been the suggestion that with the development of our modern chemical industrial society, there has been an introduction of an unknown chemical into our environment which may be the cause of the recent rapid increase in CMM, making it the second most rapidly increasing rate of cancer today. Whether this hypothesis will prove to be correct must wait for further research.[111]

A recent paper on the dysplastic nevus syndrome and sunlight suggests that in these patients there are more AN on the exposed areas (cephalad region) than on the unexposed areas (caudad); however, again there is no in-depth genetic investigation which clearly delineates the hereditary FAMMM syndrome patients from the nonhereditary dysplastic sporadic individuals.[112] The authors did not verify the medical records of all their probands. This is necessary as at least two thirds of known hereditary cancer patients will have written in their records that there is no history of cancer in their families.[113] This lack of investigation in this study does not allow us to draw solid conclusions concerning the relationship of sunlight and AN in patients with the FAMMM syndrome.

In 1982, Ramsay et al.[114] reported that lymphoblastoid cell lines from two families with multiple primary melanomas in several generations demonstrated post-UV radiation inhibition of DNA replication intermediate between controls and an excision-deficient xeroderma pigmentosum cell line; however, spontaneous and UV light-induced sister chromatid exchange frequencies were similar to control cell lines. In that same year Smith et al.[115] reported that cultured skin fibroblasts from patients with hereditary melanoma showed enhanced cell killing sensitivity as compared to normal controls following 254-nm UV irradiation. These same cell lines had essentially normal sensitivity to γ-radiation. The enhanced photosensitivity was not associated with abnormal patterns in either DNA repair synthesis or UV-induced inhibition and recovery of *de novo* DNA synthesis. In 1984, Howell et al.[116] compared fibroblasts derived from skin biopsies of several patients with hereditary cutaneous malignant melanoma and the dysplastic nevus syndrome for sensitivity to the mutagenic and/or cytotoxic effect of broad-specturm simulated sunlight and of a UV mimetic carcinogen, 4-nitroquinoline 1-oxine (4NQO). They found that the nonmalignant fibroblasts from patients with hereditary variant of malignant melanoma are abnormally susceptible to carcinogen-induced mutations which suggests that hypersensitivity to mutagens contributes to the risk of melanoma in these patients. Perera et al.[117] examined the effect of UV radiation on cultured lymphoid cells from patients with hereditary dysplastic nevus syndrome. Using mutagenesis at the hypoxanthine-guanine phosphoribosyltransferase locus as assessed by measuring the induction of resistance to thioguanine, three lymphoblastoid cell lines from patients with hereditary DNS and melanoma had a two- to three-fold greater frequency of induced mutants/clonable cells than three normal lines following exposure to UV radiation. They concluded that hereditary DNS exhibits *in vitro* hypermutability which may reflect increased susceptibility to UV-induced somatic mutations *in vivo*. Recently, Jung et al.[118] studied sister chromatid exchanges in fibroblasts from 12 patients with DNS but they did not establish whether these patients were of the hereditary or nonhereditary types. In any case, patients with DNS without CMM and with CMM both showed significant UV-C induced SCE as compared to normal persons or patients with solitary CMM without DNS. This finding is the opposite of previous reports. All of these reports suggest that the UV environment of sunlight may have a significant promoting effect on patients with AN but whether there is a difference in the effect on the hereditary vs. the nonhereditary form of AN is yet to be ascertained.

VIII. HEMOCHROMATOSIS

Hemochromatosis is a hereditary disorder of iron metabolism in which the small intestine is unable to restrain itself from absorbing unneeded iron from dietary intake.[119-120] This disorder is also known as bronze diabetes, iron storage disease, and Hanot-Chauffard syndrome. The term hemochromatosis was coined by von Recklinghausen in 1899 who erroneously believed that the discoloration of the skin and organs was caused by blood pigment (hemachroma). The color of the skin is attributed to primarily the deposition of melanin. Patients with hemochromatosis need to be treated early in their disease process to prevent damage to various tissues of the body. Niederau et al.[121] points out the necessity of early diagnosis with intensive phlebotomy for iron depletion. In terms of cancer prognosis, hepatocellular carcinoma occurs in one third of patients with cirrhosis. It has not been reported in the precirrhotic patients who have been intensively treated by phlebotomy.

The introduction of insulin and antibiotics has significantly increased the life expectancy of patients with hemochromatosis. Patients with hemochromatosis used to die of diabetes, infections, and cardiac and renal failure. Because of the increased longevity, primary carcinoma is the leading cause of death among patients.

Hemochromatosis was considered a rare disease. The frequency of occurrence of the hemochromatosis gene is estimated to be about 0.05 in the populations of the U.S., Canada, Sweden, and France;[122-127] thus, about 1 person in 20 is heterozygous for the disorder and a homozygote frequency would be about 2 or 3 persons per thousand population. In Scotland in series of 21,565 autopsies, the estimate was 0.002.[128]

Genetic studies have determined that idiopathic hemochromatosis is inherited as an autosomal recessive trait with a partial biochemical expression in heterozygotes. Individuals homozygous for the abnormal allele show severe iron overload. Those persons who are heterozygous for the normal allele and the susceptibility allele show a wide clinical variability. Many heterozygous persons have no clinical findings but do show a significant difference from normal individuals in that they have a mild iron overload as demonstrated by various clinical tests.

The abnormal gene is tightly linked to the HLA histocompatibility locus on the short arm of chromosome 6.[122,123,129,130] By means of HLA typing, we can identify normal heterozygous carriers and abnormal homozygotes among the relatives (first degree) of patients. About 70% of hemochromatosis patients have the antigen HLA-A3 (normal distribution 28%). The disease may appear to be an autosomal dominant inheritance by occurring in two or more generations but this is the result of a homozygote pairing with an unrelated heterozygote. This is more frequent than most clinicians realize as the frequency of the heterozygote in the general population is 5% which makes the 0.3% disease frequency more understandable.

The disease frequency does not correlate with the gene frequency (0.056) as florid hemochromatosis develops five times more frequently in men than in women even though the male-to-female ratio of homozygosity is 1:1. The menstrual frequency of women has been used in the past to explain this difference but in women with florid hemochromatosis, intestinal absorption of iron far exceeds the menstrual iron loss. These facts suggest that the X chromosome suppresses the expressivity of the hemochromatosis gene. To further complicate the genetics of this disorder, the pattern of which the targeted organ in the body becomes loaded with iron appears to also be under separate genetic control. Patients who have hemochromatosis have very varied patterns of which the organ is hit by excessive iron deposition. When hemochromatosis occurs in identical twins who have been separated at or soon after birth, there is identical organ iron storage patterns even though the twins were raised in separate households and have eaten very different diets.

The environment does play a significant role in the development of this disease and probably the ultimate expression of the hepatomas associated with the disorder. Iron loading is accelerated by the use of alcohol, from 2 to 10%. Also alcoholic products may contain additional iron. Alcoholism is not part of the disease process. Fatty degeneration of hepatocytes and portal inflammatory infiltrates are common in alcoholic liver disease but uncommon in hemochromatosis; thus, treated patients with hemochromatosis often regain good liver function. The dietary and health fads in the U.S. of consuming vitamins in amounts greater than the normal daily requirement poses a hazard to persons genetically marked with hemochromatosis as many preparations, especially those designed for normal adult females, contain large amounts of iron. In addition, the fad of consuming large amount of vitamin C may be detrimental as vitamin C enhances absorption of iron. The routine inclusion of iron in vitamin pills even for menstruating women should be discouraged as iron deficiency is an inconsequential syndrome when compared with the lethal nature of hemochromatosis. It should be remembered that iron overloading may develop from repeated use of blood transfusions which were given for the presence of another disorder.

The cutaneous finding of a generalized hypermelanosis varies over a spectrum of bronze, blue-gray, and brown black color. This pigmentation will be accentuated with tanning in the sun-exposed areas of the skin as the primary pigment in patients with hemochromatosis is melanin. The mucosal surface can be hyperpigmented in 15 to 25% of the patients. The hypermelanosis may precede the other clinical manifestations of the disease by several years. Other cutaneous changes include ichthyosis-like skin, palmar erythema, spider angiomas, leukonychia, koilonychia, onychonychia, alopecia, and atrophy.

Along with hypermelanosis, the systemic findings of hepatomegaly and diabetes complete the classical triad but other clinical findings of note are abdominal pain, changes in mental status, arthritis, impotence, amenorrhea, sterility, and cardiac failure. Abdominal pain is one of the most common presenting symptoms and disappears after phlebotomy is initiated. It is not necessary to have the classical triad to establish the diagnosis of hemochromatosis; the crucial reference point is the abnormal presence of iron. The determination of serum iron concentration can be a useful routine diagnostic tool especially in a multiphasic serum chemistry profile. Serum ferritin concentration is a reasonably accurate index of total body iron. The most sensitive indicator of increased body iron is the transferrin saturation index.

In advanced disease, the index is usually greater than 70% but an index of 50% or higher deserves further investigation of the iron status. The ultimate evaluation procedure for the diagnosis of hemochromatosis is a liver biopsy. The most reliable aspect of the biopsy is grading of stainable iron in the hepatic parenchymal cells which normally contain little or no stainable iron.

Because of increasing longevity from phlebotomies, the incidence of hepatomas in hemochromatosis is increasing and at present between 7 to 14% of patients develop hepatomas.[131-132] The majority of hepatomas are very vascular but hypovascularity of these tumors though uncommon has been reported.[133] Other tumors in the liver include osteogenic sarcoma,[134] cholangiocarcinoma,[135] and hemangioendothelial sarcoma.[136]

IX. EPIDERMOLYSIS BULLOSA

Epidermolysis bullosa (EB) is a group of primarily cutaneous disorders which have as their clinical characteristic the formation of blisters of varying sizes usually over bony prominances but also on any part of the cutaneous surface depending upon the particular subtype. The name is really a misnomer as the pathologic process involves not only the epidermis but the tissue in the region between the epidermis and dermis as well as the dermis itself; in fact, the classification follows this definition. The three clinical divisions of EB correlate with the level of the pathologic blister seen histologically.[137]

Because of the biologic defect(s) in these respective regions of the integument, the skin responds abnormally to topical pressure with clinical shearing of the skin after contact with external objects depending upon which of the respective genetic or acquired EB disorders is present and the amount of contact pressure between the skin and the external body. These physical stimuli would not normally cause a pathologic response in persons with normal skin but in these patients any minor form of contact, depending upon the disease subtype present, must be considered a significant traumatic experience.

Trauma covers a wide spectrum of applied pressure and forces. These traumatic experiences can become accumulative and manifestational if applied minimally over a period of time that is short enough to exceed the repair capacity of the individual's respective disease state. The disorders may also not become manifest except under unusual stress such as long distance walking. We observe under those abnormal conditions, a higher incidence of blisters in a group of these patients than in a similar age- and sex-matched group of normal individuals.

Other organs besides the skin are affected in this disease. The gastrointestinal tract in some of these disorders has sufficient loss of structural integrity due to the biologic defect(s) that passage of food or liquids/solids (hot/ice) may be sufficiently traumatic to produce damage and scarring.

In this group of disorders, there are a few hereditary subtypes which can be classified as a cancer-associated genodermatosis in that these patients develop epithelial malignancies usually of the squamous cell type. It is presumed that external environment plays a significant role in the initiation of cancer by creating chronic ulcerations and scarring in the tissues. This in turn leads to the development of the cutaneous or gastrointestional malignancies. There are three categories of EB with many of the disorders known to be hereditary (Table 4).

Each of these three major categories has its pathologic process located in a different anatomic site. These sites are the epidermis, epidermal-dermal junction, and the upper dermal papillary region. The patients who have the epidermolytic form develop their blisters within the epidermis; therefore, the pathologic degeneration which leads to the blister is due to a degradation of the basal or lower spinous cells. The second category of patients develops a blister between the basal layer of the epidermal cells and the basal lamina, i.e., in the lamina lucida. These patients have the junctional form of EB. These two previous categories do

Table 4
CLASSIFICATION OF EPIDERMOLYSIS BULLOSA

Disorder/subtype	Inheritance	Other designations
Epidermolytic (nondystrophic)		
Generalized EB Simplex	AD	Koebner
Localized EBS	AD	Weber-Cockayne
EB herpetiformis	AD	Dowling-Meara
EBS variant	AD	Ogna
EBS localized	AD	Bart's syndrome
EBS variant		Mendes de Costa
Junctional (atrophic)		
EB atrophicans generalisata gravis	AR	EB lethalis Herlitz-Pearson disease Junctional bullous epidermatosis
EB atrophicans generalisata mitis	AR	
EB atrophicans localisata		
EB atrophicans inversa		
EB atrophicans progressiva		
EB cicatricial junctional		
Dermolytic (dystrophic)		
Dominant dystrophic EB	AD	
Hyperplastic dystrophic		Cocayne-Touraine
Albopapuloid		Pasini
Recessive dystrophic	AR	
Generalized gravis		Hallopeau-Siemens
Generalized mitis		
Localized type		
Inverse type		

Note: Autosomal dominance = AD and autosomal recessive = AR.

not form scars as a sequelae of the blister formation. This may be significant in the understanding of the cancer potential of these groups of disorders. The last category which is the dermolytic form has the primary pathologic blister below the basal lamina within the papillary dermis. It is only in this category that blister formation is followed by scarring. As Table 4 demonstrates, there are several subtypes; in fact, some authors believe there are more subtypes than listed above but those listed seem to be the most readily documented and accepted.[138]

It is apparent in reviewing the clinical, histologic, immunologic, and genetic aspects of these disorders that the findings clearly hint that there must be different biochemical abnormalities in each of these disorders with some of them clearly showing autosomal dominant and recessive Mendelian traits. The immunofluoresence and electron microscopic data indicate some of the disorders have identifiable biochemical and anatomic aberrations but the exact mechanisms of the defects in all of the disorders remains unknown.[139]

In one family with generalized EB simplex, there was a deficiency of galactosylhydroxylsyl glucosyltransferase in the skin, serum, and cultured fibroblasts but this finding was not verified in three other families (different pedigrees) with the same disorder.[140] In the Ogna variant of EB simplex a genetic linkage to the erythrocyte glutamicpyruvic transaminase (GPT) locus was established but it was not found in the localized or generalized EB simplex.[141]

Electron microscopic studies of patients with the Herlitz variant of junction atrophic EB show the early blister formation in the lamina lucida.[139] The generalized atrophic benign EB has a histologic picture such that it is differentiated from the Herlitz variant only by clinical manifestations. In the Cockayne-Touraine variant of the dominant dystrophic EB, the electron microscopic photographs show the dermolytic blister below the basal lamina with decreased numbers of rudimentary anchoring fibrils. Sasai et al.[142] have demonstrated increased amounts of degraded chondroitin sulfates (nonspecific in character) in the skin of patients with EB dystrophica et albopapuloidea. Bauer et al.[143] have shown that skin fibroblasts in cell culture accumulate increased amounts of sulfated glycosaminoglycans. This increased accumulation of sulfated glycosaminoglycans both extracellularly and intracellularly seems to be from an increased synthesis as the degradation process appears to be proceeding at a normal rate. Electron microscopy shows some degradation of collagen in skin biopsies from patients with dermolytic recessive dystrophic disease. Organ cultures of skin from these patients show increased collagenase production.[144] Increased collagenase production has been demonstrated to result from increased biosynthesis rather than from absence of an inhibitor or delayed inactivation.[145] Ultrastructural studies in dystrophic disease show that the basal lamina in a fresh induced blister from the roof of the lesion has structural defects in adherence of the basal lamina to the underlying dermis (anchoring fibrils).[146] The other disorders in this subgroup have yet to have any abnormal patholoic processes elucidated.

In reviewing these diverse data, it is apparent that the only cohesive unifying characteristic of the group is the cutaneous blister formation due to physical trauma to the integument. These initiating traumatic episodes are probably within the normal range of physical contacts that are tolerated within the average daily activity of normal persons, but in the realm of these patients such events are pathological. As the mechanism of these disorders are clarified on a biochemical as well as an electron microscopic and immunologic level, these now seemingly similar disorders may become separated to different classes of disorders. The appearance of cutaneous and systemic cancer clearly is not present in all of them.

The reported cancers in EB have been restricted to the dermolytic forms in which the biochemical and anatomic damage is clearly within the dermis and not within the epidermis or at the epidermal-dermal junction. The dermolytic recessive dystrophic form is the most common form of EB leading to skin cancer. These patients develop epidermoid carcinomas especially in cutaneous sites of chronic, nonhealing ulcerations and scars.[147-149] In addition, basal cell epitheliomas and keratoacanthomas have also been reported.[150] Bullous involvement of the mucous membranes (mouth, nose, eyes, oropharynx, esophagus, and genital tract) are not uncommon and there has been instances of oral and esophageal squamous cell carcinoma with poor prognosis.[151-153] Cutaneous squamous cell carcinomas have also been reported in the Cockayne-Touraine dystrophic autosomal dominant form of epidermolysis bullosa.[154]

ADDENDUM

Since 1987, we have studied with cytogenetic techniques two large FAMMM pedigrees of several generations with our colleagues, Drs. Hecht, Hecht, and Sandberg. Preliminary data showed that these FAMMM pedigrees were a chromosome instability disorder in which cells cultured from normal skin and atypical nevi showed an elevation in chromosome rearrangements with nonrandom breakpoints and clonal proliferation marked by chromosome changes. There were consistently significant genomic alterations with translocations, duplications, and deletions seen in numerous members in each of the two pedigrees and reported by H. T. Lynch et al. at the AACR May 25th, 1988 meeting (Bergman. W., Watson, P., Fusaro, R., and Lynch, H., Non-melanoma cancer incidence in the Familial Atypical Multiple Mole Melanoma (FAMMM) syndrome, *Proc. Am. Assoc. Cancer Res.*, 29, 257, 1988). Hecht and Hecht reanalyzed a previously reported pedigree with familial melanoma (McCaw, B. K. and King, C. R., Familial melanoma in three generations, *Am. J. Hum. Genet.*, 29, 71A, 1977) which showed similar abnormalities in a father and son (Hecht, F. and Hecht,

B., Chromosome rearrangements in Dysplastic Nevus Syndrome predisposing to malignant melanoma, *Cancer Genet. Cytogenet.*, 35, 73, 1988). The FAMMM syndrome is thus the only known dominantly inherited chromosome instability disorder.

REFERENCES

1. **Emmett, E. A.,** Ultraviolet radiation as a cause of skin cancers, *Crit. Rev. Toxicol.*, 2, 211, 1973.
2. **Urbach, F., Epstein, J. H., and Forbes, P. D.,** Ultraviolet carcinogenesis: experimental, global and genetic aspects, in *Sunlight and Man,* University of Tokyo Press, Tokyo, 1974, 259.
3. **Blum, H. F.,** *Carcinogenesis by Ultraviolet Light,* Princeton Universtiy Press, Princeton, 1959.
4. **Diffey, B. L.,** Use of UV-A sunbeds for cosmetic tanning, *Br. J. Dermatol.*, 115, 67, 1986.
5. **Staberg, B., Wulf, H. C., Poulsen, T., et al.,** Carcinogenic effect of sequential artificial sunlight and UVA irradiation in hairless mice, *Arch. Dermatol.*, 119, 641, 1983.
6. **Der, C. J., Krontiris, T. G., Cooper, G. M., et al.,** Transforming genes of human bladder and lung carcinoma cell lines are homologous to the ras genes of Harvey and Kirsten sarcoma viruses, *Proc. Natl. Acad. Sci. U.S.A.*, 79, 3637, 1982.
7. **Urbach, F. et al.,** in *Advances in Biology of Skin,* Vol. 7, Montagna, W. and Dobson, R. L., Eds., Pergamon Press, Oxford, 195.
8. **Auerbach, H.,** Geographic variation in incidence of skin cancer in United States, *Public Health Rep.*, 76, 345, 1961.
9. **MacDonald, E. J.,** The epidemiology of skin cancers, *J. Invest. Dermatol.*, 32, 379, 1959.
10. **MacDonald, E. J. and Bubendord, E.,** in *tumors of the skin,* Cumley, R. W., et al., Eds., Year Book Publishers, Chicago, 1964, 23.
11. **Scotto, J., Kopf, A. W., and Urbach, F.,** Non-melanoma skin cancer among caucasians in four areas of the United States, *Cancer,* 34, 1333, 1974.
12. **World Health Organization,** *Epidemiol. Vit Stat. Rep.*, 13, 426, 1960.
13. **Hall, A. F.,** Relationships of sunlight, complexion and heredity to skin carcinogenesis, *Arch. Dermatol.*, 61, 589, 1950.
14. **Silverstone, H. and Searle, J. H. A.,** Epidemiology of skin cancer in Queensland; the influence of phenotype and environment, *Br. J. Cancer,* 24, 235, 1970.
15. **Calanchini-Postizzi, E. and Frenk, E.,** Long-term actinic damage in sun-exposed vitiligo and normally pigmented skin, *Dermatologica,* 174, 266, 1987.
16. **Kock, W. H. and Chedekel, M. R.,** Photochemistry and photobiology of melanogenic metabolites; formation of free radicals, *Photochem. Photobiol.*, 46, 229, 1987.
17. **Quevedo, W. C., Jr. et al.,** Biology of melanocytes, in *Dermatology in General Medicine,* 3rd ed., Fitzpatrick, T. B. et al., Eds., McGraw-Hill, New York, 1987, 224.
18. **Wick, M. M., Hearing, V. J., and Rorsman, H.,** Biochemistry of melanization, in *Dermatology in General Medicine,* 3rd ed., Fitzpatrick, T. B. et al., Eds., McGraw-Hill, New York, 1987, 251.
19. **Silvers, W. K.,** *The Coat Colors of Mice,* Springer-Verlag, Basel, 1979, 380.
20. **Witkop, C. J., Jr. et al.,** Albinism and other disorders of pigment metabolism, in *Metabolic Basis of Inherited Disease,* 5th ed., Stanbury, J. B. et al., Eds., McGraw-Hill, New York, 1983, 301.
21. **Pearson, K. et al.,** A monograph on albinism in man, in *Draper's Company Research Memoirs,* (Biometric Series 6, 8, and 9, Parts I, II, and IV), Dulau, London, 1911.
22. **Witkop, C. J., Jr.,** Albinism, in *Advances in Human Genetics,* Vol. 2, Harris, H. and Hirschhorn, K., Eds., Plenum Press, New York, 1971, 61.
23. **Witkop, W., Jr. and Klein, D.,** Les diverse formes hereditaires de l'albinisme, *Bull. Schweiz. Acad. Med. Weiss,* 17, 35, 1961.
24. **Witkop, C. J., Jr. et al.,** Mutations in the melanin pigment system in man resulting in features of oculocutaneous albinism, in *Pigmentation: Its Genesis and Biologic Control,* Riley, V., Ed., Appelton-Century-Crofts, New York, 1972, 359.
25. **Windhorst, D. B. et al.,** The Chediak-Higashi anomaly and the Aleutian trait in mink: homologous defects of lysosomal structure, *Ann. N.Y. Acad. Sci.*, 155, 818, 1968.
26. **King, R. A. and Witkop, C. J., Jr.,** Hair bulb tyrosinase activity in acute cutaneous albinism, *Nature,* 263, 69, 1976.
27. **Bequez, C. A.,** Neutropenia cronica maligna familare con granulociones atipicas de los leucocitos, *Bol. Soc. Cubana Pediatr.*, 15, 900, 1943.
28. **Hamilton, R. E. et al.,** The Chediak-Higashi syndrome, *Oral Surg.*, 37, 754, 1974.

29. **Stegmaier, O. C. and Schneider, L. A.,** Chediak-Higashi syndrome: dermatologic ma[illegible]on, *Arch. Dermatol.*, 91, 1, 1965.
30. **Corss, H. E. et al.,** A new oculocerebral syndrome with hypopigmentation, *Pediatri*[illegible]
31. **Lockman, L. A. et al.,** The Chediak-Higashi syndrome. Electrophysiologic and [illegible]c observation on the periphera neuropath, *J. Pediatr.*, 70, 942, 1967.
32. **White, J. G.,** The Chediak-Higashi syndrome: a possible lysosomal disease, *Blooa* [illegible]3, 1966.
33. **Windhorst, D. B. et al.,** A human pigmentary dilution based on a heritable subcell[illegible]structural defect — the Chediak-Higashi syndrome, *J. Invest. Dermatol.*, 50, 9, 1968.
34. **Moran, T. J. and Estevez, J. M.,** Chediak-Higashi disease. Morphologic studies of a patient and her family, *Arch. Pathol.*, 88, 329, 1969.
35. **Bedoya, A.,** Pigmentary changes in Chediak-Higashi syndrome, *Br. J. Dermatol.*, 85, 336, [illegible]71.
36. **Lutzner, M.,** Ultrastructure of giant melanin granules in the beige mouse during autogeny (abstr.), *J. Invest. Dermatol.*, 54, 91, 1969.
37. **Bernard, J. et al.,** Un cas de maladie de Chediak-Steinbach-Higashe: etude clinique et sytologique, *Presse Med.*, 68, 563, 1960.
38. **Bessis, M. et al.,** Etude cytologique d'un cas de maladie de Chediak, Nouv Rev *Fr. Hematol. Blood Cells,* 1, 422, 1961.
39. **Lutzner, M. A. et al.,** Giant granules and wide spread cytoplasmic inclusions in a genetic syndrome of Aleutian mink, *Lab. Invest.*, 14, 2063, 1965.
40. **Myers, J. P. et al.,** Pathological findings in the central and peripheral nervous systems in Chediak-Higashi's disease and the finding of cytoplasmic neuronal inclusions (abstr.), *J. Neuropathol. Exp. Neurol.*, 22, 357, 1963.
41. **Stossel, T. P. et al.,** Phagocytosis in chronic granulomatous disease and the Chediak-Higashi syndrome, *N. Engl. J. Med.*, 286, 120, 1972.
42. **Hermansky, F. and Pudlak, P.,** Albinism associated with hemorrhagic diathesis and unusual pigmented reticular cells in the bone marrow: report of two cases with histochemical studies, *Blood,* 14, 162, 1959.
43. **Logan, L. J. et al.,** Albinism and abnormal platelet function, *N. Engl. J. Med.*, 284, 1340, 1971.
44. **Witkop, C. J., Jr. et al.,** Oculocutaneous albinism, in *Heritable Disorders of Amino Acid Metabolism,* Nyhan, W. L., Ed., John Wiley & Sons, New York, 1974, 177.
45. **Frenk, E. and Lattion, F.,** The melanin pigmentary disorder in a family with Hermansky-Pudlak syndrome, *J. Invest. Dermatol.*, 78, 141, 1982.
46. **Witkop, C. J., Jr.,** Depigmentation of the general and oral tissues and their genetic foundations, *Ala. J. Med. Sci.*, 61, 331, 1979.
47. **Hall, A. J.,** A high frequency ablinism variant on the gulf coast of Papua, *Papua New Guinea Med. J.*, 24, 35, 1981.
48. **Walsh, A. J.,** A distinctive pigment of the skin in New Guinea indigens, *Hum. Genet.*, 34, 379, 1971.
49. **Fitzpatrick, T. B. et al.,** Oculocutaneous albinism, *Br. J. Dermatol.*, 91(suppl 10), 23, 1974.
50. **Fusaro, R. M. and Lynch, H. T.,** Cutaneous signs of cancer-associated genodermatoses, in *Cancer-Associated Genodermatoses,* Lynch, H. T. and Fusaro, R. M., Eds., Van Nostrand Reinhold, New York, 1982, 111.
51. **Kraemer, K. H.,** Heritable diseases with increased sensitivity to cellular injury, in *Dermatology in General Medicine,* 3rd ed., McGraw-Hill, New York, 1987, 1791.
52. **Clendenning, W. E.,** The basal cell nevus syndrome, in *Clinical Dermatology,* Vol. 4, 13th ed., Demis, D. J. et al., Eds., Harper & Row, New York, 1986, Sect. 21, 20.
53. **Strong, L. C.,** Theories of pathogenesis: Mutation and cancer, in *Genetics of Human Cancer,* Mulvihill, J. J., Miller, R. W., and Fraumeni, J. F., Jr., Eds., Raven Press, New York, 1977.
54. **Strong, L. C.,** Genetic and environmental interactions, *Cancer,* 40, 1861, 1977.
55. **Neblett, C. R., Waltz, T. A., and Anderson, D. E.,** Neurolgoical involvement in the nevoid basal cell carcinoma syndrome, *J. Neurosurg.*, 35, 577, 1971.
56. **Howell, J. B. and Anderson, D. E.,** The nevoid basal cell carcinoma syndrome, in *Cancer of the skin — Biology-Diagnosis-Management,* Vol. 2, Andrade, R., Gumport, S. L., Popkin, C. L., and Rees, T. D., Eds., W.B. Saunders, Philadelphia, 1976, 883.
57. **Southwick, G. J. and Schwartz, R. A.,** The basal cell nevus syndrome: disasters occurring among a series of 36 patients, *Cancer,* 44, 2294, 1979.
58. **Town, T. M. and Lagattuta, V.,** Basal cell nevus syndrome — 20 years follow-up, *J. Oral Surg.*, 32, 50, 1974.
59. **Ryan, D. E. and Burkes, E. J., Jr.,** The multiple basal-cell nevus syndrome in a negro family, *Oral Surg.*, 36, 831, 1973.
60. **Repass, J. S. and Grau, W. H.,** The basal cell nevus syndrome — report of two cases, *J. Oral Surg.*, 32, 227, 1974.
61. **Giansanti, J. S. and Bakerr, G. O.,** Nevoid basal cell carcinoma in Negroes — report of five cases, *J. Oral Surg.*, 32, 138, 1974.

62. **Ellis, D. J., Akin, R. K., and Bernhard, R.,** Nevoid basal cell carcinoma syndrome — report of case, *J. Oral Surg.*, 30, 851, 1972.
63. **Strong, L. C.,** Theories of pathogenesis: mutation and Cancer, in *Genetics of Cancer,* Mulvihill, J. J., Miller, R. W., and Fraumeni, J. F., Jr., Eds., Raven Press, New York, 1977, 401.
64. **Schwartz, S., Johnson, J. A., et al.,** Erythropoietic defects in protoporphyria: a study of factors involved in labeling of porphyrins and bile pigments from ALA-3H and glycine-14C, *J. Lab. Clin. Med.*, 78, 411, 1971.
65. **Scholnik, P., Marver, H. S., and Schmid, R.,** Erythropoietic protoporphyria: evidence for multiple sites of excess protoporphyrin formation, *J. Clin. Invest.*, 50, 203, 1971.
66. **Benedetto, A. V. et al.,** Porphyria cutanea tarda in three generations of a single family, *N. Engl. J. Med.*, 298, 358, 1978.
67. **Barnes, H. D.,** A note of porphyrinuria with a resume of eleven South African cases, *Clin. Proc.*, 4, 269, 1945.
68. **Dean, G. and Barnes, H. D.,** The inheritance of porphyria, *Br. Med. J.*, 2, 89, 1951.
69. **Dean, F.,** Prevalence of the porphyrias, *S. Afr. J. Lab. Clin. Med.*, 9, 145, 1963.
70. **Mustajoke, P.,** Variegate porphyria, *Ann. Intern. Med.*, 89, 238, 1978.
71. **Muhlbauer, J. E. et al.,** Variegate porphyria in New England, *JAMA,* 247, 3095, 1982.
72. **Deyback, J. C. et al.,** The inherited enzymatic defect in porphyria variegata, *Hum. Genet.*, 58, 425, 1981.
73. **Braun, A.,** Incidence of hepatoma in prophyria cutanea tarda, *Rev. Czech. Med.*, 298, 358, 1962.
74. **Chan, C. H.,** Primary carcinoma of the liver, *Med. Clin. North Am.*, 59, 989, 1975.
75. **Keczkes, K. and Farr, M.,** Frequencey of occurrence of hepatocellular cancer in patients with porphyria cutanea tarda in long-term follow-up, *Neoplasma,* 19, 135, 1972.
76. **Chernosky, M. E. and Anderson, D. E.,** Disseminated superficial actinic porokeratosis: clinical studies and experimental production of lesions, *Arch. Dermatol.*, 99, 401, 1969.
77. **Seghal, V. N. and Dube, B.,** Porokeratosis (Mibelli) in a family, *Dermatologica,* 134, 219, 1967.
78. **Anderson, D. E. and Chernosky, M. E.,** Disseminated superficial actinic porokeratosis:genetic aspects, *Arch. Dermatol.*, 99, 408, 1969.
79. **Chernosky, M. E. and Freeman, R. G.,** Disseminated superficial actinic porokeratosis (DSAP), *Arch. Dermatol.*, 96, 611, 1976.
80. **Guss, S. B. et al.,** Porokeratosis plantaris, palmaris, et disseminata: a third type of porokeratosis, *Arch. Dermatol.*, 104, 366, 1971.
81. **Shaw, J. C. and White, C. R.,** Porokeratosis plantaris, palmaris et disseminata, *J. Am. Acad. Dermatol.*, 11, 454, 1984.
82. **Reed, R. J. and Leone, P.,** Porokeratosis: a mutant colonal keratosis of the epidermis, *Arch. Dermatol.*, 101, 340, 1970.
83. **Bellafiore, V.,** Studio clinico sulla porocheratosi, *Ann. Ital. Dermatol. Clin. Sper.*, 24, 55, 1971.
84. **Cort, D. F. and Abdel-Aziz, A. H.,** Epithelioma arising in porokeratosis of Mibelli, *Br. J. Plast. Surg.*, 25, 318, 1972.
85. **Coskey, R. J. and Mehregan, A.,** Bowen disease associated wtih porokeratosis of Mibelli, *Arch. Dermatol.*, 11, 1480, 1975.
86. **Johnston, E. N. M.,** Porokeratosis of Mibelli with squamous cell carcinoma, *Br. J. Dermatol.*, 70, 381, 1958.
87. **Savage, J.,** Porokeratosis (Mibelli) and carcinoma, *Br. J. Dermatol.*, 76, 489, 1964.
88. **Sarkany, I.,** Porokeratosis Mibelli with basal cell epithelioma, *Proc. R. Soc. Med.*, 66, 435, 1973.
89. **Shrum, J. R. et al.,** Squamous cell carcinoma in disseminated superficial actinic porokeratosis, *J. Am. Acad. Dermatol.*, 6, 58, 1982.
90. **Lynch, H. T., Fusaro, R. M., and Pester, J. A.,** Genetic heterogeneity and malignant melanoma, in *Cancer Associated Genodermatoses,* Lynch, H. T. and Fusaro, R. M., Eds., Van Nostrand Reinhold, New York, 1982, 394.
91. **Lynch, H. T., Fusaro, R. M., Kimberling, W. J., et al.,** Familial atypical multiple mole melanoma (FAMMM) syndrome: segregation analysis, *J. Med. Genet.*, 20, 342, 1983.
92. **Lynch, H. T., Fusaro, R. M., Pester, J., et al.,** Familial atypical multiple mole melanoma (FAMMM) syndrome: genetic heterogeneity and maligant melanoma, *Br. J. Cancer,* 42, 58, 1980.
93. **Bergman, W.,** The dysplastic nevus syndrome — clinical and fundamental aspects, Offsetdrukkerij Kanters B. V., Alblasserdam, 1987, 1.
94. **Ackerman, A. B. and Mihara, I.,** Dysplasia, dysplastic melanocytes, dysplastic nevi, the dysplastic nevus syndrome, and the relation between dysplastic nevi and malignant melanoma, *Hum. Pathol.*, 16, 87, 1985.
95. **Fusaro, R. M. and Lynch, H. T.,** Melanoma and the atypical nevus, *J. Am. Acad. Dermatol.*, 16, 884, 1987.
96. **Lynch, H. T., Fusaro, R. M., and Lynch, J. F.,** the NIH consensus report on precursors to malignant melanoma — a different persepctive, *Am. J. Dermatopathol.*, 6, 177, 1984.

97. **Lynch, H. T. and Fusaro, R. M.,** Natonal Institutes of Health consensus report on precursors to malignant melanoma — a difference in opinion, *JAMA,* 252, 2872, 1984.
98. **D'Arcy, C., Holman, J., and Armstrong, B. K.,** Pigmentary traits, ethnic origin, benign nevi, and family history as risk factors for cutaneous malignant melanoma, *J. Natl. Cancer Inst.,* 72, 257, 1984.
99. **English, J. S. C., Swerdlow, A. J., MacKie, R. M., O'Doherty, C. J., Hunter, J. A. A., Clark, J., and Hole, D. J.,** Relation between phenotype and banal melanocytic naevi, *Br. Med. J.,* 294, 152, 1987.
100. **Cooke, K. R., Spears, G. F. S., and Skegg, D. C. G.,** Frequency of moles in a defined population, *J. Epidemiol. Comm. Health,* 39, 48, 1985.
101. **Holly, E. A., Kelly, J. W., Shpall, S. N., and Chiu, S.-H.,** Number of melanocytic nevi as a major risk factor for malignant melanoma, *J. Am. Acad. Dermatol.,* 17, 459, 1987.
102. **Elwood, J. M., Gallagher, R. P., Davison, J., and Hill, G. B.,** Sunburn, suntan and the risk of cutaneous malignant melanoma — western Canada melanoma study, *Br. J. Cancer,* 51, 543, 1985.
103. **Elwood, J. M., Gallagher, R. P., Hill, G. B., Spinelli, J. J., Pearson, J. C. G., and Threlfall, W.,** Pigmentation and skin reaction to sun as risk factors for cutaneous melanoma; western Canada melanoma study, *Br. Med. J.,* 288, 99, 1984.
104. **Swerdlow, A. J. and Green, A.,** Melanocytic naevi and melanoma; an epidemiological perspective, *Br. J. Dermatol.,* 117, 137, 1987.
105. **Armstrong, B. K., deKlerk, N. H., D'Arcy, C., and Holman, J.,** Etiology of common acquired melanocytic nevi; constitutional variables, sun exposure, and diet, *J. Natl. Cancer Inst.,* 77, 329, 1986.
106. **Elwood, J. M., Gallagher, R. P., Hill, G. B., and Pearson, J. C. G.,** Cutaneous melanoma in relation to intermittent and constant sun exposure — the western Canada melanoma study, *Int. J. Cancer,* 35, 427, 1985.
107. **English, D. R., Rouse, I. L., Zhong, X., Watt, J. D., D'Arcy, C., Holman, J., Heenan, P. J., and Armstrong, B. K.,** Cutaneous malignant melanoma and fluorescent lighting, *J. Natl. Cancer Inst.,* 74, 1191, 1985.
108. **Beral, V., Shaw, H., Evans, S., and Milton, G.,** Malignant melanoma and exposure to fluorescent lighting at work, Lancet, ii, 290, 1982.
109. **Stern, R. S.,** Malignant melanoma and exposure to fluorescent lighting at work, *Lancet,* ii, 1227, 1982.
110. **Beral, V. and Evans, S.,** Malignant melanoma and exposure to fluorescent lighting at work, *Lancet,* ii, 1227, 1982.
111. **Rampen, F. H. J. and Fleuren, E.,** Melanoma of the skin is not caused by ultraviolet radiation but by a chemical xenobiotic, *Med. Hypotheses,* 22, 341, 1987.
112. **Kopf, A. W., Gold, R. S., Rogers, G. S., Hennessey, P., Friedman, R. J., Rigel, D. S., and Levenstein, M.,** Relationship of lumbosacral nevocytic nevi to sun exposure in dysplastic nevus syndrome, *J. Am. Acad. Dermatol.,* 122, 1003, 1986.
113. **Lynch, H. T., Follett, K. L., Lynch, P. M., Albano, W. A., Mailliard, J., and Pierson, R. L.,** Family history in an oncology clinic: implications concerning cancer genetics, *JAMA,* 242, 1268, 1979.
114. **Ramsay, R. G., Chen, P., Imray, F. P., Kidson, C., Lavin, M. F., and Hockey, A.,** Familial melanoma associated with dominant ultraviolet radiation sensitivity, *Cancer Res.,* 42, 2909, 1982.
115. **Smith, P. J., Greene, M. H., Devlin, D. A., McKeen, E. A., and Paterson, M. C.,** Abnormal sensitivity to UV-radiation in cultured skin fibroblasts from patients with hereditary cutaneous malignant melanoma and dysplastic nevus syndrome, *Int. J. Cancer,* 30, 39, 1982.
116. **Howell, J. N., Greene, M. H., Corner, R. C., Maher, V. M., and McCormick, J. J.,** Fibroblasts from patients with hereditary cutaneous malignant melanoma are abnormally sensitive to the mutagenic effect of simulated sunlight and 4-nitroquinoline 1-oxide, *Proc. Natl. Acad. Sci. U.S.A.,* 81, 1179, 1984.
117. **Perera, M. I. R., Um, K. I., Greene, M. H., Waters, H. L., Bredberg, A., and Kraemer, K. H.,** Hereditary dysplastic nevus syndrome: lymphoid cell ultraviolet hypermutability in association with increased melanoma susceptibility, *Cancer Res.,* 46, 1005, 1986.
118. **Jung, E. G., Bohnert, E., and Boonen, H.,** Dysplastic nevus syndrome: ultraviolet hypermutability confirmed in vitro by elevated sister chromatid exchanges, *Dermatologica,* 173, 297, 1986.
119. **Cartwright, G. E., Edwards, C. O., Kravitz, K., et al.,** Hereditary hemochromatosis: phenotypic expression of the disease, *N. Engl. J. Med.,* 301, 175, 1979.
120. **Ward, J. H., Kushner, W. P., and Kaplan, J.,** Iron: metabolism and clinical disorders, *Curr. Hematol. Oncol.,* 3, 1, 1984.
121. **Niederau, C., Fischer, R., Sonnenberg, A., et al.,** Survival and causes of death in cirrhotic and in noncirrhotic patients with primary hemochromatosis, *N. Engl. J. Med.,* 313, 1256, 1985.
122. **Dadone, M. M., Kushner, J. P., Edwards, C. O., et al.,** Hereditary hemochromatosis: analysis of laboratory expression of the disease by genotype in 18 pedigrees, *Am. J. Clin. Pathol.,* 78, 196, 1982.
123. **Edwards, C. O., Skolnick, M. H., and Kushner, J. P.,** Hereditary hemochromatosis: contributions of genetic analyses, *Prog. Hematol.,* 12, 43, 1981.
124. **Olsson, K. S., Ritter, B., Rosen, U., et al.,** Prevalence of iron overload in central Sweden, *Acta Med. Scand.,* 213, 145, 1983.

125. **Bassett, M. L., Doran, T. J., Halliday, J. W., et al.,** Idiopathic hemochromatosis: demonstration of homozygous-heterozygous mating by HLA typing of families, *Hum. Genet.,* 60, 352, 1982.
126. **Bassett, M. L., Halliday, J. W., Ferris, R. A., et al.,** Diagnosis of hemochromatosis in young subjects: predictive accuracy of biochemical screening tests, *Gastroenterology,* 87, 628, 1984.
127. **Borwein, S. T., Ghent, C. N., Flanagan, P. R., et al.,** Genetic and phenotypic expression of hemochromatosis in Canadians, *Clin. Invest. Med.,* 6, 171, 1983.
128. **MacSween, R. N. M. and Scott, A. R.,** Hepatic cirrhosis: a clinico-pathological review of 520 cases, *J. Clin. Pathol.,* 26, 936, 1973.
129. **Simon, M., Alexandre, J. L., Fauchet, R., et al.,** The genetics of hemochromatosis, *Progr. Med. Genet.,* 4, 135, 1980.
130. **Simon, M., Bourel, M., Fauchet, R., et al.,** Association of HLA-A3 and HLA-B14 antigens with idiopathic haemochromatosis, *Gut,* 17, 332, 1976.
131. **Finch, S. C. and Finch, C. A.,** Idiopathic hemochromatosis, an iron storage disease, *Medicine,* 34, 381, 1955.
132. **Berk, J. E. and Lieber, M. M.,** Primary carcinoma of the liver in hemochromatosis, *Am. J. Med. Sci.,* 202, 708, 1941.
133. **Nebesar, R. A., Pollard, J. J., and Stone, D. L.,** Angiographic diagnosis of malignant disease of the liver, *Radiology,* 86, 284, 1966.
134. **Maynard, J. H. and Fone, D. J.,** Hemochromatosis with osteopenic sarcoma in the liver, *Med. J. Aust.,* 2, 1260, 1969.
135. **McLoughlin, M. J. and Hill, M. O.,** Angiography in clolangiocarcinoma complicating hemochromatosis, *J. Can. Assoc. Radiol.,* 21, 238, 1970.
136. **Sussman, E. B., Nydick, I., and Gray, G. F.,** Hemangioendothelial sarcoma of the liver and hemochromatosis, *Arch. Pathol.,* 97, 39, 1974.
137. **Gedde-Dahl, T. and Anton-Lamprecht, I.,** Epidermolysis bullosa, in *Principles and Practice in Medical Genetics,* Emory, A. E. H. and Rimoin, D. L., Eds., Livingstone, New York, 1981.
138. **Gedde-Dahl, T.,** *Epidermolysis Bullosa: A Clinical, Genetic and Epidemiological Study,* Johns Hopkins Press, Baltimore, 1971; **Gedde-Dahl, T.,** Phenotype-genotype correlations in epidermolysis bullosa, *Birth Defects,* 7, 107, 1971.
139. **Cooper, T. W., Bauer, E. A., and Briggaman, R. A.,** The mechanobullous diseases (epidermolysis bullosa), in *Dermatology in General Medicine,* 3rd ed., Fitzpatrick, T. B., Eisen, A. Z., Wolff, K., Freedberg, I. M., and Austen, K. F., Eds., McGraw-Hill, New York, 1987, 610.
140. **Savolainen, E. R., Kero, M., and Pihlajaniemi, T.,** Deficiency of galactosylhydroxylsyl glucosyltransferase, an enzyme of collagen synthesis in a family with dominant epidermolysis bullosa simplex, *N. Engl. J. Med.,* 304, 197, 1981.
141. **Olaisen, B. and Gedde-Dahl, T.,** GPT-epidermolysis bullosa simplex (Ogna) linkage in man, *Hum. Hered.,* 23, 189, 1973.
142. **Sasai, Y. et al.,** Epidermolysis bullosa dystrophica et albopapuloidea, *Arch. Dermatol.,* 108, 554, 1973.
143. **Bauer, E. A., Fiehler, W. K., and Esterly, N. B.,** Increased glycosaminoglycan accumulation as a genetic characteristic in cell cultures of one variety of dominant dystrophic epidermolysis bullosa, *J. Clin. Invest.,* 64, 32, 1979.
144. **Lazarus, G. S.,** Collagenase and connective tissue metabolism in epidermolysis bullosa, *J. Invest. Dermatol.,* 58, 242, 1972.
145. **Valle, K. J. and Bauer, E. A.,** Enhanced biosynthesis of human skin collagenase in fibroblast cultures from recessive dystrophic epidermolysis bullosa, *J. Clin. Invest.,* 66, 176, 1980.
146. **Briggaman, R. A. and Wheeler, C. E., Jr.,** Epidermolysis bullose dystrophica-recessive: a possible role of anchoring fibrils in the pathogenesis, *J. Invest., Dermatol.,* 60, 203, 1975.
147. **Edland, R. W.,** Dystrophic epidermolysis bullosa; tolerance of the bed and response of multifocal squamous cell carinomas to ionizing radiation; report of a case, *Am. J. Roentgenol.,* 105, 644, 1969.
148. **Didolkar, M. S., Germer, R. E., and Moore, G. E.,** Epidermolysis bullosa dystrophica and epithelioma of the skin, *Cancer,* 33, 198, 1974.
149. **Wechsler, H. L. et al.,** Polydysplastic epidermolysis bullosa and development of epidermal neoplasms, *Arch. Dermatol.,* 102, 374, 1970.
150. **Reed, W. B. et al.,** Epidermolysis bullosa dystrophica with epidermal neoplasms. *Arch. Dermatol.,* 110, 894, 1974.
151. **Nix, T. E. and Christianson, H. B.,** Epidermolysis bullosa of the esophagus; report of two cases and review of the literature, *South. Med. J.,* 58, 612, 1965.
152. **Sonneck, H. J. and Hantzschel, K.,** Uber eiven Fall von epidermolysis bullosa dystrophica mit oesophagus stenose und kardiocarcinom, *Hautarzt,* 12, 124, 1961.
153. **Reed, W. B., Roenigk, J., Jr., Dorner, W., Jr., et al.,** Epidermal neoplasm with epidermolysis bullosa dystrophica with the 1st report of carcinoma with the acquired type, *Arch. Dermatol.,* 253, 1, 1975.
154. **Schwartz, R. A., Birnkrant, A. P., Rubenstein, D. J., et al.,** Squamous cell carcinoma in dominant type epidermolysis bullosa dystrophica, *Cancer,* 47, 615, 1981.

Chapter 12

GENETIC FACTORS IN THE ETIOLOGY OF ESOPHAGEAL CANCER AND THE STRATEGY FOR ITS PREVENTION IN HIGH-INCIDENCE AREAS IN NORTHERN CHINA

Min Wu, Nan Hu, and Xiuqin Wang

TABLE OF CONTENTS

I. INTRODUCTION

In contrast to most developed countries, cancer of the esophagus is a very common disease in many areas of China, especially in the north.[1-3] Data collected in the period from 1975 to 1978 indicated that the number of all cancer deaths in China was 700,000 per year, among which 157,000 died of esophageal cancer.[4] It was estimated that in 1977 this malignant disease constituted 24.6% of all cancer deaths in men and 18.2% of those in women.[4] Examination of cancer mortality by county showed that cancer of the esophagus was the leading cause among all cancer deaths in China.[5] In many densely populated, administrative areas, esophageal cancer is the most commonly seen malignancy and constitutes from 20.9 to 45.1% of all cancer deaths. Henan province has the highest incidence in China.[4,6]

The vast majority of esophageal cancer patients, if not all, when diagnosed, are in an advanced state. Their prognosis is very poor. Efforts have been made by Chinese cytologists and surgeons in the past 2 decades to detect and treat patients in the early stages of cancer development. Early, asymptomatic, or subclinical cases of cancer of the esophagus were successfully detected by means of balloon cytosmear.[7-9] The 5-year survival rate of these patients after surgical treatment was quite satisfactory (89.9%).[10] However, in order to identify early cancer patients, it is necessary to carry out regular screening among the population at risk using balloon cytology. Such screening must be done once or twice a year, lest new cases would escape detection. This, of course, requires a tremendous amount of manpower and costs large sums of money which might not be provided even in developed countries. Furthermore, because of their apparent good health, patients so detected usually refuse surgery, which is the only effective treatment. Also, therapeutic facilities are not available since most of the patients suffering from esophageal cancer are living in remote rural districts of counties located in mountainous areas.

Areas with high esophageal cancer risk also have concomitantly high rates of dysplasia of epithelial cells of the esophagus.[5] Over time, the progression from mild to severe dysplasia and then to cancer has been observed (Figure 1). Studies of the inhabitants in Linxian have shown that the relative risk of developing esophageal cancer among patients suffering from epithelial dysplasia of the esophagus is about 100 times higher than in the normal population.[8] An intervention program through treatment of esophageal dysplasia is being conducted in a district of Linxian.

Primary prevention programs based solely on environmental etiology have met great difficulties. Although there is strong evidence indicating that dietary habits and food hygiene are the etiologic factors for the development of esophageal cancer, to modify the dietary habits of millions of Chinese peasants, or to change the cultivation regime in closed mountainous areas, is almost impossible in the near future. Therefore, carcinoma of the esophagus in China is a challenging problem for Chinese scientists and therapists.

In this chapter, we describe a strategy for cancer prevention in a county with a very high mortality rate of cancer of the esophagus. This strategy is based on the knowledge that most human cancers are caused by a genetic/environmental interaction, and on our experimental data obtained mainly from human populations.

II. GENETIC EPIDEMIOLOGY OF ESOPHAGEAL CANCER IN HIGH-INCIDENCE AREAS OF NORTHERN CHINA

Between 1975 and 1978, health authorities in China mobilized large numbers of people to conduct a nationwide cancer mortality survey encompassing 29 provinces, municipalities, and autonomous regions (395 cities and perfectures, and 2101 counties), with a population of 850 million. This retrospective survey of cancer deaths in China disclosed a peculiar geographic distribution of cancers, especially cancer of the esophagus. The difference in

Normal ⇄ Mild Dysplasia ⇄ **Severe Dysplasia**

? years → Early Cancer — 4 years → **Advanced Cancer**

FIGURE 1. Process of development of epithelial dysplasia and cancer of the esophagus.

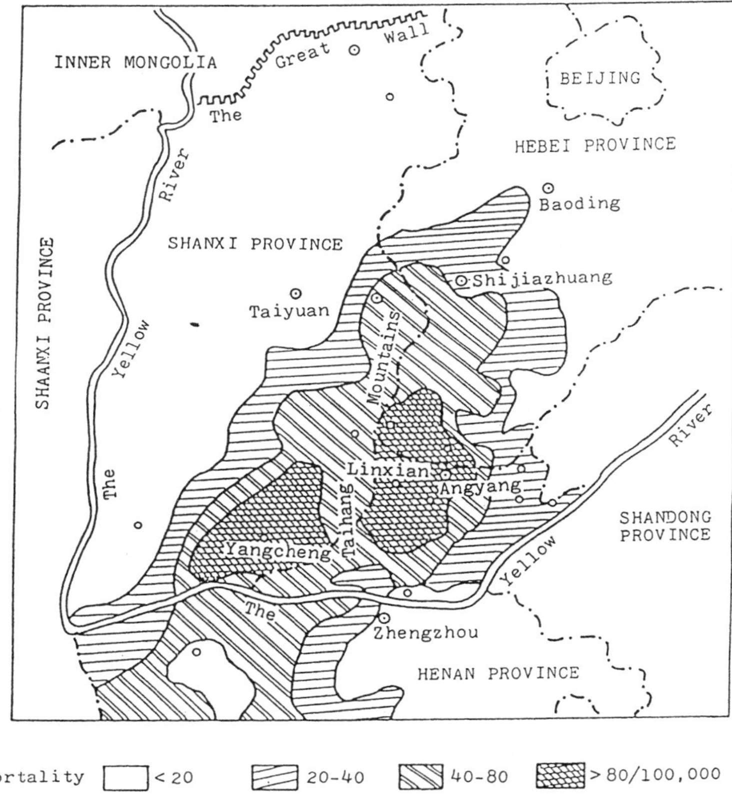

FIGURE 2. Distribution of esophageal cancer in the triprovincial areas of Hebei, Henan, and Shanxi in northern China.

esophageal cancer death rates between the different counties may be severalfold to several hundredfold. For instance, the highest county rates are 254.77/100,000 for males and 161.11/100,000 for females (Linxian county, Henan province). These rates are 670-fold higher than counties with the lowest esophageal cancer death rates for each sex (0.38/100,000 for males in Lancang county, Yunnan province; 0.24/100,000 for females in Xundian county, Yunnan province).[4] The highest mortality figures are from the counties where the borders of the three provinces (Hebei, Henan, and Shanxi) meet on the south side of the Taihang Mountains (Figure 2).[1-3] From these high incidence areas, extending outwards on all sides, the figures gradually decrease, giving an impression of irregular concentric belts. The ratio between the highest mortality rates in the innermost zone and the lowest rates in the outermost belt is approximately 100 to 1 (Figure 2).[4,6]

Esophageal cancer death rates in high-incidence areas are very stable. Historical records dating from 2000 years ago noted "dysphagia" syndromes among the inhabitants of Henan

Table 1
AGE-ADJUSTED MORTALITY RATES OF ESOPHAGEAL CANCER IN MINORITIES IN CHINA

	Rates (per 100,000)	
Nationality	**Male**	**Female**
Kazak	39.27	27.08
Hui	18.90	6.32
Mongol	12.89	5.73
Uygur	12.87	7.93
Zhuang	7.80	5.34
Korean	5.82	1.62
Yi	1.67	0.91
Miao	1.61	0.63

Note: Age adjusted to population of China, 1964.

province. In Linxian of Henan, ''difficulty in swallowing disease'' has been an endemic disease for centuries. The typical symptoms of this disease are familiar to almost every inhabitant of this county. The serious concern and fear of this disease in old times was reflected in the existence of the ''Houwang Miao'' (meaning Throat-God Temple).[3] According to the data collected in Linxian, the death rates from esophageal cancer have remained unchanged during the last 40 years.[4,6]

The rate of death from cancer of the esophagus increases with age. Mortality among patients over 35 years of age makes up 99.04% of the total, and that among those between 50 and 74 years of age accounts for 74.99%.[6] Age at death is on average about 10 years younger in high risk areas than in low risk ones.[6]

Comparative statistics from various ethnic minorities in China show that cancer of the esophagus is common among the Kazakh people of Xinjiang autonomous region, whose rate of death from this disease is 2 to 31 times higher than that among other minority groups (Table 1).[6] Living in the same county (Jingho), Kazakhs, Uygurs, and Mongolians show totally different rates of mortality. According to Doll,[11] there is a high incidence among the Turkomans and Kazakhs in the Soviet Union. In America, the incidence among blacks exceeds that among Caucasians and that among immigrant Chinese.[12] The incidence among overseas Chinese is highest in those speaking Chaozhou and Fujian dialects; that among those speaking Hakka ranks next, while that among those speaking Cantonese is the lowest.[13] This is in agreement with the findings in China.[6]

From 1967 to 1969, about 60,000 people migrated to Zhongxiang and Jimmen counties of Hubei province from Zhechuan county of Henan province. The original standardized esophageal cancer death rates in Zhongxiang and Jimmen were 15.39/100,000 and 7.13/100,000, respectively (1968 to 1978). The immigrants, however, still have rates of 75.81/100,000 and 98.30/100,000, i.e., 5 to 14 times higher than the local people. The mortality in Zhechuan is 55.40/100,000 (1970 to 1972).[6]

Esophageal carcinoma mortality in China by size of community is in the following decreasing order: village > small city > town > large city. There is a high predilection for the countryside in which the population has little tendency to migrate for very long periods of time[1,6] and tends to form genetic isolates of different sizes.

The above-mentioned epidemiologic characteristics of esophageal cancer in China were thought by most researchers to be attributed to the activity of strong carcinogens in the environment.[4] Therefore, great efforts have been and are being made to find the putative cancer-causing factors in the environment. Little, if any attention was given to the genetic factors in the pathogenesis of this human cancer. However, it has been well established that the major criterion of malignancy is uncontrolled growth of the neoplastically transformed cells, and since cell growth is under gene control, the implication is that genetic factors are involved in all cancers. Some cancers are almost predominantly the result of the genetic makeup, such as heritable retinoblastoma, Wilms' tumor, etc. Other cancers have been shown to occur because of repeated action of environmental carcinogens on the genetic material of the host.[14] Esophageal cancer could be of the latter case. The statement that 80 to 90% of cancer is caused by environmental factors and therefore is preventable[15] is too simple for understanding and controlling cancer. In fact, the epidemiologic characteristics, such as unusually high and constant mortality from esophageal carcinoma in limited and closed mountainous areas, great ethnic differences in mortality, and data obtained in immigrant studies, etc., are strong evidence for genetic factors in the etiology of this human malignancy.

Epidemiological surveys carried out in high-incidence areas of esophageal cancer in northern China during the early 1970s disclosed also a strong tendency to familial aggregation of patients (unpublished). In several reports, over 60% of esophageal cancer patients had a positive family history. The so-called "cancer families" in a village were often well known by the local inhabitants who frequently raised the question as to whether esophageal cancer was a heritable disease. In order to answer this question, a pilot study was carried out in 1 of the 15 communes in Linxian.[16] The total population of this commune, named Henshui, was 68,000. Its crude mortality of esophageal cancer calculated from the figures recorded in 1974 to 1976 was 121.32/100,000, approaching the average level for the whole county (crude mortality rate 133.07/100,000). In order to assess the genetic and environmental factors in the etiology of esophageal cancer in this commune, we assumed that living in a common household implied common exposure to putative environmental carcinogens and that kinship to the proband was an indication of a genetic factor. The procedure of this study was as follows

1. Collect data from all existing patients with esophageal carcinoma and carcinoma of the gastric cardia (all were cytologically confirmed) within the whole commune, with the help of local medical personnel
2. Trace the history of esophageal cancer among probands' relatives in four successive generations, including parents, grandparents, siblings, offspring, and their corresponding relatives, and to record their names, sex, age, relation to the proband, occupation, and cause of death
3. Calculate the standardized mortality ratio (SMR), indirect age-adjusted mortality rate (IMR) standardized to the esophageal cancer mortality for the whole population of Linxian, and the relative risk (RR), as well as the attributative risk (AR) of different populations for both the genetic and the environmental factors. Some of the data obtained are shown in Table 2.

The pilot study showed clearly that the SMR and RR for blood relatives of the 80 existing patients in this commune were significantly higher than those for nonblood relatives. A stepwise descending gradient, proportional to the remoteness of blood relationship, was also evident. The SMR for all nonblood relatives was much lower than one (0.547). This is also evidence for the uneven distribution of esophageal cancer patients among the whole population of this commune. If the families with proneness to esophageal cancer were excluded from the population, the mortality rate for the rest of the inhabitants would decrease markedly.

The next study was then carried out in a neighboring commune (Yoacun) with the highest

Table 2
STANDARDIZED MORTALITY RATIOS (SMR) AND RELATIVE RISKS (RR) AMONG PROBANDS' DIFFERENT RELATIVES IN HENGSHUI COMMUNE

Relatives	Number of relatives recorded	Number of EC observed	Number of EC expected	SMR	RR
Blood relatives					
Parents	160	30	11.229	2.671	4.88
Children	271	0	0.346	0	0
Siblings	181	14	7.097	1.973	3.61
Grandparents	320	16	15.553	1.029	1.88
Siblings of parents	224	12	12.850	0.934	1.70
Other relatives	813	17	17.830	0.953	1.74
Total	1969	89	64.905	1.371	2.50
Nonblood relatives					
Spouses	79	4	3.857	1.037	
Parents in-law	158	6	12.699	0.472	
Brother or sister in-law	164	6	9.772	0.614	
Children in-law	173	1	0.326	3.067	
Spouse's uncles and aunts	217	12	19.515	0.615	
Other nonblood relatives	516	14	32.416	0.432	
Total	1307	43	78.579	0.547	

Table 3
STANDARDIZED MORTALITY RATIOS (SMR), INDIRECT AGE-ADJUSTED MORTALITY RATES (IMR), AND RELATIVE RISK (RR) IN YAOCUN STUDY

Group	Number of relatives recorded	Number of EC observed	Number of EC expected	SMR	IMR	RR[a]
		Proband Group				
Blood relatives	6,649	401	232.889	1.722	229.147	2.005
Nonblood relatives	5,916	233	269.949	0.863	114.839	1.040
		Control Group				
Blood relatives	6,065	193	224.730	0.859	114.307	
Nonblood relatives	4,961	191	230.119	0.830	110.448	
Total	23,591	1,018				

Note: IMR = SMR X Crude Mortality Rate

[a] Compared with corresponding controls.

mortality rate for esophageal cancer in Linxian (crude mortality rate 187.85/100,000).[16] In this survey, 180 esophageal and gastric cardiac cancer patients, belonging to 180 families, were found and for each a normal control of the same sex, age group, and similar economic status living close by was identified. The blood relatives and nonblood relatives of these probands and controls in three successive generations (grandparents and their siblings excluded because of the difficulty in obtaining reliable information about this generation) were investigated. The results obtained from this case/control study are in part summarized in Tables 3 and 4.

From Table 3, one can see that the observed deaths from esophageal cancer among

Table 4
ATTRIBUTIVE RISKS FOR KINSHIP AND HOUSEHOLD LIVING IN YAOCUN STUDY

Relationship to probands	Number of EC deaths / number of relatives recorded	IMR 1/100,000	AR[a] 1/100,000
Kinship + household living (parents)	96/360	404.134	221.961
Household living only (spouses)	18/180	221.162	38.989
No kinship and no household living	171/1260	182.173	0
Controls' spouses	16/180	211.981	
Controls' parents	47/360	160.482	
Spouses' parents	56/360	188.959	
Parents of controls' spouses	52/360	189.625	

[a] AR = IMR − IMR for the "No kinship and no household living" group (182.173).

probands' blood relatives significantly exceeded the expected ones. The SMR was 1.722, and the RR, when compared with corresponding controls, reached 2.005. But the observed death numbers in the three other groups; namely, probands' nonblood relatives and controls' blood and nonblood relatives, were all less than the expected. Their SMRs were also similar to each other. This phenomenon suggests that since the environment for these inhabitants was so similar that it contributed no difference in esophageal cancer mortality among the inhabitants, the factor which made the deaths of esophageal cancer doubled in the blood relatives group might be the kinship to the probands.

When we took the parents of the probands as a group with kinship plus a common environment, probands' spouses as a group with common environment only, and compared them with a group with no kinship and different environment, including controls' spouses, controls' parents, and parents of controls' spouses, we found that the IMR only increased slightly for those living in the same household, with an AR of 38.898. However, a high IMR value of 404.134 with the corresponding AR reaching 221.961 was observed when both kinship and living in the same household were considered. Hence, these data support the hypothesis that there is a strong influence of kinship on the incidence of esophageal cancer and that the environment alone seems to be responsible for the baseline mortality (182.173) in this population (Table 4).

The data obtained from these two communes indicate that since the effect of environmental factors is the same throughout this high risk area, there seems to be unequivocal evidence of genetically determined susceptibility to esophageal cancer.

Another retrospective survey conducted by Li and He[17] in Yangcheng County, Shanxi Province, is also very informative. This ia also a mountainous county located at the southern end of the Taihang mountain range (see Figure 2) with a very high mortality of esophageal cancer (149.29/100,000). The authors and their team members visited all families in this county one by one. A family member, usually a person about 50 years of age, was interviewed. The family tree was traced back to the generation of his or her grandparents on paternal and maternal sides, and all deaths of esophageal cancer were recorded. The results revealed that among the 81,388 families in the county, 74,723 families, accounting for 91.81% of the total, had no esophageal cancer deaths over three successive generations. Death from esophageal carcinoma was concentrated in only 8.19% (6665) of the families. In these families with esophageal cancer deaths, 3871 families had only one case per family and 2794 families (3.43% of all families in the county) had multiple cases. Of all the 11,446 esophageal cancer deaths recorded, 5290 (46%) were from the families with sporadic single cases and 6156 (54%) from the families with multiple cases. It implies that more than half of the cancer deaths were from 3.43% of the families in this county.

Therefore, surveys in both Linxian and Yangcheng have disclosed a strong tendency to familial aggregation of esophageal cancer patients. This suggests a genetically determined proneness to this human cancer. These two counties are both on the slopes of the Thaihang mountains. The inhabitants have very poor transportation facilities and therefore little access to the outside world for long periods of time. They not only share some similar environmental conditions, but may also have some peculiar genetic makeup, perhaps susceptible to certain environmental carcinogens.[14]

III. LABORATORY METHODS FOR IDENTIFYING PERSONS AT HIGH RISK FOR ESOPHAGEAL CANCER

According to the genetic segregation law, the descendants from high risk families are not expected to be equally prone to esophageal cancer. In order to sharply define persons at high risk, laboratory methods must be developed.

That the origin of human cancer is a multistep process is widely accepted[18] and supported by numerous lines of evidence, including the long-term course of oncogenesis described by clinicians, pathologists,[8,19] and cytologists.[9] The statistical analysis of age-incidence cancer data suggests six to seven independent events for human epithelial cancers.[20] Cytogenetic data reveal multiple chromosome abnormalities in most tumor cells and increasingly aberrant chromosome structures that arise during tumor growth and progression.[21,22] The localization of oncogenes at translocation breakpoints in specific forms of cancer greatly strengthens the evidence that chromosome rearrangements play a causal role in oncogenesis.[23] The high probability of cancer developing in individuals with genetic diseases that increase chromosomal instability provides strong evidence for the causal role of DNA damage in cancer etiology.[24,25] Therefore, our attention was focused on decreased DNA repair capacity, increased chromosomal instability, and genetic variations in response to environmental carcinogens.

A. Unscheduled DNA Synthesis

Since all normal mammals and most other living organisms so far examined have DNA repair systems capable of dealing with many different kinds of damage, including DNA-bound carcinogens, it follows that DNA repair deficiencies or the inhibition of DNA repair should lead to increased susceptibility to chemical carcinogenesis. The discovery of defective DNA repair in cells from xeroderma pigmentosum patients (XP)[26] stimulated the examination of a variety of other diseases in which sensitivity to sunlight or X-irradiation had been noticed for evidence of DNA repair deficiencies. There are now several conditions in which some preliminary evidence of abnormalities in DNA repair or DNA replication has been discovered. Some of these are summarized in Rasmussen's review.[27] XP provides a classical mechanism for the action of a specific carcinogen (UV light) upon a clearly defined cancer-prone genotype. Each factor is necessary, but neither is a sufficient agent in carcinogenesis. If patients with XP could meticulously avoid exposure to the carcinogenic effects of solar radiation, the skin cancer could be prevented, as observed by Lynch et al.[28]

During life, there is an accumulation of damage to the DNA. Enzymatic repair is an important compensatory mechanism to decrease the severity of this damage. Reduced capability for DNA repair may be one of the factors responsible for the accumulation of DNA damage and possibly also for the neoplastic transformation of the cells.

We have studied 84 individuals in Linxian with respect to the excision repair capacity of DNA of their lymphocytes.[29] These individuals were divided into four groups: group I — esophageal cancer patients with positive family history (20 persons), group II — esophageal cancer patients with negative family history (19 persons), group III — normal subjects with family history of esophageal cancer (26 persons), and group IV — normal subjects with no

Table 5
UNSCHEDULED DNA SYNTHESIS OF LYMPHOCYTES AFTER UV IRRADIATION

Group	Number of subjects	Integrated ^{3}H-TdR (cpm/10^6 cells) X ± SD	Comparison with group IV (*t* test)
I Esophageal cancer patients with family history	20	210.4 ± 73.6	$p < 0.001$
II Esophageal cancer patients without family history	19	300.0 ± 103.4	$p > 0.05$
III Normal subjects with family history of esophageal cancer	26	257.9 ± 113.4	$p < 0.001$
IV Normal subjects without family history of esophageal cancer	19	361.3 ± 103.9	

Table 6
UNSCHEDULED DNA SYNTHESIS OF GASTRIC MUCOSAL EPITHELIA AFTER UV IRRADIATION

Source of samples	Number of samples	Integrated ^{3}H-TdR (cpm/μg DNA) X ± SD	*t* test
High-incidence areas	24	17.1 ± 29.4	$p < 0.05$
Low-incidence areas	17	44.3 ± 56.2	

family history of esophageal cancer (19 persons). The results show decreased unscheduled DNA synthesis (UDS) of blood lymphocytes after UV irradiation in groups I and III compared with normal subjects without family history (group IV). Cancer patients with negative family history (group II) also show decreased repair capacity as compared with group IV, but the difference is not statistically significant (Table 5).

Wu and colleagues[30] have recently conducted an interesting work in Fujian province. Since there are some counties with very high incidence of gastric cancer (about 110/100,000) in this province, they compared the excision repair capacity of DNA of gastric mucosal epithelia of 49 patients from a high incidence area with that of 17 patients from a low incidence area (mortality rate less than 5/100,000). They revealed that the gastric epithelium of patients from the high incidence area showed much lower UDS after UV irradiation than those from the low incidence area (Tables 6 and 7).

B. Sister Chromatid Exchanges in Lymphoyctes

Interest in sister chromatid exchanges (SCEs) has centered on their use in the detection of mutagenic-carcinogenic effects on cells[31,32] and in the characterization of chromosome fragility diseases.[33] Although the molecular basis of the SCE process is not fully established, SCE can serve as an empirically useful signature of one type of cellular response to DNA damage.[34]

The rates of SCE induced with nitroso-methylbenzylamine, a putative environmental carcinogen detected in Linxian,[35] at different doses (0, 20, 40, and 80 μg/ml), have been scored in the short-term cultivated peripheral lymphocytes taken from esophageal cancer

Table 7
UNSCHEDULED DNA SYNTHESIS OF GASTRIC EPITHELIA TAKEN FROM PATIENTS SUFFERING FROM GASTRIC CANCER OR FROM PEPTIC ULCER IN HIGH-INCIDENCE AREAS OF GASTRIC CANCER

Source of samples	Number of samples	Integrated ^{3}H-TdR (cpm/μg DNA) X ± SD	*t* test
Gastric cancer patients	25	14.4 ± 23.5	p > 0.05
Peptic ulcer patients	24	17.1 ± 29.4	

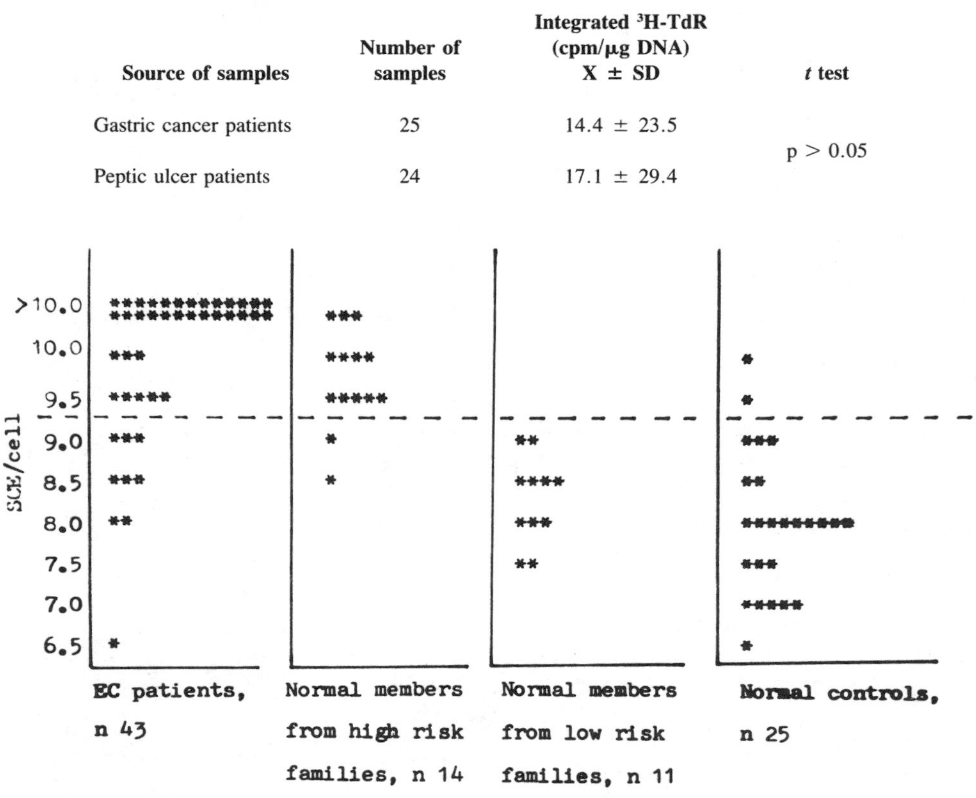

FIGURE 3. Distribution of the rates of sister chromatid exchange (SCE) among esophageal cancer patients, normal members from high- and low-risk families, and normal controls. Nitrosomethylbenzylamine at a dose of 80 μg/ml was added to the culture medium.

patients, healthy members from families with multiple esophageal cancer deaths in Yangcheng, healthy members from families with no cancer history, and normal individuals in an area with low mortality of esophageal cancer. The results showed that (1) the spontaneous SCE rates of esophageal cancer patients are significantly higher than those of the three other groups ($p < 0.01$), (2) without addition of S-9 mixture (microsome fraction of rat liver), the nitroso-methylbenzylamine was able to induce an SCE increase, and (3) at the dose of 80 μg/ml of nitroso-methylbenzylamine, the healthy members from families with high risk of esophageal cancer showed a significantly higher SCE increase than the other three groups ($p < 0.01$)(see Figure 3).[36]

C. Rate of Chromosome Aberration in Lymphocytes

It is well documented that some rare, heritable syndromes with chromosomal fragility are prone to neoplasia.[21,22,24,25] It is not yet clear whether increased chromosomal instability has any connection with increased susceptibility to frequently seen human malignancies such as esophageal cancer. In the following, we describe some of our recent works which may give hints to the answer of this important question.[37-42]

Table 8
SUMMARIZED DATA ON CHROMOSOME ABERRATION RATES OF CANCER PATIENTS

	Case (no.)	Chromosome aberration rate (%)
Cancer patients		
Esophageal cancer	45	8.41
Ovarian and uterine cancers	90	9.62
Lymphoma and ALL[a]	22	12.98
Miscellaneous malignancies	16	8.50
Total	173	9.58
Average		($p < 0.01$)
Normal controls	54	1.10

[a] Acute lymphocytic leukemia.

Table 9
SUMMARIZED DATA ON CHROMOSOME ABERRATION RATES OF 360 INDIVIDUALS

	Case (no.)	CAR (%)	CAR <2% (%)	CAR >2% (%)
Cancer patients	173	9.58	29(16.8)	144(83.2)
Normal members from cancer families	54	8.07	14(25.9)	40(74.1)
Normal members from families with high risk to EC	52	5.87	13(25.0)	39(75.0)
Normal members from families with low risk to EC	27	0.91	25(93.6)	2(7.4)
Normal individuals as control	54	1.10	48(88.9)	6(11.1)

A total of 390 cancer patients and healthy persons belonging to cancer families in accordance with the definition set by Lynch and Krush[43] — high and low risk families for esophageal cancer, and normal controls from areas with low incidence of esophageal cancer (Beijing and Taiyuan) — were studied with respect to their chromosome aberration rate (CAR). In order to get information of fragile sites from the same sample, the lymphocytes were incubated in medium with a low content of folic acid and calf serum (5%). The pH of the medium was adjusted to 7.5 and the incubation time prolonged for 24 h (to a total of 96 h). It is interesting to note that under such stress conditions, most of the cancer patients and about two thirds of the persons from cancer families or from families with high risk of esophageal cancer show an increased rate of chromosome aberrations, while most of the normal controls have a low CAR, if an arbitrary demarcation line is drawn at the value of 2% (see Tables 8 and 9 and Figure 4).[42]

D. Fragile Sites

Until recently, little was known about how recurrent chromosome defects occur in cancers and why some individuals and families have a higher incidence of malignancy. Yunis[44-46] suspects that some protooncogenes and very active genes of differentiated cells may have a hypersensitive or fragile site that facilitates such chromosomal rearrangements and may represent sites where carcinogens often attack.

The often observed chromosomal defects in malignant cells may be a reciprocal translocation,[47,48] an inversion,[49] or a partial deletion;[50-52] each involve two precise breakpoints — one of them the likely site of a protooncogene that becomes deregulated as a result of chromosomal rearrangement. What deregulates the oncogene may be its general proximity, following rearrangement, to a regulatory sequence normally used by an active gene(s) of a

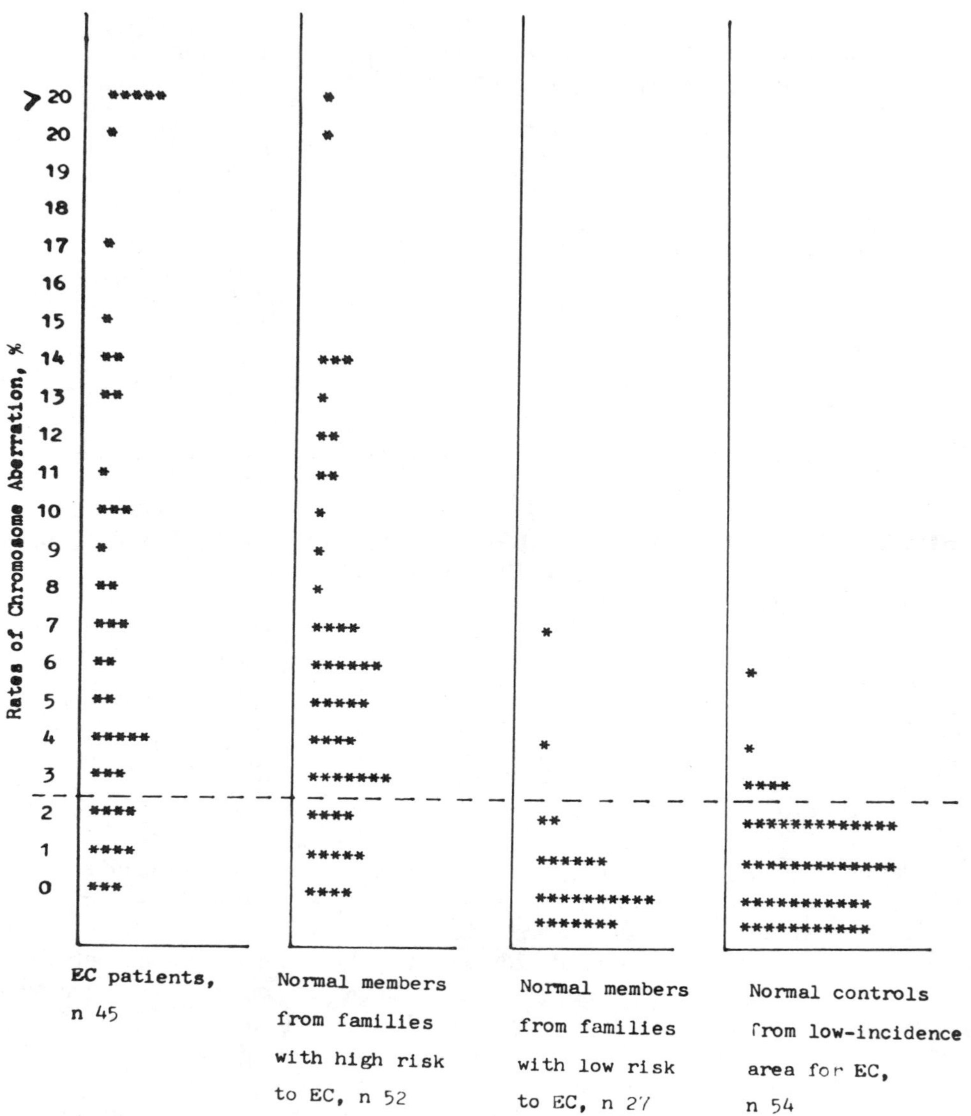

FIGURE 4. Distribution of rates of chromosome aberration among esophageal cancer patients, normal members from high- and low-risk families, and normal controls.

differentiated cell. The well-known example is the translocation of *myc* to the heavy chain immunoglobulin gene region in the t(8;14) found in Burkitt's lymphoma.[53]

Our studies on fragile sites among cancer patients, persons from high risk families, and normal controls are summarized in Tables 10 and 11.[42] Since one half to more than three fourths of the persons with some genetic background of cancer carry fragile site(s), as opposed to less than one tenth of the normal controls, the fragile sites may also be used as an additional indirect marker for proneness to cancer.

IV. STRATEGY FOR PREVENTING ESOPHAGEAL CANCER IN HIGH-INCIDENCE AREAS OF NORTHERN CHINA

Based on all aforementioned data and ideas, we are developing a strategy for the prevention of esophageal cancer in Yangcheng county.[54] The highlights are as follows. The persons

Table 10
SUMMARIZED DATA ON RATES OF THE FRAGILE SITE AMONG CANCER PATIENTS, NORMAL MEMBERS FROM CANCER FAMILIES, NORMAL MEMBERS FROM FAMILIES WITH CANCER PATIENT(S), AND NORMAL CONTROLS FROM FAMILIES WITHOUT CANCER PATIENT IN THREE OR MORE GENERATIONS

Group	Case no.	Carrier of the fras[a] (no.)	Rate of the carrier (%)
Cancer patients	87	77	88.5
Normal members from cancer families	40	33	82.5
Normal members from families with cancer patient(s)	6	3	50.0
Normal controls from families without cancer patient	71	3	4.2

[a] Fragile site.

Table 11
FRAGILE SITES DETECTED AMONG 204 PERSONS AND THE FREQUENCY OF DETECTION

Group (no.)	Fragile sites (number of carriers, frequency of detection)
Cancer patients (87)	3pl4(70,149), 16q22(10,15), 10q23(12,13), 6q26(8,12), 5q31(7,7), 2q33(6,6), 8q22(5,6), 10q25 (5,5), 14q24(5,5) 1p31(4,5),1p32(4,4), 9q22 (4,4), 1q21(3,4), 2q31(3,3), 7q31(3,3), 9q32(3,3), 11q23(3,3), 2q11(2,3), 12q13(2,3),1q44(2,2), 5pl3(2,2), 6p22(2,2), 7q22(2,2), 11q13(2,2), 13q34(2,2), Xq22(2,2), 7p13(2,2), 16p12(1,2), 1p21,[a] 1p22,[a] 1q42,[a] 2p13,[a] 2q21,[a] 2q37,[a] 4p11,[a] 4q12,[a] 6p23,[a] 6q23,[a] 7p11,[a] 7q12,[a] 7q32,[a] 8q24,[a] 10q22,[a] 11p14,[a] 11p15,[a] 11q14,[a] 14q23,[a] 15q22,[a] 17q23,[a] 18q22,[a] and 19q13[a]
Normal members from cancer families (40)	3p14(24,49), 5q31(5,5), 1p22(4,4), 2q31(3,3), 4q31(3,3), 11q13(3,3), 9q22(2,4), 6q26(2,2), 7q22(2,2), 8q22(2,2), 11p15(2,2), 1p21,[a] 1p32,[a] 1q21,[a] 2q11,[a] 2q21,[a] 3p24,[a] 4q12,[a] 5p13,[a] 6p22,[a] 6q23,[a] 7p11,[a] 7p14,[a] 7p22,[a] 7q31,[a] 10q22,[a] 10q23,[a] 11q23,[a] 12q13,[a] 14q21,[a] and 16q22[a]
Normal members from families with cancer history (6)	1q25(1,2), 3p14,[a] 4q12,[a] 4p16,[a] and 5q31[a]
Normal controls (71)	1p22(2,2) and 3p14[a]

[a] (1,1).

who are 40 to 69 years of age from the families with multiple esophageal cancer account for a total (about 3000 persons) of less than 1% of the whole population of the county (360,000). Using the previously described laboratory methods, we divided these individuals at risk into subgroups with various degrees of risk according to their individual test results. For instance, the ones with marked epithelial dysplasia of the esophagus, low DNA excision repair capacity, high chromosome aberration rate, and fragile site(s) could be considered as the subgroup with the highest risk of esophageal cancer.

Depending upon the manpower and financial support available, various preventive measures could be applied to some or all of these subgroups. Persuading them to change their harmful dietary habits and to quit smoking, supplying them with necessary vitamins (B_2, C, etc.) and/or drugs (retinoic acid derivatives, etc.) which may inhibit the malignant transformation of esophageal epithelia are some of the measures to be used (see Figure 5).[8,16] Since these persons all had esophageal cancer deaths in their families, they should be cooperative participants in such a mass prevention program and provide reliable information. Moreover, since they are near or at the age of developing esophageal carcinoma, the effectiveness of such a program could be evaluated in a relatively short period of time. Once the

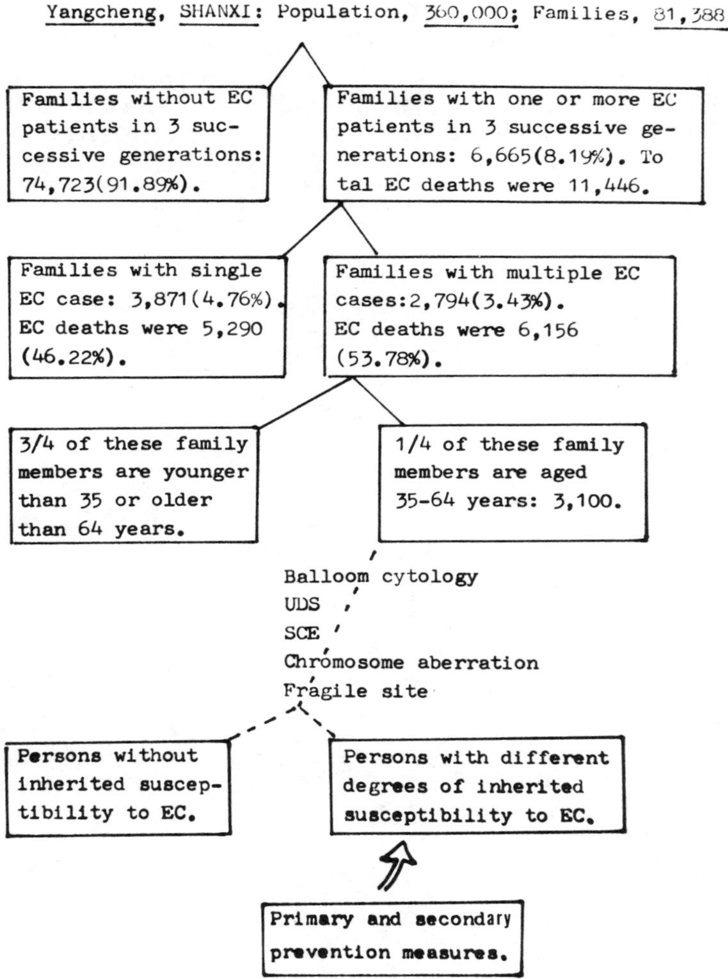

FIGURE 5. Sketch of the strategy for prevention of esophageal cancer in Yangcheng.

effect of this intervention becomes evident, the rest of the inhabitants will gradually adopt the same measures. This may well be a realistic and economic way to control cancer of the esophagus in high-incidence areas in a developing country such as China.

ACKNOWLEDGMENTS

The authors are deeply indebted to Drs. M. Liao-Law and A. B. Burdick for reading the manuscript.

REFERENCES

1. National Cancer Control Office, *Investigation of Cancer Mortality in China,* People's Health Publishing House, Beijing, 1980.
2. National Cancer Control Office, Nanjing Institute of Geography, *Atlas of Cancer Mortality in the People's Republic of China,* China Map Press, Beijing, 1980.

3. **Yang, S. C.,** Research on esophageal cancer in China: a review, *Cancer Res.*, 40, 2633, 1980.
4. **Li, J. Y.,** Epidemiology of esophageal cancer in China, *Natl. Cancer Inst. Monogr.*, 62, 113, 1982.
5. **Li, J. Y.,** Investigation of geographic patterns of cancer mortality in China, *Natl. Cancer Inst. Monogr.*, 62, 17, 1982.
6. **Liu, B. Q. and Li, B.,** Epidemiology of carcinoma of the esophagus in China, in *Carcinoma of the Esophagus and Gastric Cardia,* Huang, G. J. and Wu, Y. K., Eds., Springer-Verlag, Berlin, 1984, chap. 1.
7. Coordinating Group for the Research of Esophageal Carcinoma, Henan Province and Chinese Academy of Medical Sciences, Studies on relationship between epithelial dysplasia and carcinoma of the esophagus, *Chin. Med. J.*, 1, 110, 1975.
8. **Lin, P. Z., Lu, S. X., and Zhang, J. S.,** The present status of studies on precancerous lesions of esophagus (epithelial dysplasia), *Chin. J. Oncol.*, 5, 391, 1983.
9. **Shen, Q.,** Diagnostic cytology and early detection, in *Carcinoma of the Esophagus and Gastric Cardia,* Huang, G. J. and Wu, Y. K., Eds., Springer-Verlag, Berlin, 1984, chap. 6.
10. **Wu, Y. K. and Huang, G. J.,** Surgical treatment, in *Carcinoma of the Esophagus and Gastric Cardia,* Huang, G. J. and Wu, Y. K., Eds., Springer-Verlag, Berlin, 1984, chap. 11.
11. **Doll, R.,** The geographic distribution of cancer, *Br. J. Cancer.*, 23, 1, 1969.
12. **Clemmesen, J.,** *Statistical Studies in Malignant Neoplasm,* Vol. 1, Munksgaard, Copenhagen, 1965, 104.
13. **De hong, U. W., Breslow, N., Hong, J. G. E., Sridharen, M., and Shanmugaratnam, K.,** Etiological factors in esophageal cancer in Singapore Chinese, *Int. J. Cancer,* 13(3), 291, 1974.
14. **Mulvihill, J. J.,** Cancer control through genetics, in *Genes, Chromosomes, and Neoplasia,* Arrighi, F. E., Rao, P. N., and Stubblefield, E., Eds., Raven Press, New York, 1981, 501.
15. **Higginson, J. and Muir, C. S.,** Environmental carcinogenesis: misconception and limitations to cancer control, *J. Natl. Cancer Inst.*, 63, 1291, 1979.
16. **Ding, J. H. and Wu, M.,** Genetically determined susceptibility to esophageal cancer (EC) in high-incidence areas of North China and the genetic approach to its control, in *Genes and Disease, Proceedings of the First Sino-American Human Genetics Workshop,* Wu, M. and Nebert, D. W., Eds., Science Press, Beijing, 1986, 48.
17. **Li, G. H. and He, L. J.,** A survey on the familial aggregation of esophageal cancer in Yangcheng county, Shanxi province, in *Genes and Disease, Proceedings of the First Sino-American Human Genetics Workshop,* Wu, M. and Nebert, D. W., Eds., Science Press, Beijing, 1986, 43.
18. **Klein, G. and Klein, E.,** Evolution of tumors and the impact of molecular oncology, *Nature,* 315, 190, 1985.
19. **Foulds, L., Ed.,** *Neoplastic Development,* Academic Press, New York, 1975, 764.
20. **Farber, E. and Cameron, R.,** The sequential analysis of cancer development, *Adv. Cancer Res.*, 31, 125, 1980.
21. **German, J.,** Chromosomal breakage syndromes, *Birth Defects,* 5(5), 117, 1969.
22. **Heddle, J. A., Krepinsky, A. B., and Marshall, R. R.,** Cellular sensitivity to mutagens and carcinogens in the chromosome-breakage and other cancer-prone syndromes, in *Chromosome Mutation and Neoplasia,* German, J., Ed., Alan R. Liss, New York, 1983, 203.
23. **Rowley, J. D.,** Biological implications of consistent chromosome rearrangements in leukemia and lymphoma, *Cancer Res.*, 44, 3159, 1984.
24. **German, J.,** Genes which increase chromosomal instability in somatic cells and predispose to cancer, *Prog. Med. Genet.*, 8, 61, 1972.
25. **German, J.,** The association of chromosome instability, defective DNA repair, and cancer in some rare human genetic diseases, in *Human Genetics,* Armendares, S. and Lisker, R., Eds., Excerpta Medica, Amsterdam, 1977, 64.
26. **Cleaver, J. E.,** Defective repair replication of DNA in xeroderma pigmentosum, *Nature,* 218, 652, 1968.
27. **Rasmussen, R. E.,** Repair of chemical carcinogen-induced lesions, in *Genetic Differences in Chemical Carcinogenesis,* Kouri, R., Ed., CRC Press, Boca Raton, FL, 1980, chap. 3.
28. **Lynch, H. T., Lynch, P. M., and Guirgis, H. A.,** Host-environmental interaction and carcinogenesis, in *Genetic Differences in Chemical Carcinogenesis,* Kouri, R. E., Ed., CRC Press, Boca Raton, FL, 1980, chap. 7.
29. **Ding, J. H., Wang, X. Q., and Wu, M.,** DNA repair in esophageal cancer (EC) patients and their blood relatives in Lin Xian county, in *Abstracts of Contributed Papers, Part I, 15th International Congress of Genetics,* Oxford & IBH Publishing, New Delhi, 1983, 57.
30. **Wu, D. F., Zheng, Z., Zhang, Y., and Liu, H. L.,** DNA repair capacity of human gastric mucosal epithelia and mortality rate of gastric cancer, *Heredity Dis.*, 4(3), 133, 1987.
31. **Kato, H.,** Spontaneous and induced sister chromatid exchanges as revealed by the BUdR-labelling method, *Int. Rev. Cytol.*, 49, 55, 1977.
32. **Wolff, S., Rodin, B., and Cleaver, J. E.,** Sister chromatid exchanges induced by mutagenic carcinogens in normal and xeroderma pigmentosum cells, *Nature,* 265, 345, 1977.

33. **Chaganti, R. S. K., Schonberg, S., and German, J.,** A manyfold increase in sister chromatid exchanges in Bloom syndrome lymphocytes, in *Proc. Natl. Acad. Sci. U.S.A.*, 71, 4508, 1974.
34. **Latt, S. A., Shreck, R. R., Dougherty, C. P., Gustashaw, K. M., Juergens, L. A., and Kaiser, T. N.,** Sister chromatid exchange — the phenomenon and relationship to chromosome-fragility diseases, in *Chromosome Mutation and Neoplasia*, German, J., Ed., Alan R. Liss, New York, 1983, 169.
35. **Li, M. X. and Cheng, S. J.,** Etiology of the carcinoma of the esophagus, in *Carcinoma of the Esophagus and Gastric Cardia*, Huang, G. J. and Wu, Y. K., Eds., Springer-Verlag, Berlin, 1984, chap. 2.
36. **Xu, N. Z., Hu, N., Wang, X. Q., Wu, M., Tang, Z. Z., and He, L. J.,** Nitrosomethylbenzylamine (NMB_zA) induced increase of SCEs and the individual susceptibility to esophageal cancer, *Natl. Med. J. China*, 66, 733, 1986.
37. **Hu, N., Wang, X. Q., Wu, M., Zheng, Q. Y., Zhang, Z., Liu, Y. C., and Li, G. H.,** Chromosome fragility in 30 esophageal cancer patients, *Natl. Med. J. China*, 65, 404, 1985.
38. **Hu, N., Wang, X. Q., Wu, M., Tang, Z. Z., Kong, L. H., and Wang, Y. L.,** Chromosome fragility in patients with lymphoma and lymphocytic leukemia, *Chin. J. Hematol.*, 6, 389, 1985.
39. **Hu, N., Wang, X. Q., Xu, X., Wu, M., and Hong, W. J.,** Chromosome fragility in 70 patients with malignancies, *Heredity Dis.*, 2, 135, 1985.
40. **Hu, N.,Wang, X. Q., Li, L. Y., Wu, M., He, L. J., Zhao, M. K., and Tang, Z. Z.,** Chromosome aberration rate and genetically determined susceptibility to esophageal cancer, *Natl. Med. J. China*, 66, 593, 1986.
41. **Hu, N., Xu, X., Wang, X. Q., Li, L. Y., Fu, M., Hong, W. J., and Wu, M.,** Cancer family, chromosome aberration rate, and fragile sites, *Heredity Dis.*, 3, 134, 1986.
42. **Hu, N.,** Rate of chromosome aberration, fragile site and genetically determined susceptibility to cancer, Ph.D. Dissertation, Cancer Institute, CAMS PUMC, Beijing, 1986.
43. **Lynch, H. T. and Krush, A. J.,** The cancer family syndrome and cancer control, *Surg. Gynecol. Obste* 132, 247, 1971.
44. **Yunis, J. J. and Soreng, A. L.,** Constitutive fragile sites and cancer, *Science*, 226, 1199, 1984.
45. **Yunis, J. J.,** Genes and chromosomes in human cancer, *Prog. Med. Virol.*, 32, 58, 1985.
46. **Yunis, J. J.,** Chromosomal rearrangements, genes, and fragile sites in cancer: clinical and biologic implications, in *Important Advances in Oncology 1986*, DeVita, V. T., Jr., Hellman, S., and Rosenberg, S. A., Eds., Lippincott, Philadelphia, 1986, chap. 5.
47. **Rowley, J. D.,** A new consistent chromosomal abnormality in chronic myelogenous leukemia identified by quinacrine fluorescence and Giemsa staining, *Nature*, 243, 290, 1973.
48. **Zech, L., Haglund, U., and Nilsson, K.,** Characteristic chromosomal abnormalities in biopsies and lymphoid cell lines from patients with Burkitt and non-Burkitt Lymphomas, *Int. J. Cancer*, 17, 47, 1976.
49. **Le Beau, M. M., Diaz, M. O., Karin, M., and Rowley, J. D.,** Metallothionein gene cluster is split by chromosome 16 rearrangements in myelomonocytic leukemia, *Nature*, 313, 709, 1985.
50. **Whang-Peng, J., Kao-Shan, C. S., Lee, E. C., Bunn, P. A., Carney, D. N., Gaydar, A. F., and Minna, J. D.,** Specific chromosome defect associated with small-cell lung cancer: deletion 3p(14-23), *Science*, 215, 181, 1982.
51. **Cavenee, W., Dryla, T. P., Phillips, R. A., Benedict, W. F., Godbout, R., Gallie, B. L., Murphree, A. L., Strong, L. C., and White, R. L.,** Expression of recessive alleles by chromosomal mechanisms in retinoblastoma, *Nature*, 305, 779, 1983.
52. **Koufos, A., Hansen, M. F., Lampkin, B. C., Workman, M. L., Copeland, N. G., Jenkins, N. A., and Cavenee, W. K.,** Loss of alleles at loci on human chromosome 11 during genesis of Wilms' tumor, *Nature*, 309, 170, 1984.
53. **Leder, P., Battey, J., Lenoir, G., Moulding, C., Murphy, W., Potter, H., Stewart, T., Taub, T., and Taub, R.,** Translocation among antibody genes in human cancer, *Science*, 222, 765, 1983.
54. **Wu, M., Hu, N., and Wang, X. Q.,** Familial aggregation of esophageal cancer in high-incidence areas of North China: a strategy of control through genetic analysis, in *Familial Cancer, 1st Int. Res. Conf.*, Mueller, H. and Weber, W., Eds., Karger, Basel, 1985, 52.

Chapter 13

GENETICS OF COLON CANCER AT THE INFRA-HUMAN LEVEL

Margaret A. Tempero

In the absence of a reliable animal model for spontaneous colon cancer, carcinogen-induced models have become widely used and accepted by most as being biologically similar to the human counterpart. Although many colon carcinogens have been described such as aflatoxin, nitrosamines, nitrosamides, aryl and heterocyclic amines, the most commonly used agents are 1,2-dimethylhydrazine (DMH) and its proximate metabolites, azoxymethane (AOM) and methylazoxymethanol (MAM).

This family of carcinogens was developed following the discovery by Laqueur[1] in 1965 that cycasin, derived from the nut of the cycad tree, was a potent colon carcinogen. The structure of cycasin was shown to be the β-glucoside of MAM.[2] Druckrey[3] subsequently demonstrated that DMH was structurally related to MAM and shared organotropism with this agent. Druckrey suggested that DMH might be metabolized to MAM *in vivo* and this was later confirmed by Fiala[4] who also demonstrated that AOM was an intermediate metabolite of DMH.

The spontaneous decomposition of MAM yields formaldehyde and a methyl diazonium ion, an unstable electrophilic methyl carbonium ion capable of methylating nucleic acids.[4] However, the final steps in the metabolism of MAM have not been clearly defined and the spontaneous release of a methylating species does not explain the unusual organotropism of this compound. Weisburger[5] proposed that DMH might be metabolized to MAM in the liver, and transported to the colon via the bile. However, it has since been shown that parenterally administered DMH and MAM will produce colon tumors in parts of the colon excluded from the fecal stream,[6,7] suggesting that the carcinogen gains access to the colon mucosa via the blood supply.

Alcohol dehydrogenase may be involved in the final metabolic pathway of MAM. Grab and Zedeck[8] have suggested that MAM is metabolized by alcohol dehydrogenase to the aldehydic derivative. Indeed, pyrazole (an inhibitor of NAD+-dependent alcohol dehydrogenase) appears to block both MAM-induced acute toxicity and carcinogenesis.[8-10] However, disulfiram, an inhibitor of aldehyde dehydrogenase, also decreases the carcinogenicity of MAM,[11] and Fiala et al.[12] has demonstrated that MAM is still metabolized in mice genetically deficient in tissue alcohol dehydrogenase. Thus, neither the question of the final step in the metabolism of MAM nor the biochemical sequence explaining its organotropism have been resolved.

In experimental studies, DMH is usually given subcutaneously to rodents in multiple weekly doses. As with most carcinogens, increasing the number of doses decreases tumor latency time and increases tumor yield.[13] However, a single large dose of DMH can produce colon tumors in the majority of treated animals after a long observation period.[14] DMH and AOM occasionally produce extra colonic tumors in proximal small bowel, pancreas, and external ear canal.[15,16] Attempts to produce colon tumors with these carcinogens have failed in dogs and swine because of acute hepatotoxicity, and in guinea pigs in which only bile duct carcinomas and hepatomas were observed.[17]

MAM is an unstable compound in aqueous solution and is commercially available as an acetate ester. It is administered by intraperitoneal injection with similar scheduling as described for DMH and has also been shown to cause extra colonic tumors. In addition to proximal small bowel tumors, MAM has been shown to produce tumors of kidney, liver, and lung in rodents.[9] In guinea pigs, MAM, like DMH, has been shown to induce hepatocarcinomas and bile duct carcinomas.[18] Similar pathologic findings along with colon polyps have been demonstrated with administration of MAM acetate to old-world monkeys.[19]

In rodents, the pathology of intestinal neoplasms induced by this family of carcinogens is somewhat strain dependent. It is not clear that an adenoma-adenocarcinoma sequence exists in all models. Ultrastructural studies in colon mucosa of male Fischer 344 rats after treatment with AOM support an adenoma-adenocarcinoma sequence in that animal.[20,21] However, Maskens and Dujardin-Loits[22] have described DMH-induced microscopic invasive carcinomas in inbred male BB IX rats and in reviewing the literature, these authors conclude that *de novo* carcinogenesis can occur with this family of carcinogens and that both *de novo* carcinomas and adenomatous polyps can even occur within the same experimental model. The majority of large bowel lesions identified in Sprague-Dawley and Wistar rats appear to be adenocarcinomas although adenomas have also been described. Other examples include the appearance of distal adenomas (exophytic neoplasms) in DMH-induced colon tumors of CF_1 and random-bred ICR/Ha Swiss mice, contrasted with the appearance of predominantly adenocarcinomas in inbred ICR/Ha Swiss mice after carcinogen treatment.[23,24] Germ-free Fisher rats develop colon adenomas while conventional Fisher rats tend to develop adenocarcinomas following DMH treatment.[25] Thus, nongenetic factors may also be responsible in part for variable pathology of DMH-induced colon tumors.

Clearly, many factors independent of genetic susceptibility will modify the incidence of experimental colon tumors. These include age, sex, diet, character or presence of the fecal stream, and nonspecific injury. Young age and female sex are associated with an increased susceptibility to carcinogen treatment although rigorous trials evaluating these parameters have not yet been conducted.[16] Increased dietary fat intake appears to enhance colon carcinogenesis;[26-29] increased dietary cholesterol[30,31] and decreased dietary fiber[32-35] are sometimes associated with similar effects. Increased fecal bile acids,[36-39] especially secondary bile acids, and changes in fecal bacterial metabolic activity[40,41] are often associated with enhanced colon carcinogenesis. Germ-free rats[42] or rats with a diverted fecal stream[43] are less susceptible to carcinogen treatment. Nonspecific injury of the colon enhances tumor yield at the site of injury.[44,45] Finally, certain pharmacologic agents such as butylated hydroxyanisole,[46] indomethacin,[47] difluoromethylornithine,[48] and dihydroepiandrosterone[49] can influence colon carcinogenesis by interfering with carcinogen metabolism or poorly understood events in colon tumor promotion.

Resistence of certain rat and mouse strains to colon tumor induction has been well documented. In 1974, Evans et al.[50] demonstrated that C57BL/Ha and DBA/2 mice were resistant to DMH treatment, while inbred ICR/Ha mice were 100% susceptible to the carcinogen. These investigators studied this relationship further in F_1, F_2, and reciprocal hybrids derived from a cross between the two inbred mouse strains, ICR/Ha and C57BL/Ha.[24] In this study, tumor incidence in the F_1 hybrids was 100 and 78% in F_2 hybrids. Tumor incidence in the resistant backcross mice of genotype C57BL/Ha X F_1 was 39%. These authors concluded that sensitivity to DMH-induced colon tumors in the experimental model follows an autosomal dominant mode of inheritance.

Diwan et al.[51,52] also noted genetic differences in the induction of colorectal tumors by DMH. These investigators studied several inbred strains (SWR/J, P/J, C57BL/6J, and AKR/J). In this study, SWR/J and P/J mice demonstrated a tumor incidence of 80% or greater. Strain AKR/J appeared to be resistant although these animals died from leukemia and the shortened survival time may have interfered with the identification of colon lesions. In their report, the C57BL/6J mouse strain was not totally resistant with 48% of the animals developing colorectal tumors. This discrepancy was thought to be related to age of animals during carcinogen exposure. Because DMH is metabolized to MAM *in vivo*, Diwan et al.[53] also studied the effects of MAM acetate on some of the same mouse strains. Susceptibility to MAM acetate appeared to be greater overall with 100% of the SRW/J mice and 77% of the C57BL/6J mice demonstrating colon tumors. As in the prior studies, the AKR/J mice died early of leukemia. These studies suggest that at least one explanation for DMH resistance might be a genetic inability to metabolize the carcinogen.

The question of impaired DMH metabolism as an explanation for DMH resistance has been explored by Pollard and Zedeck.[54] In this study, Lobund Wistar rats thought to be resistant to DMH were treated with MAM acetate and surprisingly demonstrated MAM acetate sensitivity although the tumors produced were smaller in size and number than those produced in Sprague-Dawley rats treated in parallel. These findings led to the conclusion that metabolism of DMH is one probable factor in the mechanism of resistance but that other factors must be involved to explain the apparent change in tumor latency with MAM acetate treatment in certain rodents.

James et al.[23] have attempted to study the morphologic, histochemical, and proliferative changes induced in the colon of sensitive and resistant mice following DMH treatment. While macroscopic lesions were common in the ICR/Ha mice, microscopic analysis of the resistant C57BL/HA mouse also demonstrated small foci of adenocarcinomas. This supports the suggestion that the ''resistance'' of the C57BL/Ha strain is a function of tumor latency. In addition, early expansion of the zone of cell proliferation along with an earlier appearance of dysplastic foci in epithelium of large bowel mucosa was identified in the sensitive ICR/Ha strain. Deschner et al.[55,56] have subsequently evaluated the proliferative characteristics of colonic epithelial cells in sensitive and resistant mouse strains following treatment with both DMH and MAM. In these studies, the tritiated thymidine labeling index of colon mucosa and the size of the proliferative compartment showed a positive correlation with sensitivity to carcinogen treatment. These findings were not confirmed by Wargovich et al,[57] a possible result of genetic drift in the outbred CF_1 mice used for study.

Recently, Bolognesi and Boffa[62] have examined DNA damage in liver, kidney, and colon after DMH administration in resistant and sensitive mice. Although DNA damage in liver and kidney was equal in all strains, colon DNA damage showed a positive correlation with strain susceptibility. Resistant mice (AKR/J, DBA/2) showed virtually no colon DNA damage. Thus, DNA strand breakage may serve as a biomarker for DMH susceptibility in experimental carcinogenesis.

In summary, DMH and related compounds are commonly used in experimental models of colon carcinogenesis. Many nongenetic factors can influence susceptibility to these carcinogens. In certain species and strains of rats and mice, the histopathology of colon tumors resembles that seen in the human counterpart with a suggested adenoma/adenocarcinoma sequence. Resistance to treatment with DMH and its proximate metabolites has been documented in rats and mice. DMH resistance appears to follow an autosomal dominant pattern of inheritance and may be related in part to an inability to metabolize DMH. Abnormalities in colon epithelial cell proliferation or DNA damage may be useful biomarkers in predicting colon tumor susceptibility in experimental models.

REFERENCES

1. **Laqueur, G. L.,** The induction of intestinal neoplasms in rats with the glycoside cycasin and its aglycone, *Virchows Arch. Pathol. Anat.*, 340, 151, 1965.
2. **Matsumoto, H.,** Carcinogenicity of cycasin, its aglycone methlazoxymethanol, and methylazoxymethyl-glucosiduronic acid, in *Naturally Occurring Carcinogen-Mutagens, and Modulators of Carcinogenesis,* Miller, E. C., Miller, J. A., Hirono, I., Sugimuri, T., and Tarayama, S., Eds., University Park Press, Baltimore, 1979, 67.
3. **Druckrey, H.,** Production of colonic carcinomas by 1,2-diakylhydrazines and azoxyalkanes, in *Carcinomas of Colon and Antededent Epitheliaum,* Burdette, W. J., Ed., Charles C Thomas, Springfield, IL, 1970, 267.
4. **Fiala, E. S.,** Investigations in to the metabolism and mode of action of the colon carcinogens 1,2-dimethylhydrazine and azoxymethane, *Cancer,* 40, 2436, 1977.
5. **Weisburger, J. H.,** Colon carcinogens: their metabolism and mode of action. *Cancer,* 28, 60, 1971.
6. **Rubio, C. A. and Nylander, G.,** Further studies on the carcinogenesis of the colon of the rat with special reference to the absence of intestinal contents, *Cancer,* 48, 951, 1981.
7. **Matsubara, N., Mori, H., and Hirono, I.,** Effect of colostomy on intestinal carcinogenesis by methylazoxymethanol acetate in rats, *J. Natl. Cancer Inst.,* 61, 1161, 1978.
8. **Grab, D. J. and Zedeck, M. S.,** Organ-specific effects of the carcinogen methylazoxymethanol related to metabolism by nicotinamide adenine dinucleotide-dependent dehydrogenases, *Cancer Res.,* 37, 4182, 1977.
9. **Notman, J., Tan, C. H., and Zedeck, M. J.,** Inhibition of methylazoxymethanol-induced intestinal tumors in the rat by pyrazole with parodoxical effects on skin and kidney, *Cancer Res.,* 42, 1774, 1982.
10. **Moriya, M., Harada, T., and Shirasu, Y.,** Inhibition of carcinogenicities of 1,2-dimethylhydrazine and azoxymethane by pyrazole, *Cancer Lett.,* 17, 147, 1982.
11. **Wattenberg, L. W., Lam, L. K. T., Fladmoe, A. V., and Borchert, P.,** Inhibitors of colon carcinogenesis, *Cancer,* 40, 2432, 1977.
12. **Fiala, E. S., Coswell, N., Stathopoulos, C., Felder, M. R., and Weisburger, J. H.,** Non-alcohol dehyrdrogenase mediated metabolism of methylazoxymethanol (MAM), *Proc. Am. Assoc. Cancer Res.,* 24, 318A, 1983.
13. **Deschner, E. E., Long, F. C., and Maskens, A. P.,** Relationship between dose, time and tumor yield in mouse dimethylhydrazine-induced colon tumorigenesis, *Cancer Lett.,* 8, 23, 1979.
14. **Schiller, C. M., Curley, W. H., and McConnell, E. E.,** Induction of colon tumors by a single oral dose of 1,2-dimethylhydrazine, *Cancer Lett.,* 11, 75, 1980.
15. **Ward, J. M., Yamamoto, R. S., and Brown, C. A.,** Pathology of intestine neoplasms and other lesions in rats exposed to azoxymethane, *J. Natl. Cancer Inst.,* 51, 1029, 1973.
16. **Rogers, A. E., and Nauss, K. M.,** Rodent models for carcinoma of the colon, *Dig. Dis. Sci.,* 30, 875, 1985.
17. **Wilson, R. B.,** Species variation in responses to dimethylhydrazine, *Toxicol. Appl. Pharmacol.,* 38, 647, 1976.
18. **Laqueur, G. L. and Spatz, M.,** Oncogenecity of cycasin and methylazoxymethanol, in *Recent Topics in Chemical Carcinogenesis,* Gann Monogr. 17, Odashima, S., Takayama, S., and Sato, H., Eds., University Park Press, Baltimore, 1975, 189.
19. **Sieber, S. M., Conea, P., Dalgard, D. W., McIntire, K. R., and Adamson, R. H.,** Carcinogenicity and hepatotoxicity of cycasin and its aglycone methylazoxymethanol acetate in non-human primates, *J. Natl. Cancer Inst.,* 65, 177, 1980.
20. **Shamsuddin, A. K. M. and Trump, B. F.,** Colon epithelium. II. In vivo studies of colon carcinogenesis. Light microscopic, histochemical and ultrastructural studies of histogenesis of azoxymethane-induced colon carcinomas in Fischer 344 rats, *J. Natl. Cancer Inst.,* 66, 389, 1981.
21. **Shamsuddin, A. K. M.,** Carcinoma of the large intestine: animal models and human disease, *Hum. Pathol.,* 17, 451, 1986.
22. **Maskens, A. P. and Dujardin-Loits, R.,** Experimental adenomas and carcinomas of the large intestine behave as distinct entities: most carcinomas arise de novo in flat mucosa, *Cancer,* 47, 81, 1981.
23. **James, J. T., Shamsuddin, A. M., and Trump, B. F.,** Comparative study of the morphologic, histochemical and proliferative changes induced in the large intestine of ICR/Ha and C57BL/Ha mice by 1,2-dimethylhydrazine, *J. Natl. Cancer Inst.,* 71, 955, 1983.
24. **Evans, J. T., Shows, T. B., Sproul, E. E., Paolini, N. S., Mittelman, A., and Hauschka, T.,** Genetics of colon carcinogenesis in mice treated with 1,2-dimethylhydrazine, *Cancer Res.,* 37, 134, 1977.
25. **Reddy, B. S., Watanabe, K., Weisberger, J. H., and Wynder, E. L.,** Promoting effect of bile acids in colon carcinogenesis in germ-free and conventional F344 rats, *Cancer Res.,* 37, 3238, 1977.
26. **Bull, A. W., Soullier, B. K., Wilson, P. S., Hayden, M. T., and Nigro, N. D.,** Promotion of azoxymethane induced intestinal cancer by high fat diets in rats, *Cancer Res.,* 39, 4956, 1978.

27. **Reddy, B. S., Watanabe, K., and Weisberger, J. H.,** Effect of high-fat diets on colon carcinogenesis in F344 rats treated with 1,2-dimethylhydrazine, methylazoxymethanol acetate, or methylnitrosourea, *Cancer Res.*, 37, 156, 1977.
28. **Sakaguchi, M., Minoura, T., Hiramatsu, Y., Takada, H., Yamamura, M., Hioki, K., and Yamamoto, M.,** Effects of dietary saturated and unsaturated fatty acids on fecal bile acids and colon carcinogenesis induced by azoxymethane in rats, *Cancer Res.*, 46, 61, 1986.
29. **Nigro, N. D., Singh, D. V., Campbell, R. L., and Pak, M. S.,** Effect of dietary beef fat on intestinal tumor formation by azoxymethane in rats, *J. Natl. Cancer Inst.*, 54, 439, 1975.
30. **Hiramatsu, U., Takada, H., Yamamura, M., et al.,** Effect of dietary cholesterol on azoxymethane-induced colon carcinogenesis in rats, *Carcinogenesis*, 4, 553, 1983.
31. **Cruse, J. P., Lewin, M. R., Ferilano, G. P., and Clark, C. G.,** Co-carcinogenic effects of dietary cholesterol in experimental colon cancer, *Nature*, 276, 822, 1978.
32. **Barbolt, T. A. and Rajender, A.,** The effect of bran on dimethylhydrazine-induced colon carcinogenesis in the rat, *Proc. Soc. Exp. Biol. Med.*, 157, 656, 1978.
33. **Fleiszer, D., Murray, D., Macfarlane, J., and Brown, R. A.,** Protective effect of dietary fiber against chemically induced bowel tumors in rats, *Lancet*, 2, 552, 1978.
34. **Freeman, H. J., Spiller, G. A., and Kim, Y. S.,** A double-blind study on the effect of purified cellulose dietary fiber on 1,2-dimethylhydrazine-induced rat colonic neoplasia, *Cancer Res.*, 38, 2912, 1978.
35. **Wilson, R. B., Hutcheson, D. P., and Wideman, L.,** Dimethylhydrazine-induced colon tumors in rats fed diets containing beef fat or corn oil with or without wheat bran, *Am. J. Clin. Nutr.*, 30, 176, 1977.
36. **Narisawa, T., Magadia, N. E., Weisburger, J. H., and Wynder, E. L.,** Promoting effect of bile acids on colon carcinogenesis after intrarectal instillation of *N*-methyl-*N*-nitro-nitrosoguanidine in rats, *J. Natl. Cancer Inst.*, 53, 1093, 1974.
37. **Reddy, B. S. and Watanabe, K.,** Effect of cholesterol metabolites and promoting effect of lithocholic acid and colon carcinogenesis in germ-free and conventional F344 rats, *Cancer Res.*, 39, 1521, 1979.
38. **Chomchai, C., Bhadrachari, N., and Nigro, N. D.,** The effect of bile on the induction of experimental intestinal tumors in rats, *Dis. Colon Rectum*, 17, 310, 1974.
39. **Oscarson, J. A., Veen, H. F., Ross, J. S., and Malt, R. A.,** Ileal resection potentiates 1,2-dimethylhydrazine-induced colonic carcinogenesis, *Ann. Surg.*, 189, 503, 1979.
40. **Reddy, D. S., Mangat, S., Weisburger, J. H., and Wynder, E. L.,** Effect of high risk diets for colon carcinogenesis on intestinal mucosal and bacterial β-glucuronidase activity in F344 rats, *Cancer Res.*, 37, 3533, 1977.
41. **Bauer, H. G., Asp, N. C., Oste, R., Dahlqvist, A., and Fredlung, P. E.,** Effect of dietary fiber on the induction of colorectal tumors and fecal β-glucuronidase activity in the rat, *Cancer Res.*, 39, 3752, 1979.
42. **Asano, T. and Pollard, M.,** Strain susceptibility and resistance to 1.2-dimethylhydrazine-induced enteric tumors in germ-free rats (40146), *Proc. Soc. Exp. Biol. Med.*, 158, 89, 1978.
43. **Filipe, M. I., Scurr, J. H., and Ellis, H.,** Effects of fecal stream on experimental colorectal carcinogenesis. Morphologic and histochemical changes, *Cancer*, 50, 2859, 1982.
44. **Calderisi, R. N. and Freeman, H. J.,** Differential effects of surgical suture materials in 1,2-Dimethylhydrazine-induced rat intestinal neoplasia, *Cancer Res.*, 44, 2827, 1984.
45. **Pozharisski, K. M.,** The significance of nonspecific injury for colon carcinogenesis in rats, *Cancer Res.*, 35, 3824, 1975.
46. **Reddy, B. S., Maeura, Y., and Weisburger, J.,** Effect of various levels of dietary butylated hydroxyanisole on methylazoxymethanol acetate-induced colon carcinogenesis of CF_1 mice, *J. Natl. Cancer Inst.*, 71, 1298, 1983.
47. **Pollard, M. and Luckert, P. H.,** Indomethacin treatment of rats with dimethylhydrazine-induced intestinal tumors, *Cancer Treat. Rep.*, 64, 1323, 1980.
48. **Kingsnorth, A. N., King, W. W. K., Diekema, K. A., McCann, P. P., Ross, J. S., and Malt, R. A.,** Inhibition of ornithine decarboxylase with difluoromethylornithine: reduced incidence of dimethylhydrazine-induced colon tumors in mice, *Cancer Res.*, 43, 2545, 1983.
49. **Nyce, J. W., Vhagee, P. N., Hard, G. C., and Schwartz, A. G.,** Inhibition of 1,2-dimethylhydrazine-induced colon tumorigenesis in BALB/c mice by dehydroepiandrosterone, *Carcinogenesis*, 5, 57, 1984.
50. **Evans, J. T., Hauschka, T. S., and Mittelman, A.,** Brief communication: differential susceptibility of four mouse strains to induction of multiple large-bowel neoplasms by 1,2-dimethylhydrazine, *J. Natl. Cancer Inst.*, 52, 999, 1974.
51. **Diwan, B. A., Meier, H., and Blackman, K. E.,** Genetic differences in the induction of colorectal tumors by 1,2-dimethylhydrazine in inbred mice, *J. Natl. Cancer Inst.*, 59, 455, 1977.
52. **Diwan, B. A. and Blackman, K. E.,** Differential susceptibility of 3 sublines of C57BL/6 mice to the induction of colorectal tumors by 1,2-dimethylhydrazine, *Cancer Lett.*, 9, 111, 1980.
53. **Diwan, B. A., Dempster, A. M., and Blackman, K. E.,** Effects of methylazoxymethanol acetate on inbred mice: influence of genetic factors on tumor induction (40550), *Proc. Soc. Exp. Biol. Med.*, 161, 347, 1979.

54. **Pollard, M. and Zedeck, M. S.,** Induction of colon tumors in 1,2-dimethylhydrazine-resistant Lobund Wistar rats by methylazoxymethanol acetate, *J. Natl. Cancer Inst.*, 61, 493, 1978.
55. **Deschner, E. E., Long, F. C., Hakissian, M., and Herrmann, S. L.,** Differential susceptibility of AKR, C57BL/6J, and CF1 mice to 1,2-dimethylhydrazine-induced colonic tumor formation predicted by proliferative characteristics of colonic epithelial cells, *J. Natl. Cancer Inst.*, 70, 279, 1983.
56. **Deschner, E. E., Long, F. C., Hakissian, M., and Cupo, S. H.,** Differential susceptibility of inbred mouse strains forecast of acute colonic proliferative response to methylazoxymethanol, *J. Natl. Cancer Inst.*, 72, 195, 1984.
57. **Wargovich, M. J., Medline, A., and Bruce, W. R.,** Early histopathologic events to evolution of colon cancer in C57BL/6 and CF1 mice treated with 1,2-dimethylhydrazine, *J. Natl. Cancer Inst.*, 71, 125, 1983.
58. **Bolognesi, C. and Boffa, L. C.,** Correlation between incidence of 1,2-dimethylhydrazine-induced colon carcinomas and DNA damage in six genetically different mouse strains, *Cancer Lett.*, 30, 91, 1986.

Chapter 14

EPIDEMIOLOGY OF FAMILIAL PREDISPOSITION TO LARGE BOWEL CANCER

Motoi Murata and Takashi Takahashi

TABLE OF CONTENTS

I. INTRODUCTION

Large bowel cancer has been rapidly increasing in recent years in Japan. This trend is especially remarkable for colon as compared with rectal cancers. For instance, age-adjusted mortality rates of colon and rectum cancers in males were 2.3 and 4.3 per 10^5 population, respectively, in 1955, while the corresponding rate was 7.2 and 6.2, respectively, in 1984.[2] This elevation was undoubtedly brought about by rigorous changes of life styles in Japan. In particular, the pattern of nutritional intake has been quite rapidly changed from the Japanese traditional style to that of western countries, the latter being a preference for consumption of animal foods and less cereals. The national nutritional survey conducted by the Ministry of Health and Welfare demonstrated that the per capita intake of fat in 1980 was slightly more than three times as high as that of 1950 and that of carbohydrate was decreased to about 80% during the same period.[3] Thus, any epidemiologic studies on this cancer should take the chronological changes of the disease incidence into consideration.

In addition to these environmental factors, host factors may also be participating in the etiology of large bowel cancer. A probable significant role of the hereditary factor in large bowel cancer has been generally suspected from the following facts: (1) incidence rate of the same disease among blood relatives of the patients is two- to threefold higher compared with that of the general population;[4,5] (2) a dominant genetic disease, adenomatosis coli, strongly predisposes to this cancer;[6] (3) there exists families with strong clustering of patients which is called the cancer family syndrome, or hereditary nonpolyposis colon cancer (HNPCC).[7,8] As the frequency of adenomatosis coli patients is very rare in a population, it cannot account for the whole familial tendency.[9,10] The cancer family syndrome, which was first proposed by Lynch who succeeded the study of Warthin's "G" family, is also considered as being a dominant hereditary condition with proneness to nonpolyposis colon cancer. In Japan, too, case reports of possible HNPCC kindreds tended to increase in recent years.[11-13] This is probably because physicians are inclined to be more careful about the familial anamnesis of this cancer than has been the case in the past. But, unfortunately there are to date no clinical or pathological features which are exclusively found in HNPCC. Therefore, it is not possible to determine whether individual familial cases of large bowel cancer fall under this category or not. Needed is an informative pedigree.

In this study we attempted to clarify possible clinicoepidemiological characteristics of the familial large bowel cancer, and by comparing them to those of HNPCC described by Lynch,[8] to examine what proportion of this cancer is ascribable to the genetic etiology.

II. MATERIALS AND METHODS

Hospital records of 1626 patients with large bowel cancer, surgically treated at the Cancer Institute Hospital during the period of 1946 to 1979, were enrolled for the present epidemiologic analysis. Patients with familial polyposis coli were excluded. Cases were classified by their site and multiplicity of the tumor, such as (1) proximal colon cancer, (2) distal colon cancer, (3) rectum cancer, (4) double primary cancer, (5) multiple colorectal cancer (synchronous and metachronous), as shown in Table 1. The fourth category (double primary) was assigned for those who were additionally affected with cancer of other organs but not with a second colorectal cancer. One can obviously see in this table that the number of cases is rapidly increasing in successive quinquennial periods, reflecting the rise of their incidence in the Japanese general population.

Cases were also classified according to their cancer family history (FH) into four categories: (1) positive FH of colon cancer, (2) positive FH of rectal cancer, (3) positive FH of other cancers, and (4) cancer FH negative. The positive FH is defined here as an incidental occurrence of at least one cancer in the first and second degree relatives of a proband patient.

Table 1
NUMBER OF COLORECTAL CANCER PATIENTS BY SITE AND MULTIPLICITY GROUP AND BY YEARS OF HOSPITAL ADMISSION TO CIH

Site/multiplicity	Sex	1946	1950	1955	1960	1965	1970	1975	Total
Proximal colon	M	4	9	15	11	10	18	30	97
	F	2	8	11	11	20	12	17	81
Distal colon	M	7	14	7	16	30	55	53	182
	F	5	5	5	12	22	35	46	130
Rectum	M	32	50	76	65	93	98	130	544
	F	15	40	65	41	65	83	90	399
Double primary	M	0	6	5	5	10	11	16	53
	F	0	3	4	3	8	10	22	50
Multiple colorectal	M	0	10	5	6	10	18	12	61
	F	1	0	2	5	7	3	11	29
Total	M	43	89	108	103	153	200	241	937
	F	23	56	87	72	122	143	186	689

Table 2
PERCENTAGE OF POSITIVE FAMILY HISTORY OF CANCER AMONG COLORECTAL CANCER PATIENTS OF DIFFERENT SITE OR MULTIPLICITY GROUPS AT CIH

Site/multiplicity	Number of Case	Cases with FH of cancer at site (%)					
		Stomach	Colorect	Liver	Lung	Breast	Uterus
Proximal colon	178	18.0	6.2	2.3	1.1	0.6	3.9
Distal colon	312	17.3	6.1	1.9	0.6	2.6	4.5
Rectum	943	19.9	4.2	1.8	1.6	1.1	6.6
Double	103	17.5	8.7	2.9	1.9	1.9	9.7
Multiple	90	26.4	18.9	1.1	0	1.1	11.0
Total	1626	19.4	5.9	1.9	1.3	1.4	6.3

Note: Males and females are pooled.

Investigation of hospital records covered the following items; site and multiplicity of the tumor, age at surgery, the coupled organ of the double primary cancer, concurrence of intestinal polyps, and FH of cancer. The FH was documented if the patient remembered any cancer cases that occurred in their family members. Their family structure was not known. In addition, the information on cancer in the family was not medically verified, which may cause some incorrectness in our data.

III. RESULTS

A. Family History of Cancer

In Table 2, frequency of the positive FH of various cancers is presented for different groups of patients with large bowel cancer by their sites and multiplicity. Positive FH of large bowel cancer was observed, on the average, in 5.9% of the patients (96/1626), of which 2.2% was colon cancer and 3.7% was rectal cancer. The proportion of positive FH of large bowel cancer was 2.7 and 3.6%, respectively, among the breast cancer patients and lung cancer patients in the same hospital (Murata, unpublished data). Hence the presently observed percentage of FH positive for large bowel cancer was almost twice that when compared to the breast and lung cancer patients. Furthermore, among the 96 patients with positive FH 16 reported more than 1 relative as being affected with cancer of the same organ, which is significantly larger than the expected number, 3, from a Poisson distribution. These facts indicate familial aggregation of large bowel cancer in the present study population. It is apparent in Table 2 that the proportion of patients with positive FH of large bowel cancer varies among the five site/multiplicity groups, from 18.9% in the multiple colorectal group to 4.2% in the rectal group. This difference is statistically significant ($X^2 = 33.5$, df $= 4$, $p < 0.01$). However, if the group of multiple primary colorectal cancer is excluded from the analysis, the difference among the remaining four groups is reduced to a nonsignificant level. The FH of other cancers also appears to be variable among these groups, although the differences are not significant.

B. Age at Surgery

Mean age at surgery is shown in Table 3 for the different groups by sites and multiplicity of cancer, and by their cancer FH. The group of multiple colorectal cancer was further divided into synchronously and metachronously occurring cancers. For the latter group, only the age at surgery of earlier onset cancer was counted. It appears that positive FH of other cancers does not have any effect on the age at surgery. Hence this group was pooled with the group of positive FH of no cancers into the one designated as the FH negative. If not discriminating sites and multiplicity of cancer, the average age was 55.3 ± 1.3 years for the group with positive FH of large bowel cancer, the difference being not significant with Student t test. When those cases with positive FH of colon cancer were selected, the mean age of 52.2 differs significantly from that of FH negative group ($t = 2.22$, df $= 1564$, $p < 0.05$). Those with positive FH of two or more colorectal cancers showed a still younger mean age, but the difference from that of the FH negative cases was not significant with Cochran-Cox's method.

C. Double Primary and Multiple Colorectal Cancers

Frequency of double primary cancer was 6.9% (113/1626) as a whole. In approximately 60% of these cases, the extracolonic cancer was diagnosed earlier than the large bowel cancer, 30% were treated simultaneously, and 10% were treated later (Table 4). Almost one half of them manifested stomach cancer and a quarter had uterine cancer. Stomach cancer was most frequently observed in the patients with proximal colon cancer (15/200), which was significantly larger than that (40/1386) in the other groups of patients ($X^2 = 10.4$, df $= 1$, $p < 0.01$). The rate of uterine cancer incidence seemed to be unusually high: the proportion of this cancer among all female cases of double primary cancers was 53.6% (30/56) in contrast with 31.5% (52/165) obtained by a survey study of double primary cancer among stomach cancer patients, which was conducted by the Japan Research Society for Gastric Cancer[4] ($X^2 = 7.8$, df $= 1$, $p < 0.01$). However, for 12 of these 30 cases, the large bowel cancer was considered to be induced by therapeutic radiation for uterine cancer. If they are excluded, the frequency of double primary cancer among total patients become 6.2% and significantly changes among different FH groups, namely 13.5% in the group of positive FH of large bowel cancer, 7.1% in that of other cancers and 4.0% in that of negative FH ($X^2 = 18.4$, df $= 2$, $P < 0.001$).

Multiple colorectal cancer was diagnosed synchronously in 63 and metachronously in 27 patients. Of the former group, the accompanying cancer was staged as an early cancer in 36 cases, whereas in the metachronous group early cancers were rarely found. An early cancer is defined as being localized within the mucosa and submucosa, and may include precancerous lesions. Accordingly the diagnosis of multiple primary cancer may not be true in some cases of synchronously diagnosed colorectal cancer. In Table 2, the proportion of positive FH of large bowel cancer was larger in the patients of metachronous (8/27, 29.6%) than synchronous (9/63, 14.3%) multiple primary cancers. But the difference disappears after excluding those early cancer cases (8/27 vs. 6/27).

Table 3
MEAN AGE AT SURGERY OF COLORECTAL CANCER PATIENTS AT CIH BY SITE AND MULTIPLICITY GROUP AND BY FAMILY HISTORY OF CANCER

Site/Multiplicity	FH (+) of colon cancer	FH (+) of rectal cancer	FH (+) of colorectal cancer	FH (+) of ⩾ 2 colorectal cancer	FH (+) of other cancer	FH (−)
Proximal colon	51.3 ± 5.9 (6)	48.0 ± 6.5 (6)	50.8 ± 4.4 (11)	39.3 ± 5.0[a] (3)	56.6 ± 1.6 (54)	58.1 ± 1.0 (113)
Distal colon	63.6 ± 3.6 (8)	50.9 ± 2.3[a] (12)	56.8 ± 2.4 (19)	49.0 ± 4.9 (3)	56.4 ± 1.4 (88)	57.3 ± 0.8 (205)
Rectum	54.9 ± 3.2 (8)	58.9 ± 1.9 (34)	58.3 ± 1.7 (40)	61.8 ± 6.2 (4)	55.3 ± 0.8 (286)	56.1 ± 0.5 (617)
Double	46.2 ± 8.9 (5)	58.3 ± 8.5 (6)	54.3 ± 5.8 (9)	46.0 ± 28.0 (2)	61.0 ± 1.9 (36)	62.2 ± 1.3 (58)
S. Multiple	46.7 ± 6.6[a] (3)	53.3 ± 4.2 (7)	53.0 ± 4.7 (9)	35.0 (1)	59.5 ± 2.7 (19)	62.3 ± 1.6 (35)
M. Multiple	45.3 ± 4.8[a] (6)	47.5 ± 6.7 (4)	46.5 ± 3.6[a] (8)	47.0 ± 9.5 (3)	54.4 ± 3.6 (7)	56.9 ± 2.7 (12)
Total	52.2 ± 2.3[a] (36)	55.3 ± 1.6 (69)	55.3 ± 1.3 (96)	48.8 ± 4.1 (16)	56.2 ± 0.6 (490)	57.1 ± 0.4 (1040)

Note: Males and females are pooled. Number of cases in parentheses.

[a] Significantly younger compared to F.H.(+) of other cancer and F.H.(−) inclusively, with Student's t-test.

Table 4
FREQUENCY OF EXTRACOLONIC CANCER AMONG COLORECTAL CANCER PATIENTS BY SITE AND MULTIPLICITY OF COLORECTAL CANCER AND BY FAMILY HISTORY OF CANCER

Site/multiplicity	Family history	Number of cases	Double primary cancer		
			Stomach	Uterus	Others
Proximal colon	Colorectal cancer FH(+)	14	2	1	0
	Other cancer FH(+)	66	9	3	0
	FH (−)	120	4	0	3
Distal colon	Colorectal cancer FH(+)	21	1	1	1
	Other cancer FH(+)	100	8	3	1
	FH (−)	221	9	1	6
Rectum	Colorectal cancer FH(+)	44	1	1	3
	Other cancer FH(+)	289	2	4	5
	FH (−)	652	16	14	6
Multiple	Colorectal cancer FH(+)	17	1	0	1
	Other cancer FH(+)	26	1	0	0
	FH (−)	47	1	2	2

Notes: Males and females are pooled.

Table 5
FREQUENCY OF POLYP CONCURRENCE AMONG COLORECTAL CANCER PATIENTS BY SEX, AGE GROUP, SITE AND MULTIPLICITY GROUP, AND FAMILY HISTORY OF COLORECTAL CANCER

Sex	Males	0.353 (331/937)	Females	0.232 (160/698)

Age class	<40	40—49	50—59	60—69	70+
	0.17(26/156)	0.23(68/299)	0.30(135/448)	0.35(175/499)	0.38(96/251)

Site/ multiplicity	FH(+)		FH(−)	
	Age < 50	Age 50+	Age < 50	Age 50+
Proximal colon	0.33 (2/6)	0.40 (2/5)	0.17 (7/41)	0.29 (36/126)
Distal colon	0.25 (1/4)	0.60 (9/15)	0.21 (16/76)	0.32 (69/217)
Rectum	0.0 (0/9)	0.45 (14/31)	0.20 (54/276)	0.32 (202/627)
Double	0.75 (3/4)	0.20 (1/5)	0.14 (2/14)	0.26 (21/80)
S. Multiple	0.50 (2/4)	0.60 (3.5)	0.44 (4/9)	0.76 (34/45)
M. Multiple	0.40 (2/5)	0.33 (1/3)	0.0 (0/3)	0.38 (6/16)
Total	0.31 (10/32)	0.47 (30/64)	0.20 (83/419)	0.33 (368/1111)

D. Polyp Concurrence

Polyp concurrence was observed in 30% of total cases (Table 5). It was more frequently detected in males than females ($X^2 = 26.9$, df $= 1$, $p < 0.001$) and in older than in younger patients ($X^2 = 34.8$, df $= 4$, $p < 0.01$). Distal colon or rectal cancers were accompanied by polyps more frequently than proximal colon cancers. Synchronous multiple colorectal cancers were marked with an exceptionally high rate of polyp concurrence (43/63, 68%). Even after those early cancer cases as defined before were excluded, it still amounts to 56% (15/27). On the contrary, metachronous multiple colorectal cancers presented the rate (9/27, 33%) indistinguishable from that of the total cases. The discrimination between adenomatous or hyperplastic polyps was not made. Our unpublished data, however, indicates that the result would be quite similar even when confined to adenomatous polyps.

FH of colorectal cancer was also somehow associated with the intestinal polyp. In Table

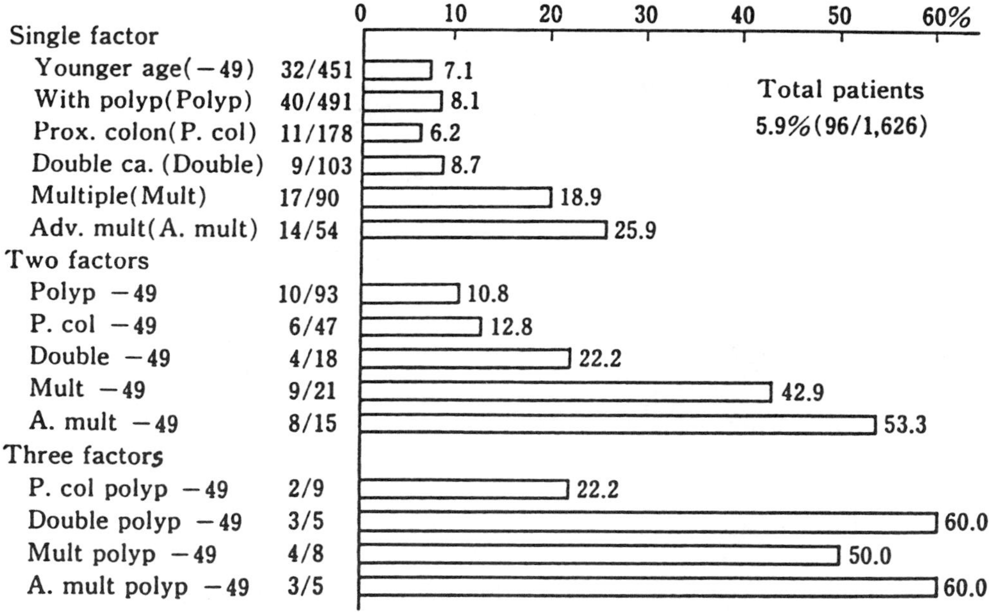

FIGURE 1. Frequency of cases with positive family history of colorectal cancer, by age, polyp concurrence and site/multiplicity differences, and their combinations. Adv. mult. means multiple colorectal cancer excepting those early cancer cases. See text for other abbreviations.

5, the difference between FH positive and negative groups is significant (X^2 = 5.8, df = 1, $p < 0.05$). However, if these cases were classified by site and/or multiplicity of cancer and also by ages, then different figures were seen among them. The higher rate of polyp concurrence in FH positive as compared with FH negative cases was significant only if age was under 50 for those of proximal colon, double primary and multiple colorectal cancers inclusively (9/19 vs. 13/67, X^2 = 4.5, df = 1, $p < 0.05$). It should be noted that these groups were the ones with the most frequent positive FH of large bowel cancer, as already mentioned (Table 2).

E. Combination of Multiple Factors

These results could further be analysed to see how certain combinations of multiple factors would give rise to stronger associations with the familial predisposition of this cancer. It is obvious in Figure 1 that the proportion of cases with positive FH is increased step by step as a patient carries more factors, such as the younger age at surgery, the polyp concurrence, and the state of being affected with proximal colon, multiple colorectal, or double primary cancers. It eventually attained around 50%, although not statistically significant because of the small number of cases. Furthermore, the proportion of familial patients who have two or more colorectal cancer relatives should also be calculated, which may represent the rate of FH duplication. It was 16.7% (16/96) of total familial patients and was slightly elevated in those aged less than 50 (9/33) as well as in those with proximal colon, multiple colorectal or double primary cancers (9/37), whereas polyp concurrence seemed to have no relation with FH duplication. Combination of multiple factors also adds no significant effect on FH duplication.

Association of FH with the other factors was statistically tested by means of a 2 × 2 × 2 factorial analysis with the logistic model.[1] If f is the proportion of positive FH, s in the binary discrimination of site/multiplicity of cancer, a is that of age at surgery, and p is that

Table 6
FACTORIAL ANALYSIS TESTING FOR ASSOCIATION OF FAMILY HISTORY OF LARGE BOWEL CANCER WITH VARIOUS DIAGNOSTIC TRAITS

	Categorization of Factor s					
	Proximal colon/ others		Double/others		Multiple/others	
Factor	Δz	t	Δz	t	Δz	t
s (site/multiple)	1.35	1.1	3.65	2.7[a]	6.92	5.6[a]
a (age −49/50+)	3.26	2.6[a]	3.94	3.0[a]	3.57	2.9[a]
p (polyp +/−)	2.62	2.1[a]	3.35	2.5[a]	0.88	0.7
s × a	2.30	1.8	2.98	2.2[a]	3.08	2.5[a]
s × p	0.33	0.3	1.40	1.1	1.26	1.0
a × p	0.39	0.3	2.22	1.7	0.85	0.7
s × a × p	0.35	0.3	2.85	2.1[a]	1.29	1.0

[a] Significant at 5% level.

of polyp concurrence, then the logistic transformation, $z = \log(f/1 - f)$, is given by $z = s + a + p + s \times a + s \times p + a \times p + s \times a \times p$. An effect of each factor can be tested with Student's *t* test, i.e., by dividing the difference of z by square root of its variance. In Table 6, combinations of site/multiplicity of cancer are given in the second row. The primary effects of single factors, such as double primary cancer, multiple colorectal cancer, younger age, and polyp concurrence, are all significant. Synergistic effect of younger age with site/multiplicity was also noted.

IV. DISCUSSION

Apart from the well-defined genetic neoplasms, it is rather difficult to obtain any evidence of genetic etiology of human common cancers. This is because we have no index traits which could discriminate between genetic and nongenetic familial clustering of the disease. Anderson[14,15] attempted to isolate a group of breast cancer patients who might be strongly genetically predisposed, by means of the FH of breast cancer, age at diagnosis, and disease multiplicity. Thus, he concluded that if the proband case was premenopausal, bilateral, and with positive FH of breast cancer in both mother and a sister, it might be regarded a hereditary breast cancer. The present study method is similar to that of Anderson. One difference is that we adopted the proportion of positive FH instead of the probability of the disease incidence among family members. The positive FH is an all-or-none variable and does not by itself represent a heritability of the disease. Nevertheless, if it was very frequently observed in certain subgroups of patients, it might be preferable to interpret it by genetic rather than nongenetic factors running in a family. The FH positive rate of more than 3% as observed in Figure 1 is about ten times higher than that observed in random samples of Japanese general population.

The present result seems to support the view that there is a subgroup of large bowel cancer characterized by (1) younger age at onset, (2) proximal colon, double primary, or multiple colorectal cancer, and (3) positive FH of the same disease. These are characteristics of HNPCC. If a certain patient is endowed with all these traits or even with any two of them, genetic predisposition could be strongly suspected. It should be a general rule that a hereditary cancer is diagnosed earlier than ages compared with nonhereditary cases of the same disease. For large bowel cancer, Anderson[16] reported about 10-years younger age at onset in familial than in nonfamilial cases in the U.S. Comparing to it, overall age reduction from the nonfamilial to familial cases is less remarkable in the present sample. But if confined to those cases of proximal colon, double primary and multiple colorectal cancers, the age difference reaches about 10 years. Thus, the above-mentioned rule would also be correct in this country. Comparing the high risk with low risk countries, the increase of incidence of this disease is mainly noted in older ages. If the excess is due to cases of nongenetic etiology, the age difference between hereditary and nonhereditary cases should be more remarkable in the western countries.

Many authors reported that familial large bowel cancer includes proximal colon and multiple colorectal cancers more frequently than nonfamilial cases. According to Utsunomiya et al.,[13] Shimada,[17] and Sadahiro et al.,[18] the proportion of positive FH of large bowel cancer is fourfold higher in multiple than in solitary cancers. We found that the proportion is 5% for the solitary and 20% for the multiple cancers. On the other hand, tumors developed at the proximal colon in 25% of familial and in 14% of nonfamilial cases, when solitary and multiple cancers were pooled. Their ratio is 1.8. Utsunomiya et al.[13] also obtained almost the same ratio (39 vs. 23%), while, according to Anderson[16] it was 2.7 (65 vs. 24%) in the U.S.

It has been stated that, except for familial polyposis coli, there should be no correlation between familiality and polyp concurrence. Recently however, Burt et al.[19] hypothesized that discrete adenomatous polyp and colorectal cancer should share the influence of an inherited autosomal dominant gene. From the points of sex-, age-, and tumor-site differences observed in the present materials (Table 5), environmental rather than hereditary factors seem to be more important for polyp development. On the other hand, familial predisposition also appeared to be associated with polyps (Table 6). These rather complex results may mean that some environmental risk factors which enhance the polyp development also cause some familial clustering of colorectal cancer.

Our primary question concerns the fraction of whole large bowel cancers which is attributable to the genetic etiology. If the three features of HNPCC, i.e., the positive FH of the same disease, the younger age of onset and proximity or multiplicity of cancer, are all required for diagnosis, 19 out of 1626 cases (about 1%) would be included in this category. But if any 1 of the 3 conditions might be relaxed, then 167 cases or about 10% should be included. A correct estimate must be situated between these two values.

REFERENCES

1. **Cox, D. R.,** *The Analysis of Binary Data,* Chapman and Hall, London, 1970.
2. **Statistics and Information Department,** Minister's Secretariat, Ministry of Health and Welfare, Mortality Statistics from Malignant Neoplasms, Special Report of Vital Statistics in Japan, 1933—1958 (1961); 1958—1971 (1973); 1972—1984 (1986).
3. **Ministry of Health and Welfare,** Current Nutritional Status in Japan, Report of National Nutritional Survey Studies, Daiichishuppan, Tokyo, 1985.
4. **Japan Research Society for Gastric Cancer,** Synchronous and metachronous double primary cancer in stomach cancer patients, *J. Jpn, Soc. Cancer Ther.,* 17, 1226, 1982.
5. **Woolf, C. M.,** A genetic study of carcinoma of the large intestine, *Am. J. Hum. Genet.,* 10, 42, 1958.
6. **Reed, T. E. and Neel, J. V.,** A genetic study of multiple polyposis of the colon, *Am. J. Hum. Genet.,* 7, 236, 1955.
7. **Anderson, D. E. and Strong, L. C.,** Genetics of gastrointestinal tumor, in *Cancer Epidemiology, Environmental Factors,* (Int. Congr. Ser. No. 351, Vol. 3), Excerpta Medica, Amsterdam, 1974, 267.
8. **Lynch, H. T., Lynch, P. M., and Lynch, J. F.,** What is hereditary colon cancer?, in *Prevention of Hereditary Large Bowel Cancer,* Ingall, J. R. F. and Mastromarino, A. J., Eds., Alan R. Liss, New York, 1983, 3.
9. **Murata, M., Utsunomiya, J., Iwama, T., and Tanimura, M.,** Frequency of adenomatosis coli in Japan, *Jpn. J. Hum. Genet.,* 26, 19, 1981.

10. **Utsunomiya, J., Murata, M., and Tanimura, M.,** An analysis of the age distribution of colon cancer in adenomatosis coli, *Cancer,* 45, 198, 1980.
11. **Nomizu, T., Watanabe, I., and Endo, S.,** Familial colorectal cancer; a case report and review of the literature, *Jpn. J. Gastroenterol. Surg.,* 14, 1499, 1981.
12. **Ohara, T. and Ihara, O.,** Non-polyposis colon cancer, *Jpn. J. Clin. Med.,* 39, 2061, 1981.
13. **Utsunomiya, J.,** Non-polyposis familial large bowel cancer, *Geka,* 43, 881, 1981.
14. **Anderson, D. E.,** A genetic study of human breast cancer, *J. Natl. Cancer Inst.,* 38, 1029, 1972.
15. **Anderson, D. E.,** Breast cancer in families, *Cancer,* 40, 1855, 1977.
16. **Anderson, D. E.,** Risk in families of patients with colon cancer, in *Colorectal Cancer: Prevention Epidemiology, and Screening,* Winawer, S. J., Schottenfeld, D., and Sherlock, P., Eds., Raven Press, New York, 1980, 109.
17. **Slimada, K.,** Multiple carcinoma of the large intestine, *Adult Dis.,* 11, 1899, 1981.
18. **Sadahiro, S.,** A clinical study of multiple carcinomas of colon and rectum, *J. Jpn. Soc. Colo-Proctol.,* 35, 524, 1982.
19. **Burt, R. W., Bishop, T., Cannon, L. A., Dowle, M. A., Lee, R. G., and Skolnik, M. H.,** Dominant inheritance of adenomatous colonic polyps and colorectal cancer, *N. Engl. J. Med.,* 312, 1540, 1985.

Chapter 15

PATHOLOGY, GENETICS, AND MANAGEMENT OF HEREDITARY GASTROINTESTINAL POLYPOSES

Joji Utsunomiya

TABLE OF CONTENTS

I. INTRODUCTION

Accumulated studies have revealed that there are several types of familial large bowel cancer which are operationally divided into the hereditary GI polyposes and nonpolyposis familial large bowel cancers. The latter include the hereditary nonpolyposis colorectal cancer (HNPCC) syndromes which include site-specific colon cancer and the cancer family syndrome (Lynch syndromes I and II).[1] (Please refer to Chapter 16 for further discussion on HNPCC.)

Morson's pathological classification of intestinal polyposis neoplastic lesions, i.e., adenomatosis coli and hamartomatous polyposes, (Peutz-Jegher's syndrome and juvenile polyposis), includes four important principal characteristics: familial occurrence, tendency to produce malignant lesions, involvement throughout the GI tract, and association with other

Table 1
CLASSIFICATION OF THE GI POLYPOSES

Classification			Site of polyposes			Cancer high risk	Mode of inheritance
Genetic	Histological	Nomenclature	st.	si.	li.		
Hereditary	Neoplastic	Adenomatosis coli	+	+	+		AD
		Familial polyposis coli					
		Gardner syndrome					
		Turcot syndrome					(AR)
		Zanca syndrome					
	Hamartomatous	Peutz-Jeghers syndrome	+	+	+	+	AD
		Juvenile polyposis	+	+	+	+	AD
		Cowden disease	+	+	+	+	AD
Nonhereditary	Inflammatory	Inflammatory polyposis	—	—	+	—	—
		Lymphoid polyposis	—	+	+	—	—
	Unclassified	Metaplastic polyposis	—	—	+	—	—
		Cronkhite-Canada syndrome	+	+	+	±	—

Note: st = stomach, si = small intestine, li = large intestine, AD = autosomal dominant, AR = autosomal recessive.

lesions (Table 1). Therefore, they can be reasonably termed the ''hereditary gastrointestinal polyposes'' (HGIP) or hereditary polyposis syndromes.[2]

Adenomatosis coli (AC) or familial adenomatous polyposis is the most important HGIP because of its extremely high risk of large bowel cancers, its relatively high incidence among HGIP, and its predominant familial occurrence, often appearing in a large kindred. Peutz-Jegher's syndrome and juvenile polyposis are less frequent compared to AC, but recent studies have disclosed that they are at high risk for large bowel cancer.

This chapter will describe pathological, genetic, and clinical aspects of HGIP, mainly based on the author's studies and on other reports from Japan.

II. CENTRAL REGISTER OF THE POLYPOSES

In 1972, the author encountered an AC case in which some of the patient's relatives had been previously reported (twice) in the literature as an independent family (42 and 13 years previously). Consequently, he had strongly realized the necessity for a central register for collecting information on AC families throughout the nation, and for continuously accessing them over generations. The Center for Analysing Familial Polyposis (the Polyposis Center) was established at the Tokyo Medical and Dental University in 1975 under the time-limited national law for 7 years.[3,4] Since 1982, when the author left there, this activity has been maintained under the name of the Research Center for Polyposes and Intestinal Diseases.

The information on the probands of HGIP as well as nonpolypotic familial cancer has been collected through five different sources, including inquiries to hospitals throughout the nation, Japanese autopsy records, published literature, voluntary visits of patients, and the Japanese Society for Large Bowel Cancer Research. On each family, an exact pedigree map, ''the working pedigree'', was constructed using the Koseki, the national family register, which has been conducted traditionally for more than 90 years. In order to identify family members, we devised a permanent coding system as seen in Figure 1.[3,5] The affected members were identified using hospital records, death certificates, and communications with their family members. The center sends the lists of these high risk people to local physicians who register the cases in order to encourage local family examinations. During this activity, the fusion of two or more pedigrees has been recognized increasingly (Table 2) and ascertainment of the pedigrees has been accelerated.

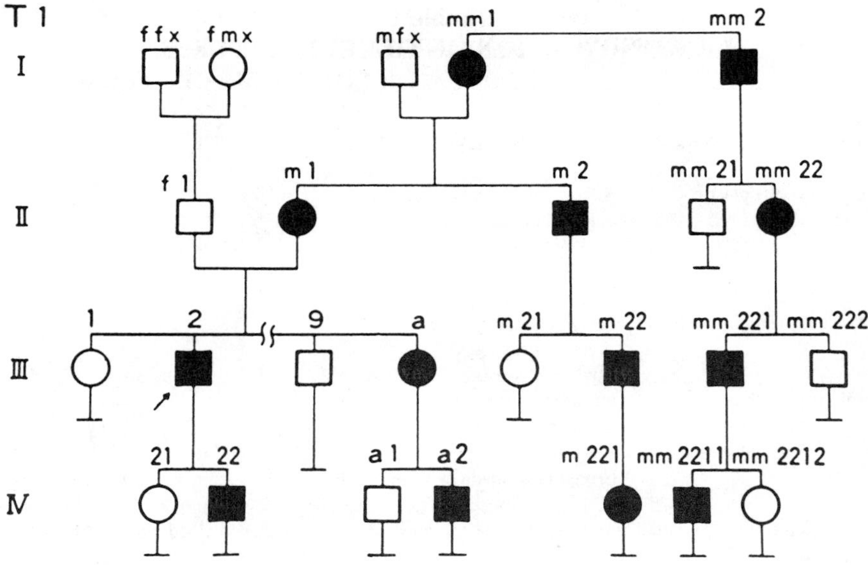

FIGURE 1. A new coding system of working pedigree. Sibships of proband are given by single numbers up to 9 and alphabet letters for double numbers (10 = a, 11 = b, 12 = c, etc.) in order of birth. Offspring are given by numbers of their parents added by a number of birth order. Father of the proband is given by f and a number of birth order, and mother by m and a number of birth order. For example, father of the proband is expressed by "fx" (grandfather on father's side), "ff x" (grandmother on mother's side), "mm x", etc.

In 1982, when the author moved from the center to the present institution, namely, the Hyogo College of Medicine, 472 families (697 cases) of AC and 146 families (131 cases) of Peutz-Jeghers syndrome and many other polyposis cases/families had been registered (Table 3).[6] The family survey has now been completed on 327 AC families with 4847 members, and has revealed the presence of 854 affected and 3545 persons at high risk for being a possible AC gene carrier. Pathological, genetic, and epidemiological analysis has been completed using some of these materials in several published reports which will be reviewed herein.

III. PATHOLOGY OF ADENOMATOSIS COLI

AC indicates the condition in which more than 100 adenomas are distributed throughout the large bowel regardless of familial occurrence or association with extracolonic lesions.[3,7]

A. Lesions of the Large Bowel

1. Polyps

a. Number of Polyps

We observed two distinct groups of patients with adenomatous polyps in the large bowel, by dividing the groups at the number of around 100[3] (Figure 2) as Bussey similarly observed.[7] Therefore, it may be reasonable to define the cases with less than 100 adenomas as "multiple adenomas", to differentiate them from AC.

In the resected specimen, there are two heterogeneous classes of AC — the profuse type and the sparse type — regarding the number of polyps.[8] The criteria for delineating these clusters were a total count of 5000 polyps or a unit amount of 10/cm^2 under macroscopic observation and microscopically, two adenomatous foci detected in one centimeter of a histological section or adenomatous foci estiamted to occupy 20% of the total area of the

Table 2
FREQUENCY OF FUSION OF PEDIGREE IN AC FAMILIES REGISTERED IN THE POLYPOSIS CENTER

	1961	1972	1976	1979	1983	Total
Registered family	45	122	168	128	99	562
Fusion of pedigree	1	12	25	14	20	72
%	2.2	7.8	14.9	10.9	20.2	12

Note: Data at 1982.

Table 3
NUMBER OF REGISTERED CASES (FAMILY) OF HEREDITARY POLYPOSES AND THE RELATED CONDITIONS IN THE POLYPOSIS CENTER, 1982[6]

Research	Adenomatosis coli	Multiple adenomas	PJ syndrome	Juvenile polyposis	Familial cancer of the colon
Jpn. Soc. LBC[a]	169(111)	82(62)	23(20)	2(1)	16(15)
Questionnaire	182(148)	92(91)	70(67)	2(2)	41(35)
Literature	82(58)	7(7)	7(7)	0(0)	7(4)
Autopsy record	23(17)	30(30)	8(8)	0(0)	0(0)
Voluntary registration	241(138)	6(6)	38(29)	6(6)	15(10)
Total	697(472)	216(196)	146(131)	10(9)	79(64)

[a] Japanese Society for Large Bowel Cancer Research.

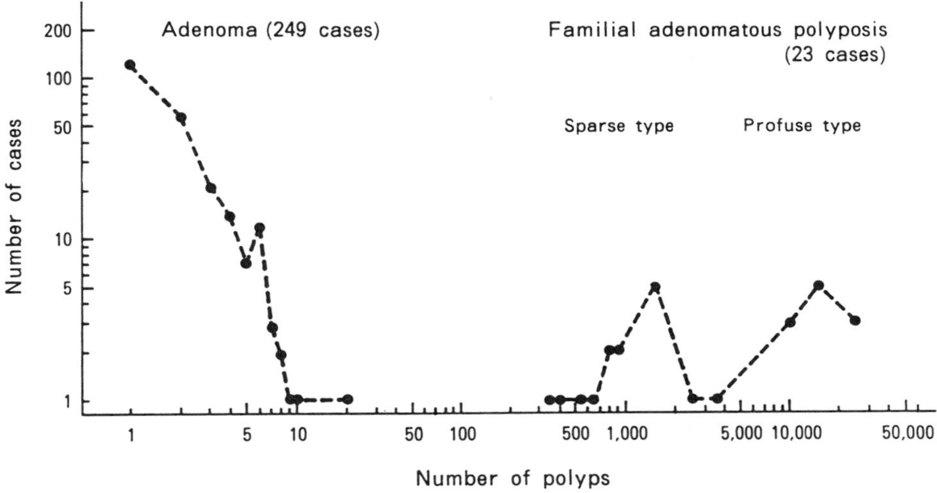

FIGURE 2. Distribution of cases with respect to number of polyps.

section (adenoma percent).[8] Radiologically, double contrast barium enema revealed that the boundary range distinguishing these two types was six to nine polyps per square centimeter in adults and 3 to 6/cm^2 in children.[9]

b. Size of Polyps

Small polyps (diameter less than 5 mm) constituted over 80% of the polyps in the specimen[8] (Table 4). The cases with one or more polyps greater than 1 cm in diameter were associated

Table 4
FREQUENCY OF CANCER IN ADENOMA IN ADENOMATOSIS COLI AND NONPOLYPOTIC ADENOMAS

	Adenomatosis Coli		Adenomas	
Size (mm)	N(%)	Cancer(%)	N	Cancer(%)
Utsunomiya et al.[11]				
0—5	3,593(90.1)	65(1.8)	189	3(1.6)
6—10	289	57(20.2)	127	19(15.0)
11—20	71	23(32.4)	49	22(44.9)
21—	31	10(32.3)	7	5(71.4)
Total	3,984	155(3.9)	372	49(13.2)
Fujiwara et al.[10]				
0—5	6,763(94.6)	7(0.1)	171	0(0)
6—10	326	9(2.8)	74	10(13.5)
11—20	44	8(18.2)	35	15(42.9)
21—	12	7(58.2)	29	20(69.0)
Total	7,145	76(1.1)	309	45(14.6)
Iwama[8]				
0—5	15,708(97.7)	7(0.04)	—	
6—10	270	1(0.3)	—	
11—20	81	6(7.4)	—	
21—	25	12(4.8)	—	
Total	16,084	26(0.2)	—	

Table 5
FREQUENCY OF LARGE BOWEL CANCER AT DIAGNOSIS[6]

	Male			Female			Total		
	Case	Ca (+)		Case	Ca (+)		Case	Ca (+)	
Group	n	n	%	n	n	%	n	n	%
Proband	197	131	66.5	127	87	68.5	324	218	67.3
Call up	87	26	29.9	43	11	25.6	130	37	28.5
Total	284	157	54.7	170	98	57.6	454	255	56.2

with advanced cancer somewhere in the large bowel by a frequency of 47%, whereas in the case in which the lesions were 5 mm or less malignancy was never detected.[9]

c. *Histology*

The malignant potential of the adenomas of AC seemed to be of no significant difference when compared to the usual solitary adenomas of the large bowel[8,10,11] (Table 4). Cytokinetic studies revealed that an abnormal cellullar proliferation pattern exists in the crypts of apparently nonadenomatous mucosa.[12] Sialomucin properties of the nonadenomatous mucosa of AC were different from those of the normal colon.[13] There was an abnormal histochemical distribution of the lectin (UEA-1) binding site in flat rectal mucosa of AC patients.[11]

2. *Cancer*

Advanced cancers of the large bowel were found in 56.2% of the total patients at the time of diagnosis. The frequency was much less in the call-up cases (28.5%) than in the probands (67.3%) (Table 5). Their subsite distribution within the bowel was similar to that of the usual colorectal cancers in both Japanese and British series (Table 6).[6,7,14] The relative incidence of cancer in the sigmoid colon vs. that in the rectum (S/R ratio) also increased in the AC patient as compared to the general colorectal cancer population in Japan (Table 6).

Table 6
SUBSITE DISTRIBUTION OF LARGE BOWEL CANCER

Subsite	Japan				England			
	Adenomatosis coli, Polyposis Centre[6] (1982)		General population, Jap. Soc. LBC[a] (1977—81)		Adenomatosis coli, St. Mark's Hosp[7] (1974)		General population Smiddy and Goligher[14] (1957)	
	No.	%	No.	%	No.	%	No.	%
Cecum	8	2.5	—	5.7	13	4.5	101	6.1
Ascending colon	31	9.9	—	7.6	4	1.4	48	2.9
Hepatic flexure	—	—	—	—	8	2.8	29	1.8
Transverse colon	39	12.5	—	7.2	18	6.3	77	4.7
Splenic flexure	—	—	—	—	16	5.6	50	3.0
Descending colon	26	8.3	—	4.5				
Sigmoid colon	82	26.2	—	24.5	63	22.0	350	24.0
Rectum	131	41.9	—	45.1	141	49.3	944	57.4
Anal canal	—	—	—	5.1				
Unclassified	—	—	—	—	23	8.0	—	—
Total	313	100.0	18.915	100.0	286	100.0	1644	100.0

[a] Report from Japanese Society of Large Bowel Cancer Research.

Table 7
MULTIPLICITY OF LARGE BOWEL CANCER

	Adenomatosis coli		General population[a]	
	No.	%	No.	%
Total	229	100.0	24,616	100.0
Single	142	63.3	23,504	95.5
Multiple	87 (100.0)	38.0	1,112	4.5
2	(40)	46.0	670	84.5
3	(21)	24.1	91	11.5
4	(4)	4.6	21	2.6
Over 5	(22)	25.3	11	1.4

[a] Meeting No. 16 of Japanese Society of Large Bowel Cancer Research.

Table 8
GASTRIC POLYPS IN ADENOMATOSIS COLI

		Incidence of Polyp				Proportion of adenoma	
		In case		In family			
Reporter	Place (year)	No.	%	No.	%	No.	%
Japanese literature							
Utsunomiya et al.[15]	Tokyo (1974)	10/15	66.7	6/6	100.0	4/6	66.7
Ushio et al.[16]	Tokyo (1976)	10/15	66.7	7/8	87.5	0/6	0
Iida et al.[17]	Kyushu (1978)	18/25	72.0	14/16	87.5	9/18	50.0
Utsunomiya et al.[18]	Hyogo (1986)	16/20	80.0	12/15	80.0	10/16	62.5
Jap. Soc. LBC Res.[a]	Japan (1986)	115/309	37.1	—	—	43/96	44.8
Literatures[b]	— (1977—1985)	99/200	49.5	—	—	—	—
Western literature							
Ranzi et al.[19]	Italy (1981)	6/9	66.7	—	—	4/6	66.7
Jarvinen et al.[20]	Finland (1983)	21/34	61.7	—	—	4/21	19.0
Burt et al.[21]	U.S. (1984)	7/11	63.6	—	—	1/7	14.3
Shemesh et al.[22]	Israel (1985)	7/14	50.0	—	—	7/7	100.0
Tonelli et al.[23]	Italy (1985)	6/24	25.0			3/6	50.0
Bulow et al.[24]	Denmark (1985)	13/26	50.0			1/13	7.7
Western total		60/118	50.8			20/60	33.3

[a] Summed data of the reports at the 26th meeting of Japanese Society for Large Bowel Cancer Research.
[b] 14 reports on gastric polyps in AC.

Multiple lesions were found in 38.0% in AC cancer. This was an extremely high frequency when compared with the 4.5% occurrence of colorectal cancer in the general population of Japan (Table 7).

B. Lesions of the Upper GI Tract

1. Gastric Polyps

We detected gastric polyps in 66.7% of our cases and assumed that they must be an integral phenotypic manifestation of the AC gene[15] because these cases with gastric polyps were distributed in all of the families studied. Similar results were reported from other institutes.[16-18] An increasing number of reports from other countries suggested that this phenomenon is not Japanese specific (Table 8).[20-24] There are two types of these polyps by histology: (1) adenomatous[15] and (2) hamartomatous ones of the fundic gland.[25] Neither are specific to AC, although the fundic gland polyp of AC was suggested to have some histo-

Table 9
DUODENAL POLYP IN ADENOMATOSIS COLI

Reporter	Place(year)	Incidence of the polyp		Proportion of adenoma	
		No.	%	No.	%
Japanese literature					
Iida et al.[17]	Kyushu(1977)	12/13	92.0	12/12	100
Ushio et al.[16]	Tokyo(1976)	9/10	90.0	5/9	55.6
Utsunomiya et al.[18]	Hyogo(1986)	18/24	75.0	18/18	100
Jap. Soc. LBC Res.[a]	—(1986)	60/253	18.8	—	—
Western literature					
Ranzi et al.[19]	Italy(1981)	6/9	66.7	6/6	100
Jarvinen et al.[20]	Finland(1983)	20/33	60.6	16/20	80
Burt et al.[21]	U.S.(1984)	8/11	72.3	7/8	89
Shemesh et al.[22]	Israel(1985)	14/14	100.0	14/14	100
Bulow et al.[24]	Denmark(1985)	13/26	50.0	12/10	92.3
Tonelli et al.[23]	Italy(1985	14/24	58.3	14/14	100
Western total		75/117	64.1	69/75	92

[a] Summed data of the reports of the 26th meeting of Japanese Society Large Bowel Cancer Research.

chemically different characteristics when compared with those found in the general population.[26] While adenomatous lesions were found in 44% of the cases with gastric polyps in the Japanese series, this was 33% in the accumulated series from western reports (Table 8). This difference may be related to intestinal metaplasia which was seen more frequently in the stomachs of the Japanese than in the western populations.[25] Although the fundic gland polyps do not seem to harbor any malignant potential, some evidence of malignant foci associated with the adenomatous lesion has been observed by us.[18]

2. Gastric Cancer

Of AC cases with gastric cancer, 15 or more have been reported in Japan. In some cases, they are multiple.[25] The incidences were estimated to be 2.1% in the Japanese series and 0.6% in the Western.[26a]

3. Duodenal Polyps

Histologically verified small adenomas were detected in virtually all of the cases examined by endoscopic biopsy or at autopsy.[17,25] The evidence has been confirmed by studies in western countries (Table 9).[16-24] They are distributed mainly in the second portion and Vater's papillae and were found in 50% of those patients who were biopsied.[17,25] We have recently observed a case with large adenomas confined both at Vaterian and accessory papillae. This finding suggests an increased neoplastic potential around the orifices of the pancreatic duct.

4. Duodenal Cancer

Duodenal carcinoma occurring in AC has been reported in 9 cases in the Japanese literature and the frequency was reported to be 0.9 or 1.9%.

5. Jejunal and Ileal Lesions

Polyps or adenomas were found in the jejunum of 8 cases and the ileum of 4 cases out of a total of 16 cases endoscopically examined at operation.[27]

As described above, it is now clear that adenomatous involvement throughout the GI tract is a consistent phenotypic manifestation of the AC gene and is not a Japanese-specific observation. On the other hand, some possibility of environmental modifying factors superimposed on the AC genotype should be considered.

Table 10
PROPORTION OF GARDNER SYNDROME

	Registered case				Personal case	
	1974		1981			
Gardner stigmata	**No.**	**%**	**No.**	**%**	**No.**	**%**
Case without GS	203	92.8	388	74.3	16	57.1
Case with one GS	15	6.8	96	18.4	10	35.7
Case with both GS	2	0.9	40	7.7	2	7.1
Total	220	100.0	522	100.0	28	100.0

Note: GS = Gardner syndrome.

C. Extragastrointestinal-Associated Lesions and Variant Syndromes

It has been recognized that AC patients could manifest various neoplastic lesions in the tissues or organs other than the GI tract and some of them are considered as the marker of genetically distinctive variants of AC.

1. Gardner Syndrome

Since Gardner[28] reported a family with superficial hard tumors (osteomas) and soft tumors (desmoid, fibroma) in association with adenomatous polyposis, this combination has been called Gardner syndrome (GS). While GS of complete type was observed in about 7% in both of the series examined personally and in that of the registry, GS of incomplete type was found more frequently (35.7%) in the former than in the latter (18.4%) (Table 10). The evidence indicates that there are a considerable number of cases with GS which might be overlooked at examination.

Panoramic X-ray examination of the jaw disclosed the radiopaque lesions (“the occult osteomatous lesion”) in 94% of AC patients.[29] Autopsy of a case revealed that these lesions were endosteomas. Their pathogenesis has been speculated to represent an excess of a “repair” process occurring in the jawbone.[30] The nature of the lesion itself was not specific to AC, but multiple occurrences were characteristic.[30] They had a positive relationship to the superficial stigmata of GS.[30] As to be discussed later in the genetic section, GS (particularly its complete form) may pose a specific, distinct genotype, but there may be many clinically indistinguishable transitional cases between complete GS and simple AC (familial polyposis coli). Therefore, these two categories can be grouped as the common subtypes of AC while Turcot and Zanca syndromes represent the rare subtypes.

2. Turcot's Syndrome

This disorder represents an association of tumors of the central nervous system and colonic polyposis.[31] It has been reported in several families in Japan. The syndrome appears to have a more heterogeneous character when compared with GS; the mode of transmission of some of the cases was apparently recessive, the age of onset was much younger, and the adenomas were larger and fewer than in other forms of AC.[32]

3. Zanca Syndrome

Zanca[33] described a nonfamilial case with two small adenomas in the colon which were associated with multiple cartilaginous exostosis (MCE) of the long bones and he believed the condition was a hereditary syndrome. Since no similar case has been reported, the combination was considered to be coincidental. A recent paper, however, has strongly suggested that it might be a genetically distinctive variant of AC.[34] This report involved a case of a 41-year-old male who had a typical course of MCE. He underwent colectomy for

Table 11
AGE-SPECIFIC INCIDENCE AND PREVALENCE OF AFFECTED INDIVIDUALS IN 53 SETS OF TOTALLY EXAMINED SIBLINGS WITH AN AFFECTED PARENT[2]

Age group	0	5	10	15	20	25	30	Total
Examined	1	15	25	25	24	16	11	117
Manifested	0	6	8	14	12	6	4	50
Incidence (%)	0	40.0	32.0	56.0	50.0	37.5	36.4	42.7
Prevalence (%)	0	37.5	34.1	42.4	44.4	43.3	42.7	42.7

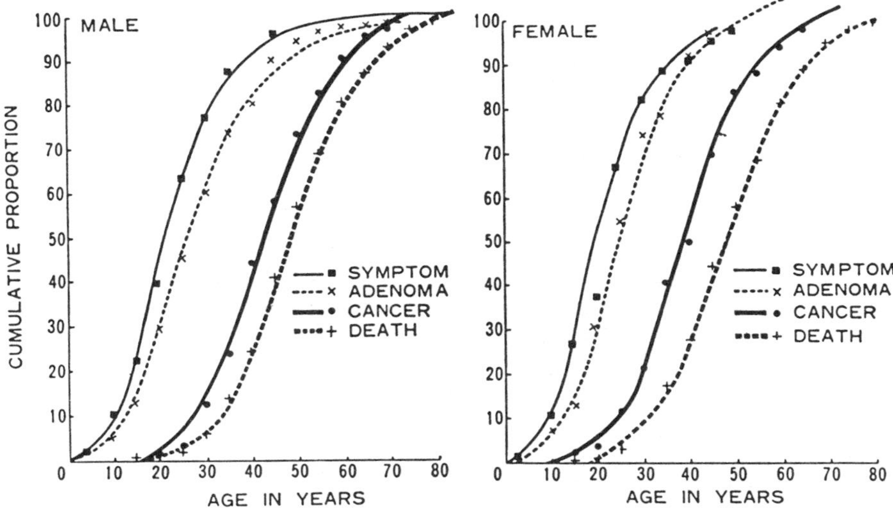

FIGURE 3. Age-specific prevalence of the stages of adenomatosis coli (familial polyposis coli).

a cancer which was associated with diffuse adenomatous polyposis of the colon. His father manifested classical MCE and died of colonic cancer associated with polyposis. One of his aunts was known to have MCE.

IV. NATURAL HISTORY AND CANCER RISK IN ADENOMATOSIS COLI

A. Stages of Disease

The natural history of AC can be divided into three stages for the large bowel lesions: latent, adenoma, and cancer.

The specific incidence and prevalence of affected individuals were calculated in 53 selected sets of siblings with affected parents, where all members were known to have been examined for polyps.[2] It was estimated that polyps of clinically detectable size started to appear in 80% of the gene carriers between 5 and 10 years of age, since polyps were detected in 40% of possible dominant gene carriers by this age (Table 11). Therefore, the latent stage was estimated to average approximately 7 years. Using well-described registered cases, where age-specific cumulative incidence rates of prevalence of symptom onset was known, diagnosis of polyposis, large bowel cancer, and death were calculated[35] (Figure 3). From these data, ages at different risk or prevalence for the various clinical stages were estimated as in Table 12.[35-37]

Table 12
AGE AT DIFFERENT RISK OR PREVALENCE OF VARIOUS STAGES[35]

	Risk (%)	Japan		England[a]	
		Male	Female	Male	Female
Symptom onset	10	10.3	9.7	10.8	12.3
	50	22.5	21.3	25.5	25.0
Adenoma diagnosis	10	12.8	12.1	12.5	11.8
	50	27.7	24.7	26.7	25.1
Large bowel cancer diagnosis	1	16.0	13.1	17.5	12.4
	10	29.5	23.8	27.3	24.6
	50	42.0	39.8	41.9	40.7
	90	58.7	65.7	55.1	56.3
Death	10	32.8	32.8	29.4	29.4
	50	50.1	49.4	45.4	44.7

[a] Modified from the data by Veale[36] and Ashley.[37]

B. Factors Affecting the Natural History and Cancer Risk

The age-specific prevalence of large bowel cancer of British patients that were calculated from the data of St. Mark's Hospital and presented in Veale's[36] article were similar to the Japanese series.[38] However, the Japanese males appear to have a slightly slower progression in their natural history compared with the males in the British series (Table 12).

By sex, the adenomas as well as cancers were manifested a few years earlier in females than in males (Table 12). Average ages of patients with cancer were 39.5 years for males, 36.8 years for females, and 38.3 for the total.

Average age of cancer occurrence in the profuse polyp type was 34.0 years. This was about 8 years younger than that of the sparse polyp type (41.8 years) (Table 13).[39] However, the sparse type with GS produced cancer at an average age of 37.1 years, which was younger by 6 years for the sparse type without GS (43.3 years old) (Table 13). Time trends in these values were not apparent during the period of study.

C. Malignancy of Other Organs

When the patient lives longer as a result of surgical treatment, malignant lesions will occur in various organs other than the large intestine. Gastric cancer was reported in 2.5 to 5.3% of the patients and duodenal cancer in 1.9%. The death rate from gastric cancer was significantly higher in the family members with AC than in the controls.[40] The actual prevalence needs to be clarified in the future, but currently available data suggests that these cancers might develop at a slightly older age than the large bowel cancer, but apparently earlier than in the general population. The average age of death due to gastric cancer is 43.6 years in 12 Japanese cases and 49.8 years in 5 non-Japanese patients. That of duodenal cancer is 41.1 years. The apparent ability of small bowel adenoma to develop many years after colectomy is one more vexing aspect of the natural history of AC.[41,42]

V. GENETICS OF ADENOMATOSIS COLI

A. Incidence

The frequency of AC patients at birth was estimated to be $0.45 \pm 0.5 \times 10^4$ or 1:22,222.[43] The comparable data from western countries was 1:23,930 in England,[36] 1:7,437 in the U.S.A.[19] and 1:7,646 in Sweden.[44]

B. Sex Ratio

Male/female ratio was significantly higher for males, being 1.38 or 352:256 in our total

Table 13
COMPARISON AMONG GARDNER AND POLYP AMOUNT SUBTYPES FOR LARGE BOWEL CANCER AND OTHER ASSOCIATED LESIONS

	GS (+)		GS (−)		Sparse		Profuse		GS (+)				GS (−)				Total	
									Sparse		Profuse		Sparse		Profuse			
	136		529		236		104		63		18		173		86		665	
Case no.	**No.**	**%**	**No.**	**%**	**No.**	**%**	**No.**	**%**	**No.**	**%**	**No.**	**%**	**No.**	**%**	**No.**	**%**	**No.**	**%**
Large bowel cancer																		
Case	67	49.3	285	53.9	113	47.9	56	53.8	27	42.9	10	55.6	86	49.7	46	53.5	352	52.9
Age of Dx	38.30		39.06		41.8		34.0		37.1		37.3		43.3		33.3		38.9	
Multiple cancers	(16 24.6)		(99 35.9)		(34 30.6)		(20 26.4)		(6 23.1)		(2 20.0)		(28 32.9)		(18 40.0)		(115 33.7)	
Extracolonic lesion																		
Gastric polyps	62	45.6	104	19.7	73	30.9	32	30.8	28	44.4	10	55.6	45	26.0	22	25.6	166	25.0
Duodenal polyps	25	18.4	51	9.6	38	16.1	16	15.4	13	20.6	5	27.8	25	14.5	11	12.8	76	11.4
Gastric-duodenal cancer	5	3.7	12	2.3	5	2.1	2	1.9	1	1.6	2	11.1	4	2.3	0	0	17	2.6
OO[a] of jaw	63	46.3	57	10.8	65	27.5	22	21.2	37	58.7	7	38.9	28	16.2	15	17.4	120	18.1
Other tumor	26	19.1	36	6.8	32	13.6	7	6.7	15	24.8	3	16.7	17	9.8	4	4.7	62	9.3

[a] OO = occult osteoma.

From Tanimura, M., *Ochanomizu Med.*, 33, 83, 1985. With permission.

series. This was similar to the 1.31 ratio at St. Mark's[36] and 1.48 in Reed's series.[48] In call-up cases, however, there was no significant sex difference; the ratios were 1.18 or 73:62 in ours[45] and 1.08 in the St. Mark's series,[36] respectively. The decreasing trend of the ratio in the recent case indicated an increased chance of detecting female patients.

The infant death rate among the siblings of the affected patients was found to be significantly higher than that in controls. This increase in mortality was more predominant in females than in males.[45] This phenomenon indicated that female gene carriers might be less resistant to various diseases at infancy and suggested that it might be related to the earlier manifestation of the disorder in females.

C. Nonfamilial Cases

The proportion of nonfamilial (or sporadic) cases was 41.5% in our series of 1981 and 45% or 90 out of 200 families in the St. Mark's study.[36] The value has been decreasing since the beginning of our study in 1968, when it was 64%, suggesting improved progress in the ascertainment of family members through activity of the Center.[46]

D. The Relative Fitness

It was calculated to be 0.88 in our series as shown below[47] while it was 0.8 in Veale's[36] and 0.78 in Reed's.[48]

$$F = \frac{\text{Average number of offspring of 18 years or older of affected member}}{\text{Average number of offspring of 18 years or older of nonaffected member}}$$

$$= \frac{\frac{134}{54}}{\frac{212}{75}} = \frac{2.48}{2.87} = 0.88$$

E. Penetrance

There were 126 pedigrees selected in which parents of the proband were determined to be an obligate gene carrier by family analysis. In 111 pedigrees, or 88.1% of these, 1 of the parents was ascertained to be affected. If parents who had died of suspected GI malignancy were included in the analysis, the penetrance of our series was 93.7%. The remaining four parents were dead by accidental or unknown causes before 52 years of age. If they are included as affected, the actual value may be almost 100%![40] The comparative value was 80% in Veale's[36] and 90% in Reed's series.[48]

F. Segregation Ratio

The families which were selected for analysis were those in which all offspring of affected parents had been examined. The observed segregation ratio (θ) was 0.427 in our series. The data of Veale was 0.361[36] and that of Reed was 0.400.[48] The segregation ratio adjusted (A) for penetrance (P) was calculated in our series as follows:

$$A = \frac{\theta\ 0.427}{P\ 0.937} = 0.456$$

G. Genetic Heterogeneity

1. Age

Veale demonstrated that there were two peaks in the distribution of the age of diagnosis.[36] He speculated that there existed two heterogeneous forms based on the onset of lesions: the

Table 14
CORRELATION IN RELATIVES FOR AGE OF DEATH

Sib/sib	n	r	Parent/child	n	r	Uncle/nephew, etc.	n	r
Brother/brother	27	0.63[a]	Father/son	15	0.34	Uncle/nephew	12	0.47
Brother/sister	16	0.47	Father/daughter	13	0.09	Uncle/niece	6	0.55
Sister/brother	17	0.48	Mother/son	12	0.48	Aunt/nephew	14	0.27
Sister/sister	7	0.58[a]	Mother/daughter	5	0.39	Aunt/niece	10	0.08
Total	67	0.53		45	0.09		42	0.30

Note: n = number of pair and r = correlation index.

[a] Significant.

From Utsunomiya, J., Tanimura, M., Iwama, T., Tanaka, K., and Tonomura, A., *Jpn. J. Hum. Genet.*, 24, 202, 1979. With permission.

Table 15
CORRELATION BETWEEN PROBAND AND AFFECTED RELATIVES FOR POLYP AMOUNT TYPE

Proband	Affected relatives: Profuse	Affected relatives: Sparse	Total
Profuse	24	1	25
Sparse	2	26	28
Total	26	27	53

From Tanimura, M., *Ochanomizu Med.*, 33, 83, 1985. With permission.

early-onset and the late-onset cases. Our results were less clear regarding this aspect. However, age of death was significantly correlated between affected sibs of the same sex (Table14),[46] suggesting there are some genetic heterogeneous subsets regarding progression of the disease.

2. Polyp Amount Type

Each of the profuse and sparse types were found separately in families by 98.1% (Table 15), suggesting they are genetically heterogeneous.[39]

3. Gardner stigmata

The propositi with GS had GS-positive relatives in 35.1%, while GS-negative propositi had positive relatives in 14.9% (Table 16).[39] This familial concentration of GS was not due to consanguinity. The evidence indicates that GS may be controlled by a single gene and is not multifactorial.

There was a significant correlation between the number of polyps and GS type. Of the sparse-type cases, 33.9% or 19 out of 56 were associated with GS, while only 1 out of 22 of the profuse-type cases showed this association. Sparse GS-positive probands showed a 40% GS-positive rate in the relatives which was apparently a higher rate compared to that of the sparse GS-negative-type and profuse-type families.

There may be three major subtypes present in the common subtypes of AC: simple familial polyposis with sparse polyps, those with diffuse polyps, and GS-type with sparse polyps.[39]

Table 16
CORRELATION BETWEEN PROBAND AND AFFECTED RELATIVES FOR GARDNER STIGMATA

Proband		Parents or offspring		GS in Affected Relative[a]				Total	
				Siblings		Others			
Gardner stigmata	Family no.	No.	%	No.	%	No.	%	No.	%
+	28	5/13	38.46	8/22	36.36	7/22	31.80	20/57	35.09
—	87	9/51	17.65	9/72	12.50	8/52	15.36	26/175	14.86
Total	115	14/64	21.88	17/94	18.09	15/74	20.27	46/232	19.83
r		0.2026		0.2625		0.1868		0.2184	
		$0.1 < p < 0.2$		$0.01 < p < 0.05$		$0.1 < 0.2$		$p < 0.001$	

[a] Excluding proband.

From Tanimura, M., *Ochanomizu Med.*, 33, 83, 1985. With permission.

VI. MANAGEMENT OF ADENOMATOSIS COLI

The present policy of AC management is prophylactic removal of the large bowel. In practice, however, there are many problems to be solved.

A. Detection of the Patient

1. Identification of the Candidates for Examination

All of the first and second degree relatives of the proband are identified as possible gene carriers by means of constructing a working pedigree. Persons of 10 years of age or older are selected as candidates for examination. The author surveyed 34 families, including 330 members at the Polyposis Center, which revealed 273 possible gene carriers and 258 were candidates for examination.

2. Contacting the Candidates for Examination

Out of the 189 candidates who were contacted by various methods, 84 or 44.5% did not respond to the initial communication, but after repeated attempts, 26 or 13.8% responded later, yielding an overall 69.3% response rate. Colonic examinations were performed on 109 or 83.2% of the 131 who responded. Polyps were found in 39 patients. Within a year, 75% of the responders came to us and 25% finally received the examination after repeated contacts, the longest time lag being 7 years.[50] These experiences revealed the efficacy of continuous attempts to educate the family members through various means. We compiled an educational booklet which explained the general factual content about the natural history of the disease, the necessity of examination, and an outline of management. It was sometimes efficient for accelerating the family survey to select the key person(s) who could help to educate the family members on the necessity of the examination. Occult blood test paper sent by mail provided a chance to initially contact the family members in distant places.[50] The response rate was not influenced by age of the candidate but the rate was 1.2 times higher in the males than in the females.[50]

3. Examination and Diagnosis

Initial examination of the called-up person was made both by sigmoid fibrescope and double-contrast barium enema. Diagnosis of the patient with full-blown characteristic features of multiple minimum adenomatous polyps distributed throughout the large bowel was not difficult. In the beginning of the adenoma stage, a few minimum-sized elevations of the mucosal surface could be the only sign of the manifestation and can often be overlooked even by an experienced examiner. The use of a mucosal vital staining method or a magnifying endoscope was useful in the suspected cases.

The finding of occult osteomatous changes in an orthopantomogram[30] and/or congenital hypertrophy of the retinal pigment epithelium[51] may provide additional information for identifying the gene carrier before the appearance of colonic manifestation. The examinations were repeated every year until the age of 30 in order to exclude patients who were gene carriers.

Identification of location and stage of cancer in the large bowel and determination of the number and type of polyps, profuse or scarce, are essential for selection of the type of operation.[9]

The extracolonic neoplastic lesions such as the gastric and duodenal lesions are screened by upper GI series and endoscopy.

B. Surgery

1. Age to Perform Prophylactic Operation

The optimal timing of surgery for the patient with adenomas should be between 15 and 25 years of age. The risk of developing cancer reached 1% at the age of 16 years for males and 13 years for females, and rapidly increased after 20 years of age (Table 12). The nonsymptomatic patient might not accept surgery at an older age when he is involved in an active social life.

2. Type of Operation for Prophylactic Surgery

Total colectomy with ileorectal anastomosis (IRA) followed by surveillance of the retained rectum, which was proposed by Lockhart-Mummery et al.[52] is accepted as the procedure of choice by most surgeons at present. The operation provides natural anal function with a good quality of life but presents the question of whether the remaining rectum could really be prevented from an occurrence of cancer for long enough to achieve the aim of the cancer preventive surgery.

The incidence of cancer in the retained rectum showed considerable differences among the reports[7,53-60] (Table 17). There are two options — one supporting this policy of treatment and one insisting on the more radical surgery for it. Bussey[55] of St. Mark's Hospital reported that the incidence of cancer in the retained rectum is only 13% over 25 years of follow-up after IRA. In contrast, the Mayo Clinic group reported that 60% of the IRA patients suffered rectal cancer after 20 years.[54] The author's personal experience of a 10-year follow-up of IRA was discouraging with observed rectal cancer in 3 or 25% of 12 cases operated.[53] The overall results of multiple institutions in Japan was quite similar to the Mayo series (Table 17). The discrepancy may be created by different factors which influence the actual results, such as duration of follow-up, criteria for selection of patients, length of the retained rectum, age at operation (Figure 4), number of polyps, and postoperative follow-up compliance of the patients. The favorable results of St. Mark's Hospital may be due to their successful postoperative follow-up system. This is, however, not always realistic in many of the other institutions. About half of my patients with IRA never received regular checkups during 7 years of follow-up in spite of intensive urging. No surgeon can guarantee surveillance of the retained rectum throughout his patient's lifetime.

In Japan, we are facing a serious problem of an ever-increasing number of colectomized patients at high risk of rectal cancer who have escaped from the continuous follow-up. For a solution to this problem, there are three possible approaches: first, the provision of central surveillance system for abnormal gene carriers before and after surgery; second, the establishment of a practical procedure for total removal of colorectal mucosa without an abdominal stoma; and third, research on the chemoprevention of cancer and adenoma in the rectum.[61]

Table 17
PREVALENCE OF CANCER IN RETAINED RECTUM AFTER ILEORECTAL ANASTOMOSIS

Reporters		Age	Follow up term (year)					
			All over	5	10	15	20	20<
Iwama[53a]	1980	30.9 (9—67)	4/19 (21.1%)	1/16 (6.3%)	3/12 (25.0%)	—	—	—
Jpn. Soc. L. B. C. Res.	1987[a]	34.6(17—65)	14/115 (12.2%)	8/79 (10.1%)	4/30 (13.3%)	0/9 (0%)	2/2 (100.0%)	0/1 (0%)
Moertel et al.[54]	1971	36.0 (8—68)	31/143 (21.7%)	7/132 (5.3%)	14/105 (13.3%)	8/72 (11.1%)	16/38 (42.1%)	0/17 (0%)
Bussey[55]	1984	—	11/166 (6.6%)	—	— (6.0%)	—	— (10.0%)	— (18.0%)
Schaupp and Volpe[56]	1984	—	1/36 (2.8%)	1/30 (3.3%)	—	0/5 (0%)	—	—
Harvey et al.[57]	1978	28.6 (7—53)	4/35 (11.4%)	—	1/19 (5.3%)	1/10 (0%)	1/5 (20.0%)	1/4 (25.0%)
Gingold et al.[58]	1979	28.0 (—)	0/26 (0%)	0/26 (0%)	0/12 (0%)	0/5 (0%)	0/4 (0%)	0/4 (0%)
Watne et al.[59]	1983	24.0(10—54)	7/32 (21.9%)	7/32 (21.9%)	1/9 (11.1%)	2/10 (20.0%)	3/6 (50.0%)	—
Jarvinen[60]	1985	41.0(20—76)	0/52 (0%)	0/52 (0%)	0/13 (0%)	0/8 (0%)	0/2 (0%)	0/1 (0%)

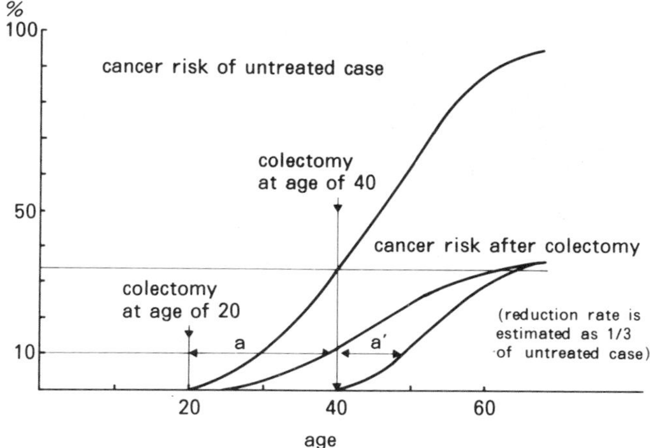

FIGURE 4. Expected effect on reduction of cancer risk in the large bowel by colectomy and ileorectal anastomosis for familial polyposis.

For the surgeon, the second approach is feasible at present while others must be continuously researched through collaborations with other fields, such as epidemiology and biochemistry.

The total removal of the diseased large bowel mucosa, with preservation of normal anal continence, is achieved by total colectomy, rectal mucosectomy with ileoanal anastomosis (IAA). The first clinical trial of IAA was performed on a boy with AC in Nissen in 1932,[62] but without success. Ravitch and Sabiston[63] achieved the first clinical success on ulcerative colitis patients in 1947 and Devine and Webb[64] performed it on AC patients in 1951. The procedure, however, did not gain favor with surgeons because of three major problems: (1) the technical difficulty, (2) the often serious postoperative complications, and (3) the sub-optimal functional results. Its potential role and value, however, are being reappraised as exemplified by the recent increase in the number of reports on IAA. The author began his search for a practical procedure of IAA for this challenging problem in 1977 when he was discouraged with the poor result of IRA and incidentally faced the treatment of a family with many patients who had profuse polyps. Recently, the problems of IAA have been largely solved by improvements in operative technique and surgical materials. The most important achievement in the development of modern IAA is clinical application of the pelvic ileal pouch of various types such as the S of Parks,[65] J of the author,[66-69] W of Nicholles,[70] and H of Fonkalsrud[71] to reduce fecal frequency (Figure 5). The J-pouch devised by the author is now most widely used because of its technical simplicity and better function when compared to other types of pouches (Table 18).[69-77] By our operative technique currently in use, the functional result is comparable with that of IRA, and surgical intervention and technical complexity is more or less equal to Kock's abdominal pouch (Table 19).[78,79] This procedure can be performed on all patients on whom colectomy and IRA are currently indicated. These patients are potential candidates for IAA unless they are older than 60 years of age.[78] This operation, however, is recommended to be performed in the central institute for this disease because it requires technical skill and expert postoperative management based on a considerable amount of experience.

3. Follow-up after Operation

The remaining rectum of the patient after IRA is observed through a fiber sigmoidoscope or rigid sigmoidoscope every 6 to 12 months. All visible polyps are destroyed by means of

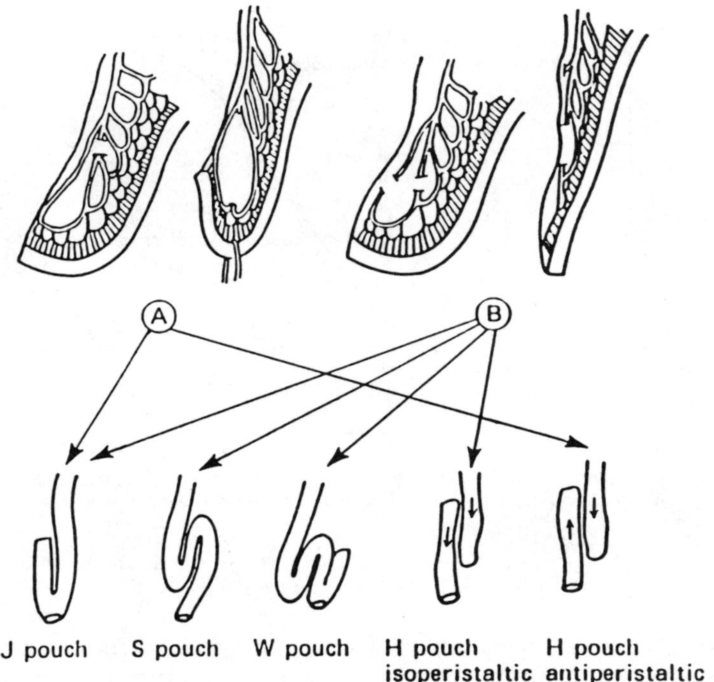

FIGURE 5. Different methods of pelvic ileal pouch.

electrocoagulator or laser coagulator not only for eliminating adenomas but also for easier detection of flat early cancer.

Out of 45 patients on whom the author personally performed IAA over the last 9 years, 1 recently died of a duodenal cancer 6 years after the operation. The evidence strongly suggests that we must expect to more frequently encounter cancers in other organs than the large bowel when more patients survive longer because they had prophylactic surgery to prevent colorectal cancer. The stomach and duodenum should be examined through X-ray as well as endoscopy every year after surgery.

Gastric polyposis itself is not an indication for prophylactic surgery but the stomach with multiple adenomatous lesions with severe dysplasia may be an indication for partial gastrectomy. Vater's papillae should always be biopsied to detect invisible adenomatous involvement which may be a risk factor for cancer development.

Intraperitoneal desmoid tumor is closely observed by means of US and CT and removed when it tends to grow.

VII. PEUTZ-JEGHER'S SYNDROME

A. General Concepts and Definitions

Peutz-Jegher's syndrome (PJS) is a hereditary condition comprised of GI hamartomatous polyps associated with a characteristic mucocutaneous pigmentation.[80,81] The mode of transmission is autosomal dominant.[81] At one time, the risk of malignancy was thought to be negligible,[82] but it has recently been reevaluated[83] and considered to be a cancer high risk condition.

B. Polyposis

Polyps are distributed fairly evenly throughout the digestive tract, with the exception of the esophagus. They are sessile and pedunculated. They have a characteristic surface ap-

Table 18
CURRENT STATUS OF ILEOANAL ANASTOMOSIS IN THE WORLD

			Disease		Pouch					
Institute	Reporter	Year	UC	AC	J	S	W	H	N	Total
Tokyo Medical Dental University	Utsunomiya	1983	11	37	32	0	0	2	10	48
Hyogo College of Medicine	Utsunomiya	1987	12	11	23	0	0	0	0	23
Mayo Clinic	Metcalf[69]	1985	177	—	183	5	0	0	0	188
St. Mark's Hospital	Nicholls[70]	1984	70	18	13	68	23	0	0	104
Lahey Clinic	Scholtz[72]	1986	71	13	63	21	0	0	0	84
UCLA	Fonkalsrud[71]	1985	78	8	0	0	0	86	0	86
Sanfose Medical Center	Peck[73]	1980	17	12	0	0	0	29	0	29
University of Toronto	Grant[74]	1986	76	6	65	15	0	0	0	82
University of Goteborg	Hulten[75]	1985	—	—	30	0	0	0	0	30
University of Cophenhagen	Hansen[76]	1985	19	3	0	22	0	0	0	22
Hennepin County Medical Center	Bubrik[77]	1986	21	2	0	23	0	0	0	23

Note: J = J pouch, W = W pouch, H = H pouch, N = nonpouch, UC = ulcerative colitis, and AC = adenomatosis coli.

Table 19
CHOICE OF SURGICAL PROCEDURE FOR STAGE AND TYPE OF FAMILIAL POLYPOSIS

Cancer	Adenoma	Age	Colectomy, ileorectal anastomosis	Proctocolectomy: Abdominal ileostomy	Proctocolectomy: Ileoanal anastomosis
Non	Sparse	20—60	O	X	O
		60 or more	O	O	X
	Profuse	—	X	O	O
Colon			O	O	O
Rectum					
Upper			X	O	O
Lower			X	◎	O
Early			X	◎	O
Advanced					

Note: X = contraindications, O = relative indication, and ◎ = absolute indication.

pearance with lobulation or cerebellar gyrus-like construction. The number of polyps varies from one to 10 to 20 per subsite segment of the GI tract, and carpeting is never seen as occurs in AC. The growth rate of the polyps shows considerable differences from each other when observed by sequential examination.

The characteristic feature is a branching forth overgrowth of the muscularis mucosa, on which epithelial cells composed of normal cellular and structural components are arranged. No cytokinetic disorder is observed in the cells as seen in adenomas. Everted growth into the muscular layer is sometimes observed, and can be mistaken for malignant invasion.[82]

C. Pigmentation

These are cutaneous signs which are characterized by an accumulation of minute, flat, dark brown or black macules. They are symmetrically distributed in specific anatomic locations, including the lips or perioral region (94.1%), buccal mucosa (65.8%), and distal portion of the limbs (73.9% in the upper and 62.2% in the lower extremities).[84] Histologically, an accumulation of melanin pigment and an increased number of melanocytes are seen in the basal layer of the epidermis, particularly in the stratum spinosum, but not in the straum germinativum of the palmar and plantar surfaces. Usually, the parent first notices the appearance of pigmentation on the lower lip as a few small, solitary, dark macules when the affected child is 1 to 2 years of age. In some patients, the pigmentation was not present on the lips, but occurred on other parts of the body. These patients were over 45 years of age, indicating that fading of the lip pigmentation may occur with age as reported by Peutz.[80]

D. Malignant Changes in the Polyps

An important clinical issue is the possibility of malignant transformation of the polyps. At the very beginning of the study of PJS, it was considered that the polyps could undergo malignant transformation.[81] Bartholomew et al.[82] indicated that the typical polyps are hamartomatous and that the presence of mitotic figures or heterotropic accumulation of glandular structures in the mucosal layer should not be necessarily considered as evidence of malignant transformation of the polyps. Recently however, malignant and adenomatous transformation in the polyps is again being acknowledged, although it is quite a rare event. The author has observed a microfocus highly suspicious of malignancy of polyps from two cases,[79] and similar evidence was reported by other researchers.[86,87]

E. Natural History and Cancer Risk

The survival rate of PJS cases was found to be shorter than that of the control population

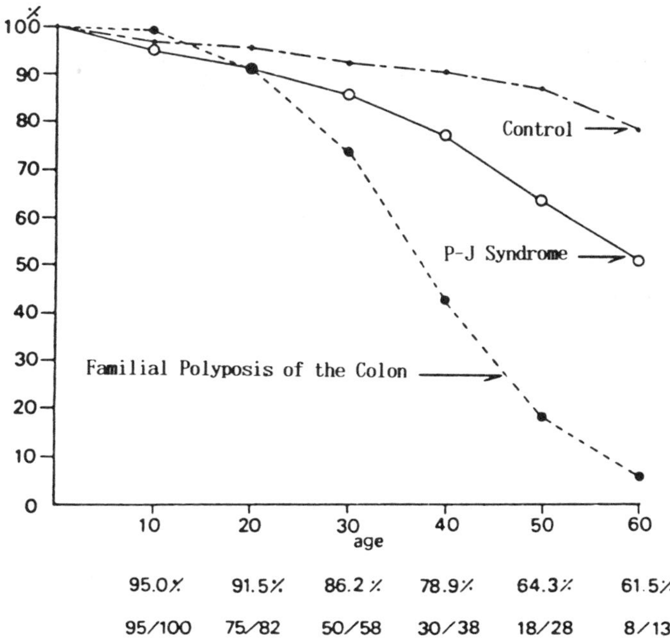

FIGURE 6. Survival rate of 102 followup cases of Peutz-Jegher's syndrome. (From Utsunomiya, J., Gocho, H., Miyanaga, T., Hamaguchi, E., Kashimura, A., and Aoki, N., *Johns Hopkins Med. J.*, 36, 71, 1975. With permission.)

(Figure 6). Of the deaths occurring before age 30, 42.9% were due to acute complications of the polyposis, such as intussusception. Of the deaths occurring after age 30, approximately 60% were attributed to neoplastic disease.[83] Analysis of the type of neoplastic lesions causing death in 23 patients revealed that cancer of the colon occurred with the highest frequency, in 8 patients altogether, but that tumors of a variety of other sites also occurred, including the small intestine, stomach, liver, gallbladder, pancreas, lung, uterus, ovary, and bone[83] (Table 20). Predominance of large bowel cancer as the cause of death of PJS was confirmed in the Johns Hopkins Hospital series.[84] In females, ovarian tumers[88] well-differentiated adenocarcinoma of the cervix,[89] and bilateral breast cancer[90] are attracting special attention.

F. Heredity and Clinicoepidemiological Factors

1. Age and Sex

The average age of diagnosis is 23.0 years in males and 26.0 years in females. This should be contrasted with AC, which manifests earlier in females than in males. The male to female ratio is 1.0:1.1.

2. Familial Occurrence[83]

Familial cases accounted for 45.1% of the 127 cases in whom a family history was obtained. The average number of affected individuals per pedigree is 1.51, much smaller than the 2.37 of AC. This may possibly be due to earlier manifestation of PJS than AC.

3. Mode of Transmission[83]

It is consistent with autosomal dominant inheritance. The observed segregation ratio was estimated to be 0.333. No consanguinity was detected.

Table 20
MALIGNANT TUMOR ASSOCIATED WITH PEUTZ-JEGHER'S SYNDROME

	Utsunomiya[83]	Hood[84]	Rodu[85]
Gastrointestinal			
Stomach	3	2	
Duodenum	1		8
Small intestine	1	2	
Large intestine	8	6	
Liver	1	—	—
Biliary tract	1	—	—
Pancreas	1	2	—
Breast	0	2	5
—	1		
Cervix		—	5
Ovary	2	1	28 (sex cord tumor)
Lung	2	3	—
Bone	1	—	—
Leukemia	—	1	—
Other	—	1	1 (sertoli cell tumor)

G. Management

Insofar as possible, this disease should be treated conservatively because the patient will necessarily have many intestinal operations during his life and prophylactic surgical removal of the organ is not justified since site of occurrence of malignant lesions cannot be predicted and the risk is not as great as in AC. The main concern of surgeons in this disease is prevention of intestinal intussusception. If operative measures are required, every effort should be made to avoid peritoneal adhesions which would complicate the inevitable later surgical procedures.

The patient should be advised to see a physician knowledgeable about this disease at regular intervals or immediately upon the occurrence of symptoms. If intussusception should occur, polypectomy is mandatory, for with repeated attacks, intussusception becomes more severe and at times ischemic damage necessitates intestinal resection. After reduction of intussusception, the base of the advancing polyp is detected by a dimple produced when the intestinal wall is stretched. Through a small, longitudinal incision adjacent to the dimple, the polyp is extracted and, if the dimple is large, a spindle-shaped section of wall including the base of the stalk is removed with the polyp. This maneuver removes the lesion and possible invasion of the base of the stalk, yet minimizes the defect in the intestinal wall. When polyps of considerable size are detected elsewhere in the small bowel, these can also be removed through the same opening by everting oral and anal intestine. Segmental resection of the intestine should be avoided so far as possible to prevent malnutrition disorders. Polyps in the stomach should be removed endoscopically. The authors experienced gastroduodenal intussusception in one case.

VIII. JUVENILE POLYPOSIS

A. General Concepts and Definition

The rare condition of multiple occurrences of juvenile polyps in the GI tract is termed juvenile polyposis. In this disorder, familial occurrence, association of congenital abnormalities, and a positive relationship of the occurrence of adenomas and cancer have recently been disclosed. Since the first report by Ravitch[91] in 1948, 153 cases including 18 Japanese cases have been reported up to 1986.

B. Subclasses

Sachatello et al.[92] prefer to classify juvenile polyposis (JP) into three subgroups on the basis of site of involvement and age: (1) JP of the infant, (2) generalized JP of the GI tract, and (3) JP coli. This classification was based primarily on clinical grounds. The occurrence of both generalized and colonic JP in the same kindred[93] suggests that these are different expressions of the same disorder rather than distinct syndromes. In 153 reported cases, the polyposis involved the colon and rectum in 104 cases or 75%, the entire GI tract in 34 cases or 23%, and only 2 cases in the stomach. Though the generalized types are observed in younger patients and less frequently with familial occurrence than in others, no final conclusion can be reached for supporting the existence of these distinct varieties.

C. Polyposis

A general impression of the individual polyp is that of an irregular shape, sometimes oval with a pointed top, sessile or pedunculated, of uneven size, scattered or sometimes occurring in groups in the lower rectum or the gastric antrum. The number of the polyps is much less than in AC and similar to PJS. There were 15% of cases which had less than 10 polyps, 70% had more than 11, and another 15% had more than 100.

Juvenile polyps have characteristic histologic features that include proliferation and cyst formation of nonatypical, normal-appearing epithelial cells, and an abundant stroma with edema and round cell infiltration. Morson[94] considered it a hamartoma, while others[95,96] believe their orgin to be inflammatory. Goodman et al.[96] speculated that they occurred as inflammatory modifications of hyperplastic polyps. Kachula[97] described a case with numerous colonic polyps of three types: adenomatous, juvenile, and an intermediate form having features of both juvenile and adenomatous polyps. The findings have been readily confirmed by others[93,97-99] and the occurrence of villous adenomas has been reported.[100] The evidence suggests that this condition has a close etiologic relationship with adenomas and can present possible diagnostic confusion with AC.

D. Cancer Risk

The malignant potential of JP had been considered negligible until Stemper et al.[93] described a high incidence of GI carcinomas in a kindred with ten members with multiple or solitary juvenile polyps. Goodman et al.[96] speculated that a focal adenomatous area of a juvenile polyp would develop carcinoma. Malignant lesions were described in 13 cases or 10.5% of the reported series; 13 cases within the colorectum, 2 cases in the pancrease, and 1 in the stomach. The fact that colorectal cancer was documented by family history in 14 families or 20.8% out of 67 families suggests the condition is apparently hereditary. Stemper et al.[93] comment that malignancy in association with hamartomatous conditions can occur, as is known in tuberous sclerosis, neurofibromatosis, and Cowden's syndrome.

E. Associated Nonmalignant Lesions: Congenital Anomalies

The association of various congenital anomalies in patients with JP was found in 73.3% of nonfamilial cases and in 3.2% of the familial. Congential anomalies include macrocephalus and other conditions of the CNS in 28%, cardiovascular such as Fallot tetralogy in 20%, and others such as malrotation of the gut, Meckel's diverticulum, bipolar uterus, umbilical fistula, megacolon, etc. Schwartz and McCauley[100] indicated that the anomalies were usually associated with the generalized GI type of JP.

F. Genetics

Familial occurrence of JP was first described by Veale et al.[101] Subsequently, familial occurrence has been demonstrated in 33% of the reported cases. The mode of inheritance is possibly autosomal dominant. Veale et al.[101] described two cases of JP belonging to two AC families and hypothesized an intimate genetic relationship to AC. These families, however, are now considered to have JP mixed with adenomatous polyps, rather than AC.[102]

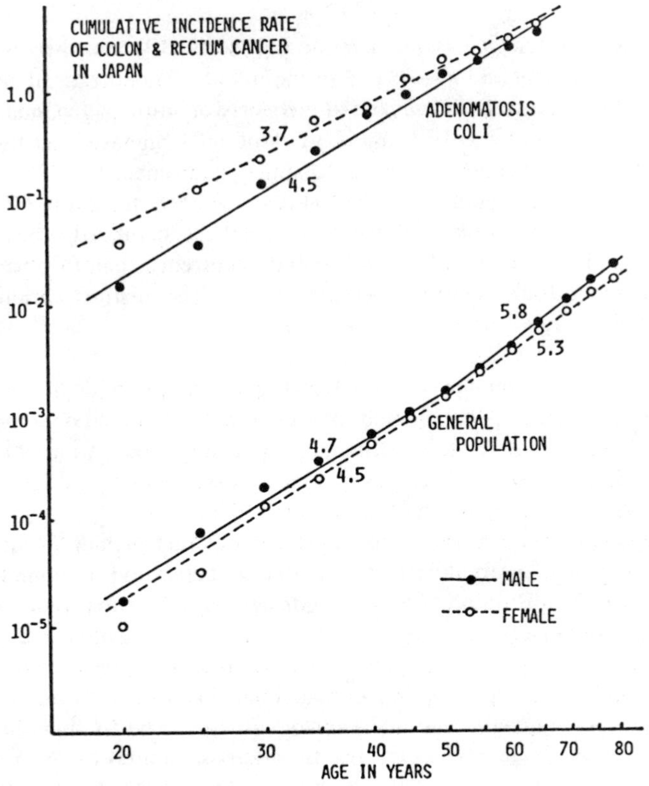

FIGURE 7. Age specific prevalence of colorectal cancer in Japanese and English AC patients and in the general population as presented by Knudson's method. (From Utsunomiya, J., Iwama, T., Murata, M., and Tanimura, M., *Taishya (Metabolism)*, 17, 183, 1980. With permission.)

G. Clinicoepidemiological Factors

Male/female ratio was 83:69 by an analysis on the reported cases. Average age of diagnosis was 14.4 years in males and 16.9 years in females.[99] Of the patients, 95% complained of anorectal bleeding.

H. Management

Preventive colectomy with IRA could be justified because in the majority of cases in which polypectomy or segmental colectomy had been performed, subsequent surgery was necessary for recurrent polyposis in the remaining colon.

IX. ETIOLOGY OF CARCINOGENESIS IN HEREDITARY GASTROINTESTINAL POLYPOSES

A. Multihit Theory

The age-specific incidence of almost all cancer showed a straight line if placed in a logarithmic scale. Armitage and Doll[103] presented a theory that cancer develops from sequential multiple hits and that the number of necessary hits can be calculated from the age-specific incidence of the cancer. The number of hits for colorectal cancer in the general population is estimated to be six, whereas Ashley[37] estimated one hit or more for cancer in AC. We have obtained essentially the same result using the Japanese series of AC[38] (Figure 7). According to Knudson,[105] the implication is that these individuals have received a prezygotic or genetic hit and fewer postzygotic hits or environmental effects, as compared to the general population.

The specific characteristics of familial large bowel cancer can be partially explained by this theory. In AC, a very early appearance and an even distribution of multiple adenomas suggest that very few hits are required to produce the adenomatous lesion. However, the distal occurrence of large bowel cancer in polyposis (Table 6), which is similar to that seen in the general population, suggests that cancer requires additional environmentally derived hits.

The observation of different grades of dysplasia in adenomas may represent the sequential changes evolving toward cancer from multiple hits. The cytokinetic disorder observed in the flat mucosa may represent the genetic abnormality that is responible for producing deficient control of DNA synthesis in the mucosal cells. The autosomal mode of transmission suggests that the abnormality is localized in a single gene. The series of subclinical or *in vitro* abnormalities observed in the skin fibroblasts of AC patients[106] are characterized as a phenotypically initiated preneoplastic state and suggest that all somatic cells of the AC patient have been affected by a prezygotic change. This assumption has been supported in a study by Kopelovich[107] who showed that AC skin fibroblasts transformed from administration of tumor-promoting factor alone.

B. Future Projections: Advances in Molecular Genetics

As this chapter was undergoing completion, certain advances in molecular genetics appeared in the literature which could aid significantly in the understanding of etiology of colorectal cancer in general and those syndromes associated with multiple colonic polyps in particular. Specifically, Herrera et al.[108] observed two possible sites on chromosome 5, namely, 5q13-q15 vs. 5q15-q22, as a constitutional deletion in an AC patient. Following this observation, Bodmer et al.[109] observed close linkage to FAP of a genetic marker mapped to the 5q21-q22 region of an alternative site for this putative deletion. Of further interest is the work of Solomon et al.,[110] who observed tumor-specific allele loss in 23% of sporadic colon cancer through analysis of two loci which were mapped to the terminal third of 5q(5q31 and 5q34-qtr). Wildrick and Boman (personal communication, 1987) have shown allele loss at the glucocorticoid receptor gene (GRL) locus which is mapped at the proximal region of 5q. These latter observations suggest that in many occurrences of colorectal carcinoma, either a large portion of the 5q, the entire arm, or the entire chromosome may be lost. This work is of significance in that the observed tumor-specific allele loss in the area of proximity of the GRL locus to the region 5q suggests that this genetic alteration may be etiologic in colon carcinogenesis. Further credence to the possibility that steroid hormones may be important in the growth of carcinoma cells has been the subject of a review by Boman et al.[111] The work of Boman is now being extended to the HNPCC syndromes (Lynch syndromes I and II) in collaboration with Lynch and colleagues. It is hoped that this research may provide elucidation to the heterogeneity of colorectal cancer and that, ultimately, it may provide important clues to colon carcinogenesis and its control.

REFERENCES

1. **Lynch, H. T., Kimberling, W., Albano, W., Lynch, J. F. Biscone, K., Schuelke, G. S., Sandberg, A. A., Deschner, E. E., Mikol, Y. B., Elston, R. C., Bailey-Wilson, J. E., and Danes, B. S.,** Hereditary nonpolyposis colorectal cancer. I and II, *Cancer,* 56, 934, 1985.
2. **Utsunomiya, J. and Iwama, T.,** Clinical and population genetics of the hereditary gastrointestinal polyposis, *Heterogeneity and Genetics of Common Gastrointestinal Disorders,* Rother, J. I., Samloff, and Rimoin, D. L., Eds., Academic Press, New York, 1980, 351.
3. **Utsunomiya, J.,** Present status of adenomatois coli in Japan, in *Pathophysiology of Carcinogenesis in Digestive Organs,* Farber, E. et al., Eds., University of Tokyo Press, Tokyo, 1977, 305.

4. **Utsunomiya, J. and Iwama, T.,** Studies of hereditary gastrointestinal polyposes, *Asian Med. J.,* 21, 76, 1978.
5. **Tanimura, M. and Utsunomiya, J.,** A new coding method for "working pedigree", *Jpn. J. Hum. Genet.,* 26, 148, 1981.
6. **Utsunomiya, J.,** Hereditary gastrointestinal polyposis, *Nihon Iji Shinppo,* 3044, 126, 1982.
7. **Bussey, H. J. R.,** *Familial Polyposis Coli,* Johns Hopkins Press, Baltimore, 1975.
8. **Iwama, T.,** Pathological study on adenomatosis coli, *J. Jpn. Surg. Soc.,* 79, 10, 1978.
9. **Maeda, M., Iwama, T., Utsunomiya, J., Aoki, N., and Suzuki, S.,** Radiological features of familial polyposis coli: grouping by polyp profusion, *Br. J. Radiol.,* 57, 217, 1984.
10. **Fujiwara, A., Yanagisawa, A., Koto, H., and Sugano, H.,** Malignant potential of adenoma in adenomatosis coli, *Igaku No Ayumi,* 132, 442, 1985.
11. **Kuroki, T. and Utsunomiya, J.,** unpublished data.
12. **Iwama, T., Utsunomiya, J., and Sasaki, J.,** Epithelial cell kinetics in the crypts familial polyposis of colon, *Jpn. J. Surg.,* 7, 230, 1978.
13. **Muto, T., Kamiya, J., Sawada, T., Agawa, S., Morioka, Y., and Utsunomiya, J.,** Mucin abnormality of colonic mucosa in patients with familial polyposis coli, *Dis. Colon Rectum,* 28, 147, 1985.
14. **Smiddy, F. G. and Goligher, J. C.,** Results of surgery is the treatment of cancer of the large intestine, *Br. Med. J.,* 1, 793, 1957.
15. **Utsunomiya, J., Maki, T., Iwama, T., Matsunaga, Y., Ichikawa, T., Shimomura, T., Hamaguchi, E., and Aoki, N.,** Gastric lesions of familial polyposis coli, *Cancer,* 34, 745, 1974.
16. **Ushio, K., Sasagawa, M., Doi, H., Yamada, T., Ichikawa, H., Hojo, K., Koyama, Y., and Sano, R.,** Lesions associated with familial polyposis coli: studies of lesions of the stomach, duodenum, bones, and teeth, *Gastrointest. Radiol.,* 1, 67, 1976.
17. **Iida, M. and Ohmae, T.,** Extra-colonic tumor-like lesions in familial polyposis of the colon and in Gardner's syndrome, *Fukuoka Igaku Zasshi,* 69, 169, 1981.
18. **Utsunomiya, J.,** to be published.
19. **Ranzi, T., Castagnone, D., Velio, P., Bianchi, P., and Polli, E. E.,** Gastric and duodenal polyps in familial polyposis coli, *Gut,* 22, 363, 1981.
20. **Jarvinen, H., Nyberg, M., and Peltokallio, P.,** Upper gastrointestinal tract polyps in familial adenomatosis coli, *Gut,* 24, 333, 1983.
21. **Burt, R. W., Berenson, M. M., Lee, R. G., Tolman, K. G., Preston, J. W. and Gardner, E. J.,** Upper gastrointestinal polyps in Gardner's syndrome, *Gastroenterology,* 86, 295, 1984.
22. **Shemesh, E., Pines, A., and Bat, U.,** Spectrum of extracolonic gastrointestinal tract involvement in Gardner syndrome, *Isr. Med. Sci.,* 21, 973, 1985.
23. **Tonelli, F., Nardi, F., Bechi, P., Taddei, G., Gozzo, P., and Romagnoli, P.,** Extracolonic polyps in familial polyposis coli and Gardner's syndrome, *Dis. Colon Rectum,* 26, 295, 1985.
24. **Bulow, S., Lauritsen, K. B., Johansen, A., Svendsen, L. B., and Sondergaard, J. O.,** Gastroduodenal polyps in familial polyposis coli, *Dis. Colon Rectum,* 28, 90, 1985.
25. **Watanabe, H., Enjoji, M., Yao, T., and Ohsato, K.,** Gastric lesions in familial adenomatosis coli, *Hum. Pathol.,* 9, 269, 1978.
26. **Nishimura, M., Hirota, T., Itabashi, M., Ushio, K., Yamada, T., and Oguro, Y.,** A clinical and histochemical study of gastric polyps in familial polyposis coli, *Am. J. Gastroenterol.,* 79, 98, 1984.

26a. **Utsunomiya, J., Miki, V., and Kuroki, T.,** Phenotypic expression of patient with familial adenomatous polyposis in Japan, in *Familial Adenomatous Polyposis,* Herrera, L., Ed., Allan R. Liss, New York, to be published.

27. **Ohsato, K., Yao, T., Watanabe, H., Iida, M., and Itoh, H.,** Small intestinal involvement in familial polyposis diagnosed by operative intestinal fiberoscopy, *Dis. Colon Rectum,* 20, 414, 1977.
28. **Gardner, E. J.,** A genetic and clinical study of intestinal polyposis, a predisposing factor for carcinoma of the colon and rectum, *Am. J. Hum. Genet.,* 3, 167, 1951.
29. **Utsunomiya, J. and Nakamura, T.,** The occult osteomatous changes in the mandible in patients with familial polyposis coli, *Br. J. Surg.,* 62, 45, 1975.
30. **Ida, M., Nakamura, T., and Utsunomiya, J.,** Osteomatous changes and tooth abnormalities found in the jaws of patients with adenomatosis coli, *Oral Surg.,* 52, 2, 1981.
31. **Turcot, J., Desperes, J. P., and St. Pierre, F.,** Malignant tumors of the central nervous system associated with familial polyposis of the colon: report of two cases, *Dis. Colon Rectum,* 2, 465, 1959.
32. **Itoh, H. and Ohsato, K.,** Turcot syndrome and its characteristic colonic manifestations, *Dis. Colon Rectum,* 28, 399, 1985.
33. **Zanca, P.,** Multiple hereditary cartilaginous exostosis with polyposis of the colon, *U.S. Armed Forces Med. J.,* 6, 116, 1953.
34. **Miura, O., Inoue, K., Matsuda, S., Adachi, Y., Hukutome, A., Soga, K., and Aoki, M.,** A case of familial polyposis coli associated with hereditary multiple cartilaginous exostosis: the so-called Zanca's syndrome, *Naika,* 56, 592, 1985.

35. **Utsunomiya, J., Tanimura, M., Iwama, T., and Murata, M.,** Natural history of adenomatosis coli, *Cancer Chemother.*, 7(Suppl.), 16, 1980.
36. **Veale, A. M. O.,** *Intestinal Polyposis,* Cambridge University Press, Cambridge, England, 1965.
37. **Ashley, D. T. B.,** Colonic cancer arising in polyposis coli, *J. Med. Genet.*, 6, 376, 1969.
38. **Utsunomiya, J., Murata, M., and Tanimura, M.,** An analysis of the age distribution of colon cancer in adenomatosis coli, *Cancer,* 45, 198, 1980.
39. **Tanimura, M.,** Study on genetic heterogeneity of adenomatosis coli, *Ochanomizu Med. J.*, 33, 83, 1985.
40. **Tanaka, K., Utsunomiya, J., Tanimura, M., and Iwama, T.,** Genetic analysis of adenomatosis coli: on affection of parents of the affected, unpublished article.
41. **Stryker, S. J., Carney, J. A., and Dozois, R. R.,** Multiple adenomatous polyps arising in a continent reservoir ileostomy, *Int. J. Colorect. Dis.*, 2, 43, 1986.
42. **Nakahara, S., Itoh, H., Iida, M., Iwashita, A., and Ohsato, K.,** Ileal adenomas in familial polyposis coli: differences before and after colectomy, *Dis. Colon Rectum,* 28, 875, 1985.
43. **Murata, M. and Utsunomiya, J.,** Carcinogenesis in familial polyposis coli and cancer family syndrome, *J. Clin. Sci.*, 19, 175, 1983.
43a. **Murata, M., Utsunomiya, J., Iwama, T., and Tanimura, M.,** Frequency of adenomatous coli in Japan, *Jpn. J. Hum. Genet.*, 26, 19, 1981.
44. **Ȃlm, T. and Licznerski, G.,** The intestinal polyposes, *Clin. Gastroenterol.*, 2, 577, 1973.
45. **Utsunomiya, J., Iwama, T., Suzuki, H., Tanaka, T., Tonomura, A., Sasaki, M., Nakamura, T., Hamaguchi, H., Mori, W., and Komatsu, I.,** Clinical and genetic studies on familial polyposis coli: sex ratio, *Jpn. J. Hum. Genet.*, 20, 283, 1976.
46. **Tanimura, M., Utsunomiya, J., Iwama, T., and Komatsu, I.,** Sporadic cases in adenomatosis coli, *Jpn. J. Hum. Genet.*, 27, 178, 1982.
47. **Utsunomiya, J., Iwama, T., and Suzuki, H., Hamaguchi, H., Tonomura, A., Sasaki, M., Tanaka, K., Mori, W., Nakamura, T., and Komatsu, I.,** Genetics of adenomatosis coli, *Stom. Intestine,* 9, 1146, 1974.
48. **Reed, T. E. and Neel, J. V.,** A genetic study of multiple polyposis of the colon (with an appendix deriving a method of estimating relative fitness), *Am. J. Hum. Genet.*, 7, 236, 1955.
49. **Utsunomiya, J., Tanimura, M., Iwama, T., Tanaka, K., and Tonomura, A.,** Clinical genetic study of familial polyposis coli: correlation of the age at onset of cancer between relatives, *Jpn. J. Hum. Genet.*, 24, 202, 1979.
50. **Utsunomiya, J., Iwama, T., and Tanimura, M.,** Result of family survey on adenomatosis coli, *Ryn Kenkyu,* 57, 2161, 1980.
51. **Lewis, R. A., Crowder, W. E., Eierman, L. A., Nussbaum, R. L., and Ferrell, R. E.,** The Gardner syndrome: significance of ocular features, *Ophthalmology,* 91, 916, 1984.
52. **Lockhart-Mummery, H. E., Dukes, C. E., and Bussey, H. J. R.,** The surgical treatment of familial polyposis of the colon, *Br. J. Surg.*, 43, 476, 1956.
53. **Iwama, T. and Mishima, Y.,** Postoperative followup of familial polyposis, *Stom. Intestine,* 19, 659, 1984.
54. **Moertel, C. G., Hill, J., and Adson, H. R.,** Management of multiple polyposis of the large bowel, *Cancer,* 28, 160, 1971.
55. **Bussey, H. J. R.,** Result of treatment for familial polyposis: St. Marks' experience, *Dis. Colon Rectum,* 27, 572, 1984.
56. **Schaupp, W. C. and Volpe, P. A.,** Management of diffuse colonic polyposis, *Am. J. Surg.*, 124, 218, 1972.
57. **Harvey, J. C., Quan, S. H., and Stearn, M. W.,** Management of familial polyposis with preservation of the rectum, *Surgery,* 88, 476, 1978.
58. **Gingold, B. S., Jagelman, D. G., and Turnbull, R. B., Jr.,** Surgical management of familial polyposis and Gardner's syndrome, *Am. J. Surg.*, 137, 54, 1979.
59. **Watne, A. H., Carrier, J. M., Durham, J. P., et al.,** The occurrence of carcinoma of the rectum following ileoproctestomy for familial polyposis, *Ann. Surg.*, 197, 550, 1983.
60. **Jarvinen, H. J.,** Time and type of prophylactic surgery for familial adenomatosis coli, *Ann. Surg.*, 202, 93, 1985.
61. **Bussey, H. J. R., DeCosse, J. J., Deschner, E. E., Eyers, A. A., Lesser, M. L., Morson, B. C., Ritchie, S. M., Thomson, J. P. S., and Wadsworth, J.,** A randomized trial of ascorbic acid in polyposis coli, *Cancer,* 50, 1434, 1982.
62. **Nissen, R.,** Berlin surgical society, *Chirung,* 15, 888, 1933.
63. **Ravitch, M. M. and Sabiston, D. C.,** Anal ileostomy with preservation of the sphincter: a proposed operation in patients requiring total colectomy for benign lesions, *Surg. Gynecol. Obstet.*, 84, 1095, 1947.
64. **Devine, J. and Webb, R.,** Resection of the rectal mucosa, colectomy, and anal ileostomy with normal continence, *Surg. Gynecol. Obstet.*, 92, 437, 1951.
65. **Parks, A. G., Nicholls, R. G., and Belliveau,** Proctocolectomy with ileal reservoir and anal anastomosis, *Br. J. Surg.*, 67, 533, 1980.

66. **Utsunomiya, J., Iwama, T., Imajo, M., Matsuo, S., Sawai, S., Yaegashi K., and Hirayama, R.,** Total colectomy, mucosal proctectomy, and ileoanal anastomosis, *Dis. Colon Rectum,* 23, 459, 1980.
67. **Utsunomiya, J. and Iwama, T.,** The J ileal pouch-anal anastomosis: the Japanese experience, *Alternatives to Conventional Ileostomy,* Dozois, R. R., Ed., Year Book Medical Publishers, Chicago, 371, 1987.
68. **Utsunomiya, J., Ohta, M., and Iwama, T.,** Recent trends in ileoanal anastomosis, *Ann. Chir. Gyn.,* 75, 56, 1986.
69. **Metcalf, A. M., Dozois, R., Kelly, K. A., et al.,** Ileal ''J'' pouch-anal anastomosis, *Ann. Surg.,* 202, 735, 1985.
70. **Nicholls, R. J. and Pezim, M. E.,** Restorative proctocolectomy with ileal reservoir for ulcerative colitis and familial adenomatous polyposis: a comparison of three reservoir designs, *Br. J. Surg.,* 72, 470, 1985.
71. **Fonkalsrud, E. W.,** Endorectal ileal pull-through with isoperistaltic ileal reservoir for colitis and polyposis, *Ann. Surg.,* 202, 145, 1985.
72. **Scholtz, D. J., Jr., Coller, D., and Veidenheimer, M. C.,** Ileoanal reservoir for ulcerative colitis and familial polyposis, *Arch. Surg.,* 121, 404, 1986.
73. **Peck, D. A.,** Rectal mucosal replacement, *Ann. Surg.,* 191, 294, 1980.
74. **Grant, D., Cohen, Z., McHuge, S., McLead, R., and Stern, H.,** Restorative proctocolectomy clinical results and manometric findings with long and short rectal cuffs, *Dis. Colon Rectum,* 29, 27, 1986.
75. **Hulten, L.,** The continent ileostomy (Kock's pouch) versus the restorative proctocolectomy (pelvic pouch), *World J. Surg.,* 9, 952, 1985.
76. **Hansen, L. K., Olsen, P. R., and Simonsen, L.,** Total colectomy, mucosal proctectomy, and an ileal reservoir to an anal anastomosis: a comparison of short and long efferent legs, *Scan. J. Gastroenterol.,* 20, 1091, 1985.
77. **Bubrik, M. P., Jacobs, D. M., and Levy, M.,** Experience with the endorectal pull through and S-pouch for ulcerative colitis and familial polyposis in adults, *Surgery,* 98, 689, 1985.
78. **Utsunomiya, J.,** The J-ileal pouch-anal anastomosis, operative technique, in press.
79. **Utsunomiya, J.,** Evolution of technique and result of the J-ileal pouch anal anastomosis, *Dig. Surg.,* in press.
80. **Peutz, J. L. A.,** A very peculiar familial polyposis of the mucous membrane of the digestive tract and the nasopharynx together with peculiar pigmentation of the skin and mucous membranes, *Ned. Maandschr. Geneesk.,* 10, 134, 1921.
81. **Jeghers, H.,** Pigmentation of skin, *N. Eng. J. Med.,* 231, 88, 1944.
82. **Bartholomew, L. G., Dahlin, D. C., and Waugh, J. M.,** Intestinal polyposis associated with mucocutaneous melanin pigmentation (Peutz-Jeghers syndrome), *Gastroenterology,* 30, 434, 1957.
83. **Utsunomiya, J., Gocho, H., Miyanaga, T., Hamaguchi, H., Kashimura, A., and Aoki, N.,** Peutz-Jeghers syndrome, *Johns Hopkins Med. J.* 36, 71, 1975.
84. **Hood, A. B. and Krush, A. J.,** Clinical and dermatologic aspects of the hereditary intestinal polyposes, *Dis. Colon Rectum,* 26, 546, 1983.
85. **Rodu, B. and Martinez, M. G.,** Peutz-Jeghers syndrome and cancer, *Oral Surg.,* 58, 584, 1984.
86. **Pergin, K. and Bridge, M. F.,** Adenomatous and carcinomatous polyps of the small intestine (Peutz-Jeghers syndrome), *Cancer,* 49, 971, 1982.
87. **Miller, L. L., Bartholomew, L. G., Dozois, R. R., and Dahlin, D. C.,** Adenocarcinoma of the rectum arising in a hamartomatous polyp in a patient with Peutz-Jeghers syndrome, *Dig. Dis. Sci.,* 28, 1047, 1983.
88. **Young, R. H., Welch, W. R., Dickersin, R., and Scully, R. E.,** Ovarian sex cord tumor with annular tubules, review of 74 cases including 27 with Peutz-Jeghers syndrome and 4 with adenoma malignant 9th cervix, *Cancer,* 50, 1384, 1982.
89. **Kaku, T., Hachisuga, T., Toyoshima, S., et al.,** Extremely well differentiated adenocarcinoma (''adenoma malignum'') of the cervix in a patient with Peutz-Jeghers syndrome, *Int. J. Gynecol. Pathol.,* 4, 266, 1985.
90. **Trau, H., Schewach-Millet, M., Fisher, B. K., and Tsur, H.,** Peutz-Jeghers syndrome and bilateral breast carcinoma, *Cancer,* 50, 788, 1982.
91. **Ravitch, M. M.,** Polypoid adenomatosis of the entire gastrointestinal tract, *Ann. Surg.,* 128, 283, 1948.
92. **Sachatello, C. R., Pickren, J. M., and Grace, J. T.,** Generalized juvenile gastrointestinal polyposis, *Gastroenterology,* 58, 699, 1970.
93. **Stemper, T. J., Kent, T. H., and Summers, R. W.,** Juvenile polyposis and gastrointestinal carcinoma — a study of a kindred, *Ann. Intern. Med.,* 83, 639, 1975.
94. **Morson, B. C.,** Some peculiarities in the histology of intestinal polyps, *Dis. Colon Rectum,* 5, 337, 1962.
95. **Roth, S. I. and Helwig, E. B.,** Juvenile polyps of the colon and rectum, *Cancer,* 16, 468, 1963.
96. **Goodman, Z. D., Yardley, J. H., and Milligan, F. D.,** Pathogenesis of colonic polyps in multiple juvenile polyposis: report of a case associated with gastric polyps and carcinoma of the rectum, *Cancer,* 43, 1906, 1979.
97. **Kachula, R. O. C.,** Mixed juvenile adenomatous and intermediate polyposis coli, report of a case, *Dis. Colon Rectum,* 14, 368, 1971.

98. **Sawada, T., Muto, T., Kusama, S., et al,** Juvenile polyposis coli in two sibs in a family, *Stom. Intestine,* 13, 411, 1978.
99. **Ichikawa, T. and Utsunomiya, J.,** Two cases of juvenile polyposis coli, *Stom. Intestine,* 17, 1009, 1982.
100. **Schwartz, A. M. and McCauley, R. G. K.,** Juvenile gastrointestinal polyposis, *Radical,* 121, 441, 1976.
101. **Veale, A. M. O., McColl, I., and Bussey, H. J. R.,** Juvenile polyposis coli, *J. Med. Gent.,* 3, 5, 1966.
102. **Bussey, H. J. R.,** personal communication.
103. **Armitage, P. and Doll, R.,** The age distribution of cancer and a multistage theory of carcinogenesis, *Br. J. Cancer,* 8, 1, 1954.
104. **Utsunomiya, J., Iwana, T., Murata, M., and Tanimura, M.,** The hereditary gastrointestinal polyposis and cancer research, *Taishya,* 17, 183, 1980.
105. **Knudson, A. G.,** Genetic and environmental interaction in the origin of human cancer, in *Genetics of Human Cancer,* Mulvihill, J. J., Miller, R. W., and Fraumeni, J. F., Eds., Raven Press, New York, 1977.
106. **Miyaki, M., Akamatsu, N., Sato, C., and Utsunomiya, J.,** Chemical and viral transformation of cultured skin fibroblasts from patient with familial polyposis coli, *Mutat. Res.,* in press.
107. **Kopelovich, L.,** Phenotypic manner in human skin fibroblasts as possible diagnostic indice of hereditary adenomatosis of the colon and rectum. *Cancer,* 39, 2534, 1977.
108. **Herrera, L., Kakati, S., Gibas, L., et al.,** Gardner's syndrome in a man with interstitial deletion of 5q, *Am. J. Med. Genet.,* 25, 473, 1986.
109. **Bodmer, W. F., Bailey, C. J., Bodmer, J., et al.,** Localization of the gene for familial adenomatous polyposis on chromosome 5, *Nature,* 328, 614, 1987.
110. **Solomon, E., Voss, R., Hall, V., et al.,** Chromosome 5 allele loss in human colorectal carcinomas, *Nature,* 328, 616, 1987.
111. **Boman, B. M., Lointier, P., and Wildrick, D. M.,** Chromosome 5 allele loss at the glucocorticoid receptor locus in human colorectal carcinomas, in *Gastrointestinal Cancer: Current Approaches to Diagnosis and Treatment,* University of Texas Press, Austin, in press.

Chapter 16

GENETIC EPIDEMIOLOGY OF COLON CANCER

Henry T. Lynch, Jane F. Lynch, and Giuseppe Cristofaro

TABLE OF CONTENTS

I. INTRODUCTION

Colorectal cancer is second in indicence only to lung cancer in many of the western industrialized nations.[1] Its incidence has shown a steady increase since the turn of the century, a trend which has been attributed by some to changes in dietary patterns.[2] While environmental factors are of unquestionable significance in the etiology of colorectal cancer, the role of genetic factors, as in all forms of human diseases, must be considered. Unfortunately, in the case of colorectal cancer, with the exception of familial multiple adenomatous polyposis coli (FPC), the importance of genetics has been severely neglected. Recently, this entire subject has been extensively reviewed.[3-5]

Colon cancer survival has not improved in the last 2 decades.[6] A major problem is its early detection. Surveillance programs that focus on high risk groups would logically show a higher cancer yield and thereby become more cost-effective. Identification of high risk groups, of which genetics is of particular importance, should therefore become a high priority to our national cancer effort.[3,6]

II. GEOGRAPHIC VARIATION IN INCIDENCE

Cancer of the colon shows marked geographic variation throughout the world. It is particularly common in North America, the U.K., Australia, New Zealand, and other industrialized countries, and contrastingly, it occurs infrequently in countries such as India, Colombia, and Senegal, areas noteworthy for being economically poorly developed. For example, there is a 50-fold variation in the frequency of cancer of the colon between Connecticut (32.3 per 100,000) and Dakar in Senegal, West Africa (0.6 per 100,000). These remarkable differences in incidence have been attributable in a major way to dietary factors, wherein there are characteristic highly refined diets comprised of high animal fat and low fiber in the high colon cancer incidence industrialized nations. In those less affluent areas of the world where colon cancer is infrequent, diets are low in animal fat and protein but are rich in fiber.[7]

In spite of these striking contrasts in environmental exposures, one must be cognizant of the fact that only a relatively small fraction of individuals exposed to the affluent, highly refined, western low fiber-high animal fat diet develop colon cancer. The obvious question is ''What *predisposes* some individuals to colorectal cancer and, contrariwise, what *protects* others, similarly exposed, from developing colorectal cancer?'' We believe that primary genetic factors are an important etiologic parameter which significantly modulate the deleterious carcinogenic environmental mileu and thereby partially explain the differences in susceptibility to colorectal cancer throughout the world.[3]

III. PRECANCER LESIONS OF THE GASTROINTESTINAL TRACT

The etiology of any form of cancer must necessarily be viewed in the context of a multifactorial cascade of events. As in the case of breast cancer (Chapter 18), this would embrace diet, socioeconomic status and geographical background, hormonal and endocrine factors, medications of all varieties, ionizing radiation, and a plethora of other environmental carcinogenic exposures, all within the context of host (genetic) factors. While we remain ignorant about the precise causal events in cancer, it is clear that malignant transformation is a multistep process which involves an *initiation* event which may occur as long as 3 decades prior to the detection of the primary tumor mass, *promotional* events which precede phenotypic transformation, the *transformation* event per se, wherein cells manifest typical histologic and biologic features of cancer, and finally, both early and late *progression* events wherein local tumor spread and widespread metastases are evidenced.

When considering cancers of the GI tract (or for that matter, any other organ system), it is helpful for the cancer geneticist and cancer epidemiologist to be cognizant of precancerous lesions and their histological classification. In the case of the colon, as will be seen shortly, the adenomatous polyp becomes the hallmark example of a precancerous lesion. We define a precancerous lesion as a histpathological aberration of tissue wherein a malignant neoplastic lesion is more likely to become manifested as opposed to its apparently normal histological counterpart. The use of the term precancer does not imply that ultimate cancer occurrence is mandatory. What we are stating is that a precancerous lesion has an increased probability for undergoing a malignant neoplastic change.

In the typical precancer setting, we see an epithelial alteration which is consonant with what is referred to as "dysplasia". In this particular context, the reason for malignant neoplastic transformation depends upon the grade or severity of the dysplasia. Problems which obfuscate the diagnosis of dysplasia are concerned with the distinction between regenerative, inflammatory, and reactive changes as well as the separation between severe dysplasia and so-called early invasive carcinoma. Another problem pertains to the histologic recognition of dysplasia and its clinical significance wherein there is often limited knowledge relevant to the statistical risk which the dysplastic lesion has for ultimate progression to carcinoma in any individual patient.

With respect to the GI tract, certain precancerous lesions have been clearly identified as follows:

1. Oral cavity — leukoplakia, dysplasia
2. Esophagus — Barrett's esophagus, chronic esophagitis, dysplasia, and carcinoma *in situ*
3. Stomach — intestinal metaplasia, dysplasia, hyperplastic polyps, gastric ulcer, adenoma, chronic atrophic gastritis, and dysplasia in Menetrier's disease
4. Duodenum and small intestine — dysplasia as in Peutz-Jegher's polyps, dysplasia in Crohn's disease, and adenomas
5. Appendix — adenomas
6. Colorectum — adenomas, juvenile polyps with dysplasia, hyperplastic or metaplastic polyps with dysplasia, dysplasia in Crohn's disease and in ulcerative colitis, as well as dysplasia in *Schistosomiasis japonica,* transitional mucosa, lesions which simulate dysplasia, and finally, dysplasia following ureterosigmoidostomy
7. Anal canal — dysplasia in leukoplakia and in carcinoma *in situ*
8. Anal margin — condyloma acuminatum, Bowden's disease, Paget's disease, and dysplasia

IV. CLASSIFICATION OF HEREDITARY COLORECTAL CANCER

We have operationally classified hereditary colonic cancer into four major categories:[3] (1) multiple polyposis coli syndromes (FPC), (2) hereditary *non*polyposis colorectal cancer syndromes (HNPCC), (3) familial inflammatory bowel disease syndromes (IBD), and (4) miscellaneous hereditary cancer aggregations and/or syndromes, of which isolated (common) hereditary adenomatous polyp is the latest member.[8]

We shall survey problems in colon cancer genetics and focus our major attention on hereditary *non*polyposis colorectal cancer syndromes (HNPCC), also referred to as Lynch syndromes I and II.[9]

As seen in Figure 1, HNPCC constitutes at least 5 to 6% of all occurrences of colorectal cancer, as opposed to approximately 1% or less in the case of FPC. In spite of the disparity in frequency between FPC and HNPCC, the bulk of research to date has been devoted to FPC. Part of this disproportionate effort is due to the relatively recent identification of the significance of HNPCC.

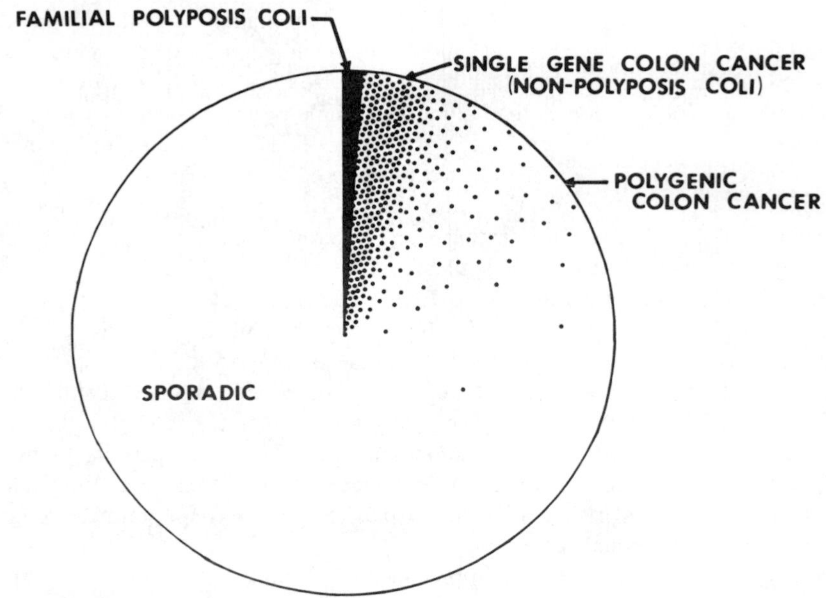

FIGURE 1. Distribution of hereditary colon cancer and heterogeneity. (From Lynch, H. T., Rozen, P., and Schuelke, G. S., *Cancer*, 35, 95, 1985. With permission.)

The full impact of primary genetic factors in the etiology of colorectal cancer remains enigmatic. Only a paucity of investigations have been directed toward the interactions between environment and genetic factors in its etiology.[3]

V. FREQUENCY OF GENETIC FACTORS IN COLORECTAL CANCER BURDEN

Primary genetic factors are estimated to account for between 5 to 10% of the total cancer burden. By this, we mean that Mendelian inheritance patterns will be observed and that cancer expression within *hereditary* cancer-prone kindreds will be highly predictable. Given the estmate of 985,000 (495,000 male, 490,000 female) new incident cancers (all sites) in the U.S. based on rates from the NCI SEER program[10] between 44,750 and 98,500 patients can be expected to have hereditary cancer this year. Each of these patients will therefore represent a family which will be inordinately predisposed to cancer. In the case of cancer of the colorectum, 147,000 patients will manifest this disease in 1988, of which approximately 10% (14,700 patients) will have an etiology attributable to primary genetic factors.[3] An additional 15 to 20% (22,050 to 29,400) of colorectal cancer-affected individuals will have one or more affected primary or secondary relatives but otherwise lack criteria to fit the hereditary category.[3] These individuals will fit our operational definition of *familial colonic cancer*.

VI. FAMILIAL MULTIPLE ADENOMATOUS POLYPOSIS COLI

Probably no genetic disorder of the colon has been more extensively investigated than familial polyposis coli (FPC). For recent reviews of this subject, please refer to Lynch and Lynch[3] and Lynch et al.[5]

Historically, interest in the heritability of colon cancer was focused primarily on FPC.[3] In 1882, Cripps provided the first description of familial multiple adenomatous polyposis coli; its cancer association was established in 1890 by Handford. More than a quarter of a century later (1925), the St. Mark's group under the direction of Lockhart-Mummery established the first registry of FPC families — a registry that has been expanded by his successors until the present time. These pioneering efforts yielded significant etiologic insights. They also showed that this disease could be controlled through knowledge of its natural history and genetics, and through prophylactic colectomy in persons manifesting the phenotype (colonic polyposis). The necessity of vigilant programs for case detection and surveillance was demonstrated early on. Because of its premonitory cancer sign (multiple colonic polyps), FPC remains the undisputed model for colon cancer genetic investigations. However, as already alluded to, HNPCC poses a more significant public health problem.

As knowledge accrued, it became apparent that FPC was not the simple disease it was originally thought to be. A major breakthrough was made by Gardner in the early 1950s when he recognized the significance of extracolonic signs in FPC. Initially considered a distinct entity, Gardner's syndrome and perhaps even the polyposis-glioma complex (Turcot's syndrome), have come to be considered by many to be a continuous phenotypic expression of the FPC gene. The present controversy shows no sign of early resolution.[3]

VII. A NEW CLINICAL SIGN IN GARDNER'S SYNDROME: CHRPE

Traboulsi et al.[11] studied 134 members of 16 families with Gardner's syndrome (GS) for congenital hypertrophy of the retinal pigment epithelium (CHRPE). They observed that 41 of these patients had documented findings of GS of whom 37 (90.2%) had CHRPE. These lesions were found to be bilateral in 32 (78.1%) and 2 of 42 controls (4.8%). Among 43 first degree relatives at 50% risk, a bimodal distribution for presence of bilateral CHRPE was observed, consonant with the autosomal dominant mode of inheritance of GS. The authors concluded that ". . . the presence of bilateral lesions, multiple lesions (more than 4), or both appeared to be a specific (specificity 0.952) and sensitive (sensitivity 0.780) clinical marker for Gardner's syndrome."

CHRPE is most probably congenital, as had also been inferred by Blair and Trempe[12] and Lewis et al.[13] who made the original descriptions of CHRPE in GS, and confirmed by Traboulsi et al.[11] who observed CHRPE in a 3-month-old baby at risk. As mentioned, Traboulsi et al. found retinal lesions in at least 1 member from each of the 16 families with GS which they examined, as opposed to only 3 of the 7 GS families examined by Lewis et al.,[13] leading to the assumption that one should not consider any family with documented GS as failing to show CHRPE until a sufficiently large number of affected and at-risk individuals have been evaluated. Variable expressivity of this and other traits in autosomal dominantly inherited diseases must be expected to occur and this may well explain the different numbers and sizes of the lesions within and between families. Importantly, the absence of CHRPE should not be used to conclusively infer the absence of the disease (Gardner's syndrome), and thereby such individuals should still remain under colonic surveillance in accord with recommended protocols.

Traboulsi and Maumenee[14] studied two families with Peutz-Jegher's syndrome and did not observe these ocular lesions. Lynch et al,[16] wondered about the possibility of CHRPE being present in patients manifesting FPC in the absence of Gardner's stigmata. We therefore performed ophthalmologic examinations on two FPC families with complete absence of Gardner's osseous or cutaneous stigmata. All four of the patients from these two families with FPC have shown the CHRPE phenotype, an example of which is depicted in Figure 2. This should now be investigated in other FPC kindreds as well as in HNPCC families.[17] Such research could aid in the clarification of the nosology of hereditary colon cancer wherein heterogeneity has been found to be extant.[18-21]

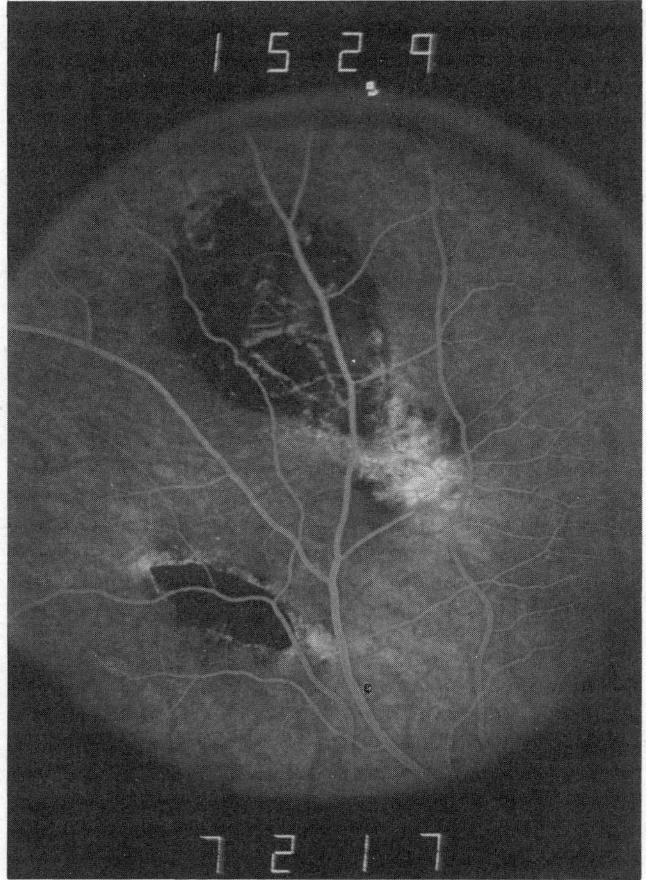

FIGURE 2. Congenital hypertrophy of the retinal pigment epithelium (CHRPE) seen in members of families with familial polyposis coli.

VIII. EXTRACOLONIC CANCER IN FPC

A variety of extracolonic cancers have been described in patients with FPC. These were originally thought to be linked primarily with so-called Gardner's syndrome variant wherein the predominant tumors have included desmoids, sarcomas, brain tumors, and tumors of the small bowel and stomach. However, extracolonic tumors have been found in kindreds with FPC which did not show the osseous and cutaneous stigmata of Gardner's syndrome.[3-6]

Li et al.[22] have recently reported hepatoblastoma in four unrelated children with positive family histories of FPC. In their review of the literature, they noted the same association in ten other FPC kindreds. We have recently encountered an FPC kindred wherein a 2-year-old child manifested hepatoblastoma. CHRPE was found in our kindred, and this was also reported in the patients studied by Li et al.[22]

The classification of patients with FPC in terms of whether they fit Gardner's syndrome, Turcot's syndrome, or FPC without extracolonic findings (in which there might be a variety of subcategories), will require elucidation of their underlying molecular biology. Linkage analyses and cytogenetic investigations thus far have not been informative,[23,24] although promise for resolution of these issues may be nearing (Ray White Ph.D., personal communication, 1987). A recent report of chromosome 11p13 deletion in hepatoblastoma[25] may hold clues in that this region of the genome might also predispose to FPC. Finally, Bodmer et al.[26] and Solomon et al.[27] have provided data purporting that the gene for FPC is located on chromosome 5, most probably near bands 5q21-q22. Their research was aided by a case report of an interstitial deletion of chromosome 5 in a mentally retarded individual with multiple developmental abnormalities in context with FPC. Solomon et al.[27] examined sporadic colorectal adenocarcinomas in the search for loss of alleles on chromosome 5. They used a highly polymorphic "minisatellite" probe which maps to chromosome 5q. They found that ". . . at least 20% of this highly heterogeneous set of tumors lose one of the alleles present in matched normal tissue. This parallels the assignment of the FAP (same designation for FPC) gene to chromosome 5. . . and suggests that becoming recessive for this gene may be a critical step in the progression of a relatively high proportion of colorectal cancers."

We are currently involved in similar investigations on patients with hereditary nonpolyposis colorectal cancer (HNPCC) and will include particular attention to a search of chromosomme 5 and the area of bands 5q21-q22.

IX. HEREDITARY DISCRETE (COMMON) COLONIC POLYPS AND CANCER

Burt et al.[8] have recently studied a large Utah kindred containing over 5000 members who manifested common or discrete colorectal polyps and colonic cancer. While there were multiple cases of common colorectal cancer in this family, the inheritance pattern was not recognizable. However, following systematic screening for colonic polyps in members of the pedigree, and using spouse controls, an autosomal dominant inheritance pattern with respect to both colonic polyps and cancer was identified. A feature of keen interest in this huge pedigree was the fact that colon cancer was typical of the common variety which appears in the general population relevant to its age at onset and general site distribution within the colorectum. Cancer of extracolonic sites did not occur in excess in this family. These investigators suggested that hereditary factors, possibly in interaction with environmental factors, may account for a much larger proportion of colorectal cancers in the general population. Thus, many past examples thought to have represented familial occurrences of colonic cancer, wherein specific patterns of inheritance were not readily apparent, may in fact represent families showing hereditary transmission of colonic cancer similar to this huge Utah pedigree. These authors therefore suggested that common or discrete adenomatous polyps are inherited and that they comprise a vital component of these colon cancer-prone pedigrees.

This study is exceedingly important because of the increasing risk for development of adenomatous polyps in association with increasing age, and the known relationship between adenomatous polyps and carcinoma of the colon, namely, the so-called "adenoma-polyp-cancer sequence". One therefore wonders about the role of environmental effects on polyp development and/or cancer in this disorder. To date, there is no evidence for the frequency of hereditary discrete (common) polyposis coli. This disorder could pose a problem of immense concern to the understanding of the genetic epidemiology of cancer.

X. HEREDITARY NONPOLYPOSIS COLORECTAL CANCER (HNPCC)

The HNPCC syndromes may be further divided into two subcategories: (1) Lynch syndrome I — hereditary site-specific nonpolyposis colonic cancer and (2) Lynch syndrome II — HNPCC in association with *other* forms of cancer, particularly endometrial and ovarian carcinoma. This has also been termed the cancer family syndrome (CFS). In both of the hereditary nonpolyposis colorectal cancer syndromes, there is *proximal* predominance of nonpolyposis colonic cancer (making sigmoidoscopy an ineffective screening tool), vertical transmission, early age at cancer onset, an excess of multiple primary cancer, and significantly improved survival when compared stage for stage with the American College of Surgeons Audit Series.[28] In Lynch syndrome I, the multiple primary cancers are restricted to colonic mucosa, and herein, about one third will involve the distal colon inclusive of the rectum. In Lynch syndrome II, cancers will involve the entire colon, including the rectum, as in the former category, but *other* anatomic sites can be involved, including the endometrium and ovaries.[3,28]

XI. NATURAL HISTORY OF COLORECTAL CANCER IN HNPCC

We investigated colorectal cancer expression from a survey of ten extended HNPCC kindreds. Colorectal cancer affected members of these kindreds were found to differ significantly ($p < 0.05$) from sporadic colorectal cancer patients with respect to several parameters. Specifically, the mean age of colon cancer diagnosis was 44.6 years. Of initial colon cancers, 72% were located in the right colon; 18% had synchronous colon cancer, while 24% developed metachronous colon cancer. The actuarial risk for metachronous colon cancer over a 10-year period from initial colon cancer was found to be 40%. These facets of the natural history of HNPCC have been employed for us in our surveillance/management recommendations. Specifically, we recommend that affecteds and their first degree relatives should undergo early, intensive education and surveillance, with baseline colonoscopy by age 25 and biannually thereafter, and Hemoccult testing of the stool semiannually. Concurrently, women should have endometrial aspiration biopsies (office procedure) instituted at age 25 and annually thereafter. Patients presenting with initial colon cancer require subtotal colectomy as opposed to a more limited resection since the remaining colonic mucosa will be inordinately predisposed to malignant transformation. Women presenting with initial colon cancer should be considered as candidates for prophylactic total hysterectomy and bilateral salpingo oophorectomy, with due consideration to their psychological status and whether or not they have completed their families.

Figure 3 depicts an example of a hereditary site-specific nonpolyposis colonic cancer pedigree (Lynch syndrome I), while Figure 4 shows a pedigree with CFS findings (Lynch syndrome II).

XII. CLINICAL EXAMPLES OF GHENETIC HETEROGENEITY IN HNPCC

A kindred has recently been described (Figure 5, F-673) with vertical transmission of cancer through five generations which showed features of Lynch syndrome II in concert with pancreatic cancer.[29] The proband was a 55-year-old white male with verified pancreatic cancer. Interestingly, as seen in the figure, all of the family members manifesting colon cancer showed proximal location in the colon, and none had evidence of multiple adenomatous polyposis coli by history or pathological verification (III-3, III-5, III-6, III-8, IV-3, IV-5). There was early age of onset of colorectal cancer (mean 52 years, $n = 6$), although the number of affected individuals was not large enough for assessment of statistical significance. Adenocarcinoma of the pancreas was identified in three genetically informative relatives (II-2, III-7, IV-2). Multiple primary cancers occurred in the proband's mother and in the proband's maternal uncle (III-3, III-5) in this remarkable kindred.

Genetic heterogeneity with respect to variation in tumor spectrum has become increasingly more evident in Lynch syndrome II.[30] The etiologic significance of pancreatic carcinoma in Lynch syndrome II kindreds remains enigmatic. There are several possible explanations

1. Occurrence in this particular family may be fortuitous.
2. Pancreatic carcinoma may be integral to the Lynch syndrome II genotype, but heretofore, it may have been underreported because of incomplete pathology documentation of patients with intraabdominal cancer.
3. Due to extant heterogeneity, Lynch syndrome II may be attributable to a different allele at the same locus in a manner consonant with other hereditary colon cancer syndromes which also may be associated with pancreatic carcinoma, such as FPC and Gardner's syndrome.[29]
4. Pancreatic cancer may be a pleiotropic manifestation of the Lynch syndrome II cancer-prone genotype which is being expressed as a result of temporal changes in environmental exposures perturbing this deleterious genotype.

An interesting finding in this kindred was that of neuroblastoma (Figure 5, V-2) in a patient at age 22. This lesion is more characteristic of childhood and its occurrence in this patient is puzzling. While this could be fortuitous, it is also possible that it represents a pleiotropic manifestation of the Lynch syndrome II genotype. For example, Sorensen et al.[31] reported a familial aggregation of adult onset GI tract tumors, including carcinoma of the colon. Four members of that particular family manifested childhood cancer; two were neuroblastomas, one was bilateral retinoblastoma, and one was an unconfirmed brain tumor. Love[32] has described a kindred with features of Lynch syndrome II but which showed certain rare cancers which have not ordinarily been associated with this syndrome. Specifically, in addition to the typical tumor presentations of Lynch syundrome II, patients in the direct genetic lineage also manifested small bowel cancers and B-cell lymphatic leukemia. One patient in this family manifested six primary cancers; the first, a cystadenocarcinoma of the ovary, was diagnosed at age 32 years. She was subsequently diagnosed with adenocarcinoma of the colon (splenic flexure) at age 35, mucinous adenocarcinoma of the colon (hepatic flexure) at age 45, two primary adenocarcinomas of the rectum at age 54, and an infiltrating ductal carcinoma of the breast at age 63. She had evidence of metastases, namely, a hepatic nodule found to be an adenocarcinoma, over the years, yet at the time of Love's publication, she was 64 years of age, in good health, and without clinical evidence of cancer.

Budd and Fink[33] described a black American kindred with features consistent with Lynch syndrome II. Of particular interest was the finding of mucoid colon adenocarcinoma in 7 of 14 patients with colonic cancer.

We have reported a unique Navajo Indian HNPCC kindred (Figure 6) that manifested a tumor pattern at some variance with Lynch syndromes I and II.[34] Pathologic study was unable to determine whether the proband's initial cancer originated in the ovary or in the endometrium. So far as we have been able to determine, this represents the first description of HNPCC among American Indians. Although nonpolyposis colorectal cancer is relatively rare in this American Indian population, its occurrence in this family is consonant with a significant cancer-prone genotype that may be expressed in an otherwise low environmental carcinogenic milieu. Longitudinal study of this family will be required for classification of this hereditary cancer syndrome.

XIII. MUIR-TORRE CUTANEOUS SIGNS IN HNPCC

Muir-Torre syndrome (MT) is characterized by the occurrence of sebaceous hyperplasia, adenoma and carcinoma, basal cell carcinoma with sebaceous differentiation, and/or keratoacanthoma in association with visceral cancer (often multiple), and improved survival. Family studies of MT have been either wholly lacking or too incomplete to elucidate hereditary etiology.

We initially proposed that MT was integral to Lynch syndrome II.[35] More recently, we

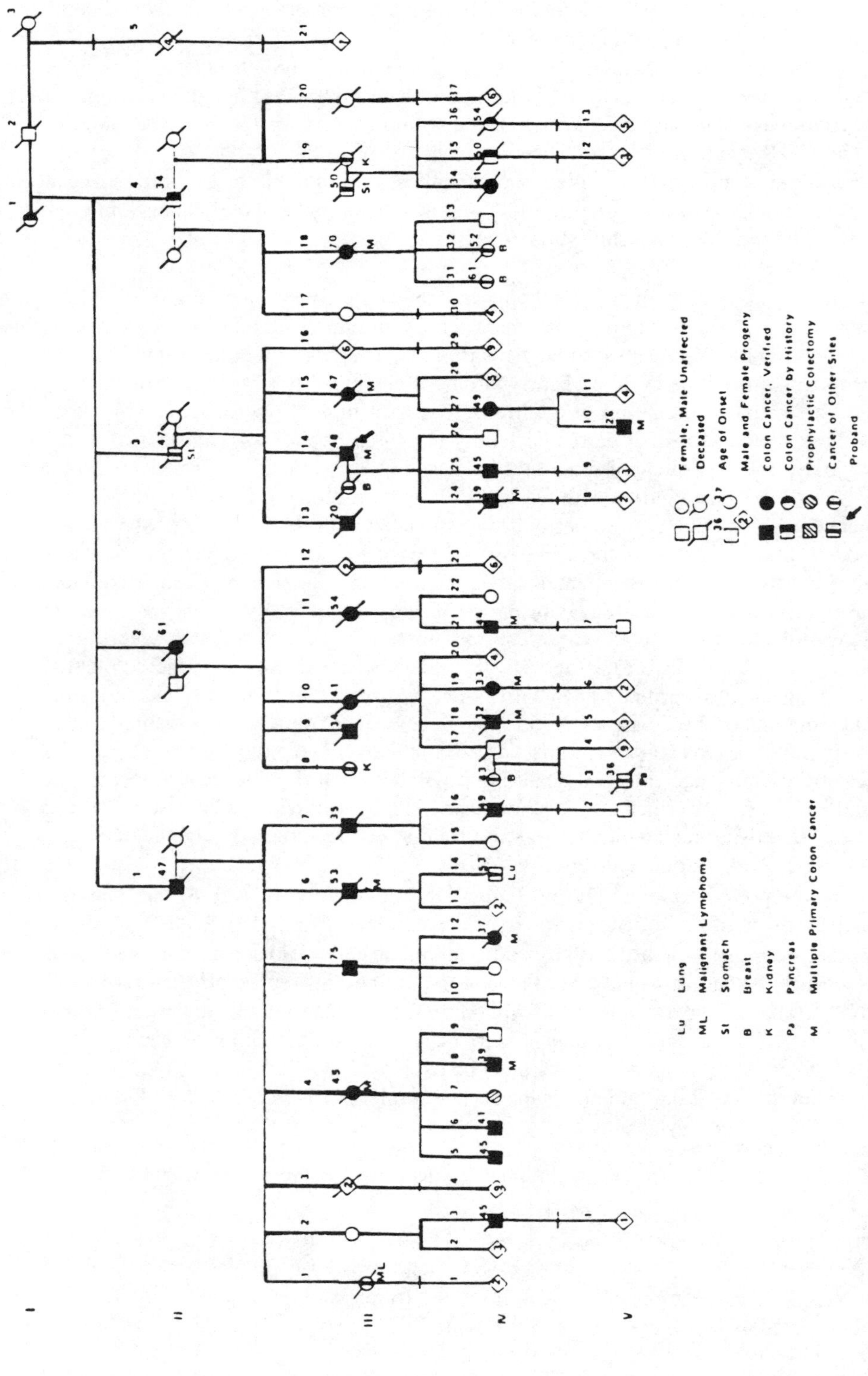

FIGURE 3. Pedigree of a family with site-specific colon cancer (Lynch syndrome I). (Modified from Lynch, H. T. et al., *Arch. Surg.* 112, 170, 1977.)

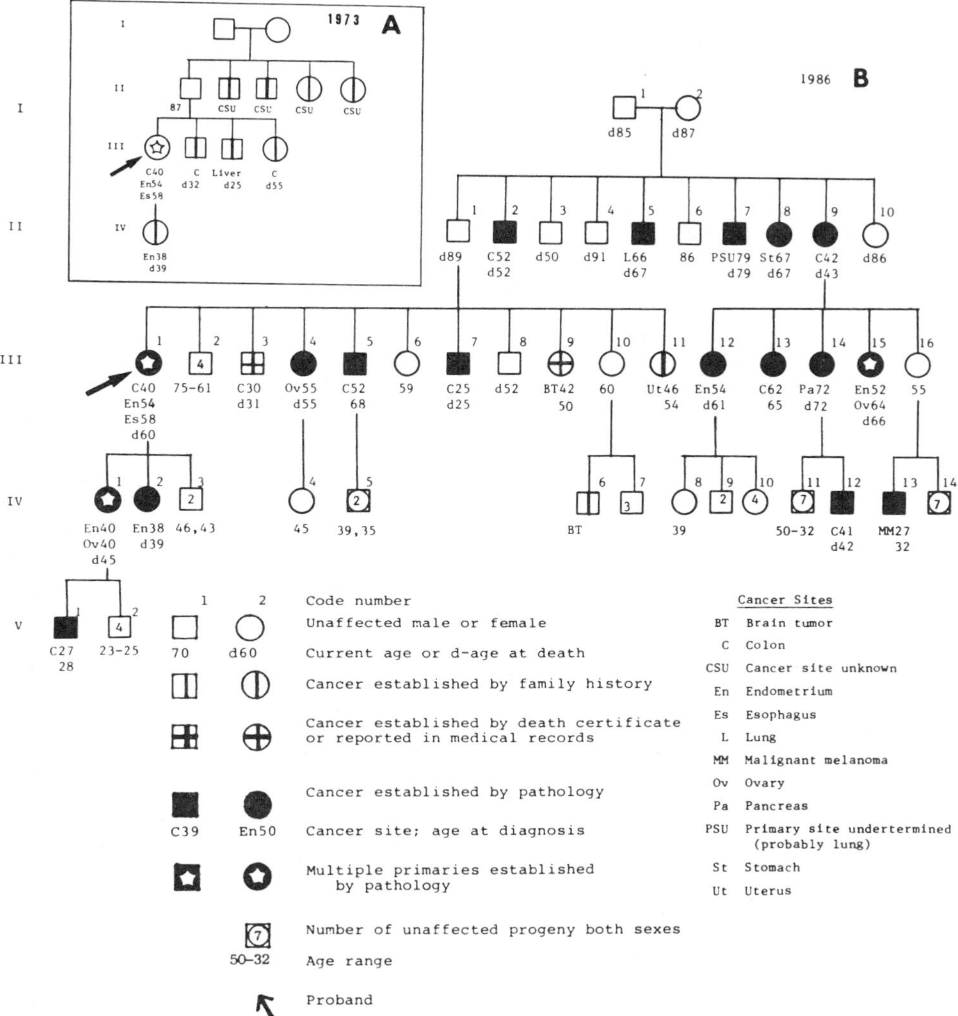

FIGURE 4. Pedigree of a family with the Cancer Family Syndrome (Lynch syndrome II). Inset A shows the preliminary pedigree as obtained in 1973 and inset B as it appeared in 1986. Note the occurrence of endometrial and ovarian carcinomas in addition to colon cancer. (From Lynch, H. T. et al., *Dis. Colon Rectum,* 30, 243, 1987. With permission.)

described the cutaneous phenotype of MT in an extended kindred with a possible variant of Lynch syndrome II (Figure 7, Table 1).[36] We emphasize the need for more thorough documentation of family histories and cancer association in this cancer-associated genodermatosis in order to clarify hereditary syndrome identification, and to improve cancer control through employment of cutaneous signs as a beacon for highly targeted forms of visceral cancer.

XIV. HISTOPATHOLOGIC FEATURES OF COLONIC MUCOSA IN HNPCC

Although the origins of colon carcinoma are complex and multifactorial, relevant histologic observations are known for some specific clinicopathologic settings. Adenomatous epithelial changes, especially those occurring in polypoid configurations of larger size, have long been

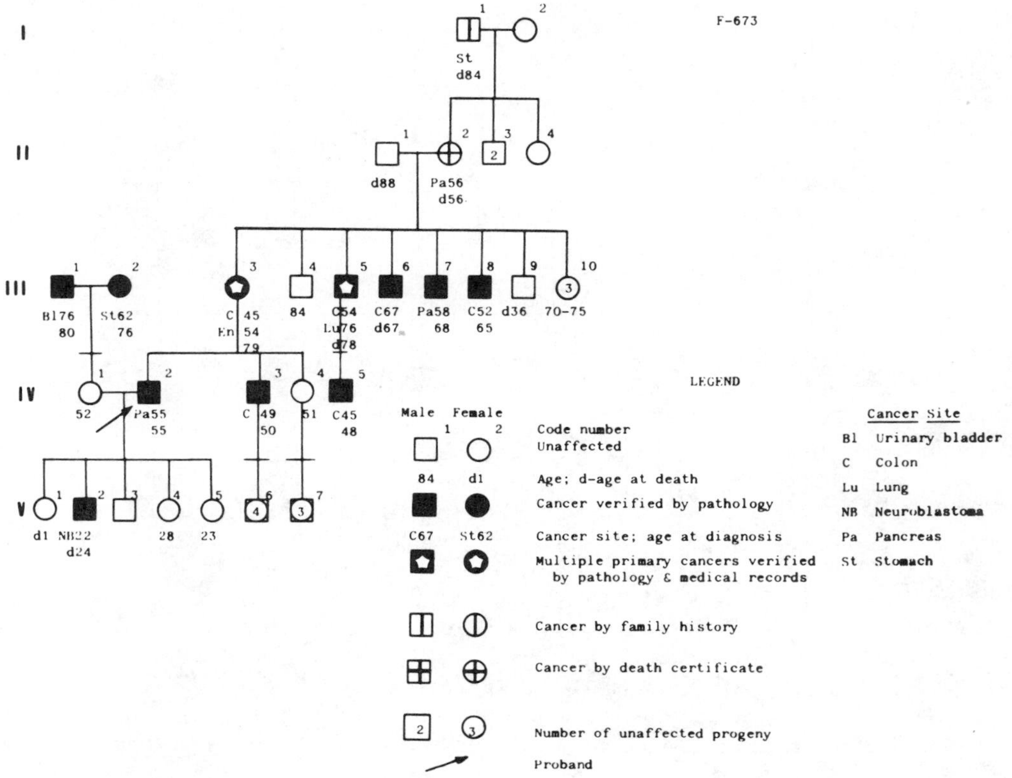

FIGURE 5. A kindred showing clinicopathologic features of hereditary nonpolyposis colorectal cancer in association with carcinoma of the pancreas. (From Lynch, H. T., Voorhees, G. J., Lanspa, S. J., McGreevy, P. S., and Lynch, J. F., *Br. J. Cancer*, 52, 71, 1985. With permission.)

implicated in the genesis of colon carcinoma. Although this relationship is known, the factors that stimulate, promote, permit, or precede the growth of this adenomatous epithelium are most likely a complex interaction of genetic as well as environmental factors.[37] The spectrum of atypical epithelial changes or dysplasia in these lesions encompasses a continuum, from benign to clearly malignant, even within the same lesion.

Dysplastic changes in colonic mucosa, and their structural and cytologic features, have been studied in greatest detail with inflammatory bowel disease.[38] Once again, a spectrum of changes occurs, from benign to malignant to indefinite, and not infrequently, these changes occur in flat, nonpolypoid mucosa.

Lynch syndromes I and II, as emphasized throughout this chapter, are associated with hereditary colon cancer, unassociated with adenomatous polyps.[9] A systematic, prospective evaluation has never been previously attempted on consecutively ascertained individuals from HNPCC kindreds whose colon carcinomas apparently do not fall into the ademona-carcinoma sequence, although we speculate that they may show dysplasia-carcinoma (in flat mucosa) sequences. The total absence of data in this regard necessitates a multidisciplinary approach. Through employment of colonoscopy, observations of the gross appearance of the mucosa can be made in order to document the presence or absence of polyps or other subtler mucosal variations. The microscopic evaluation will document the presence or absence of the known types of premalignant (adenomatous, dysplastic) changes while assessing for other epithelial or stromal alterations. In this regard, histochemical differential stains for epithelial mucins can be used to compare HNPCC patients with high risk groups studied

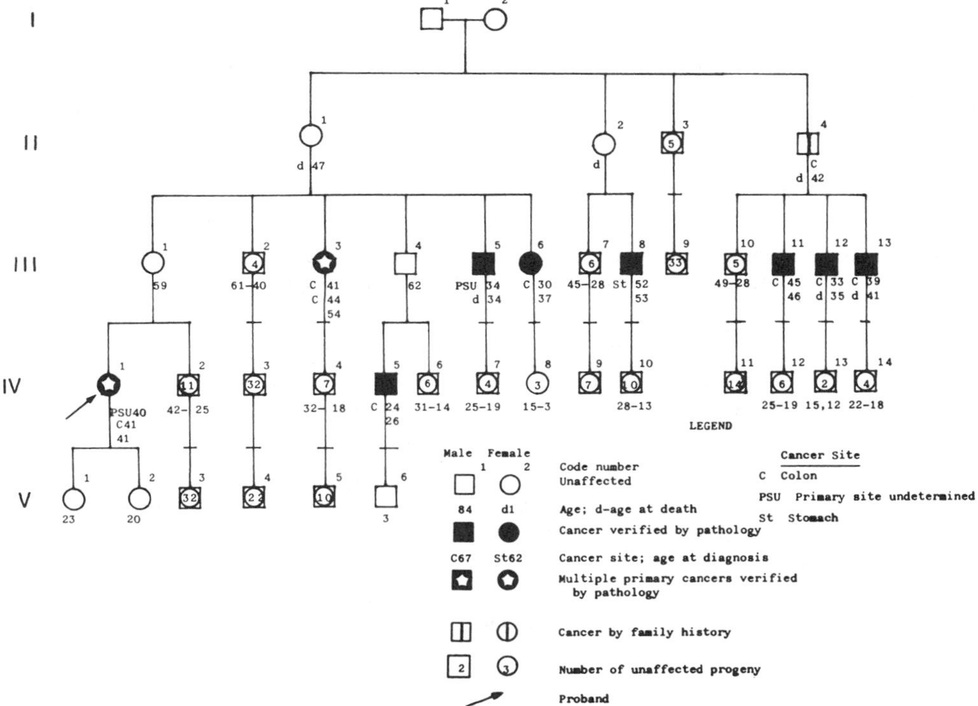

FIGURE 6. HNPCC, Navajo Indian family pedigree. (From Lynch, H. T., Drouhard, T. J., Schuelke, G. S., Biscone, K. A., Lynch, J. F., and Danes, B. S., *Cancer Genet. Cytogenet.*, 15, 209, 1985. With permission.)

using similar techniques.[39-41] Through the statistical analysis of these various parameters, delineation of the transitional or premalignant colonic mucosal changes in these patients may be possible.

Cristofaro et al.[42] have reported new phenotypic findings in a large extended kindred with Lynch syndrome II (Figure 8 and Table 2). These findings were based on meticulous attention to pathology aspects of the GI tract in affected and high genetic risk patients from this informative kindred.

The features which characterize Lynch syndrome II, namely, an excess of early onset nonpolyposis colorectal cancer with proximal predominance, endometrial cancer and other adenocarcinomas, multiple primary cancers, and vertical transmission consonant with an autosomal dominant factor, characterized this family. However, this study also revealed an excess of gastric carcinoma, complete intestinal metaplasia, and chronic atrophic gastritis restricted to the antrum, an apparent excess of colonic mucosal macrophagia, which by special stain appeared to be positive for mucin with a constant content of both sialo and sulfomucin, a lack of iron, and an inconstant positivity for lysosyme obtained by immunoperoxidase technique, and findings of crypt atrophy of the colonic mucosa.

These findings of complete intestinal metaplasia are consonant with their known association with chronic atrophic gastritis (CAG). This is pertinent in this kindred in light of the precancerous facets of this pathology. It is therefore of interest that Correa's[43] epidemiologic classification of CAG includes three major divisions: autoimmune, hypersecretory, and environmental. We considered our data to be sufficient to exclude an autoimmune cause, leaving the other two classifications as primary considerations. We favor the hypersecretory etiology as being more likely in this kindred.

Very little is known about the colonic mucosa in HNPCC. Thus, the findings of colonic mucosal macrophage excess and crypt atrophy (Figures 9a to c) are important preliminary observations, the significance of which remains enigmatic. We hypothosize that the crypt atrophy may induce a feedback proliferative mechanism. Thus, instead of rebuilding the crypt, an anomalous stimulus may invoke malignant transformation in a manner which may be comparable to the phenomenon which is linked to carcinoids in the stomach, concurrent with atropic gastritis in association with hypergastonemia.

It is important to note that macrophages containing mucoproteins are rarely recognizable in the lamina propia of the colon. While they have been observed occasionally in normal biopsy specimens, they are found more commonly in association with mucosal damage produced by prior inflammatory processes. The findings in our patients showed the macrophages to be scattered throughout the lamina propia (Figure 9b). They were not limited to the muscularis mucosa. We postulate that the atrophy may be an epiphenomenon and thereby may represent part of the poorly clarified damage source of crypt epithelium, a phenomenon which may be confirmed by an increasing number of macrophages, which in their role as "scavenger cells" may be attempting to digest the mucinous material being dispersed in the lamina propia. In turn, the atrophy may stimulate the epithelial proliferative mechanism, leading to reconstruction of the disturbed crypts. It may therefore follow that ". . . an abnormality might be present in both the immunologic and control mechanism of the proliferative process for this genetically predetermined condition, so that stimulation of the regenerative mechansim can more readily flow into the neoplastic growth pathway." It logically follows that it will now be necessary to verify these pathology observations in additional members of this family as well as in affected and at-risk members of other families since these observations harbor important implications for elucidation of etiology and carcinogenesis. Indeed, they may eventually provide the basis for a marker for prediction of cancer in either the hereditary or sporadic settings. In order to accomplish these objectives, it will be important to characterize all potentially important environmental factors which may be impacting upon host factors in a genetic-epidemiologic approach toward elucidation of this newly described pathology phenotype in Lynch syndrome II.

XV. MUCOID COLON CANCER

Mecklin et al.[44] studied the histologic characteristics of carcinomas and adenomatous polyps in 75 colorectal carcinoma patients (100 separate cancers) with HNPCC. Their comparison group comprised patients with colorectal cancer who lacked a hereditary background. In the HNPCC group, there were significantly more mucinous carcinomas (35 to 39% vs. 20%; $p < 0.05$ to 0.01) and, in addition, more poorly differentiated tumors (24 vs. 12%) as opposed to the control group. Of interest was the fact that these differences were not explicable by either site or stage of the tumors, nor by age or sex of the patients. Adenomas occurred quite often in the HNPCC patients (19%) as well as in the controls (16%). In the HNPCC patients, more adenomas with moderate or severe dysplasia ($p <$ 0.01) and more adenomas with villous features ($p < 0.05$) were observed when compared to the control group. A finding of keen significance was ". . . Mucinous histologic features in colorectal carcinoma, although not fully specific, might be characteristic of cancer family syndrome, and thus serve as one sign in the identification of the syndrome. The presence of the adenoma-carcinoma sequence in cancer family syndrome was also supported, and the histologic aggressivity of the associated adenomas might signify an accelerated advancement of this phenomenon in cancer family syndrome." We are currently investigating all of these aspects of colorectal cancer and polyp histology in our extensive HNPCC resource. Preliminarily, we have also found an excess of mucinous carcinomas, and noteworthy, we have found these to aggregate significantly in selected HNPCC kindreds.

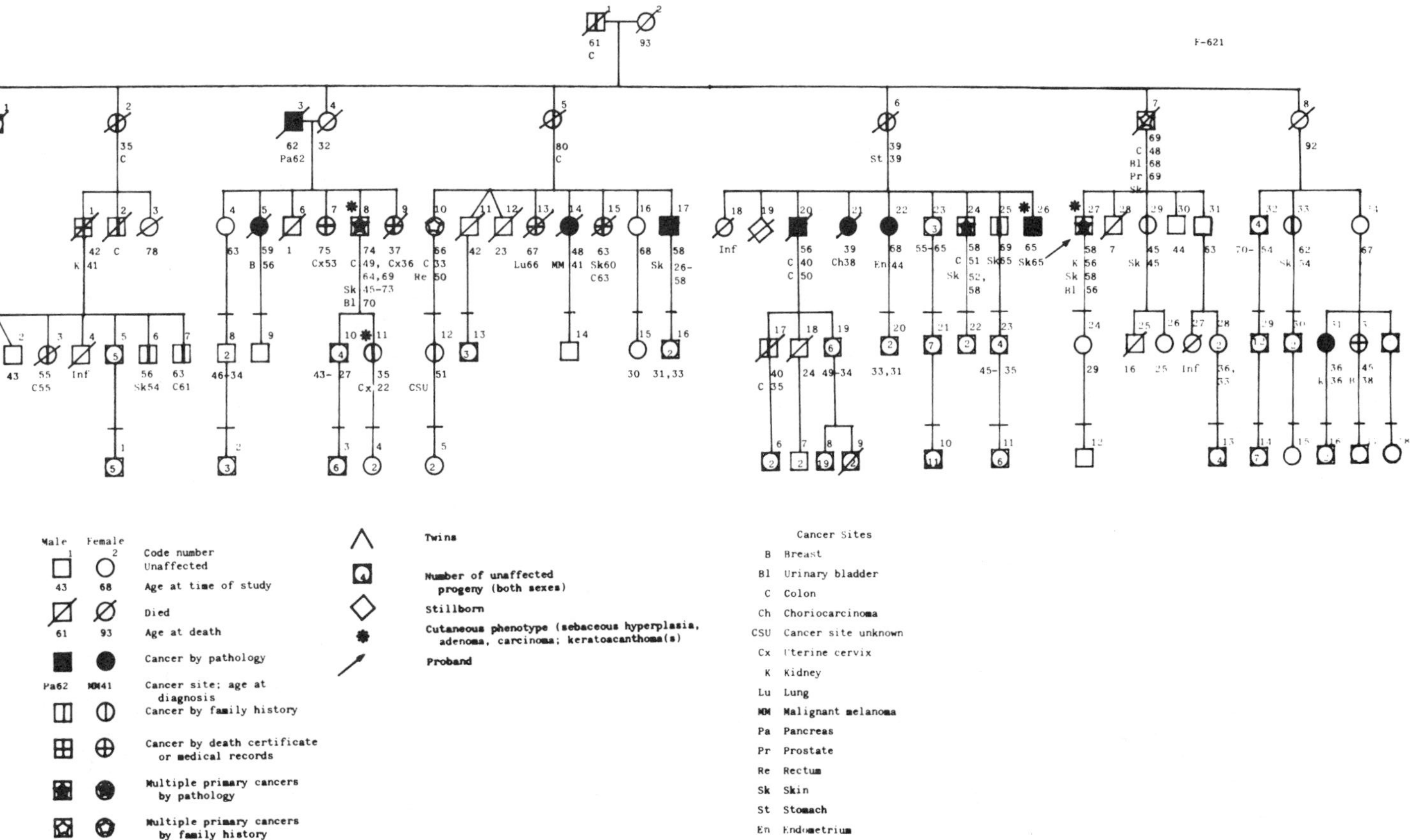

FIGURE 7. Pedigree of family with tumor spectrum consonant with Muir-Torre cutaneous phenotype in association with Lynch syndrome II variant. (From Lynch, H. T., Fusaro, R. M., Roberts, L., et al., *Br. J. Dermatol.*, 113, 295, 1985. With permission.)

Table 1
FAMILY TUMOR REGISTRY

Pedigree Number	Tumor Diagnosis: Visceral	Tumor Diagnosis: Cutaneous
I-1	Colon cancer (H-61)[2]	
II-2	Colon cancer (H-?)	
II-5	Colon cancer (H-?)	
II-6	Stomach cancer (H-39)	
II-7	Colon cancer (H-48)	
	Papillary cancer of bladder (P-68)	
	Prostate cancer (H-69)	
		Skin cancer (H-?)
III-1	Kidney cancer (C-41)	
III-2	Colon cancer (H-?)	
III-5	Breast cancer duct cell (P-56)	
III-7	Uterine cervical cancer (R-53)	
III-8		Skin, squamous cell cancer × 2 (P-45)
		Skin, squamous cell epithelioma (P-49)
	Colon cancer (sigmoid) (P-49)	
		Basal cell epithelioma (P-49)
		Sebaceous gland hyperplasia (P-49)
		Basal cell epithelioma involving a sebaceous gland (P-49)
		Skin, squamous cell epithelioma × 2 (P-54)
	Colon cancer (transverse) (P-64)	
		Sebaceous gland hyperplasia (P-64)
		Keratoacanthoma (P-67)
		Sebaceous adenoma × 2 (P-67)
		Skin, squamous cell carcinoma (P-68)
		Keratoacanthoma (P-69)
	Colon cancer (P-69)	
	Adnexal tumor (most consistent with eccrine acrospiroma) (P-70)	
	Papillary transitional cell cancer of bladder (P-70)	
		Basal cell cancer (P-71
		Keratoacanthoma (P-72)
		Sebaceous hyperplasia (P-73)
		Sebaceous epithelioma (P-73)
		Keratoacanthoma (P-73)
III-9	Uterine cervical cancer (C-36)	
III-10	Colon cancer (H-33)	
	Rectal cancer (H-50)	
III-13	Lung cancer (R-66)	
III-14		Malignant melanoma (P-41)
III-15	Colon cancer (R-63)	Basal cell cancer (R-60)
III-17		Basal cell cancer (P-26)
		Basal cell cancer (P-39)
		Basal cell cancer (P-40)
		Basal cell cancer (P-44)
		Basal cell cancer (P-45)
		Basal cell cancer (P-56)
		Basal cell cancer (P-58)
III-20	Colon cancer (R-40)	
	Colon cancer (hepatic flexure) (P-50)	
III-21	Choriocarcinoma of uterus (P-38)	
III-22	Papillary adenocarcinoma of endometrium (P-44)	

Table 1 (continued)
FAMILY TUMOR REGISTRY

Pedigree Number	Tumor Diagnosis	
	Visceral	Cutaneous
III-24	Colon cancer (ascending) (P-51)	
		Skin, squamous cell carcinoma (P-52)
		Skin, squamous cell carcinoma (P-58)
III-25		Skin cancer (H-65)
III-26		Sebaceous epithelioma (P-65)
III-27		Keratoacanthoma × 2 (P-55)
		Keratoacanthoma with sebaceous gland hyperplasia (P-55)
	Papillary transitional cell Cancer of renal pelvis (P-56)	
	Transitional cell cancer of bladder (R-56)	
		Sebaceous adenoma × 3 (P-56)
		Keratoacanthoma (P-58)
		Skin, squamous cell cancer (P-58)
		Sebaceous hyperplasia (P-58)
		Sebaceous adenoma × 2 (P-59)
III-29		Skin cancer (H-45)
III-33		Skin cancer (H-54)
IV-3	Colon cancer (H-55)	
IV-6		Skin cancer (H-54)
IV-7	Colon cancer (H-61)	
IV-11	Uterine cervical cancer (H-22)	
		Keratoacanthoma (P-33)
IV-12	Cancer, site unknown (H-?)	
IV-17	Colon cancer (H-35)	
IV-31		Basal cell cancer (P-36)
IV-32	Intraducal cancer of right breast (R-38)	

Note: H = family history, P = pathology, C = death certificate, and R = medical record.

[a] (H-61) = (basis of diagnosis — age at diagnosis).

XVI. HETEROGENEITY OF COLON CANCER RISK

A variety of methods have been employed in an attempt to determine the genetic component underlying the liability to colorectal cancer. Such analyses have compared the observed number of affected with that expected on the basis of published cancer incidences or mortality rates. However, in the case of family studies, it is clear that individual family members are drawn from several different eras and live to differing ages so that, due to secular factors, expected rates are often difficult to evaluate with precision. For example, persons born in the early 1900s show a different lifetime risk for colon cancer when compared to those individuals born in the 1930s. In the ideal situation, comparison of proband families should be made with control families selected through age- and sex-matched probands unaffected with cancer. While such an approach would be ideal from the experimental standpoint, on a practical basis, such control families are rarely available. In addition, a confounding problem is the fact that a risk analysis does not answer the question as to whether or not there is familial heterogeneity with regard to risk. In this context, heterogeneity of risk pertains to the fact that some members of families have a different risk for development of colorectal cancer than members of other families. Thus, when heterogeneity is present, one might logically conclude that some families have a higher risk than others. The origin of heterogeneity, when it exists, may be significantly perturbed by environmental or genetic

○ □ female or male without cancer
⊗ ⊠ gastrointestinal cancer, unconfirmed
◐ ◨ colorectal cancer
◑ ◪ gastric cancer
◒ endometrial cancer
↗ proband

⊛ ▣ multiple cancer sites
Cancer site and age at diagnosis
C = colon
E = endometrium
S = stomach
VC = vocal cords

? Sex unknown
B = born 19____
d = died · age

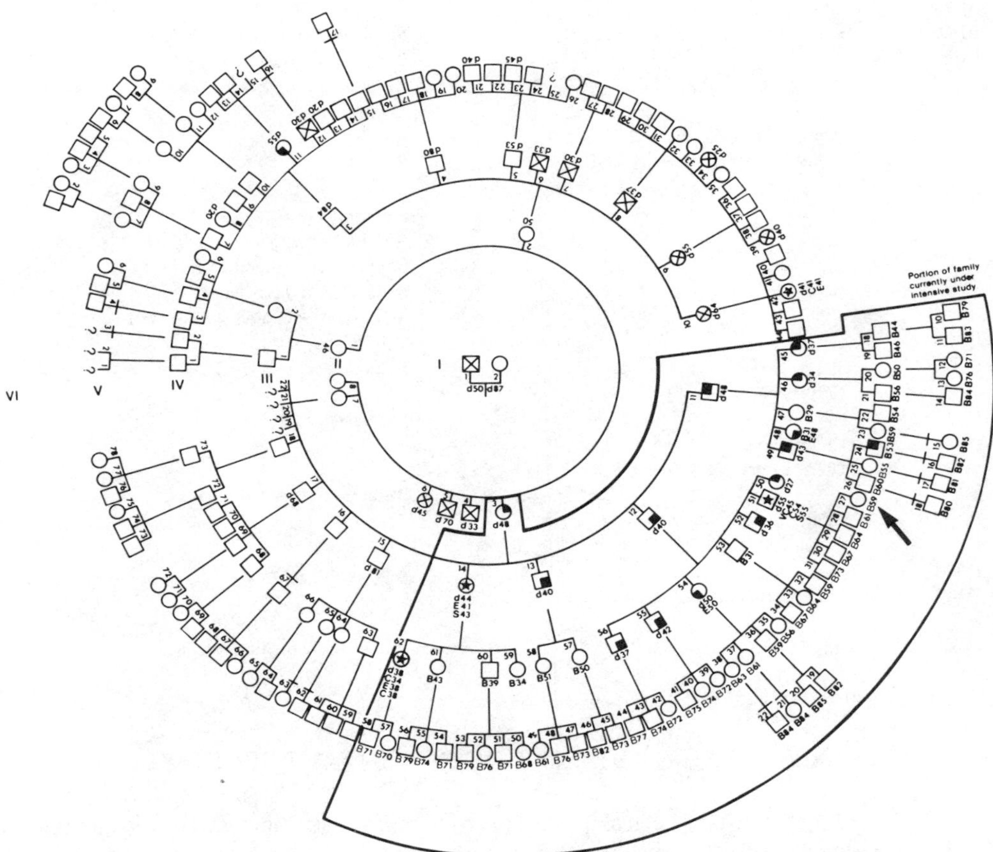

FIGURE 8. Pedigree of extended Lynch syndrome II Italian kindred showing apparent excess of gastric cancer and unique pathologic findings. (From Cristofaro, G., Lynch, H. T., Caruso, M. L., et al., *Cancer,* 60, 51, 1987. With permission.)

factors and/or their interaction. Nevertheless, it is crucial to understand the origin of heterogeneity in that this may provide cogent clues to the colon cancer etiology. When families at high risk for the development of colon cancer can be identified in an unbiased manner, then linkage analysis may be employed with those families so that the validity of specific genetic hypotheses might be tested.[45]

Lynch et al.[45] have assembled detailed family histories of cancer on 857 consecutively ascertained cancer probands from a single oncology clinic, of whom 180 manifested colorectal carcinoma. A permutation test was employed and a Z score was estimated for each family in the sample. Variance for the colon cancer group was significantly increased, while heterogeneity of risk was not observed for any of the other groups. There were 10.6% of

Table 2
CLINICAL/PATHOLOGIC FINDINGS IN 18 OUT OF 25 SUBJECTS UNDER ENDOSCOPIC SURVEILLANCE

Patient number	Birth date	Sex	Clinical findings	Histologic findings	Date of ascertainment
IV-47	1929	F	Rectal polyp removal	CAG[a] with incomplete intestinal metaplasia; metaplastic polyp; excess of macrophages in the lamina propria	April 1985
IV-48	1931	F	Gastritis	CAG with complete intestinal metaplasia; colonic mucosal hyperplasia	April 1985
IV-51	1928	M	Cauliflower-like mass lesion, stomach	Poorly differentiated adenocarcinoma	May 1984
IV-53	1931	M	Normal	CAG with complete intestinal metaplasia; colonic mucosal crypt atrophy	Nov 1984
IV-59	1934	F	Gastric polyp removal; gastritis	Hyperplastic polyp; CAG with intestinal metaplasia	January 1985
IV-60	1939	M	Erosive gastritis and duodenitis; rectal polyp removal	Chronic superficial gastritis of the gastric antrum; tubular adenoma with mild dysplasia of the rectum	January 1985
IV-61	1943	F	Normal	Excess of macrophages in the lamina propria; mucosal crypt atrophy	July 1984
			Gastritis; prophylactic hysterectomy/oophorectomy	Chronic superficial gastritis of the antrum	January 1985
				Adenomatous hyperplasia	May 1985
IV-62[b]	1946	F	Hysterectomy, bilateral oophorectomy; right hemicolectomy for ileocecal mass	Poorly differentiated adenocarcinoma of the uterine corpus and ovary;	October 1984
				Moderately differentiated mucinous adenocarcinoma (Duke's B1)	November 1984
V-21	1956	M	Normal	Chronic superficial gastritis with incomplete intestinal metaplasia	September 1985
V-22	1954	M	Normal	Excess of macrophages in the lamina propria; mucosal crypt atrophy	April 1985
V-24	1953	M	Cauliflower-like mass lesion of ascending colon	Mucinous adenocarcinoma, Duke's C	February 1985
V-27	1959	F	Normal	Chronic superficial gastritis of the antrum	September 1984
				Excess of macrophages in the lamina propria; mucosal crypt atrophy	October 1984
V-28	1961	M	Normal	Chronic superficial gastritis of the antrum	September 1984
				Mucosal crypt atrophy	October 1984
V-29	1964	M	Normal	Chronic superficial gastritis of the antrum	September 1984
V-35	1956	F	Normal	Excess of macrophages in the lamina propria; mucosal crypt atrophy	December 1984

Table 2 (continued)
CLINICAL/PATHOLOGIC FINDINGS IN 18 OUT OF 25 SUBJECTS UNDER ENDOSCOPIC SURVEILLANCE

Patient number	Birth date	Sex	Clinical findings	Histologic findings	Date of ascertainment
V-36	1959	M	Normal	Excess of macrophages in the lamina propria; mucosal crypt atrophy	December 1984
V-37	1961	F	Normal	Excess of macrophages in the lamina propria; mucosal crypt atrophy	December 1984
V-38	1963	F	Normal	Excess of macrophages in the lamina propria; mucosal crypt atrophy	December 1984

[a] CAG = chronic atrophic gastritis.
[b] This patient was an exception to the endoscopic series and is discussed separately as an anecdotal case.

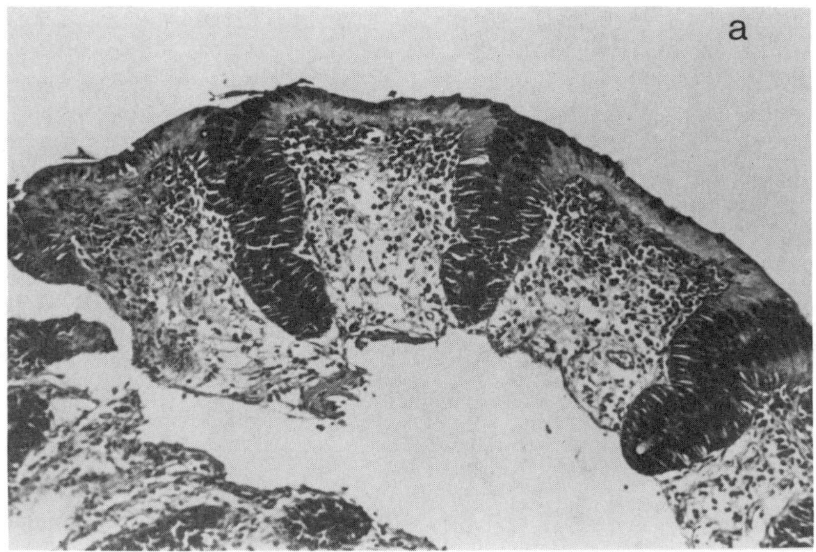

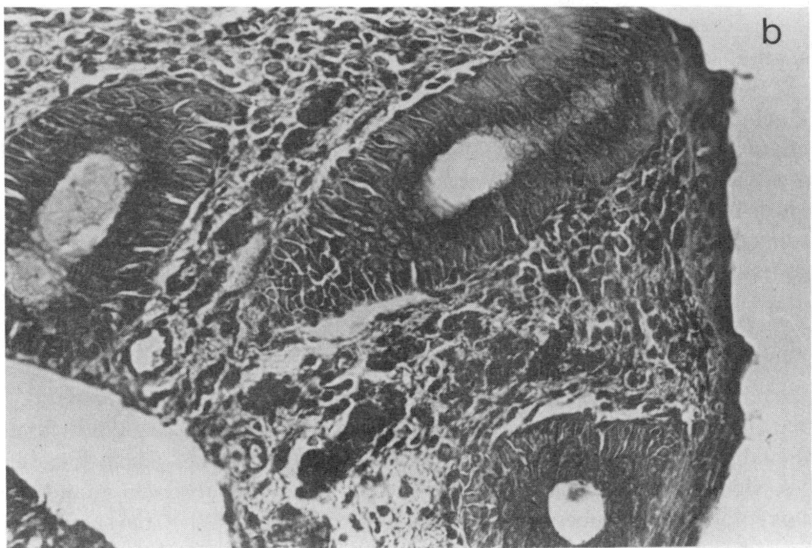

FIGURE 9. Histologic findings from colonic mucosal biopsies obtained from the patients of the Italian family in figure 8. (a) Reduction of crypts and excess of lamina propria which contains a mild increase of chronic inflammatory cells. (b) Macrophages are scattered in the lamina propria, particularly near the muscularis mucosa. (c) Concentration of macrophages in the lamina propria near the lumenal surface. (From Cristofaro, G., Lynch, H. T., Caruso, M. L., et al., *Cancer,* 60, 51, 1987. With permission.)

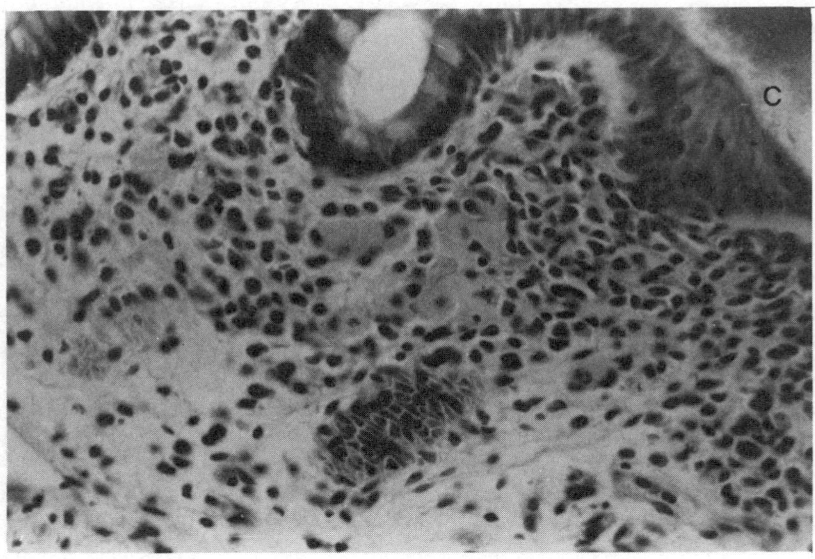

FIGURE 9c.

the colon group and 5.56% of the rectal cancer families which fell into the high risk category, but only 3.95% of the other groups combined were at high risk. Anatomic sites with the highest Z scores and variances were sigmoid and transverse colon, while the lowest variances were seen for cecum and descending colon. Risk status may therefore be partially dependent upon exact anatomic sites within the colon. The effect of *age* of diagnosis was not significant, but did show the possibility of an effect on risk for both the younger and older groups. Our findings of colon cancer heterogeneity warrant intensive genetic-laboratory epidemiologic investigations to determine why certain families express high vs. low risk for colorectal cancer.

XVII. COLON CANCER IN ISRAEL

We investigated family history of colon cancer in 38,823 individuals (2129 families) from Tel-Aviv and nearby areas which were derived from a control and an oncology patient series.[46] A significantly increased risk for colon cancer was observed among first degree relatives of colon cancer probands when compared to controls. When the sample was divided into two groups based on country and continent of birth of probands, European (Ashkenazim) and other (non-Ashkenazim), the relatives of the non-Ashkenazim probands showed a greater relative risk for colon cancer than did relatives of Ashkenazim probands ($p < 0.05$). Colon cancer was found to be less frequent in non-Ashkenazim vs. Ashkenazim controls. These findings suggest that although the colon cancer frequency in the non-Ashkenazim group is lower, the genetic omponent may be more important than for the Ashkenazim sample. The non-Ashkenazim Jews may represent distinctive subgroups which differ with respect to either primary genetic susceptibility to colorectal cancer and/or they may have been subjected to peculiar environmental carcinogenic exposures when compared to their Ashkenazim brethren. A summary of this study is presented in that it shows the approach which can be taken to population studies within a defined geographic area. While descriptive at this point in time, the stated differences in familial colon cancer expression in the Ashkenazim vs. the non-Ashkenazim probands could profit from laboratory epidemiologic investigations of a comparison of these two groups with particular attention given to studies within and between families showing proneness to vs. those showing a paucity of cancer. In addition, detailed environmental investigations, with a search for exposures which are in common vs. those which are dissimilar in the respective populations, could provide valuable clues to etiology, particularly when these are investigated in concert with familiy history determinations.

XVIII. SERUM CHOLESTEROL AND COLORECTAL CANCER

Cholesterol levels are under control of primary genetic factors in interaction with a plethora of endogenous (particularly endocrine) and exogenous (predominantly dietary) events. Given the longstanding interest in the putative role of diet in colorectal cancer, it was logical that investigators would express interest in relationships between cholesterol and colorectal cancer. It is therefore not surprising that such a readily available laboratory measure as serum cholesterol, a chemical with important physiologic function and which is associated with cardiovascular and cerebrovascular disease, should be studied as a possible risk factor in a disorder as common as carcinoma of the colorectum.

This subject has been reviewed by Sidney et al.[47] and by Neugut et al.[48] These investigators also performed case/control studies as tests for the hypothesis that low serum cholesterol levels posed a risk for colorectal cancer. However, in both of these investigations, it was concluded that low serum cholesterol levels, which had been previously believed to be etiologically associated with colon cancer, in fact represented a consequence as opposed to a cause of the cancer. Therefore, these studies did not support the findings of other investigators who proposed an inverse relationship between serum cholesterol and cancer of the large bowel.

XIX. CHEMOPREVENTION AND HNPCC

Hereditary forms of colorectal cancer provide powerful models for the study of genetic/ environmental interaction in cancer expression. In certain circumstances, knowledge from these investigations may have practical implications for the chemoprevention of cancer.

Lipkin and colleagues[49-51] have developed methods for the identification of individuals with an increased susceptibility to carcinoma of the colon as well as other areas of the GI tract. These investigations focused upon modifications of cell proliferation and differentiation at the level of the colonic mucosa which enabled the characterization of affected and at risk individuals vs. low risk individuals from populations showing an increased genetic susceptibility to cancer. Specifically, investigations identified a common hypoproliferative abnormality in preneoplastic colonic mucosa employing tritiated thymidine labeling of colonic mucosal crypts[50] in individuals with familial multiple adenomatous polyposis coli[49,51] and in HNPCC.[17]

These observations have enabled the development of short-term investigations for evaluation of the findings from dietary intervention in patients at increased genetic risk for colorectal cancer. Specifically, following the administration of 1250 mg of calcium carbonate per day, as supplemental dietary calcium, epithelial-cell proliferation was significantly reduced, with findings of an altered colonic crypt profile consonant with the pattern of tritiated thymidine labeling of the colonic mucosa in subjects at low risk for colonic cancer. These findings suggested that the oral calcium supplementation perturbed the colonic mucosa of individuals at high risk for colonic cancer so that a more quiescent proliferative equilibrium of the colonic mucosa was revealed. Thus, the findings following calcium supplementation were, as mentioned, similar to those observed for subjects at low risk for colon cancer.[52]

The leading theory for promotion of colonic carcinogenesis has strongly suggested that dietary fat may be irritating and toxic to the colon. In turn, dietary fat leads to a compensatory increase in the proliferation of colonic epithelial cells, thereby producing damaging effects.

It is therefore of interest that the oral administration of calcium in rodent models[53,54] demonstrated a reduction in these damaging effects. Thus, the animal work has provided an important stimulus for the subsequent investigations by Lipkin and Newmark of calcium carbonate supplementation in high risk patients.[52]

We have therefore come "full circle" in genetic epidemiology of colonic cancer. The first part of the equation involves descriptive epidemiology and genetics for the identification of individuals at high risk, i.e., genetic (FPC, Gardner's syndrome, HNPCC), racial, ethnic and geographic. Animals models, as mentioned, can then be capitalized upon for phase I intervention studies. Hypotheses developed from these investigations can then be tested in the clinical setting on an epidemiologic/genetic basis followed by appropriate intervention, as in the calcium carbonate story of Lipkin and Newmark.[52]

XX. SURVEILLANCE FOR HEREDITARY COLORECTAL CANCER

As in all forms of hereditary cancer, the most important measure for assuring full compliance is a meticulous educational program. Premonitory clinical signs in FPC, including extracolonic signs (osseous and cutaneous) in so-called Gardner's syndrome, and possibly occular (CHRPE), are beacons for recognition of these disorders. The key to early colonic cancer prevention in the FPC syndromes is the recognition of the multiple adenomatous coli polyp phenotype. We recommend that screening, preferably by colonoscopy, be performed late in the 1st decade of life in patients who are at increased risk, as judged from their position in the pedigree. Thus, the screening should be done before symptoms develop. Management includes total colectomy with several surgical options, including rectal mucosectomy and ileoanal anastomosis. Preservation of the anal sphincter function can be achieved with new advances in these procedures.[55,56] We recommend that in HNPCC, patients be informed of the natural history of this disease, including their risk status, by their mid- or late teens. It is important that they develop a full understanding about this problem and that they form a relationship of confidence and trust with the family physician who will coordinate the screening activities. Ideally, this physician should be knowledgeable about the genetic and natural history of HNPCC.

We recommend that colonoscopy be initiated by age 25 years and thereafter every other year. Should expertise for colonoscopy be lacking, then double air contrast barium enema may be offered. Should polyps be observed, they should be removed at the time of colonoscopy. Hemoccult testing of stool should be performed biannually. Unfortunately, in the absence of premonitory signs and/or biomarkers of acceptable sensitivity and specificity, one must await phenotypic (cancer) expression for HNPCC diagnosis. When colonic cancer is manifested, the operation of choice is subtotal colectomy. Followup of the remaining rectal segment is then mandated. Women who are sisters or progeny of HNPCC syndrome affecteds who present with colonic cancer, in addition to subtotal colectomy, may be considered for prophylactic hysterectomy and bilateral oophorectomy since they are candidates for development of cancer of the endometrium or ovaries.

Needed are investigations showing a high yield in screening of HNPCC kindreds. In a recent investigation, Mecklin et al.[57] screened 236 asymptomatic relatives in 22 Finnish HNPCC kindreds. Of these individuals 58%[137] entered the screening program. Double air contrast barium enema and sigmoidoscopy or colonoscopy was employed. Of the 137 subjects (aged 20 to 65 years) who entered the screening program, a colonic neoplasm was observed in 12 (9%). Two of these individuals manifested colonic cancer (Duke's A and B), and ten individuals showed one or more adenomas. Two of the subjects who were not screened developed Duke's C colon carcinomas during the study period, and one of them expired from metastatic cancer. Ongoing screening of 34 patients who had been previously identified with HNPCC indicated that 12 (35%) of these cases manifested metachronous colorectal tumors. These investigators considered their preliminary findings in this screening program to be encouraging. This is a promising area for research in cancer control strategies.

XXI. STRATEGIES FOR CANCER CONTROL

How can genetic knowledge expedite colon cancer control? There are certain strategies which could effectively address this question:

1. Compile a detailed family history, recording cancer of *all* anatomic sites through a minimum of second degree relatives (i.e., grandparents, aunts, uncles). These relatives are genetically more informative because of their older ages.
2. Develop appropriate surveillance/management protocols which are responsive to the particular hereditary cancer syndrome natural history (i.e., earlier initiation of highly organ-targeted surveillance, prophylactic subtotal colectomy in multiple adenomatous polyposis coli). Ideally, these protocols should extend to all available at-risk relatives.
3. Establish computerized registries of such kindreds, with capability of dissemination of risk and surveillance/management knowledge to physicians of all high risk relatives.
4. Give priority attention to research on biomarkers which correlate with cancer-prone genotypes.
5. Assess reduction in cancer morbidity and mortality in order to influence physician, patient, and societal policy, including demonstration of cost-benefit advantage to third party carriers for defraying cost of surveillance, all of which will hopefully evolve into a more positive philosophy about cancer prevention.

The Creighton Hereditary Cancer Institute's primary mission is devoted primarily to all of these objectives, and consultation is readily at hand.

REFERENCES

1. **Silverberg, E.,** Cancer statistics 1984 (American Cancer Society), *Cancer-Cancer J. Clin.,* 34, 7, 1984.
2. **Byers, T. and Graham, S.,** The epidemiology of diet and cancer, *Adv. Cancer Res,* 41, 1, 1984.
3. **Lynch, P. M. and Lynch, H. T.,** *Colon Cancer Genetics,* Van Nostrand Reinhold, New York, 1985.
4. **Lynch, H. T., Rozen, P., and Schuelke, G. S.,** Hereditary colon cancer: polyposis and nonpolyposis variants, *Cancer,* 35, 95, 1985.
5. **Lynch, H. T., Rozen, P., Schuelke, G. S., and Lynch, J. F.,** Hereditary colorectal cancer review: colonic polyposis and nonpolyposis colonic cancer (Lynch syndrome I and II), *Surv. Dig. Dis.,* 2, 244, 1985.
6. **Moore, J. R. L. and Lamont, J. T.,** Colorectal cancer: risk factors and screening strategies, *Arch. Int. Med.,* 144, 1819, 1984.
7. **Howe, G. M.,** *Global Geocancerology: A World Geography of Human Cancers,* Churchill-Livingstone, Edinburgh, 1986.
8. **Burt, R. W., Bishop, D. T., Cannon, L. A., Dowdle, M. A., Lee, R. G., and Skolnick, M. H.,** Dominant inheritance of adenomatous colonic polyps and colorectal cancer, *N. Engl. J. Med.,* 312, 1540, 1985.
9. **Boland, C. R. and Troncale, F. J.,** Familial colonic cancer in the absence of antecedent polyposis, *Ann. Intern. Med.,* 100, 700, 1984.
10. **Silverberg, E. and Lubera J.,** Cancer statistics, 1988, *Cancer-Cancer J. Clin.,* 38, 5, 1988; 37, 2, 1987.
11. **Traboulsi, E. I., Krush, A. J., Gardner, E. J., Booker, S. V., Offerhaus, G. J. A., Yardley, H. J., Hamilton, S. R., Luk, G. D., Giardiello, F. M., Welsh, S. B., Hughes, J. P., and Maumenee, I. H.,** Prevalence and importance of pigmented ocular fundus lesions in Gardner's syndrome, *N. Engl. J. Med.,* 316, 1987.
12. **Blair, N. P. and Trempe, C. L.,** Hypertrophy of the retinal pigment epithelium associated with Gardner's syndrome, *Am. J. Ophthalmol.,* 90, 661, 1980.

13. **Lewis, R. A., Crowder, W. E., Eierman, L. A., Nussbaum, R. L., and Ferrell, R. E.,** The Gardner syndrome: significance of ocular features, *Ophthalmology,* 91, 916, 1984.
14. **Traboulsi, E. I. and Maumenee, I. H.,** Periocular pigmentation in Peutz-Jeghers syndrome, *Am. J. Ophthalmol.,* 102, 126, 1986.
15. **Lynch, H. T., Priluck, I., and Fitzsimmons, M. L.,** Congenital hypertrophy of the retinal pigment epithelium (CHRPE) in non-Gardner's polyposis kindreds, Letter to the Editor, *Lancet,* ii, 333, 1987.
16. **Lynch, H. T., Schuelke, G. S., and Lynch, J. F.,** Genetics of rectal cancer, *Bull. Cancer,* 71, 1, 1984.
17. **Lynch, H. T., Kimberling, W. J., Schuelke, G. S., et al.,** Hereditary nonpolyposis colorectal cancer. I and II, *Cancer,* 56, 934, 1986.
18. **Bulow, S.,** Colorectal polyposis syndromes, *Scan. J. Gastroenerol.,* 19, 289, 1984.
19. **Bulow, S., Sondergaard, J. O., Witt I., et al.,** Mandibular osteomas in familial polyposis coli, *Dis. Colon Rectum,* 27, 105, 1984.
20. **Sondergaard, J. O., Svendsen, L. B., Witt, I. N., et al.,** Mandibular osteomas in colorectal cancer, *Scan. J. Gastroenterol.,* 20, 759, 1985.
21. **Sondergaard, J. O., Svendsen, L. B., Witt, I. N., et al.,** Mandibular osteomas in the Cancer Family Syndrome, *Br. J. Cancer,* 52, 941, 1986.
22. **Li, F. P., Thurber, W. A., Seddon, J., and Holmes, G. E.,** Hepatoblastoma in families with polyposis coli, *JAMA,* 257, 2475, 1987.
23. **Barker, D., McCoy, M., Weinberg, R., et al.,** A test of the role of two oncogenes in inherited predisposition to colon cancer, *Mol. Biol. Med.,* 1, 199, 1983.
24. **Gardner, E. J., Woodward, S. R., and Hughes, J. P.,** Evaluation of chromosomal diagnosis for hereditary adenomatosis of the colorectum, *Cancer Genet. Cytogenet.,* 15, 321, 1985.
25. **Koufos, A., Hansen, M. F., Copeland, N. G., et al,** Loss of heterozygosity in three embyryonal tumors suggests a common pathogenetic mechanism, *Nature,* 316, 330, 1985.
26. **Bodmer, W. F., Bailey, C. J., Bodmer, J., et al.,** Localization of the gene for familial adenomatous polyposis on chromosome 5, *Nature,* 328, 614, 1987.
27. **Solomon, E., Voss, R., Hall, V., et al.,** Chromosome 5 allele loss in human colorectal carcinomas, *Nature,* 328, 616, 1987.
28. **Albano, W. A., Recabaren, J. A., Hunch, H. T., Campbell, A. S., Mailliard, J. A., Organ, C. H., and Kimberling, W. J.,** Natural history of hereditary cancer of the breast and colon, *Cancer,* 50, 360, 1982.
29. **Lynch, H. T., Voorhees, G. J., Lanspa, S. J., McGreevy, P. S., and Lynch, J. F.,** Pancreatic carcinoma and hereditary nonpolyposis colorectal cancer: a family study, *Br. J. Cancer,* 52, 71, 1985.
30. **Lynch, H. T., Lynch, P. M., Albano, W. A., and Lynch, J. F.,** The Cancer Family Syndrome: a status report, *Dis. Colon Rectum,* 24, 311, 1981.
31. **Sorensen, S. A., Jensen, O. A., and Klinken, L.,** Familial aggregation of neuroectodermal and gastrointestinal tumors, *Cancer,* 52, 1977, 1983.
32. **Love, R. R.,** Small bowel cancers, B-cell lymphatic leukemia, and six primary cancers with metastases and prolonged survival in the Cancer Family Syndrome of Lynch, *Cancer,* 55, 499, 1985.
33. **Budd, D. C. and Fink, D. L.,** Mucoid colonic carcinoma as an autosomal-dominant inherited syndrome, *Arch. Surg.,* 116, 901, 1981.
34. **Lynch, H. T., Drouhard, T. J., Schuelke, G. S., Biscone, K. A., Lynch, J. F., and Danes, B. S.,** Hereditary nonpolyposis colorectal cancer in a Navajo Indian family, *Cancer Genet. Cytogenet.,* 15, 209, 1985.
35. **Lynch, H. T., Lynch, P. M., Pester, J., and Fusaro, R. M.,** The Cancer Family Syndrome: rare cutaneous phenotypic linkage of Torre's syndrome, *Arch. Intern. Med.,* 141, 607, 1980.
36. **Lynch, H. T., Fusaro, R. M., Roberts, L., Voorhees, G. J., and Lynch, J. F.,** Muir-Torre syndrome in several members of a family with a variant of the Cancer Family Syndrome, *Br. J. Dermatol.,* 113, 295, 1985.
37. **Hill, M. J., Morson, B. C., and Bussey, H. J. R.,** Aetiology of adenoma-carcimona sequences in large bowel, *Lancet,* i, 245, 1978.
38. **Riddell, R. H., Goldman, H., Ransohoff, D. F., et al.,** Dysplasia in inflammatory bowel disease: standardized classification with provisional clinical applications, *Hum. Pathol.,* 14, 931, 1983.
39. **Filipe, M. I., Edwards, M. R., and Ehsanullah, M.,** A prospective study of dysplasia and carcinoma in the rectal biopsies and rectal stump of eight patients following ileorectal anastomosis in ulcerative colitis, *Histopathology,* 9, 1139, 1985.
40. **McFadden, D. E., Owen, D. A., Reid, P. E., and Jones, E. A.,** The histochemical assessment of sulphated and nonsulfated sialomucin in intestinal epithelium, *Histopathology,* 9, 1129, 1985.
41. **Rothery, G. A. and Day, D. W.,** Intestinal metaplasia in endoscopic biopsy specimens of gastric mucosa, *J. Clin. Pathol.,* 38, 613, 1985.
42. **Cristofaro, G., Lynch, H. T., Caruso, M. L., et al.,** New phenotypic aspects in a family with Lynch syndrome II, *Cancer,* 60, 51, 1987.

43. **Correa, P.,** The epidemiology and pathogenesis of chronic gastritis: three etiologic entities, *Fron. Gastrointest. Res.*, 6, 98, 1980.
44. **Mecklin, J.-P., Sipponen, P., and Jarvinen, H. J.,** Histopathology of colorectal carcinomas and adenomas in cancer family syndrome, *Dis. Colon Rectum,* 29, 849, 1986.
45. **Lynch, H. T., Kimberling, W. J., Biscone, K. A., Lynch, J. F., Wagner, C. A., Brennan, K., Mailliard, J. A., and Johnson, P. S.,** Familial heterogeneity of colon cancer risk, *Cancer,* 57, 2089, 1986.
46. **Rozen, P., Fireman, Z., Figer, Z., Legum, C., Ron, E., and Lynch, H. T.,** Family history colorectal cancer as a marker of potential malignancy within a screening program, *Cancer,* 60, 248, 1987.
47. **Sidney, S., Friedman, G. D., and Hiatt, R. A.,** Serum cholesterol and large bowel cancer: a case/control study, *Am. J. Epidemiol.*, 124, 33, 1986.
48. **Neugut, A. I., Johnsen, C. M., and Fink, D. J.,** Serum cholesterol levels in adenomatous polyps and cancer of the colon: a case/control study, *JAMA,* 255, 365, 1986.
49. **Lipkin, M., Blattner, W., Frameni, J., et al.,** Tritiated thymidine labeling distributions in the identification of hereditary predisposition to colon cancer, *Cancer Res.*, 43, 1899, 1983.
50. **Lipkin, M.,** Method for binary categorization of individuals with familial polyposis based on (3H)dThd labeling of epithelial cells in colonic crypts, *Cell Tissue Kinet.*, 17, 209, 1984.
51. **Lipkin, M., Blattner, W. A., Gardner, E. J., et al.,** Classification and risk assessment of individuals with familial polyposis, Gardner syndrome, and familial nonpolyposis colon cancer from (3h)H dThd-labeling patterns in colonic epithelial cells, *Cancer Res.*, 44, 4201,1984.
52. **Lipkin, M. and Newmark, H.,** Effect of added dietary calcium on colonic epithelial-cell proliferation in subjects at high risk for familial colonic cancer, *N. Engl. J. Med.*, 313, 1381, 1985.
53. **Wargovich, M. J., Eng, V. W. S., and Newmark, H. L.,** Calcium inhibits the damaging and compensatory proliferative effects of fatty acids on mouse colon epithelium, *Cancer Lett.*, 23, 253, 1984.
54. **Newmark, H. L., Wargovich, M. J., and Bruce, W. R.,** Colon cancer and dietary fat, phosphate, and calcium: a hypothesis, *J. Natl. Cancer Inst.*, 72, 1323, 1984.
55. **Forbes, D., Rubin, S., Trevenen, C., Gall, G., and Scott, B.,** Familial polyposis coli in childhood, *Clin. Invest. Med.*, 10, 5, 1987.
56. **Bulow, S.,** Familial polyposis coli, *Dan. Med. Bull,* 34, 1, 1987.
57. **Mecklin, J.-P., Jarvinen, H. J., Aukee, S., Elomaa, I., and Karjalainen, K.,** Screening for colorectal carcinoma in Cancer Family Syndrome kindreds, *Scan. J. Gastroenterol.*, 22, 449 1987.

Chapter 17

GENETIC EPIDEMIOLOGY OF LUNG CANCER

Henry T. Lynch and Jane F. Lynch

TABLE OF CONTENTS

I. INTRODUCTION

In their review of genetic predisposition to lung cancer, Iannuzzi and Miller[1] state that "no organ system is more dependent on the interaction of environment and heredity than the lungs. Although this interaction is complex, progress has been made in understanding the relationship of environmental factors and genetic predisposition to lung cancer."

Lung cancer is a major public health problem in most of the world. It has overtaken carcinoma of the colon as the leading cause of death in males and is second only to cancer of the breast in females in the U.S. Cigarette smoking has been considered one of the primary causes of this desease. However, cigarette smokers appear to show significant variation in susceptibility to lung cancer and other cigarette smoking-associated disorders, such as chronic obstructive pulmonary disease. Host factors appear to play an important role in this variation in susceptibility to smoking associated disease.

An increasing body of evidence indicates that there is tremendous variation of lung cancer risk, as well as risk for cancer at *all* anatomic sites, in relatives of lung cancer probands. These observations may be a reflection of underlying genetic susceptibility to malignancy in these families.[2]

The pioneering work of Harris and colleagues[3,4] dealing with interindividual variation in carcinogen metabolism, their activation, and DNA repair at both the infrahuman and human levels, at the Laboratory of Human Carcinogenesis of the National Cancer Institute (Bethesda, MD), has provided many insights into the genetic epidemiology of lung and other forms of cancer. Central to these biomedical research efforts has been the extrapolation of data on mechanisms of etiology and carcinogenesis from experimental animals to humans. When considering the enormous complexity of humans, particularly from the standpoint of individual differences, then one can readily appreciate the effort that has gone into the development of *in vitro* models for studies of carcinogenesis. Comparative investigations at the *in vitro* level employing specimens from experimental animals and humans, performed under the same controlled experimental setting, provide invaluable opportunities for elucidation of mechanisms of carcinogenesis.[5]

A. Epidemiology

While cigarette smoking has received primary attention in lung cancer etiology during the past several decades,[6,7] it is now becoming clear that lung cancer incidence rates are also influenced by rural/urban differences, racial factors as evidenced by elevated lung cancer risk in black men[8] and in Mexican-American[9] and Chinese women,[10] migratory patterns, and even the socioeconomic and educational status of the patient.[11] Specific underlying occupational and environmental factors must be given careful scrutiny.[12] Such agents as asbestos, chromium, nickel, inorganic arsenic, iron ore (hematite), wood dust, isopropyl alcohol, halo-ethers, mustard gas, radioisotopes, polycyclic aromatic hydrocarbons (gas workers and those working with coal carbonization products and coke ovens), and possibly vinyl chloride (known agent for liver angiosarcoma), provide examples of nontobacco-related carcinogens.[13,14] Yet even here, their role as promoters of the carcinogenic effect of tobacco must be reckoned with, thus introducing problems of synergism in lung cancer etiology.[11,14,15] The role of certain iatrogenic exposures such as immunosuppressive agents and possibly Thorotrast (a known agent in liver hemangioendothelioma), must also be integrated into an encompassing lung cancer carcinogenesis model.[15]

The context in which the environmental agents act, namely, host susceptibility or resistance, has been receiving increasing attention in lung cancer epidemiology.[16,17] For example, a heightened empirical familial risk for lung cancer was initially reported by Tokuhata and Lilienfeld,[18] where 2.4 times more lung cancer was observed among relatives of patients than controls. As we might expect, the familial factor was more pronounced among lung cancer patients who were nonsmokers than among smokers, although the combination of smoking and family history of lung cancer appeared to have multiplicative effects.

B. Study of Genetic Isolates: Canadian Eskimos (Inuites)

On occasion, certain rare natural events occur involving genetic isolates which provide investigators with field epidemiology laboratory opportunities; they often harbor a potential for the elucidation of environmental events in context with host factors. The Canadian Eskimos (Inuites) provide such a clinical example in that they have been relatively isolated for many years, and until recently, their environment has been homogeneous in their nomadic existence. However, recent events in their acculturation has subjected them to certain general environmental variations, including significant changes in their personal habit patterns. Specifically, tobacco was introduced to the Eskimos by whalers and traders, and this habit pattern became rather ubiquitous in the Canadian Arctic at the turn of the present century. However, as money and supplies to these individuals became more plentiful, commensurate with increased financial affluence and urbanization during the past several decades, this habit pattern has accelerated; at the present time, Canadian Eskimos now rank as heavy smokers of factory-made cigarettes.[19]

It is of interest that until around 1920, cancer was extremely rare in Eskimos.[20] However, as cancer epidemiology studies of Eskimos began to accrue, it was found that salivary gland and renal neoplasms showed an excess which has now been displaced by cancer of the lung and uterine cervix. Breast cancer occurs rarely. Cancer of the lung in Eskimo women is now known to be exceedingly high. Schaefer and associates[20] suggest that the epidemiology of lung cancer in this population may be exceedingly complex and may be due to multiple confounding factors. These include tobacco, tuberculosis, isoniazid, and chronic nonspecific lung disease, as well as other exposures, including that of seal oil lamps. Host factors should be added to this listing.

Eskimos are known to have an unusual susceptibility to tuberculosis. So far as the relationship between tuberculosis and lung cancer is concerned, there have been conflicting results in studies from other areas of the world. For example, reports from Israel[21] and Australia[22] suggest that people who have pulmonary tuberculosis, particularly women, are at greatly increased risk for development of lung cancer. On the other hand, Berroya and associates[23] did not find any significant association between tuberculosis and lung cancer.

Isoniazid is the the most commonly used drug in the treatment of tuberculosis. It is therefore of interest that this drug and its main metabolite have been shown to cause lung tumors in mice, with the greater predominance in female than male mice.[24] However, Schaefer[20] did not find an increased association between lung tumors in the isoniazid-treated Eskimos.

Chronic nonspecific lung disease has been observed by Dutch investigators[25] to predispose to the development of lung cancer in smokers. Eskimos appear to be particularly prone to chronic nonspecific lung disease.[19] Indeed, patients with chronic bronchitis may be particularly susceptible to inhaled carcinogenic pollutants and it has been suggested that this may result from impairment in the normal physiologic mechanisms for removal of such pollutants from the lungs. Therefore, Schaefer[20] suggested that the fact that Eskimo women were traditionally exposed to high concentrations of bronchial irritants, particularly from the mentioned exposure to seal oil lamps which, incidentally, they frequently keep lit both day and night, deems this particular association worthy of greater perusal. Of possible added pertinence is the fact that increased pigmentation of the lungs has been noted at autopsy in elderly Eskimo women. It is therefore possible that the emission from seal oil lamps in concert with other environmental effects, including cigarette smoking, may have effects which differ from those generally innocuous associations with anthracosis.

Finally, Schaefer[20] suggests that additional carcinogenic factors may relate to the prior dietary habits of the Eskimos, which had been primarily centered around the consumption of caribou meat. This is of interest in that, following the Hiroshima and Nagasaki atomic bomb explosions in 1945, there has been a relatively heavy fallout in the Arctic of radioactive substances from these nuclear explosions in the atmosphere. Such radioactive elements as strontium and cesium have therefore become incorporated into the lichen-caribou-Eskimo food chain. While this obviously would not pose an inhalation risk, it might nevertheless provide a background carcinogenic effect which, in concert with other mentioned effects, could either irritate or promote pulmonary carcinogenesis.

C. Consecutive Oncology Clinic Series

Lynch et al.[2] studied detailed cancer family histories on 254 consecutively ascertained probands with histologically verified lung cancer and 231 probands with other smoking related cancers who were under medical evaluatioon at the Creighton oncology clinic. Results disclosed a lack of any strong statistical evidence for an increased risk in lung cancer per se when only lung cancer in relatives was considered. Confounding factors, particularly the effect of cigarette smoking, variation of secular trends, and the heritability of the smoking phenotype itself, tended to obfuscate identification of an inherited effect presenting itself exclusively as lung cancer liability. However, a significant increase was observed in cancers of *all* anatomic sites among the relatives of lung cancer probands ($p < 0.001$). Most of these neoplastic lesions were not associated with smoking and were not greatly influenced by secular trends. There was no significant excess of cancer at *all* antomic sites in relatives of probands with other smoking associated cancers. It was concluded that the observation of an increased risk for cancer at all anatomic sites in relatives of cancer probands may be a reflection of an underlying susceptibility to malignancy in these kindreds.

The risk showed significant heterogeneity between families. The only other group showing a more significant heterogeneity was that drawn from breast cancer probands. These observations suggested a potent familial effect as being of etiologic importance in carcinogenesis in certain of these families. The differences in cancer expression by sites, namely, that of lung cancer in some and cancer of all antomic sites in others, was in accord with genetic heterogeneity. The data were insufficient to enable the investigators to ascribe modes of genetic transmission of cancer in these families. However, studies of segregation analysis of the kindreds are currently in progress in order to test hypotheses of Mendelian patterns of inheritance. Finally, there was a nonsignificant lung cancer excess in smoking relatives of lung cancer probands when compared with smoking relatives of probands with nonsmoking related cancers. The observations of excess of lung cancer in relatives was compatible with Fisher's hypothesis which postulates that cigarette smoking behavior is due to a host factor effect and that lung cancer expression is linked to this habit pattern.[26] Alternatively, this phenomenon may be interpreted in terms of genotypic susceptibility for lung cancer which is promoted by cigarette smoking.[17]

D. Case/Control Study

Sellers et al.[27] have recently reported a retrospective case/control study of 337 southern Louisiana families. A deceased lung cancer patient was used as the proband in this cohort and a comparison of first degree relatives of proband families with spouse (control) families was performed. The findings showed a significantly greater overall risk of cancer (odds ratio, OR = 2.0; $p < 0.0001$) in the proband group. Logistic regression techniques were employed in order to control for the confounding effects of age, sex, and cigarette smoking, as well as for occupational and industrial exposures. Findings showed that lung cancer probands maintained an increased risk of nonlung cancer ($p < 0.05$). Observations showed that ". . . the crude odds ratio of a proband family having one family member with cancer was 1.67 compared with control families. Proband families were 2.16 times more likely to have two other family members with cancer. For three cancers and four or more cancers, the risk increased to 3.66 and 5.04, respectively. Each risk estimate was significant at the 0.01 level. The most striking differences in cancer prevalence between proband and control families were noted for cancer of the nasal cavity/sinus, mid-ear, and larynx (OR = 4.6); trachea, bronchus, and lung (OR = 3.0); skin (OR = 2.8); and uterus, placenta, ovary, and other female organs (OR = 2.1). These data support the hypothesis of a genetic susceptibility to cancer in families with lung cancer.'' Thus, many features of the Sellers et al.[27]study employing a retrospective case/control (spouse family as control) provide strong confirmation of our own oncology clinic series.[2]

E. Case/Control Family Studies

Ooi et al.[28] investigated demographic and morbidity/mortality data, as well as occupational experiences, in concert with tobacco use among family members of 336 deceased lung cancer probands and 307 controls (spouses of the probands). They compared the first degree relatives of the probands with first degree relatives of the controls. A strong excess risk for lung cancer was observed among the probands. Male realtives of probands showed greater risk for lung cancer than their female counterparts. There was a fourfold risk for cancer among parents of probands when compared to parents of spouses. Interestingly, female relatives of probands over 40 years of age showed a nine-times higher risk than comparably aged female controls. This risk was present even among those nonsmokers who had not reported any excessive exposure to occupations noteworthy for carcinogenic risk. There was a four- to six-fold risk for heavy smokers. These investigators found that ''. . . after control for the confounding effects of age, sex, cigarette smoking, and occupational and industrial exposures, relationship to proband remained a significant determinant of lung cancer, with a 2.4-fold greater risk among relatives of probands.''

Finally, it was of interest that cancers of the larynx, brain and nervous system, bone, endocrine glands, ovary, kidney, bladder, esophagus, and stomach, and leukemias/lymphomas (as a group) were found to be more prevalent among first degree relatives of probands which led these investigators to hypothesize a susceptibility to cancer in general or to a particular set of specific cancers.[28]

F. Chronic Obstructive Pulmonary Disease, Host Susceptibility, and Lung Cancer

Samet et al.[29] investigated lung cancer risk in context with family and personal history of respiratory diseases in a population-based case/control study. The findings showed that physician diagnoses of chronic bronchitis, emphysema, asthma, and other chest disorders were reported more often for cases than for control subjects. Specifically, they noted that 6.9% of the cases had at least one parent with a diagnosis of lung cancer, while only 2.2% of the control subjects' parents were similarly affected ($p < 0.001$). Employing multiple logistic regression models which excluded never-smokers and which included variables to control for the effects of cigarette smoking, these investigators noted ''. . . significantly increased risks for a personal history of chronic bronchitis or emphysema (odds ratio = 2.0; 95% confidence interval, 1.4 to 2.8) and a parental history of lung cancer (odds ratio = 5.3; 95% confidence interval, 2.2 to 12.8). The present study complements the results of previous investigations which demonstrated that lung cancer in smokers is modified by characteristics of the smoker and by family history.''

Cohen[30] observed that first degree relatives of lung cancer patients, like first degree relatives of chronic obstructive pulmonary disease (COPD) patients, had significantly higher rates of impaired pulmonary function than the corresponding relatives of nonpulmonary patients, more than neighborhood controls, teachers, or other nonpatients. Lynch[31] observed a similar trend between lung cancer and COPD. Specifically, there was a decline in the frequency of COPD with decreasing coancestry to lung cancer probands. These observations suggest the presence of a common familial component of COPD and lung cancer, and are in accord with Cohen's hypotheseis that lung cancer and COPD share a common familial pathogenetic component associated with pulmonary dysfunction.[30] This observation is also consonant with emerging evidence suggesting that airway obstruction, irrespective of cigarette smoking, is associated with an increased risk of neoplasms of the lung and bronchus.[32] This hypothesis also explains the manner in which inhaled carcinogens would lead to prolonged exposure to the airways as well as to other organs and tissues through their absorption. Their potential effectiveness as carcinogens would then be enhanced. In addition, tissue deterioration resulting from pulmonary dysfunction would mean that the carcinogens would be acting on damaged, and thereby primed, tissue. This tissue injury concept is important in explaining lung cancer association in certain diseases such as familial fibrocystic pulmonary dysplasia.[33]

G. Genetic Malformations and Lung Cancer

Landing and Dixon[34] have reviewed the problem of genetic malformations and genetic diseases of the respiratory tract, inclusive of the larynx, trachea, bronchi, and lungs, and identified about 70 distinct anomalies involving the system. It is prudent to consider certain of these disorders as providing the "fertile soil" for interrelationships between environmental carcinogens, genetics, and carcinogenesis. Certain of these disorders such as pulmonary lynphangiomatosis,[35] pulmonary blastomas, and hamartomas or ectopic tissues in the lung, which are considered to be the pulmonary counterparts of nephroblastoma (Wilms' tumor) and hepatoblastoma[36,37] and familial fibrocystic pulmonary dysplasia and other familial pulmonary fibroses[38,39] have shown cancer association. These disorders would therefore provide excellent models for the investigation of cancer genetic epidemiology phenomenon in lung carcinogenesis.

H. Family Studies

Goffman et al[40] reported two families with lung and other respiratory tract cancers. The influence of smoking and possible radiation sensitivity (in one of the families) suggested an environmental cancer-prone genotype interaction in accord with the concept of ecogenetics.[17] One of the families may represent a newly recognized syndrome of limb and dental anomalies.[41] Independently, two of the family members were carriers of a balanced translocation between chromosomes 13 and 14. Multiple primary cancers and nonrespiratory tract cancers were also observed, but their significance cannot be fully assessed due to limitations in family size.

Brisman and associates[41] reported a sibship in which bronchogenic carcinoma of the same histologic type occurred in four siblings. However, chance must be considered in such anecdotal reports.

Individual family investigations[30,40-42] have provided clues about the etiology of cancer development, but studies on large numbers of extended kindreds will be required in order to comprehend the significance of the variable cancer components of putative hereditary cancer-prone syndromes. For example, a complex spectrum of cancer (SBLA syndrome) has been observed to be transmitted as an autosomal dominant trait in certain kindreds wherein lung cancer has been an integral lesion.[43-45]

I. Twin Studies

Twin studies have, for the most part, been unrewarding in the elucidation of lung cancer etiology. One possible noteworthy exception is that of Joishy et al.[46] who described 58-year-old identical twin males who manifested alveolar cell carcinoma with nearly synchronous onset and similar histologic features. Both showed metastases to the brain. Each twin had had a two to three pack per day smoking history beginning at age 17. It was postulated that the genotype shared by these twins determined not only the susceptibility of pulmonary cells to malignant transformation, but moreover, the character of the resultant neoplasm, including its histologic features and metastatic behavior.

II. LUNG CANCER: LABORATORY GENETIC EPIDEMIOLOGY

A. Aryl Hydrocarbon Hydroxylase (AHH) Inducibility and Smoking-Associated Cancer

Aryl hydrocarbon hydroxylase (AHH) is a major activator of carcinogens which belong to the polycyclic aromatic hydrocarbon (PAH) group. This enzyme is a genetically determine intracellular cytochromome p450 mixed function oxygenase (MFO).

Kellerman et al.[47] were the first investigators to demonstrate high AHH inducibility and an underrepresentation of low AHH inducibility in patients with lung cancer. Other investigators have corroborated these findings in retrospective studies of patients with laryngeal,[48] oral,[49] and pulmonary carcinoma.[50] Guirgis et al.[50] confirmed the observations of Kellerman et al.[47] in a case/control study of AHH in lymphocytes from lung cancer patients and normal controls. Gelboin,[51] in a recent review has suggested that AHH has a complex role in many smoking-related human cancers.[52] In a still more recent review of the subject, Trell et al.[53] suggests that studies to date support the concept of AHH as ". . . a potential activator of tobacco smoke carcinogens of PAH type mainly when these affect the respiratory tract and/or oral cavity."

In spite of these observations, the evidence is insufficient to prove a cause-effect relationship. Thus, in spite of more than a decade of investigation of AHH, its promise as a marker for genetic susceptibility to cancer remains to be proven. We believe that prospective investigations of well-defined lung cancer-prone kindreds and cancer-free families with AHH inducibility comparisons among low risk individuals (members of cancer-free kindreds) with high risk patients (members of lung cancer-prone families) could provide valuable information about the interrelationships between genetics, environment, and carcinogenesis.

B. Debrisoquine Hydroxylase and Lung Cancer Susceptibility

The investigation of host factors which may perturb susceptibility to cigarette smoking-associated cancer, particularly lung cancer, has received priority attention. This has led to the search for a polymorphic gene which might play an important role in the control of metabolic oxidative activation of chemical carcinogens. Ayesh et al.[54] have recently focused attention upon debrisoquine 4-hydroxylation. This enzyme separates into two human phenotypes, each of which harbors characteristic metabolic capability. They investigated the frequency of debrisoquine 4-hydroxylation phenotype in age-, sex-, and smoking history-matched lung cancer patients and controls. Of interest was the finding that ". . . lung cancer patients showed a preponderance of probably homozygous dominant extensive metabolizers (78.8%) with few recessive poor metabolizers (1.6%) compared with smoking controls (27.8% and 9.0%, respectively). We conclude that the gene controlling debrisoquine 4-hydroxylation may be a host genetic determinant of susceptibility to lung cancer in smokers and that it represents a marker to assist in assessing individual risk." These data merit further investigation, ideally in the context of the same methodologic design as suggested above for AHH; namely, its identification in lung cancer-prone vs. lung cancer "resistant" kindreds.

C. Cytogenetics: Sister Chromatid Exchange

Dosaka et al.[55] have studied the inducibility of sister chromatid exchanges (SCE) by benzo(a)pyrene (BP) in cultured peripheral blood lymphocytes from 15 untreated lung cancer patients and 25 healthy persons. The controls were divided into 11 high and 14 low cancer risk categories which were tentatively classified by their family history of lung cancer as well as other neoplasms.

SCE frequency in cultured lymphocytes was found to be significantly high in the lung cancer patients when compared with the total group of healthy individuals or those who were in the low cancer risk category. Following exposure to BP, the lymphocytes among the lung cancer affecteds, as well as the patients in the high cancer risk category, demonstrated significantly increased SCE yields when compared to those individuals who were assigned to the low risk category. However, a significant difference was not observed in the lymphocyte SCE yields when the levels of lung cancer patients were compared with the total group of all healthy individuals. When a comparison was made of the net SCE increase in BP-exposed lymphocytes among the respective study groups, a significant difference in the SCE increased values was found between the high and low cancer risk patients. The authors concluded that the observed SCE yields and the net SCE increased values suggested that ". . . lymphocytes of high-risk individuals may be more susceptible to BP-induced DNA damage than those of persons at low-risk, and that such a chromosomal hypersensitivity to genotoxins may be associated with a high risk of neoplasms."

Dosaka et al.[55] suggested that the observed greater SCE response in lymphocytes of high cancer risk individuals ". . . may be associated with a defective repair of BP-induced damage in such cells. In fact, an impaired DNA repair capacity has been implicated in an increased frequency of basal and genotoxin-induced chromosome aberrations or SCEs in cells of patients with cancer-prone 'chromosome breakage syndromes'. Moreover, an association of DNA repair impairment and chromosomal instability has recently been stressed in relation to genetic instability in human populations. Further studies employing some other genotoxins, each with a different mode of action, such as an alkylating agent, DNA-intercalator, ionizing radiation, and UV light, may yield a better understanding of the mechanisms underlying the observed differences in lymphocyte SCE responses."

These investigations have clearly tested hypotheses of genetic/environmental interactive phenomenon through a laboratory epidemiologic approach employing modern technology of SCE in context with the employment of a well defined carcinogen (BP). The model utilizing lung cancer patients in context with a comparison of individuals who are, albeit, healthy but assigned to high and low familial cancer risk categories, thereby harbors a powerful potential for testing hypotheses relevant to cancer susceptibility in humans through a noninvasive approach. Furthermore, this phenomenon is of particular interest in light of recent observations by Hsu et al.[56] wherein cultured lymphocytes or fibroblasts of patients with differing types of familial cancer showed an enhanced sensitivity to chemical or physical genotoxins, as revealed by differences in chromosome aberrations.

III. SUMMARY

In this short chapter, we have traced the genetic epidemiology of lung cancer, with focus upon a variety of chemical carcinogens, geographic migratory patterns, lifestyle, a specific genetic isolate (Inuites-Canadian Eskimos), and family studies involving a consecutive series of lung cancer probands, case/control family studies, and COPD and lung cancer association. We also discussed lung cancer in a laboratory genetic epidemiologic approach employing aryl hydrocarbon hydroxylase, debrisoquine hydroxylase, and sister chromatid exchange studies. These investigations clearly indicate the need for a multidisciplined approach to this most common form of cancer death in most areas of the world, namely, carcinoma of the lung.

REFERENCES

1. **Iannuzzi, M. C. and Miller, Y. E.,** Genetic predisposition to lung cancer, *Semin. Resp. Med.,* 7, 327, 1986.
2. **Lynch, H. T., Kimberling, W. J., Markvicka, S. E., et al.,** Genetics and smoking associated cancers: a study of 485 families, *Cancer,* 57, 1540, 1986.
3. **Harris, C. C., Autrup, H., Vahakangas, K., and Trump, B. F.,** Interindividual variation in carcinogen activation and DNA repair, in *Genetic Variability in Responses to Chemical Exposure,* Cold Spring Harbor, Cold Spring Harbor, NY, 1984, 145.
4. **Vahakangas, K., Autrup, H., and Harris, C. C.,** Interindividual variation in carcinogen metabolism, DNA damage, and DNA repair, in *Methods of Monitoring Human Exposure to Carcinogenic and Mutagenic Agents,* IARC Scientific Publications, Lyon, 1984, 85.
5. **Harris, C. C., and Trump, B. F.,** Human tissue and cells in biomedical research, *Surg. Syn. Pathol. Res.,* 1, 165, 1983.
6. **Doll, R. and Peto, R.,** Mortality in relation to smoking: 20 year's observations on male British doctors, *Br. Med. J.,* ii, 1525, 1976.
7. **Hammond, E. C.,** Smoking habits and air pollution in relation to lung cancer, in *Environmental Factors in Respiratory Disease,* Lee, H. K., Ed., Academic Press, New York, 1972.
8. **Burbank, F. and Fraumeni, J. F.,** U.S. cancer mortality: nonwhite predominance. *J. Natl. Cancer Inst.,* 49, 649, 1972.
9. **Buell, P. E., Mendez, W. M., and Dunn, J. E.,** Cancer of the lung among Mexican immigrant women in California, *Cancer,* 22, 186, 1968.
10. **Fraumeni, J. F. and Mason, T. J.,** Cancer mortality among Chinese Americans, *J. Natl. Cancer Inst.,* 52, 659, 1974.
11. **Fraumeni, J. F.,** Respiratory carcinogenesis: an epidemiologic appraisal, *J. Natl. Cancer Inst.,* 55, 1039, 1975.
12. **Blot, W. J. and Fraumeni, J. F.,** Geographic patterns of lung cancers: industrial correlations, *Am. J. Epidemiol.,* 103, 539, 1976.
13. **Blot, W. J. and Fraumeni, J. F.,** Arsenical air pollution and lung cancer, *Lancet,* ii, 142, 1975.
14. **Bechlake, M. R.,** Asbestos related diseases of the lung and other organs: their epidemiology and implications for clinical practice, *Am. Rev. Resp. Dis.,* 114, 187, 1976.
15. **Doll, R.,** Strategy for detection of cancer hazards to man, *Nature,* 265, 589, 1977.
16. **Lynch, H. T.,** *Cancer Genetics,* Charles C Thomas, Springfield, IL, 1976.
17. **Mulvihill, J. J.,** Host factors in human lung tumors: an example of ecogenetics in oncology, *J. Natl. Cancer Inst.,* 57, 3, 1976.
18. **Tokuhata, G. K. and Lilienfeld, A. M.,** Familial aggregations of lung cancer in humans, *J. Natl. Cancer Inst.,* 30, 289, 1963.
19. **Beaudry, P. H.,** Pulmonary function survey of the Canadian eastern Arctic Eskimo, *Arch. Environ. Health,* 17, 524, 1968.
20. **Schaefer, O., et al.,** The changing pattern of neoplastic disease in Canadian Eskimos, *Can. Med. Assoc.,* 112, 1399, 1975.
21. **Steinitz, R.,** Pulmonary tuberculosis and carcinoma of the lung, *Am. Rev. Resp. Dis.,* 92, 758, 1965.
22. **Campbell, A. H. and Guilfoyle, P.,** Pulmonary tuberculosis, isoniazid, and cancer, *Br. J. Dis. Chest,* 64, 141, 1970.
23. **Berroya, R. B. et al.,** Concurrent pulmonary tuberculosis and primary carcinoma, *Thorax,* 26, 384, 1971.
24. **Toth, B. and Toth, J.,** Investigation on the tumor producing effect of isonicotinic acid hydrazide in ASW/Sn mice and MRC rats, *Tumori,* 36, 315, 1970.
25. **Van Der Wal, A. M. et al.,** Cancer and chronic nonspecific lung disease (CNSLD), *Scan. J. Resp. Dis.,* 47, 161, 1966.
26. **Fisher, R. A.,** *Smoking: the Cancer Controversy. Some Attempts to Assess the Evidence,* Oliver and Boyd, Edinburgh, 1959.
27. **Sellers, T. A., Ooi, W. L., Elston, R. C., Chen, V. W., Bailey-Wilson, J. E., and Rothschild, H.,** Increased familial risk for non-lung cancer among relatives of lung cancer patients, *Am. J. Epidemiol.,* 126, 237, 1987.
28. **Ooi, W. L., Elston, R. C., Chen, V. W., Bailey-Wilson, J. E., and Rothschild, H.,** Increased familial risk for lung cancer, *J. Natl. Cancer Inst.,* 76, 217, 1986.
29. **Samet, J. M., Humble, C. G., and Pathak, D. R.,** Personal and family history of respiratory disease and lung cancer risk, *Am. Rev. Resp. Dis.,* 134, 466, 1986.
30. **Cohen, B. H.,** Chronic obstructive pulmonary disease: a challenge in genetic epidemiology, *Am. J. Epidemiol.,* 112, 274, 1980.

31. **Lynch, H. T.,** Clinical, epidemiologic, and genetic considerations in lung cancer, Pulmonary Disease: Defense Mechanisms and Populations at Risk, Wyatt, J. P., Harris, T. O., and Clarks, M. A., Eds., Proc. THRI Symposium-2, Lexington, April 12 to 14, 1977.
32. **Davis, A. L.,** Bronchogenic carcinoma in chronic obstructive pulmonary disease, *JAMA,* 235, 621, 1976.
33. **Beaumont, F., Jansen, H. M., Elema, J. D., Ten Kate, L. P., and Sluiter, H. J.,** Simultaneous occurrence of pulmonary interstitial fibrosis and alveolar cell carcinoma in one family, *Thorax,* 36, 252, 1981.
34. **Landing, B. J. and Dixon, L. G.,** Congenital malformations and genetic disorders of the respiratory tract, *Am. Rev. Resp. Dis.,* 120, 151, 1979.
35. **Sheft, D. J. and Moskowitz, H.,** Pulmonary muscular hyperplasia, *Am. J. Roentgenol. Radium Ther. Nucl. Med.,* 93, 836, 1965.
36. **Kodaira, Y., Akiyama, H., Morikawa, M., and Shimiza, K.,** Pulmonary blastoma in a child, *J. Ped. Surg.,* 11, 239, 1976.
37. **Cavin, E., Masters, H. J., and Moody, J.,** Hamartoma of the lung: report of one malignant and three benign cases, *J. Thorac. Cardiovasc. Surg.,* 35, 816, 1958.
38. **Koch, B.,** Familial fibrocystic pulmonary dysplasia: observations in one family, *Can. Med. Assoc. J.,* 92, 801, 1965.
39. **McKusick, V. A. and Fisher, A. M.,** Congenital cystic disease of the lung with progressive pulmonary fibrosis and carcinomatosis, *Ann. Intern. Med.,* 48, 774, 1958.
40. **Goffman, T. E., Hassinger, D. D., and Mulvihill, J. J.,** Familial respiratory tract cancer: opportunities for research and prevention, *JAMA,* 247, 1020, 1982.
41. **Brisman, R., Baker, R. R., Elkins, R., and Hartmann, W. H.,** Carcinoma of the lung in four siblings, *Cancer,* 20, 2048, 1967.
42. **Jones, F. L., Jr.,** Bronchogenic carcinoma in three siblings, *Bull. Geisinger Med. Cent.,* 29, 23, 1977.
43. **Lynch, H. T., Mulcahy, G. M., Harris, R. E., Guirgis, H. A., and Lynch, J. F.,** Genetic and pathologic findings in a kindred with hereditary sarcoma, breast cancer, brain tumors, leukemia, lung, laryngeal, and adrenal cortical carcinoma, *Cancer,* 41, 2055, 1978.
44. **Li, F. P. and Fraumeni, J. F.,** Soft-tissue sarcomas, breast cancer, and other neoplasms: a familial syndrome?, *Ann. Intern. Med.,* 71, 747, 1969.
45. **Li, F. P. and Fraumeni, J. F.,** Familial breast cancer, soft-tissue sarcomas, and other neoplasms, *Ann. Intern. Med.,* 83, 833, 1975.
46. **Joishy, S. K., Cooper, R. A., and Rowley, P. T.,** Alveolar cell carcinoma in identical twins: similarity in time of onset, histochemistry, and site of metastases, *Ann. Intern. Med.,* 87, 447, 1977.
47. **Kellerman, G., Shaw, C. R., and Luyten-Kellerman, M.,** Aryl hydrocarbon hydroxylase inducibility and bronchogenic carcinoma, *N. Engl. J. Med.,* 289, 934, 1973.
48. **Trell, E., Korsgaard, R., Hood, B., Kitzing, P., Norden, G., and Simonsson, B. G.,** Aryl hydrocarbon hydroxylase inducibility and laryngeal carcinomas, *Lancet,* ii, 140, 1976.
49. **Trell, E., Bjorlin, G., Andreasson, L., Korsgaard, R., and Mattiasson, I.,** Carcinoma of the oral cavity in relation to aryl hydrocarbon hydroxylase inducibility, smoking, and dental status, *Int. J. Oral. Surg.,* 10, 93, 1981.
50. **Guirgis, H. A., Lynch, H. T., Mate, T., et al.,** Aryl hydrocarbon hydroxylase activity in lymphocytes from lung cancer patients and normal controls, *Oncology,* 33, 105, 1976.
51. **Gelboin, H. V.,** Editorial retropsectives: carcinogens, drugs, and cytochromes p-450, *N. Engl. J. Med.,* 309, 105, 1983.
52. **Arnott, M. S., Yamauchi, T., and Johnston, D. A.,** Aryl hydrocarbon hydroxylase in normal and cancer populations, in *Carcinogens: Identification and Mechanisms of Action,* Griffin, A. C. and Shaw, C. R., Eds., Raven Press, New York, 1979, 145.
53. **Trell, L., Korsgaard, R., Janzon, L., and Trell, E.,** Distribution and reproducibility of aryl hydrocarbon hydroxylase inducibility in a prospective population study of middle-aged male smokers and nonsmokers, *Cancer,* 56, 1988, 1985.
54. **Ayesh, R., Idle, J. R., Ritchie, J. C., Crothers, M. J., and Hetzel, M. R.,** Metabolic oxidation phenotypes as markers for susceptibility to lung cancer, *Nature,* 312, 169, 1984.
55. **Dosaka, H., Abe, S., Sasaki, M., Miyamoto, H., and Kawakami, Y.,** Sister chromatid exchange induction by benzo(a)pyrene in cultured peripheral blood lymphocytes of lung cancer patients and healthy individuals with or without familial history of neoplasms, *Int. J. Cancer,* 39, 329, 1987.
56. **Hsu, T. C., Cherry, L. M., and Samaan, N. A.,** Differential mutagen susceptibility in cultured lymphocytes of normal individuals and cancer patients, *Cancer Genet. Cytogenet.,* 17, 307, 1985.

Chapter 18

GENETIC EPIDEMIOLOGY OF BREAST CANCER

Henry T. Lynch, Joseph M. Marcus, Patrice Watson, Theresa Conway, Mary Lee Fitzsimmons, and Jane F. Lynch

TABLE OF CONTENTS

I. INTRODUCTION

Familial clustering of breast cancer had been recognized in the Roman medical literature of 100 A.D.[1] In spite of this long, historical experience, surprisingly little knowledge has emerged with respect to its biological significance and its frequency in the general population. Elucidation of fundamental pathogenetic phenomena which might explain its distinctive natural history when compared to its sporadic counterpart should be given high priority. Problems which clearly confound the search for breast cancer etiologic oncogenic events, both genetic and environmental, or their interaction, are the very common occurrence of breast cancer, its extant heterogeneity (particularly with respect to the potential for differing tumor combinations in certain breast cancer-prone families) and the present lack of any consistent biomarker(s) which have high sensitivity and specificity to breast cancer-prone genotype(s).

A. Animal Studies

Animal studies[2] have suggested that breast cancer may be due to a combination of genes and/or introduction of the mouse mammary tumor virus (MTV). Controversy has surrounded the subject of comparing the etiology of breast cancer in mice and man, and for the most part, these have pertained to the putative role of MTV.[3-6] It is important in this context to realize that not all mice that harbor MTV develop mammary tumors. This fact compels one to consider other factors, including hormones (particularly estrogens), immunological factors, diet, composition of the target organ per se, as well as host of genetic factors in mammary carcinogenesis.[1-9]

B. Human Studies

Broca,[10] the famed French surgeon, published the first significant report of a pedigree depicting familial breast cancer and associated malignant neoplasma. He traced the cause of death in 38 members of his wife's family through 5 generations between 1788 and 1856. Of the 24 women in the family, 10 died of breast cancer (Figure 1). Dr. Broca had recognized the importance of documenting cancer of *all* anatomic sites, and noted an excess of cancer of the gastrointentinal tract as well. He expressed his concern about the possibility of the inheritance of a general diathesis for cancer in this family. The significance of cancer of all anatomic site and the tumor site heterogeneity in hereditary breast cancer genetics was not

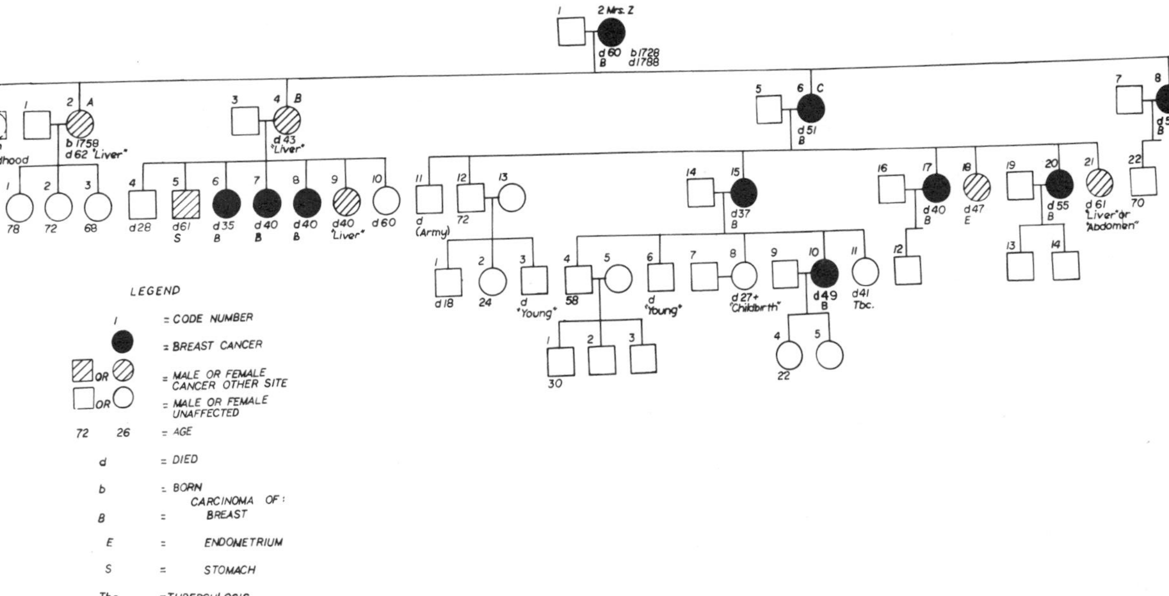

FIGURE 1. Pedigree of Broca's family constructed from a review of his original paper. (From Lynch, H. T., Krush, A. J., Lemon, H. M., et al., *JAMA*, 222, 1631, 1972. With permission.)

given any systematic attention until Lynch et al.[11] described tumor associations in breast cancer-prone families. These kindreds were then classified in terms of specific cancer-prone genotypes. Evidence has accumulated rapidly since this report in support of the contention that heterogeneity, as reflected by consistent patterns of differing tumor aggregations within certain families, is mandatory for the evaluation of patients at risk for hereditary breast cancer.[1] This matter will be discussed in greater detail subsequently.

Macklin[12] published a study on breast cancer familiality in 1959. She described a series of 295 breast cancer probands, a corresponding number of patients with "other cancer", and a third group of patients who lacked a positive history of cancer. This study focused upon the family history involving siblings, parents, and paternal as well as maternal grandparents, aunts, uncles, and cousins of these patients and controls. Breast cancer rates, based on person-years of observation for the respective classes of relatives, were compared to age-specific mortality data for the state of Ohio, where the investigation took place, as well as for the entire U.S. Although the rates for relatives of "other cancer" and "unaffected" patients corresponded very closely to expectations for the state and country as a whole, differences were noted for various classes of relatives of breast cancer-affected women, compared with statewide rates. Specifically, rates were elevated among grandmothers, mothers, aunts, and married sisters, indicating that female relatives of breast cancer patients were, on the average, more susceptible to breast cancer than were female relatives of unaffected women or women with "other cancer".

When considering breast cancer etiology in humans, just as at the infrahuman level, one of the biggest hurdles we must leap is its profound heterogeneity. Thus, when considering this pervasive problem, it would be quite short-sighted to insist on searching for the specific cause of the disease(s). Such a journey would be not unlike the proverbial problem of comparing oranges and apples. Central to this entire problem is the very concept espoused throughout this book — namely, genetic epidemiology — which compels us to search for the interaction of multiple factors, genetic and nongenetic, each of which must interact to a variable degree in order for the phenotype (cancer) to become manifest. A schematic (Figure 2) depicts our hypothesis of variable genetic and environmental interactions in cancer etiology.

II. PATHOLOGY

A. Precancer Mastopathies

Elucidation of the etiology of precancer mastopathies should aid in providing a fuller comprehension of those multiple etiologic events which contribute to frank breast cancer. The etiology of any type of cancer must be viewed in the context of a multifactorial cascade of events. In the case of breast cancer, factors related to these events include diet, socioeconomic status, geographical/residential background, endocrine factors, medications of all varieties, ionizing radiation, and other carcinogenic exposures, all occurring in concert with host (genetic) factors. While we remain ignorant about the specific details of breast (cancer) carcinogenesis, it is clear that malignant transformation requires a multistep process which involves (1) an *initiation* event which may occur as long as 2 or 3 decades prior to the detection of the primary tumor mass, (2) *promotional* events which precede phenotypic transformation, (3) the *transformation* event per se, after which cells manifest typical histologic and biologic features of cancer, and (4) both early and late *progression* events, manifest by local tumor spread and widespread metastases.

When considering "precancer" lesions and frank cancers of the breast (or cancer of any other organ), it is essential for the cancer geneticist and epidemiologist to be fully cognizant of histological variations and their significance to genetic epidemiology. We define a "precancerous" lesion as a histpathological aberration of tissue associated with increased cancer

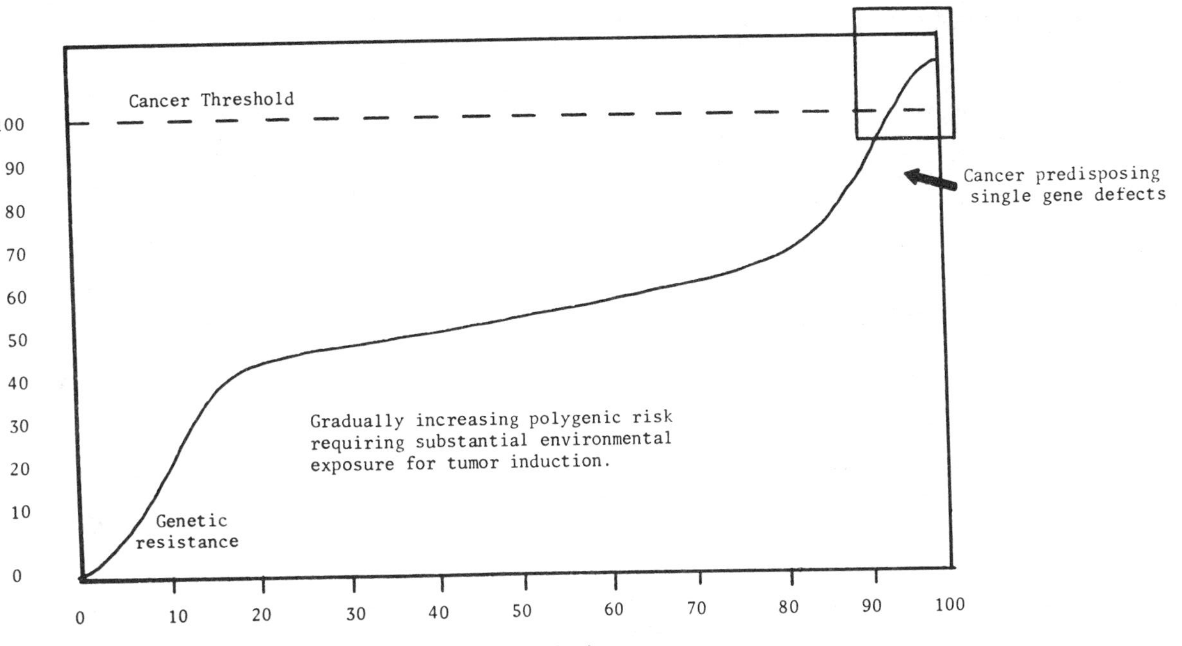

FIGURE 2. Schematic showing genetic/environmental interaction in human carcinogenesis based on variation in degree of inborn cancer susceptibility to cancer in single-gene determined diseases. (From Lynch, H. T., et al., *Prev. Med.*, 9, 231, 1980. With permission.)

risk. This definition neither implies that ultimate cancer occurrence is by any means mandatory, nor that a necessary cause/effect relation between the precancer lesion and the cancer exists. We only state that a breast with a precancerous lesion has an increased probability for undergoing a malignant neoplastic change.

Precancer mastopathies have been identified as proliferative diseases that include typical and atypical ductal and lobular hyperplasias and ductal and lobular carcinoma (neoplasia) *in situ*.[13-15] These exist on a spectrum of increasing risk for subsequent development of breast cancer. Thus, if the hyperplasia is moderate or florid (with the epithelium piling up to more than four cell layers thick), or a papilloma is present with a fibrovascular core, the increased risk is only slight, about 1.5 to 2 times, compared to a normal population. If the hyperplasia is "atypical" — i.e., with some features of carcinoma *in situ*, but not enough to make the actual diagnosis — then the risk is moderately increased to roughly fivefold. Patients with ductal or lobular carcinoma *in situ* are at a high (eight- to tenfold increased) risk of developing invasive carcinoma. Lobular carcinoma (neoplasia) *in situ* is regarded more as a marker for the development of subsequent invasive carcinoma and is associated with a high incidence of bilaterality, while ductal carcinoma *in situ* is more a determinate lesion with a high chance of invading. Even so, there does not appear to be proof than any more than 50% of ductal carcinomas *in situ* in the clinical setting are precursors of invasive carcinoma.[16,17]

The concept of graded risks, based substantially on the recent work of Page and Dupont,[13,14] represents an evolution in thinking that has been adopted by the College of American Pathologists in its Consensus Statement on precancerous breast lesions.[15] Of particular interest is the interaction of positive family history of breast cancer with the hyperplasias and atypical hyperplasias of proliferative breast disease. Thus, patients with atypical hyperplasias, but without a family history, have a 3.5-fold increased risk for developing breast cancer (95% confidence interval, 2.3 to 5.5), while for those with a family history, the increased relative risk is 8.9 (95% confidence interval, 4.8 to 17),[13] nearly the same as for carcinoma *in situ* in women without a family history. Of equal significance is the assessment of risk in women with proliferative disease without atypia, which represents a much larger group (26.7% of benign breast biopsies compared to 3.6% for proliferative disease with atypical hyperplasias). Those without a family history have a 1.5-fold increased risk (95% confidence interval, 1.2 to 1.9), while those with a family history are at a 2.1-fold increased risk (95% confidence interval, 1.2 to 3.7).[13] This represents hardly any difference, and should be some reassurance to those women with and without family histories whose biopsies fall into this disease category. Similarly, in the even larger group (69.7%) with benign biopsies without proliferative disease, family history does not increase breast cancer risk.[13]

Rosen et al.[18] have recently described juvenile papillomatosis as a special type of hyperplasia (Figure 3). Of the 180 patients in their registry, 9 presented concurrently or subsequently with *in situ* or invasive carcinoma, and of these, 5 (56%) had a positive family history, compared to a 26% positive family history in juvenile papillomatosis patients without cancer.[19] While these numbers are suggestive, they appear too small as yet to statistically associate juvenile papillomatosis and family history of breast cancer, and as the authors point out, further cases are needed.[19]

B. Significance of Breast Cancer Morphology and Genetic Epidemiology

Page and Anderson[20] have extensively reviewed the subject of breast cancer pathology and its correlates with clinical expression. They note that particular histologic subsets differ widely in prognosis, ranging from tubular cancers with 5-year survival approaching 95% to "ductal" or no special type (NST), a histologically and prognostically heterogeneous group that averages a 60% or less 5-year survival.

Questions of immediate concern to these histopathology subsets are "Do primary genetic factors play a role in determining this histopathologic variance?" and "How do environ-

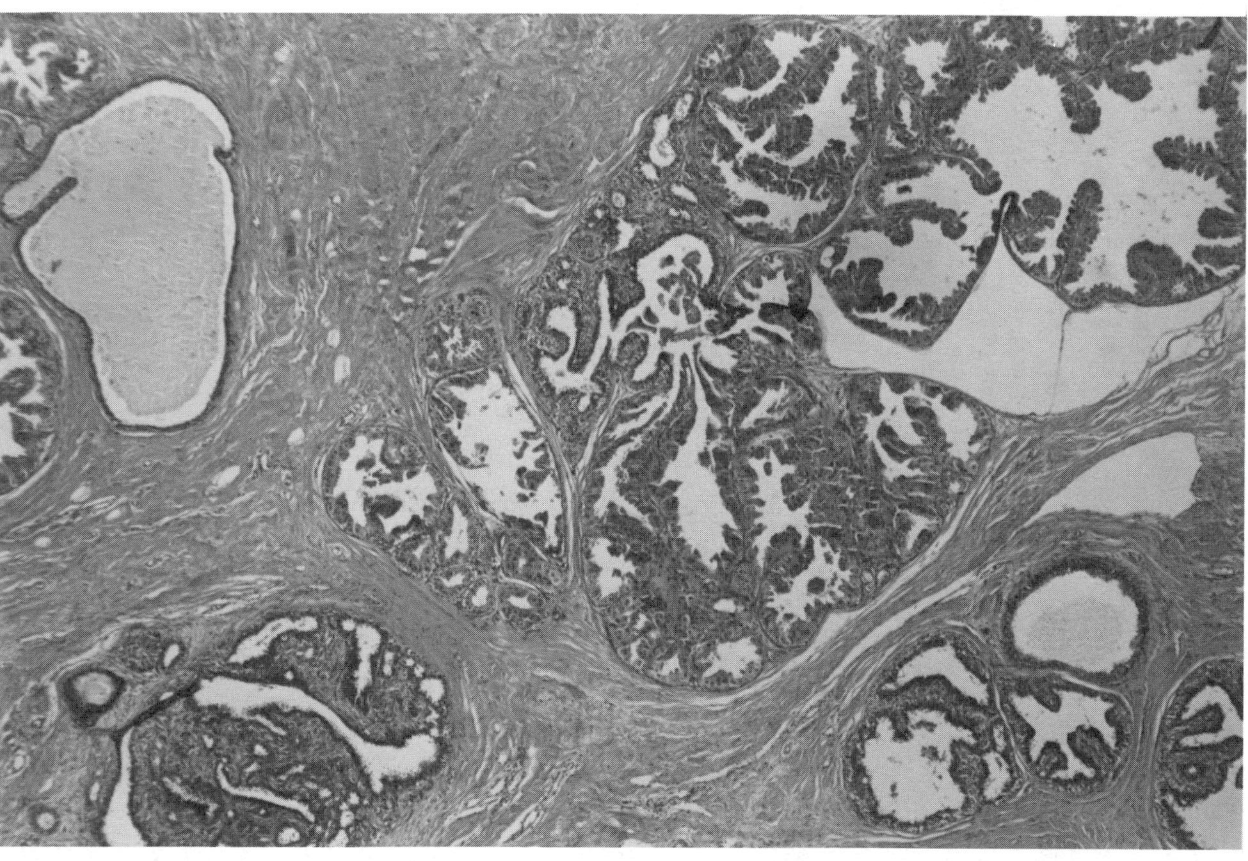

FIGURE 3. Juvenile papillomatosis in a breast biopsy from a 21-year-old woman. Fibrosis, cystic duct dilatation, papillary ductal hyperplasia, and apocrine metaplasia are present. Some evidence suggests a possible association of this recently described lesion with family history of breast cancer. H & E stain, magnification × 30.

mental factors such as diet, alcohol consumption, cigarette smoking, exogenous hormones, and irradiation exposures interact with host factors in determining breast cancer phenotype?'' Genetic linkage markers will aid immeasurably in the identification of genotypic status for studies of the etiologic of histologic differences which will be particularly important in the light of prognostic and survival differences for these differing histologies.[1,21]

Preliminary evidence is emerging in support of our hypothesis for etiologic association between primary genetic factors and these putative histopathology discriminants.[1,22] For example, an association between tubular carcinoma histology (Figure 4) and several parameters associated with HBC was identified in the investigation of 211 consecutive mastectomies.[23] Based on these results, it was suggested that ''...tubular carcinoma may be a histologic marker for a subpopulation of patients with mammary carcinoma strongly associated with multicentricity, bilaterality, and familial history of mammary carcinoma.''

In a study of the breast cancer family resource at Creighton University School of Medicine, Mulcahy and Platt[22] performed microscopic examinations of female breast cancers in pedigrees with two or more first degree relatives. The study was blinded, with the concurrently studied comparison group comprised of nonage-matched sporadic (nonfamilial), breast cancer-affected patients. Their results showed that tumors occurring in the familial subset were not confined to a single histopathologic category, but rather, encompassed a wide spectrum of histopathologic diagnoses. Although there was no high morphologic specificity in the familial breast carcinomas as a group, there nevertheless were suggestions in the data that (1) the familial tumors showed an increased frequency of medullary histologic type (Figure 5), either with or without lymphoid stromas and (2) within individual breast cancer pedigrees, there were concentrations of histologically similar tumors. Other workers have also found suggestions of excess medullary histology in familial breast carcinomas in which the hereditary nature of the pedigrees was not ascertained in the manner set forth in this chapter. Earlier, Anderson[24] had shown an excess of medullary carcinoma in patients with sisters, but not mothers, with breast cancer, while Rosen et al.[25] have observed that women with medullary carcinoma are more likely to have mothers with breast cancer.

The Mulcahy and Platt[22] finding of excess medullary carcinoma in hereditary breast cancer is tantalizing, but the control group was not age matched and there is some indication that medullary carcinoma may be more common in young age groups.[22] Marcus and colleagues[26] have been performing a double-blinded case/control study of breast cancer histology from among affected individuals from clearly defined hereditary breast cancer-prone kindreds with comparison of both age- and race-matched breast cancer controls from kindreds with sporadic breast cancer (an absence of breast cancer through second degree relatives). Slides from mastectomies are being reviewed and the tumors classified histologically according to the WHO system[27] modified to include invasive cribriform carcinoma as a separate category, and to subdivide invasive lobular carcinoma into subtypes.[20] Medullary carcinoma was classified as ''typical'' or ''atypical'' according to the criteria of Ridolfi et al.[28]

Preliminary results[26] do not show an association between medullary carcinoma histology and hereditary breast cancer in the age-matched cases but the small size of the current study (31 hereditary and 31 nonhereditary breast cancers) may obscure possible trends. On the other hand, when the data are looked at without age matching, the Mulcahy and Platt finding of excess medullary carcinoma in the hereditary group is confirmed. Further, when compared with age-specific proportions of medullary breast cancer histology in the Surveillance Epidemiology and End Results (SEER) program conducted by the National Cancer Institute (J. L. Young, NCI, personal communication), we find an excess of medullary histology in our hereditary breast cancer group but not in the nonhereditary cancer group. However, since the SEER data did not have central pathology review, it is not clear that the medullary or atypical medullary histologies entered into our and the SEER studies are exactly equivalent. A further finding of interest is a higher mitotic grade (Figure 6) in the NST (infiltrating ductal) carcinomas in the hereditary breast cancer group.

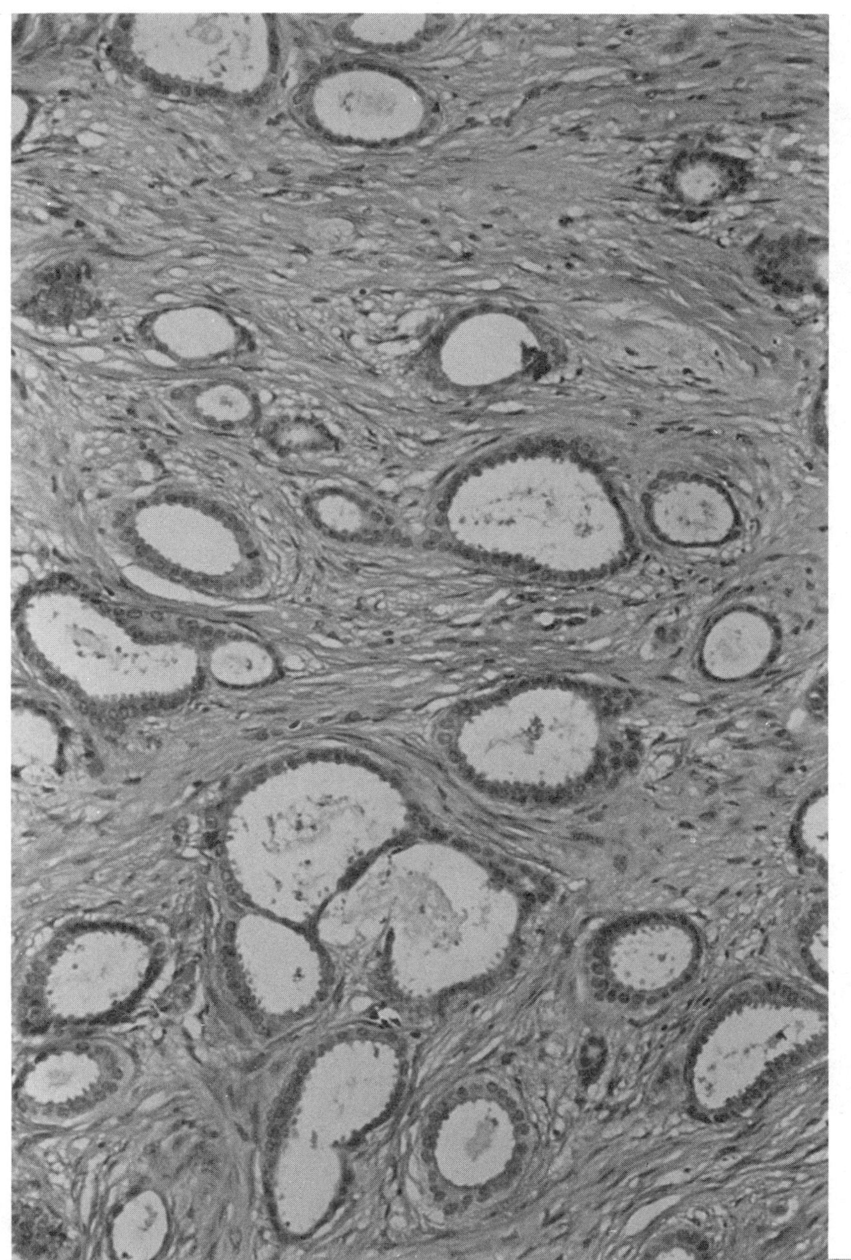

FIGURE 4. Tubular carcinoma of the breast. Tubules are very well formed, and nuclei are small land even-sized. Lagios et al.[23] found an association of this histology to familial breast cancer. H & E stain, magnification $\times$ 30.

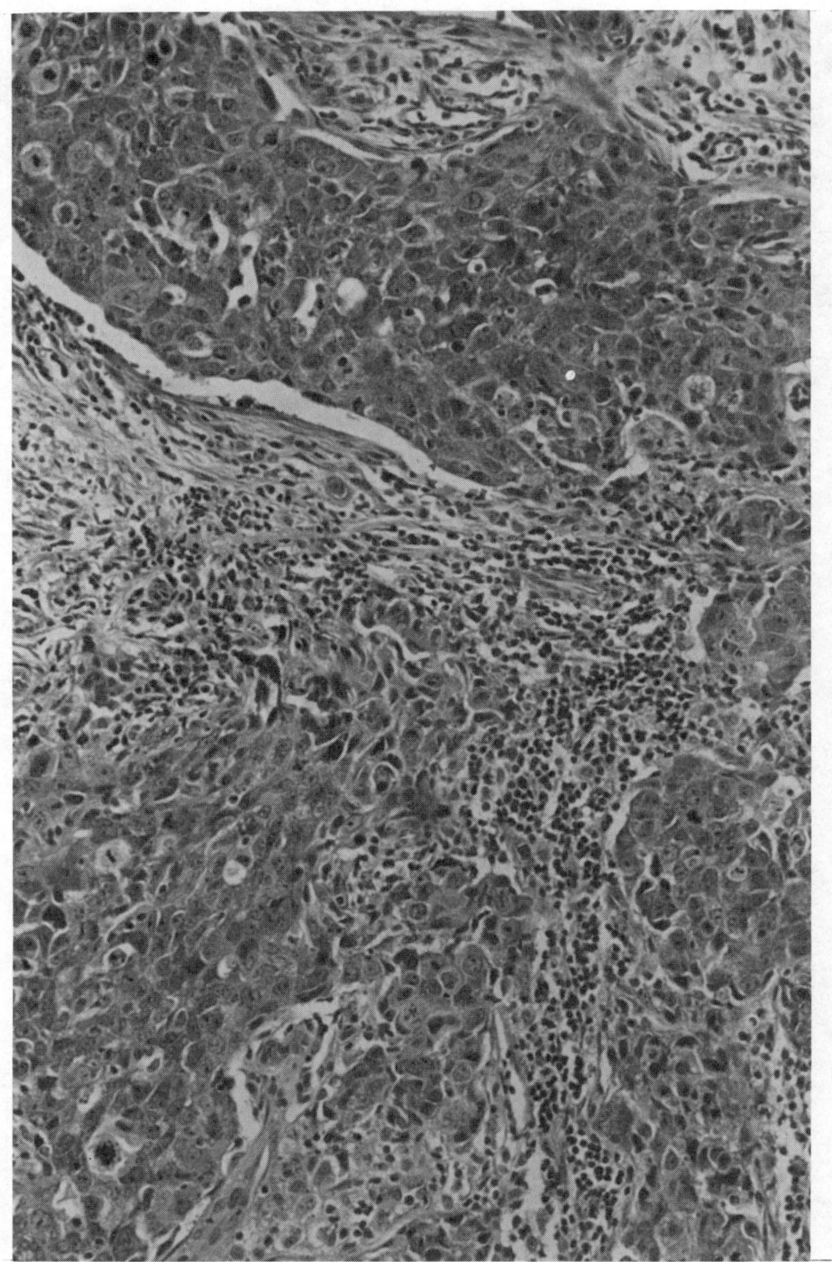

FIGURE 5. Medullary carcinoma of the breast. Interanastomosing islands of large, poorly differentiated cells with a high mitotic rate are present amidst a stroma of lymphocytes. Our ongoing studies continue to show an excess of this histologic type in hereditary breast cancer, which may be age dependent. H & E stain, magnification × 125.

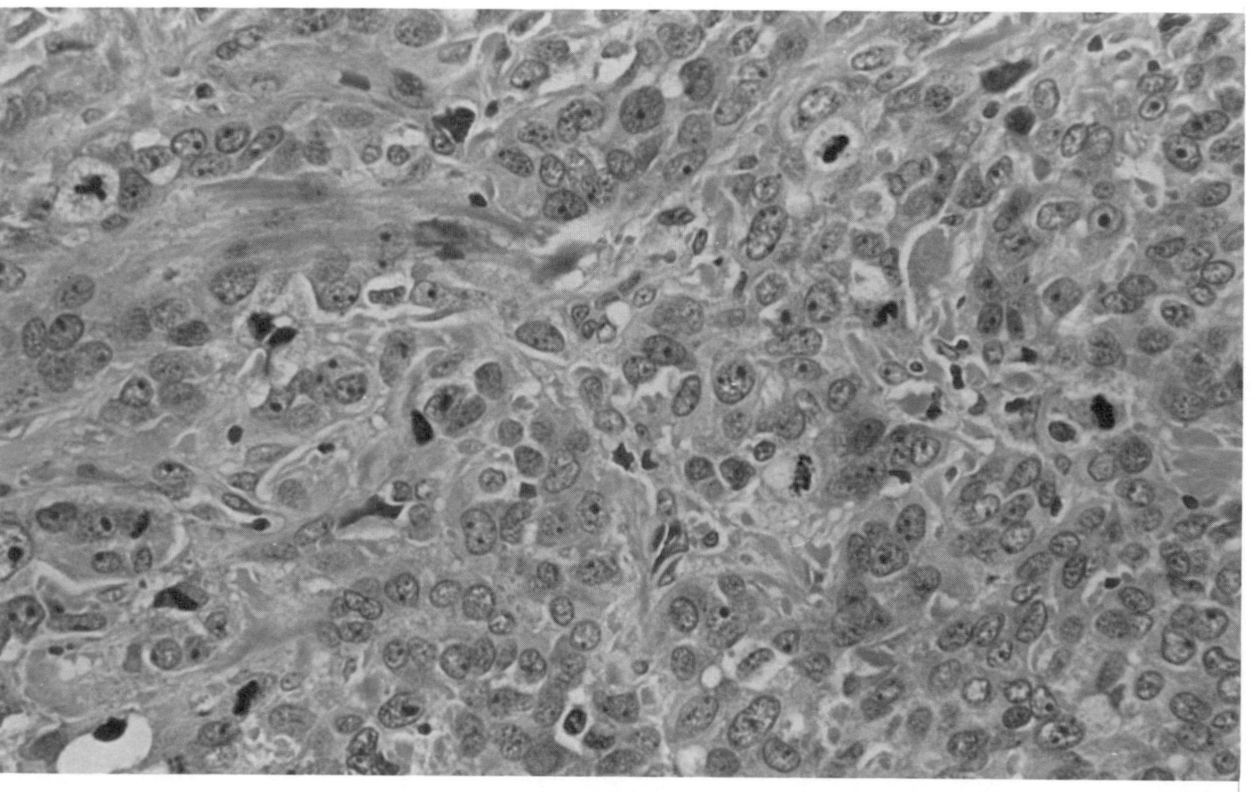

FIGURE 6. Invasive breast carcinoma of ''no special type'' (NST or infiltrating ductal) in the daughter of the patient in Figure 5. The tumor is poorly differentiated with numerous mitoses. Our studies are showing a higher mitotic grade in hereditary breast cancers. H & E stain, magnification × 300.

The question of increased frequency of medullary breast cancer is of further interest because it, as well as certain other tumor types, appear to show a slight increase in frequency in countries of low breast cancer incidence.[29-31] It is possible that in certain areas of the world, the relatively low overall incidence rates of cancer at a specific site may indicate a relatively noncarcinogenic environment, with a consequent increase in the frequency of hereditary cancer *relative* to sporadic cancer.

III. EPIDEMIOLOGY AND BREAST CANCER

A primary objective of epidemiology is to delineate disease distribution in populations and to explain these variations in incidence for differing geographic areas. This knowledge may then be useful for the identification of high risk groups so that appropriate surveillance and management measures might be developed for these target populations. Lifestyle differences between high and low risk groups have been found to be useful for development of hypotheses relevant to etiologic factors. Identification and characterization of populations at high risk have been generally considered to be in the realm of *descriptive epidemiology*. The testing of etiologic hypotheses constitutes *analytical epidemiology*.

Breast cancer has probably received greater attention from the standpoint of both descriptive and analytical epidemiology than any other form of cancer in humans.[1] These have included the study of migrant populations wherein breast cancer incidence has shown remarkable changes in successive generations of immigrants to the U.S. For example, significant excesses of breast cancer have occurred among the descendents of migrants from Japan and other areas of the Orient.

Hormonal factors have also received intensive scrutiny, including an increased risk for breast cancer among women with early onset of menarche and a late natural menopause. Early age at first full-term pregnancy (particularly before age 20) has been shown to be *protective* in that the breast cancer risk is only about one third for these women as opposed to women whose age at first pregnancy occurred after age 30. However, in hereditary breast cancer families, early age at onset of pregnancy did not show any effect on breast cancer occurrence.[32]

In an attempt to test the significance of age at first pregnancy in an HBC setting, Lynch et al.[32] studied age at onset of breast cancer among 162 women at 50% genetic risk, 72 of whom had already developed breast cancer. A comparison was then made to 154 consecutively ascertained breast cancer patients from the Creighton Cancer Center. The findings in the hereditary subset were extremely interesting and are summarized as follows:

1. Early first term pregnancy did not alter the frequency of breast cancer.
2. Early age at first term pregnancy was not associated with an earlier age at cancer diagnosis.
3. Age at breast cancer onset in nulliparous females was not significantly lower than in females having at least one term pregnancy.

Figure 7 shows that those patients with breast cancer from the consecutive series did show a significantly earlier age at diagnosis with an earlier age at first pregnancy. However, among those women from the hereditary population who eventually developed breast cancer, early age at first term pregnancy was not correlated with an earlier onset of breast cancer (t = 1.6, NS), as shown in Figure 8. It is of interest that Woods et al.[33] reported an earlier age at breast cancer diagnosis with an earlier age of first term pregnancy and an earlier age of diagnosis in nulliparous than parous females. However, as discussed, these relationships were not observed in our hereditary population. Thus, the observations demonstrate greater credence to our hypothesis of distinct biological differences between hereditary and sporadic

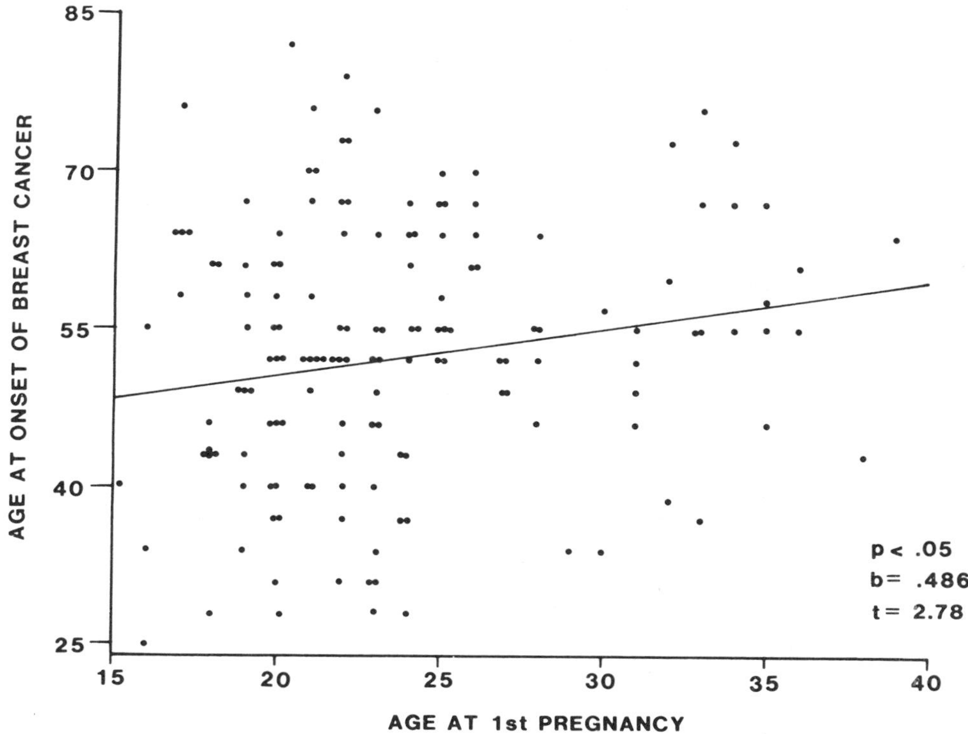

FIGURE 7. Age of diagnosis of breast cancer as a function of age at first term pregnancy in our consecutively ascertained series. (From Lynch, H. T., Albano, W. A., Layton, M. A., et al., *J. Med. Genet.*, 21, 96, 1984. With permission.)

forms of breast cancer, and that pregnancy in the hereditary breast cancer setting does not appear to influence tumorigenesis in the same manner that it does in the so-called sporadic population. The etiologic significance of these observations remains enigmatic. It is possible that differing steriod patterns predispose to oncogenesis in the hereditary population, irrspective of pregnancy status, while the fluctuating levels of estrogens in the sporadic population during pregnancy may influence carcinogenesis to a high degree. It is for this reason that we have suggested pursual of an endocrine hypothesis for elucidation of hereditary breast cancer etiology.[34,35]

Using the rat as an experimental model, chemically induced tumors provided an interesting parallel to our findings in humans. For example, previous pregnancy rendered rat mammary tissue less susceptible to chemical carcinogenesis.[36] However, when the pregnancy followed exposure to the carcinogen, the interval between exposure and the presentation of tumors was shortened.[37,38] This seems to parallel findings in the sporadic population.[33,39]

Finally, we admonish our readers to interpret our data cautiously pending their confirmation in a larger number of well-documented kindreds and giving due attention to the heterogeneity which characterizes HBC. Thus, heterogeneous forms of this disease such as the SBLA syndrome, site-specific hereditary breast cancer, and breast cancer in combination with ovarian cancer, among others, should be investigated in order to see whether stratification for these syndromes might reveal differing results so far as the role of early first term pregnancy as a protective factor in HBC is concerned.

Because of the intense interest in dietary and hormonal factors in breast cancer epidemiology, these matters will now be discussed in relatively greater detail. For a more detailed description of breast cancer epidemiology, please refer to the discussion by Lynch.[1]

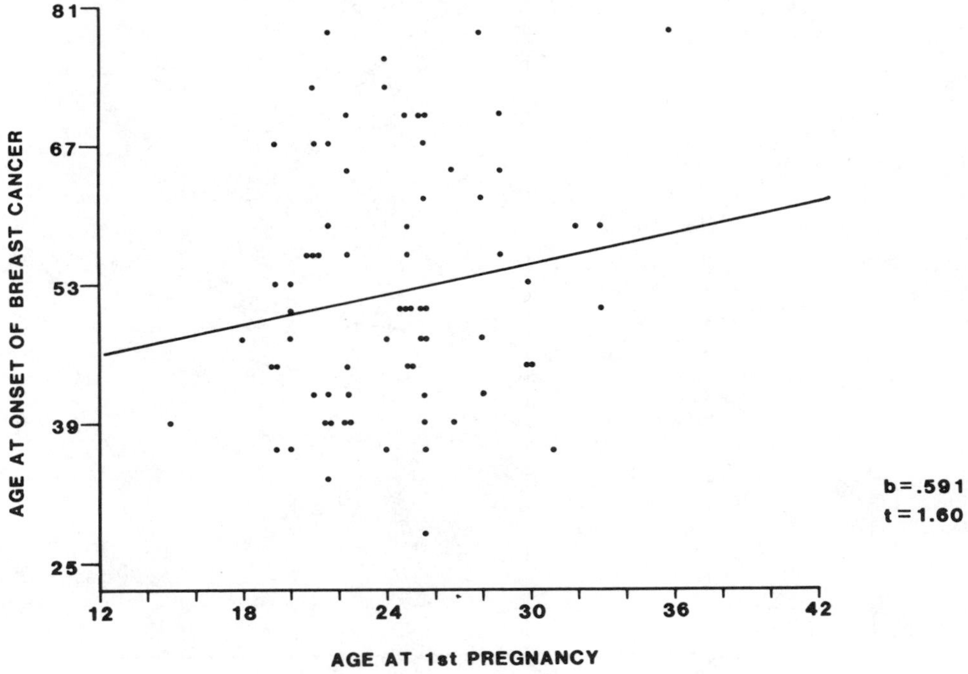

FIGURE 8. Age of diagnosis of breast cancer as a function of age at first term pregnancy in the hereditary subset. (From Lynch, H. T., Albano, W. A., Layton, M. A., et al., *J. Med. Genet.*, 21, 96, 1984. With permission.)

A. Diet, Epidemiology, and Breast Cancer

Unfortunately, genetic-epidemiology concepts have not been applied systematically to the study of diet in breast cancer etiology. Since only a fraction of patients consuming differing diets (discussed below) develop breast cancer, the crucial question regarding the possible role of specific dietary variables in the perturbation of host factors can only be broached in the context of a well-defined dataset which embraces genetic and environmental variables. Thus, the persistent concern of ours, "Why do some women on a given diet (or with other carcinogenic exposures) develop breast cancer while other women on the same diet do not?", cannot be answered in the absence of data pertaining to both endogenous and exogenous factors which may be contributing to carcinogenesis. In other words, are there host factor variables which *lower* the patients' threshold to specific dietary (or other carcinogens) events in breast carcinogenesis?

Diet, particularly high animal fat and protein consumption, has been given strong consideration in the etiology of breast cancer, as well as other forms, particularly colorectal cancer. Dietary hypotheses have been of particular importance in attempts to explain changes in breast cancer risk among migrants such as Japanese who have moved to Hawaii and the west coast of mainland U.S. This subject has been extensively reviewed by Hirohata and associates.[40] These investigators call attention to animal studies which showed that saturated[41,42] and unsaturated[43,44] fat had promoted mammary tumors in rodents. Herein, when both sources of fats were employed in the same study[45-47] polyunsaturated fats showed a tendency to produce higher tumor yields than did saturated fats. In the study by Carroll and Hopkins[48] it was observed that a combination of a large amount of polyunsaturated fats in concert with a small amount of saturated fats resulted in a greater number of mammary tumors in animals when compared to either source of fat alone.

At the human level, a positive association between breast cancer morbidity or mortality and per capital availability of total fat in the form primarily of animal fat in most of the western countries, and animal protein has been observed.[49,50] A similar association with vegetable fat, i.e., primarily unsaturated fats, however, was not observed.[51] There has been a relative paucity of case/control studies which have related the diet of individuals to breast cancer incidence.[52-55]

Because of these problems, Hirohata et al.[40] initiated a case/control study to evaluate the association of dietary fat and animal protein with breast cancer. Attention was focused upon Hawaiian/Caucasian women, who have a high risk for breast cancer, and Japanese women, who have a moderate risk for this disease.[56] This matter was evaluated in concert with the study of breast cancer and diet among Japanese women in Fukuoka, Japan, who were at low risk for breast cancer.[57]

This case/control study involved Japanese and Caucasian women whose ages ranged from 45 to 74 and who were residents of Hawaii. Each case was matched to a hospital and a neighborhood control. There were 183 sets of Japanese and 161 sets of Caucasian individuals. Of interest was the absence of any statistically significant difference between cases and controls relevant to their mean intake of total fat, saturated fat, oleic acid, linoleic acid, animal protein, and cholesterol. This investigation therefore failed to provide strong support for the hypothesis that a high fat diet is a risk factor for breast cancer. This investigation is extremely important for the comprehension of the genetic-epidemiology of diet in breast cancer, and clearly indicates the need for more research in this area, particularly when considering the popular view among the public as well as the research community that dietary factors are the major etiologic components in breast cancer.

The problem of fat consumption, its fat metabolism, and the manner in which it influences breast cancer is exceedingly complex. Other environmental factors, including host susceptibility, must undoubtedly be important. However, insufficient attention has been given to the role of genetic factors. Therefore, we know very little about the way in which genetics might interact with dietary variation, particularly dietary fat in concert with breast cancer risk.[58]

Increased body weight and height have been considered by some investigators to be associated with an increased risk for breast cancer.[59,60] This is important since it is clear that nutrition is an essential limiting factor in height and weight. Genetic factors also play an important role in determining the individual's ultimate height and weight in context with environmental factors. When assessing the role of diet in weight as risk factors, it is important to give careful consideration to the woman's previous body weight and her prior fat consumption history. For example, in prior decades, was her weight above the ideal body weight? Had she achieved her current weight, if below her past or present weight, through vigorous dieting? One should also assess her past and present physical activity since there is evidence suggesting that long-term, regular physical activity may be associated with a lower risk of breast cancer as well as cancers of the reproductive system.[61]

Willet et al.[62] note that the body weight in the adolescent years is important since heavier girls show an earlier age at menarche.[63] Early age at menarche appears to be an important breast cancer risk factor.[64] Given this brief account of those variable exogenous breast cancer risk factors, including diet, one can readily see how genetic factors may be an important etiologic determinant in each of these issues. Primary genetic factors may be important in determining height and weight wherein diet is also a prime factor. Thus, it is short-sighted to view genetics, diet, height, or weight in isolation when considering breast cancer etiology. We have discussed diet at length in order to provide the reader with background into this important area of consideration in breast cancer etiology. It will be essential that future investigations dealing with dietary risk factors in breast cancer give careful consideration to genetic factors and their interaction in the cause of breast cancer.

B. Ethyl Alcohol

Specific dietary habit patterns, such as coffee, tea, or alcohol consumption, as well as other idiosyncratic features of lifestyle of women, must be scrutinized. Recent attention has been focused upon alcohol consumption and the risk of breast cancer.[65,66] These investigations were based upon cohort studies involving about 100,000 women whose alcohol consumption was evaluated before the diagnosis of breast cancer. Other risk factors, including age at first pregnancy, number of pregnancies, and family history of breast cancer (mother affected) were evaluated concurrently and appropriately adjusted for alcohol consumption. In the study by Schatzkin et al, the relative risks associated with alcohol were between 1.4 and 2.0 following the adjustment for the above-mentioned risk factors. Dose-response findings emerged. However, in a review of this study by Graham[67] it was noted that the number of cases was so small that "...even statistically significant estimates need to be viewed cautiously: just a small change in the numbers could affect the estimate of risk per family."

Willet et al.[66] found that the risk of breast cancer in women who had one drink or more per day was 60% higher when compared to the risk in women who did not drink. As in the study by Schatzkin et al.,[65] a dose-response relationship was suggested. An interesting facet of these investigations was that the breast cancer risk was more pronounced in those women with earlier age of breast cancer onset and only moderate drinking was required. For example, in the study of Willet et al.,[66] for those women consuming 5 to 14 g of alcohol daily, which translates into approximately three to nine drinks per week, the age-adjusted relative risk of breast cancer was 1.3 (95% confidence limits — 1.1 and 1.7). When consumption was increased to 15g of alcohol or more per day, the relative risk became 1.6 (95% confidence limits — 1.3 and 2.0; MANTEL extension, X^2 for linear trend = +4.2; $p < 0.0001$) and adjustment for known breast cancer risk factors and a variety of nutritional variables failed to materially alter this relation.

For purposes of understanding genetic/environmental contributions to etiology, it should be noted that nowhere in these investigations were there indications that in-depth family studies were performed. Rather, importance of family history is inferred, apparently only on the basis of disease status in mothers of affected daughters. It would therefore be of value for future investigations to determine the manner in which alcohol might perturb breast cancer risk in the context of hereditary breast cancer. Will it lower the age of onset of breast cancer even more than expected in hereditary breast cancer? Will it increase the incidence of bilaterality? Will it increase the penetrance of the deleterious genotype?

Graham[67] suggests that, given the importance of other risk factors for breast cancer, "...one might recommend, then, that women at especially high risk for breast cancer, such as those who are obese, who have had few children, who were first pregnant when they were older than 25, or *whose mothers had breast cancer* (our emphasis), should curtail their alcohol ingestion.."

IV. HORMONAL STUDIES

A. Historical Background

Clues to the potential importance of hormonal studies in breast cancer etiology began to emerge more than 2 centuries ago through the studies of this disease in nuns in Europe.[68] Herein, an unusually high prevalence of breast cancer was noted in a group of nuns relative to women from the general population. Specifically, initial leads from these studies which revealed a high incidence of breast cancer in nuns centered around the subject of pregnancy and nulliparity. The breast cancer excess among the nuns was attributed to some factor associated with celibacy.

Subsequent studies revealed an excess of cancers of the endometrium and ovary in addition to an excess of breast cancer, with a predilection to onset during middle age among a nun cohort, a phenomenon which also contrasted strikingly with a lower frequency of cancer of the uterine cervix among the nuns.[68] Cervical carcinoma, of course, is now known to be related to early sexual intercourse and intense promiscuity, a lifestyle completely opposite to celibacy.

B. Estrogens as Carcinogens

Hertz[69] has reviewed the history dealing with the relationship between estrogens and cancer, with particular attention given to diethylstilbestrol (DES). This review disclosed a longstanding documentation of the etiologic relationship of estrogens to cancer. This knowledge emanated from the work of Beatson,[70] who showed that ovariectomy ameliorated the clinical manifestations of breast cancer in women. Loeb[71] identified the ovarian dependence of breast cancer in mice. Subsequently, estorgen administration was found to be etiologically linked to cancer involving eight organ sites (breast, cervix, endometrium, ovary, pituitary, testicle, kidney, and bone marrow) in five species of animals (mice, rats, rabbits, hamsters, and dogs).[69] This background clearly indicated prolific activity in experimental carcinogenesis in the 1930s and 1940s, with attention restricted to estrogen compounds. DES, first synthesized by Dodds and associates in 1938,[72] was also significantly linked to carcinogenesis studies in animals[73] and subsequently in humans.[69] In commenting on all available evidence at the infrahuman level, Hertz stated that he knew of "...no other pharmacological effect so readily reproducible in such a wide variety of species which had been generally regarded as potentially inapplicable to man."[69]

It is important that the estrogen-cancer link in animals be cast in proper historical perspective since it clearly should have provided important clues to the potential carcinogenicity of DES. Indeed, on the strength of these early estrogen studies, the search for carcinogenic effect of DES should have been given the highest possible priority, considering the pharmacologic, biochemical, and physiologic similarities between estrogen and DES.[74]

Some of the earliest investigators to pursue this line of reasoning were Shimkin and Grady[74] who began their carcinogenesis studies of DES the same year that the compound was discovered (1938) and published their findings 2 years later. They identified the carcinogenic potency of both estrone and DES in C3H mice, a strain known to have been prone to mammary cancer. They also reviewed numerous papers on DES, uniformly confirming its estrogenic activity and affirming that it was similar to the natural estrogens in all its diverse effects. In demonstrating the carcinogenic potency of DES and estrone in susceptible (C3H) mice, they concluded that "...stilbestrol possesses the property common to all estrogens of eliciting mammary carcinoma in mice of susceptible strains..."[74] They also discussed mammary carcinogenesis in mice treated with massive doses of natural estrogens. While documenting the carcinogenicity of estrogens in mice, Shimkin[75] also defined experimental procedures and emphasized the importance of host factors in the process.

In 1939, Gardner[76] reviewed mammary carcinogenesis in genetically susceptible mice. In mice strains with low incidences of spontaneous mammary cancer, few mammary tumors were produced by estrogen administration, while the converse held in strains (C3H) susceptible to mammary cancer. Of interest was the occurrence of mammary cancer in 11 of 12 *male* mice from a susceptible strain following estrogen administration. On the other hand, tumor development following estrogen administration occurred in excess in males and females from two strains where the incidence of spontaneous neoplasms in the untreated females was less than 2%. Carcinogenicity of stilbestrol had been concurrently advanced by Lacassagne[77] and Geschickter[78] who produced mammary cancer in C3H mice and in rats, respectively.

Carcinogenesis studies were not restricted to breast cancer. For example, in 1938, Gardner et al.[79] described uterine cervical carcinoma following estrogen administration in mice, and in 1956, Gardner and Ferrigno[80] described unusual varieties of cancers of the uterine horns among estrogen-treated mice. These included subserosal uterine adenomas, adenocarcinomas, and epidermoid carcinomas. The subserosal neoplasms were believed to have arisen either from proliferation of Mullerian rests persisting along the serosa, possibly from the serosa per se, or from endometriosis. In 1959, Gardner[81] observed a high incidence of uterine cervical carcinoma, and more frequently, vaginal epidermoid carcinomas, in mice that had been exposed to intravaginal pellets of stilbestrol-cholesterol. Placebos did not incite vaginal cancers in these mice.

Another classic paper on the subject of estrogens and cancer in animals was that of Loeb[82] published in 1940. Again, the importance of heredity was stressed, but drug dosage effect was also clearly recognized. Loeb wrote, "...a strain possessing a strong tendency to the development of mammary gland cancer shows a reaction to a relatively small amount of estrogen similar to that which a strain with a lesser hereditary tendency shows to a larger quantity of estrogen. An added amount of stimulation by estrogens can compensate for a certain difference in hereditary predisposition." This is a crucial commentary, since by using larger doses in less susceptible strains, the same carcinogenic endpoint can be achieved. This observation clearly counters the claims of those investigators who found extrapolations from inbred animal strains to be inappropriate. Loeb[82] also reviewed data dealing with estrogen administration to specific strains leading to the production of carcinoma of the cervix. In addition to carcinoma or precancerous lesions in the cervix, he also noted that corresponding changes may be induced over wide areas of the vagina. For example, "The formation or lack of formation of cancerous changes depends upon quantitative differences in tissue response, and these differences may apply to individuals, strains, and species. In the latter, they are, as a rule, greater than between different strains of the same species, and these species differences apply to tissue reactions in general."[82]

In summary, Loeb[82] provided an extensive review of the literature supporting a direct association between hormone administration (estrogens and stilbestrol) and cancer production in susceptible strains. While emphasis was given to mammary carcinoma, carcinoma of the cervix and vagina in susceptible strains was also discussed. These findings therefore show a spectrum of estrogen and DES-induced tumors in animals.

Hertz[69] noted that substantial skepticism was raised about the extrapolation of carcinogenesis studies in nonprimate species to primates (and ultimately, humans) because of the failure to induce malignant transformation by estrogen in monkeys. However, Gardner[76] noted that while cancer had not been observed in monkeys, there were changes in the tissues of monkeys following estrogen administration:

1. Many mitotic figures in the breast of one monkey following prolonged estrogen treatment.
2. Proliferation of the mammary ducts and epithelium in a Rhesus monkey after injection of small amounts of estrone. The ductal epithelium was described as being hyperplastic and poorly organized and was compared to clinical gynecomastia.
3. Cystic hyperplasia of the endometrium was described following daily estrogen injections in monkeys.
4. Epithelial metaplasia of the uterine cervical glands occurred in monkeys following daily administration of estrogen for 16 to 90 days.

Attention was also given to the morphologic similarity of the cervix of the monkey to that of the human being.[76]

The question of endocrine involvement in the etiology of breast cancer has been investigated intensively in many laboratories.[39,83-97] These studies have focused primarily on identifying possible differences in endocrine profiles between women with breast cancer and normal controls. The results obtained have been conflicting, and have failed to reveal any consistent differences which could be related to the presence of disease. A valid argument can be made that the initiation of events which result in subsequent clinical manifestation of the disease occurs in the hormonal milieu of the early premenopausal and postpubertal period, and that therefore, this is the relevant age at which possible endocrine differences need to be examined.[88,97-101] For prospective studies of this type, evaluating individuals from the general population presents major technical problems in view of the large numbers of subjects required and the long time span before the results can be correlted with the disease.

An alternative to studying larger populations, where breast cancer etiology may be considerably heterogeneous, would be the study of premenopausal unaffected women who are at a predictable hereditary risk for breast cancer. They could then be compared with carefully matched controls who do not have a positive family history of breast cancer. Such an approach was employed by Fishman et al.[34,35] It involved an in-depth study in which hormone levels throughout the menstrual cycle in 30 young women at high risk for familial breast cancer were compared with 30 matched controls. No significant differences between these populations were observed in the plasma levels of prolactin, luteinizing hormone, follicle-stimulating hormone, estrone, estradiol, or estriol at any stage of the menstrual cycle, although a consistent trend toward lower values in all of these except estriol was noted in the high risk population.[34] Analysis of urinary metabolites on the other hand revealed highly significant differences in estrone and estradiol glucuronides, with the high risk individuals excreting lower amounts of these metabolites than the controls.[35] These investigations have now been extended to include differences in urinary estrone sulfate and in plasma androsterone sulfate content. Plasma androsterone sulfate was significantly lower in the high risk subjects. A compensatory increase in the urinary estrogen sulfates was observed. Day-by-day analysis of these differences showed that they were most pronounced in the periovulatory period of the cycle. It was concluded that the genetic risk for breast cancer is associated with an abnormality in estrogen conjugation at a specific time of the ovulatory cycle.[102]

Increasing attention has been focused on estrogen-16 α-hydroxylase and its products, 16 α-hydroxyestrone and estriol, because of evidence that 16 α-hydroxylation is increased in women with breast cancer.[103] In addition, there are preliminary data indicating that this reaction is increased prior to the onset of breast cancer and that the increase is not a result of the disease. Dr. H. Leon Bradlow (Rockefeller University) has observed that this reaction is elevated in mice that develop malignant mammary tumors (C3H/OuJ) and is quite low in mice that do not develop mammary tumors (C57/Br/J). These findings were present when the mice were 6 weeks of age, well before the onset of tumor development (personal communication).

16 α-Hydroxyestrone, the initial product of 16 α-hydroxylation, possesses a combination of unusual biological properties. It is highly estrogenic in spite of only minimal binding affinity for the classical estrogen receptor.[104] In addition, it circulates free in blood because it does not bind to the sex hormone binding globulin and most importantly it possesses the unique property of forming covalent bonds with primary amino groups of proteins.[105] This latter property provides a mechanism for their long-term presence in target cells either by linking to the receptor itself or the chromatin regulatory proteins. It is possible that the decrease in the excretion of E_1 and E_2 glucuronides which have been described[34,102] is compensated for by an increase in urinary α16-OH-estrone present as either the glucuronide or the sulfate. Suggestive data for increased sulfation of the parent hormone in the high risk patients may account, in part, for increased 16 α-hydroxylation since it has been reported that estrone sulfate is a preferential precursor for 16 α-hydroxylation over the free compound.[106]

The issue of the role of exogeneous estrogens in breast cancer has been a vexing one, as evidenced by conflicting findings from one study to the next. We discuss it in the present setting because it is possible that patients at genetic risk for breast cancer may be predisposed either to direct effects of exogeneous estrogen or they may have inherited benign breast disease which, given the presence of additional risk factors (including estrogen), could cause them to undergo a complex set of interactions. For example, exogeneous estrogen + other risk factors such as oophorectomy + specific forms of benign breast disease may interact to produce epithelial hyperplasia or papillomatosis, which may then lead toward the production of breast cancer.

For example, recent data by Thomas et al.[107] showed a very complex relationship between multiple factors and association with exogeneous estrogen. The risk of breast cancer was found in their study of 1439 white women who were initially treated for biopsy-proved benign breast disease from 1942 to 1975, and who were followed through 1976 for development of breast cancer. The so-called traditional risk factors as age at menarche and birth of first child, nulliparity, and to a lesser extent, age at artificial menopause, were related to the risk of breast cancer. Of interest was the fact that exogeneous estrogen, when taken prior to the initial benign breast disease, did not alter breast cancer risk. However, subsequent use (here primarily involving conjugated estrogens) eliminated the protective effect of artificial menopause and "...appeared to act synergistically with epithelial hyperplasia or papillomatosis in the initial lesion and calcification of that lesion to increase the risk of breast cancer." Another interesting finding was that of a marked increase in risk of breast cancer in succeeding breast cancer cohorts, a phenomenon which could not be explained by simple changes in any of the other risk factors which were under consideration. Unfortunately, the role of genetics was not investigated in this interesting study.

Needed will be a painstaking effort at prospective studies of patients from breast cancer-prone families who are users of oral contraceptives (OCs), and ideally, biopsies where benign breast disease is suspected. In context with this approach, a systematic study of all known risk factors, with meticulous recording of estrogen usage (with quantity and type, as well as duration) will be essential in order to determine whether or not a particular risk is present, and if so, a quantitative determination of the full impact of the subject risk and/or its interaction with other risks will be required. Confounding the issue will be problems of genetic heterogeneity: the risk may vary in patients and families prone to carcinoma of the breast and ovary vs. those with site-specific hereditary breast cancer vs. those with the SBLA syndrome, or other hereditary variants of breast cancer.

Epidemiologic evidence suggests that the endocrine milieu in the early reproductive years of a woman's life determines the risk for the development of breast cancer many years later.[108] If one accepts this assertion, then endocrine studies conducted following the diagnosis of breast cancer could be misleading relevant to the etiologic role of hormonal factors in the onset of breast cancer. It logically follows that prospective studies of endocrine profiles obtained well in advance of the onset of breast cancer would be more meaningful. An example of such a study is one which has been ongoing on the Isle of Guernsey. Results form this study suggest the existence of endocrine differences related primarily to the androgenic hormones which appear to correlate with increased risk for breast cancer.[109,110]

Black and Zachrau[111] have studied relationships between environmental and genetic factors in breast cancer etiology, collecting data on a variety of endogenous and exogenous characteristics among breast cancer patients. Information included age, parity characteristics, menstrual history, the use of exogenous estrogens in the form of OCs as well as replacement estrogens and family history of breast cancer, among both maternal and paternal family members. They assumed that mammary carcinogenesis involved a stepwise process which includes precancer mastopathy and *in situ* carcinoma. They observed that when age, complete family history, and OC usage were considered, the findings showed that OC usage was preferentially associated with young patients with invasive breast cancer whose grandmothers or aunts had breast cancer.[112-114] More specifically, Black and Zachrau[111] found that OC usage promoted the development of invasive breast cancer among the grandmother- (paternal or maternal) and aunt- (paternal or maternal) positive women in the age range of 20 to 39 years. Furthermore, these investigators found that among such women, OC usage was preferentially associated with cancerous breast lesions of more agressive nuclear grade. They use a nuclear grading system with grade I as most agressive and grade III as least agressive (whereas most workers today use grade I and grade III in the opposite sequence). "...with poorly differentiated nuclei, i.e., nuclear grade (NG) I...the proportions of patients using oral contraceptives were similar among those patients whose breast tumors were rated NG II-III regardless of their FH characteristics, namely, 33 — 47%. On the other hand, among young patients with NG I breast cancer, OC usage was observed significantly more frequently in the grandmother/aunt-positive than the FH-negative series. In the NG I series overall, OC usage was found in 31 (69%) of 45 FH-positive patients in contrast to 15 (32%) of 47 FH-negative patients ($p < 0.001$). A tendency toward selective association between OC usage, FH, and NG was also observed among 40 — 49 year old patients."

These investigators concluded that there are subpopulations of women whose mammary parenchyma is particularly susceptible to malignant transformation during their youth, and that such susceptibility is more pronounced among women whose grandmothers or aunts manifested breast cancer. Thus, these observations imply that the familial association "...appears to involve an unusual sensitivity to female sex hormones in the form of oral contraceptives. It further appears that such sensitivity is genetically, rather than socially, determined, since the involved relatives are equally likely to be paternal as well as maternal."

Thus, the work of Black and Zachrau are fully in accord with an ecogenetic explanation for at least one subset of the breast cancer population, namely, those women with early onset breast cancer who have positive family histories of breast cancer and who use OCs. There is certainly a preventive note in this line of reasoning. Specifically, Black and Zachrau urge investigators of mammary carcinogenesis to intensify their efforts on endogenous and exogeneous variables relevant to the development of precursor lesions as well as the precursor-to-invasive cancer progression. With respect to precursor-to-invasive cancer progression, it may be possible to identify factors which enable retardation of progression in addition to those phenomenon that promote progression. They suggest that such an approach may also aid in the identification of endogenous and/or environmental variables "...whose manipulation will reduce the incidence of breast cancer. Finally, we suggest that the creation of a database pertinent to the above goals would be most efficiently accomplished by the *routine* collection of epidemiologic data and by precise classification of breast lesions at the time of diagnosis. As suggested previously, such practices should be an integral part of the responsibility of physicians charged with the diagnosis and treatment of breast lesions."

The study of estrogen metabolism, while influenced by host factors (as already discussed), may be significantly perturbed by other agents, including cigarette smoking. For example, Michnovicz et al.[115] recently described the mechanism responsible for smoking-induced changes in 2-hydroxylation and postulated that this may be useful in the development of strategies to reduce the risk of hormone-dependent tumors. We therefore see a highly complex process involving host factors, cigarette smoking, and their influence upon estrogen metabolism. The next vexing problem to be resolved pertains to whether or not there is an interaction between host factors and cigarette smoking effect upon estrogen metabolism and, if so, whether this effect is additive or multiplicative. These would be fruitful areas for research, particularly using breast cancer-prone kindreds as investigational models.

V. GENETIC CONSIDERATIONS

A. Operational Definition of Sporadic, Familial, and Hereditary Breast Cancer

There have been a plethora of studies by investigators from all parts of the world showing so-called *familial* aggregations of breast cancer.[1,116] Consensus suggests that the presence of breast cancer in a first degree relative increases a woman's risk of developing breast cancer two- to threefold.[1,117] Sattin et al.[118] recently found that the relative risk (RR) to a woman with an affected first-degree relative was 2.3; to women with an affected second degree relative, it was 1.5; and to women with both an affected mother and sister, the RR was 14. Ottman et al.[119] studied breast cancer risk to sisters of breast cancer patients in a population-based series of patients diagnosed in Los Angeles County between 1971 and 1975. They observed that sisters of patients with bilateral breast cancer diagnosed at 50 years or younger had an RR = 5 and the risk increased for sisters of bilateral patients diagnosed at age 40 years or younger (RR = 10.5). Sisters of unilateral patients diagnosed at 50 years or younger did not show a significantly increased breast cancer risk. However, sisters of unilateral patients diagnosed at age 40 years or younger had an RR = 2.4. These studies clearly indicate the existence of families in the general population which show a statistical predisposition to breast cancer.

These epidemiological studies of risk associated with a positive family history have not assumed any specific type of genetic mechanism to account for these results. However, an alternative approach has been taken which assumed that some of the familial aggregation was caused by segregation of major breast cancer susceptibility gene(s). Thus, a search has been made for family histories consistent with this hypothesis. In our own investigations, we have classified families as sporadic, familial, or hereditary, using the following operational definition.

1. Sporadic

A pedigree is tentatively classified as sporadic if the proband or index case is the only case of breast cancer among the members of the modified nuclear family of the proband — the offspring, siblings, parents, aunts, uncles, and grandparents of the proband. In other words, these are cases with a negative family history of breast cancer. It will be recognized that this definition does not rule out hereditary factors in the cancer of the proband. A new germinal mutation is always possible. Also, some pedigrees are quite uninformative, e.g., those with no female relatives on the paternal side of the proband family, preventing expression of the breast cancer phenotype. However, with present technology, any such hereditary cases are undetectable.

2. Familial

All nonsproadic cases are tentatively classified as familial, in which the breast cancer-affected proband has a positive family history of breast cancer in a daughter, sister, mother, aunt, or grandmother. Inclusion in this category does not imply that hereditary factors are involved in the cancer of the proband. Multiple cases of breast cancer can occur completely by chance within a simple family. Also, there may be shared environmental exposures among family members which increase cancer risk.

3. Hereditary

Pedigrees are selected, mainly from the familial category, for inclusion in the hereditary category if the pattern of cancer occurrence within the family is consistent with Mendelian inheritance of an autosomal dominant susceptibility gene. Factors which support this classification include the occurrence of early onset cancer, bilateral breast cancer, multiple primary cancer, and diagnoses of cancer at certain nonbreast sites which have been observed in association with breast cancer in hereditary breast cancer syndromes, such as the combination of breast and ovarian cancer. Usually an extended pedigree is required for this decision to be made, especially since in the case of breast cancer, the males in the pedigree are presumed to be able to transmit but generally not to express the trait. Occasionally, cases with a negative breast cancer family history are classified as hereditary when the family history of other cancers combines with the breast cancer in the proband in a pattern consistent with a known hereditary syndrome which includes breast cancer susceptibility, such as SBLA (described subsequently). Notice that this definition focuses on the pattern of inheritance produced by a dominant major gene (very high rates of cancer in offspring of affecteds and carriers; very low rates in offspring of unaffecteds) rather than a recessive major gene, as this is the usual pattern for previously documented, inherited cancer susceptibility disorders.[120] Note also that this definition cannot be made objectively (as can the tentative decision of sporadic vs. familial) but must be made by expert judgment of multiple factors in a situation of incomplete information. We acknowledge the fallibility and difficulty of such a system, but know of no better one in lieu of identified biomarkers of breast cancer-prone genotypes of sufficient sensitivity and specificity.

B. Segregation Analysis

Our genetic hypothesis for cancer has been tested by Go et al.[121] on 18 families from our hereditary breast cancer family resource. Each family had been ascertained on the basis of its containing a cluster of breast cancer cases. In two of these families, the familial cancer aggregation appeared to be of nongenetic origin, while in two others, mean age of breast cancer diagnosis was very early (31.3 and 32.0 years), and the families were characterized by an excess of childhood cancers rather than breast cancers. These particular families fit the diagnosis of the SBLA syndrome, discussed subsequently. The remaining 16 families were divided into 2 groups: group I comprised 12 families (1548 individuals) with mean age at diagnosis ranging from 44.9 to 52.0 years; group II comprised 4 families (463 individuals) with mean age at diagnosis ranging from 54.4 to 68.4 years. It was hypothesized that in the group I families, there was a dominant gene segregating that increased susceptibility to either breast or ovarian cancer. Female carriers of the gene in these families had an estimated lifetime risk of 0.9 to either of the two cancers, whereas noncarriers of the gene had a trivially small risk to either cancer. Furthermore, the age of onset was hypothesized to be lognormally distributed. In the group II families, on the other hand, it was hypothesized that female carriers of the dominant gene were completely susceptible, i.e., they had a lifetime risk of unity, if they lived long enough, to either breast cancer or endometrial cancer.

Goldstein et al.[122] performed complex segregation analyses on breast cancer in 200 families with bilateral breast cancer. Two analyses of these data were performed. The first was restricted to premenopausal cases of breast cancer affecteds. Results showed that Mendelian transmission of a single locus was not sufficient to explain the observed distribution of premenopausal breast cancer. The authors concluded that the major locus plus other transmission, i.e., a mixed model (genetic and/or cultural factors), was necessary to explain the distribution.

The second analysis combined postmenopausal cases with the premenopausal cancer occurrences and considered that all of the breast cancer patients were affected with the same disorder. Findings from this "all cases" analysis could not reject the mixed model "...with no generation differences in heritability when tested against the general model which allows for generation differences (i.e., the likelihoods for the two models were not significantly different)." The authors concluded that the ultimate resolution of genetic and environmental etiologies for explaining familial aggregation will only be achieved when environmental variables are measured and incorporated into genetic epidemiologic analyses. They concluded that "...future studies on breast cancer need to carefully define affection and to incorporate the findings from various disciplines into studying this disorder. Epidemiologists, geneticists, and clinicians need to collaborate on research and discuss the different methodologies used to begin to develop more informative ways of studying complex disorders like breast cancer. Without adequately combining information from all of these disciplines, the etiologies of human breast cancer will remain unfathomable."

C. Early Age of Onset of Hereditary Breast Cancer

A prior review of age at onset of breast cancer in Creighton's hereditary breast cancer resource showed the average age to be 44 years.[123] In certain of the families, a trend toward virtually all premenopausal onset occurred, while in others, postmenopausal onset predominated. Occasional families were encountered, however, wherein the pattern of extraordinarily early age of onset occurred. These families may represent an ascertainment selection bias because of the very fact that cancer is occurring at such an early age, that is, this is the very reason the families came to our attention. On the other hand, this may represent a true biological phenomenon and merit surveillance programs geared to the extraordinarily early age of onset within the specific kindreds.

At the present time, we lack a biomarker(s) of sufficient sensitivity and specificity to determine who *is* vs. who is *not* an obligate breast cancer-prone gene carrier. Thus, we cannot resolve the issue as to whether or not such families represent a statistical artifact or whether they in fact indicate a severe early onset biological variant of hereditary breast cancer.

There is a serious dilemma revolving around the best possible surveillance/management program to be employed when a high risk relative and/or the managing physician recognizes a familial aggregation of profound early age of onset of breast cancer in his practice. If this is a statistical artifact, we may unnecessarily cause alarm, anxiety, or apprehension among high risk patients. In addition to this emotional burden, we will be subjecting these patients to enormous expense, inconvenience of lifelong intensive surveillance, including extra radiation exposure from mammography. Contrariwise, should this be a genetically determined phenomenon, then at-risk women who are not under intensive surveillance may unnecessarily sustain severe morbidity and early mortality because of the lack of attention to a disease which is wholly unexpected to occur at such a very eary age.

D. Early Age of Onset as a Discriminant of Familial/Hereditary Breast Cancer Risk

We studied age of breast cancer onset among 328 consecutively ascertained patients with breast cancer who were undergoing treatment in our oncology clinic. These patients were classified by our operational definition of sporadic, familial, or hereditary breast cancer. The findings from this study were extremely interesting. Specifically, we noted breast cancer to occur more frequently in the relatives of young (< 40) breast cancer probands as opposed to the relative of older (≥ 40) breast cancer probands ($p < 0.001$; RR = 2.2). A statistically nonsignificant trend ($p < 0.09$; RR = 1.6) for an excess occurrence of breast cancer among the relatives of young hereditary breast cancer probands was found when compared to relatives of older hereditary breast cancer probands. Early onset breast cancer occurred more frequently among relatives of young breast cancer than among relatives of older breast cancer probands ($p < 0.001$; RR = 24). Finally, we noted early onset of breast cancer to occur more frequently among the relatives of older hereditary breast cancer probands ($p < 0.003$; RR = 27). These findings harbor important implications for initiation of surveillance in hereditary breast cancer-prone kindreds wherein early onset (< 40) of this disease occurs. Given the estimate of about 7 to 8 years lead time for breast cancer development from the time of its initial mitotic event to a malignant transformed cell, it would seem prudent that daughters or sisters of breast cancer-affected individuals from the direct line of descent in the hereditary breast cancer setting begin mammography by age 20 years. We recommend that these patients continue with mammography annually thereafter. In addition, we recommend that they practice self breast examination by their late teens, at which time, they should begin to undergo biannual examinations of their breasts by a physician who is skilled and knowledgeable about the natural history of hereditary breast cancer, including the indications for this very early surveillance strategy.[124]

E. Earlier Age of Breast Cancer Onset in Daughters of Breast Cancer-Affected Mothers

We have observed an earlier age of onset of breast cancer in the daughters of breast cancer-affected mothers (Table 1).[125] Our source of families wherein female relatives are

Table 1
BREAST CANCER RATES AMONG SISTERS OF MOTHER-DAUGHTER PAIRS

	Cumulative totals		Number with			
Age	Number	Person years	Breast cancer	Other cancer	Living unaffected	Breast cancer risk (%)
Mother's sisters						
50—79	46	843	8	3	16	28
20—49	50	1436	2	2	0	4
20—79	—	—	—	—	—	31
Daughter's sisters						
50—79	23	182	1	2	20	16
20—49	44	1051	6	2	12	17
20—79	—	—	—	—	—	31

prone to breast cancer contains 33 kindreds ascertained by mother-daughter proband pairs with verified breast cancer. The mothers in this group were born on the average in 1894 and their daughters in 1920. The mean age at cancer diagnosis for these parent-offspring pairs was 57.1 years for mothers and 44.0 years for daughters, which constitutes a highly significant ($p < 0.01$) 13-year intrapair difference. Notably, comparable generation differences in the onset of familial breast cancer have been previously reported.[126] However, comparisons such as these have been discounted by some as "fallacies in numerical reasoning"[127] (the fallacy being that a requirement of occurrence of breast cancer in both mother and daughter is deliberately selective for daughters who are affected at an early age, thereby resulting in an artifactual intrapair difference).

To obviate problems related to incomplete follow-up and/or ascertainment, age-specific cancer rates among sisters of the mother-daughter probands were computed and compared (see Table 1). While these data indicate that the cumulative breast cancer rates in the 20 to 79 age bracket are approximately equal for both generations (31%), they also clearly reflect a significantly ($p < 0.05$) higher rate of premenopausal breast cancer (onset before age 50) among sisters of the daughters than sisters of the mothers. On the assumption that random members of these two sister groups have comparable genetic susceptibilities to breast cancer, our data indicate that genotype/environment interactions have resulted in earlier expression of carcinoma of the breast in the later generations of women from these families.

The trend to earlier onset of familial breast cancer shown by our data may be a consequence of changes in the lifestyles of women in western cultures, e.g., the use of estrogens for treatment of menopausal and postmenopausal symptoms which began in the late 1930s, estrogens in oral contraceptives beginning in the 1960s, and many other drugs, including tranquilizers, amphetamines, and antihistamines, which are now being used frequently. In addition, significant changes in nutrition (i.e., overnutrition via increased consumption of meat protein and fats) occurred during this era, producing taller, heavier women with earlier menarche, factors which have been implicated as breast cancer risk milestones.[128] Finally, additional factors such as changes in habits (i.e., cigarette smoking and alcohol consumption) and new occupational exposures relating to technological advances should be considered etiologically in the earlier expression of this disease in genotypically susceptible women.[129]

Since no significant trend in incidence or onset of breast cancer can be substantiated from the data available for large populations,[130,131] we suggest that the alleged carcinogenic effect(s) may be operative primarily in familial breast cancer which comprises a relatively small fraction (perhaps 20 to 25%)[1,132] of the total incidence of the diseased.

It is important to understand that at one time, an earlier age of onset of a disease and/or increased severity in certain hereditary diseases, when appearing in successive generations of families, were considered to be the primary consequences of gene-determined events.

The phenomenon was referred to as "anticipation". However, scientific evidence now clearly shows that the so-called biological implication of anticipation was in error[133] and that a better explanation of earlier onset in hereditary diseases relates either to more sophisticated diagnositc techniques, greater patient awareness of signs and symptoms, or to changing environmental events which influence expression.[134] Thus, we addressed ourselves to the latter set of circumstances as a possible explanation for the earlier onset of breast cancer in our high risk families.[11,124,133]

In summary, earlier age of onset of familial breast cancer may constitute an early warning for specific carcinogenic exposures, some of which may be an accompaniment of the changing lifestyles of women in the 20th century.

F. Extended Breast Cancer-Prone Kindreds

Detailed medical-genetic studies of breast cancer-prone families with meticulous pathology correlation were initiated by Lynch and colleagues[135,136] in the mid-1960s. These investigations have been continuous over the years and now involve several hundred extended kindreds. They have aided in the comprehension of breast cancer genetics. Lynch[1] has emphasized the distinctive natural history of hereditary breast cancer, which is characterized by an earlier age of onset, excess bilaterality, vertical transmission (consonant with an autosomal dominantly inherited factor), heterogeneous tumor associations, and improved survival when compared to its sporadic counterpart.[1,137,138] The literature on hereditary breast cancer has been increasing at a remarkable rate during the past decade. Surprisingly, however, most investigators fail to recognize the clinical nuances of hereditary breast cancer when compared to its sporadic counterpart.[1,137,138] This also includes those already-mentioned familial aggregations of this disease which fail to fulfill creteria for hereditary breast cancer.[138] In addition, there is a paucity of information dealing with interrelationships between environmental breast cancer risk factors and genetics.

Hereditary breast cancer poses a significant public health problem in many of the western industrialized nations. Nevertheless, screening programs for breast cancer are almost invariably based upon general population age-adjusted rates for this disease and fail to consider the *hereditary* issue where the mean age at onset is 44 years. For example, most guidelines for surveillance initiation are somewhere between 40 and 50 years[1] and, consequently, they fail to stratify for the hereditary subset which requires *earlier* screening intervention.

There is a marked paucity of information dealing with the *incidence* of hereditary cases among breast cancer-affected individuals.[116,137] Based upon intensive follow-up of a cohort of 328 consecutively ascertained breast cancer patients from our oncology clinic, our most recent estimates are familial — 26%, hereditary — 8%, and sporadic — 66%.[139]

VI. CLASSIFICATION OF HETEROGENEOUS VARIANTS OF HEREDITARY BREAST CANCER

A. Site-Specific Hereditary Breast Cancer

Site-specific breast cancer infers that the particular pedigree shows a predominance of breast cancer in the *absence* of other histologic varieties of cancer (Figure 9). This is an exceedingly difficult breast cancer genetic diagnosis since it is based primarily upon the *exclusion* of integral patterns of other forms of cancer. For example, if we are dealing with a relatively small kindred, it is then possible that other forms of cancer were not represented simply because of the limited number of at risk subjects. One must therefore be cautious when designating a given family as fitting the so-called site-specific variant of hereditary breast cancer. As a general rule, we consider the possibility that all patients who are first degree relatives of breast cancer affecteds from so-called site-specific breast cancer-prone kindreds may be at some excess risk for cancer of differing anatomic sites.

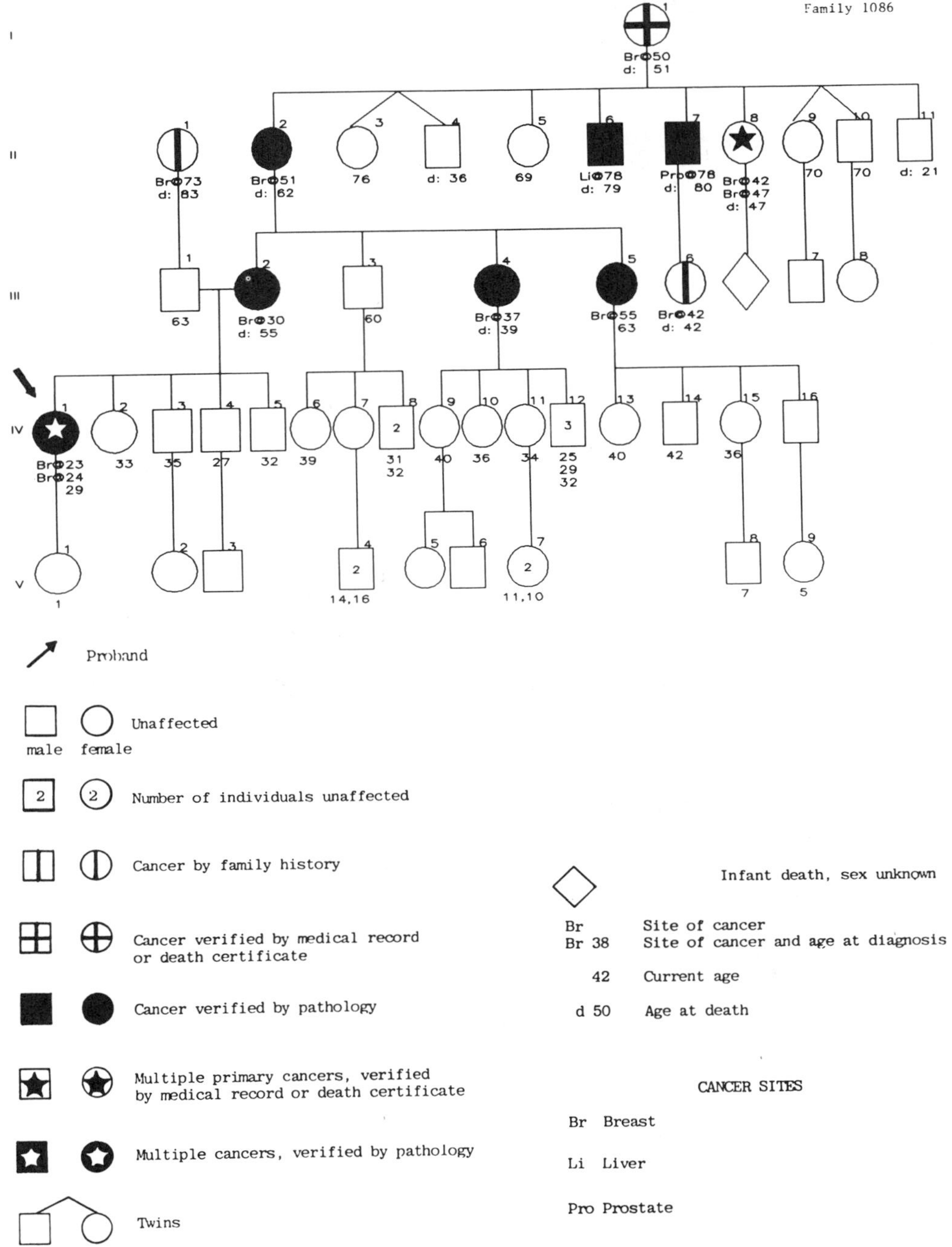

FIGURE 9. Pedigree of a site-specific breast cancer-prone family.

B. Breast/Ovarian Cancer

Based upon the evaluation of 12 breast/ovarian cancer-prone kindreds, Lynch et al.[140] concluded that the findings did not allow discrimination of an exact mode of genetic transmission. However, the findings were compatible with the assumption of transmission of a dominant trait with sex-dependent penetrance, either autosomal or X-linked.

Additional studies of informative pedigrees, such as those seen in Figure 10, will be

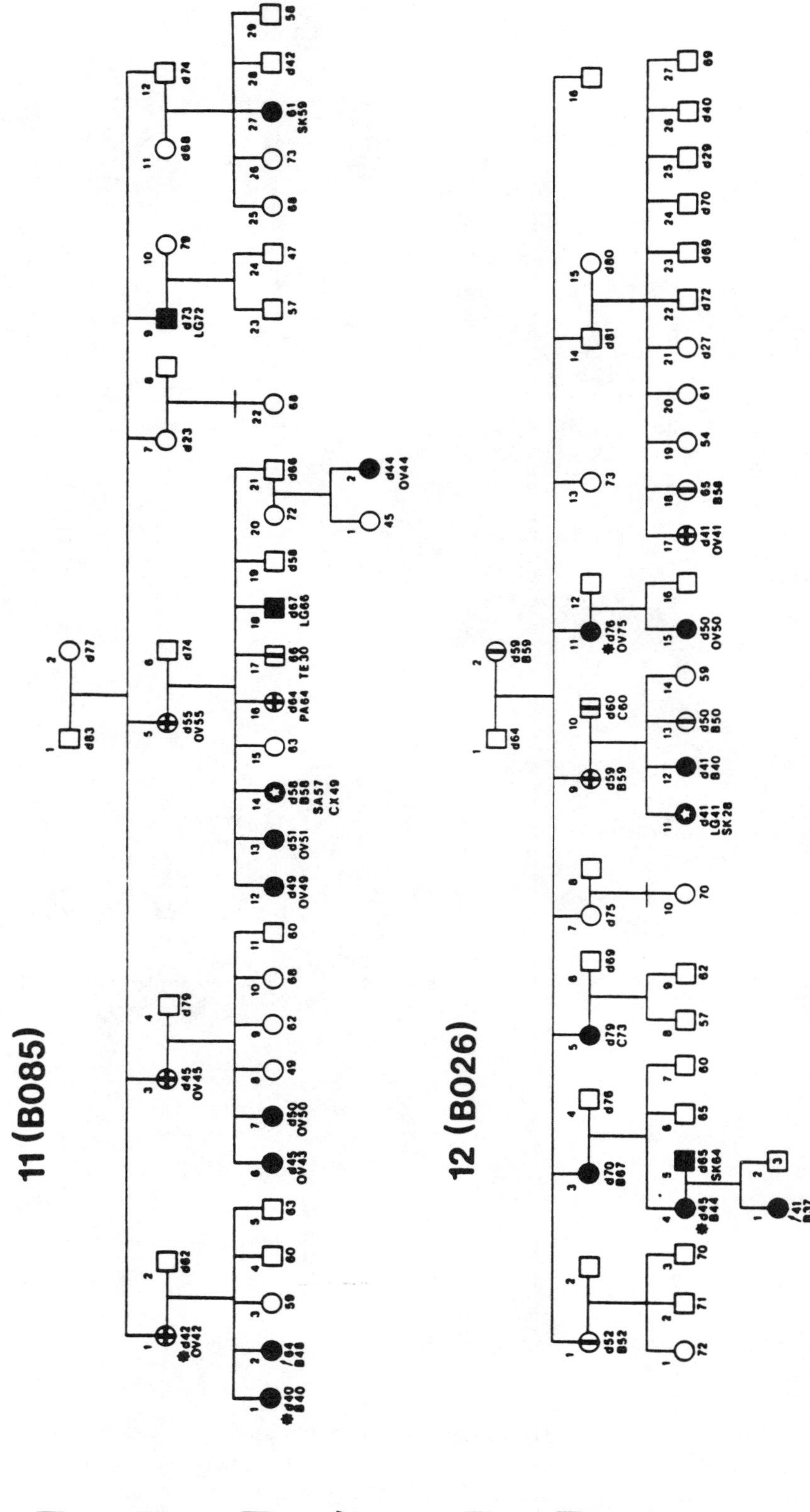
11 (B085)
12 (B026)
I
II
III
IV
I
II
III
IV

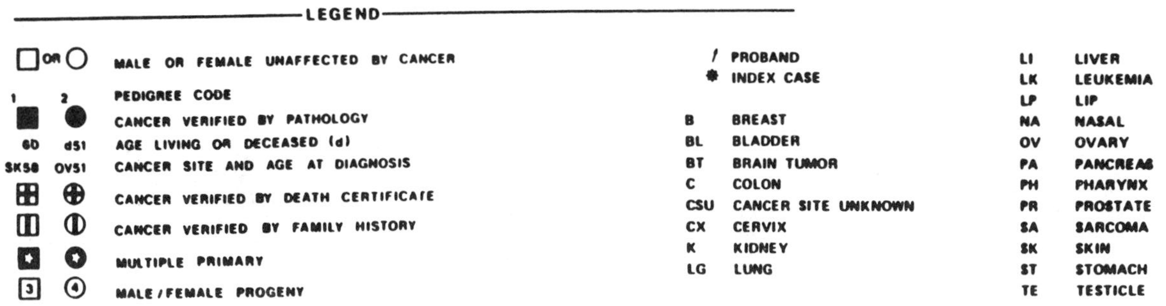

LEGEND

□ OR ○ MALE OR FEMALE UNAFFECTED BY CANCER
1 2 PEDIGREE CODE
■ ● CANCER VERIFIED BY PATHOLOGY
60 d51 AGE LIVING OR DECEASED (d)
SK58 OV51 CANCER SITE AND AGE AT DIAGNOSIS
⊞ ⊕ CANCER VERIFIED BY DEATH CERTIFICATE
◫ ⦶ CANCER VERIFIED BY FAMILY HISTORY
MULTIPLE PRIMARY
[3] ④ MALE / FEMALE PROGENY

/ PROBAND
✱ INDEX CASE

B BREAST
BL BLADDER
BT BRAIN TUMOR
C COLON
CSU CANCER SITE UNKNOWN
CX CERVIX
K KIDNEY
LG LUNG

LI LIVER
LK LEUKEMIA
LP LIP
NA NASAL
OV OVARY
PA PANCREAS
PH PHARYNX
PR PROSTATE
SA SARCOMA
SK SKIN
ST STOMACH
TE TESTICLE

FIGURE 10. Pedigrees of families who are prone to breast and ovarian carcinoma. (From Lynch, H. T., Harris, R. E., Guirgis, H. A., et al., *Cancer*, 41, 1543, 1978. With permission.)

needed to more fully clarify the exact mode(s) of inheritance in this familial tumor association. More importantly, intensified cancer surveillance focusing upon the breasts and ovaries must be implemented in high genetic risk patients/families such as these for effective cancer control.

C. The Sarcoma, Breast Cancer, Brain Tumor, Lung and Laryngeal Cancer, Leukemia, and Adrenal Cortical Carcinoma (SBLA) Syndrome

A remarkable familial cancer aggregation comprising sarcoma, breast cancer, brain tumors, leukemia, and adrenal cortical carcinoma was first reported by Bottomley and Condit[141] and by Bottomley et al.[142,143] These investigators suggested that an autosomal dominant factor was of etiologic importance in this large kindred. In addition, they reported an increased percentage of aneuploid cells in cultured peripheral blood leukocytes in certain relatives. Li and Fraumeni[144,145] subsequently proposed an interactive genetic etiologic hypothesis involving exogenous factors (putative oncogenic virus?) and the cancer-prone genotype to describe etiology for what we now refer to as the SBLA syndrome.[146] Figure 11 shows an informative kindred with this complex assortment of cancers. This syndrome is mentioned in this particular context in that breast cancer is an integral tumor. It is relevant that Birch et al.[147] studied the health status or cause of death in the mothers of 143 children with soft tissue sarcomas. Interestingly, six of these mothers had premenopausal onset of breast cancer, two of whom had bilateral disease. This represented a threefold excess risk of breast cancer. When considering the SBLA syndrome, it is clear that one must meticulously document cancer of all anatomic sites, inclusive of those in children, in order to elucidate etiology.

D. Breast Cancer and Gastrointestinal Tract Cancer

Breast cancer has also been associated with gastrointestinal tract cancer. The first significant report of familial breast cancer was that of Broca.[10] In addition to breast cancer, an excess of cancer of the gastrointestinal tract occurred in this family.

Lynch et al.[11] studied 34 families with breast cancer (2 or more first or second degree relatives who had breast cancer). In 22 of these families, 1 or more members of each family had a diagnosis of gastrointestinal tract cancer. Colon cancer was the most frequent tumor followed by carcinoma of the stomach and pancreas. However, when interpreting this type of an association, it must be realized that carcinoma of the colon is the second most common visceral tumor affecting Americans. There is some question as to whether or not breast cancer may be an integral tumor in the Cancer Family Syndrome (Lynch syndrome II) (Figure 12). This disorder is characterized by significant early age of onset of *non*polyposis colorectal carcinoma with *proximal* predominance, carcinoma of the endometrium and ovary, multiple primary cancer excess, and autosomal dominant mode of inheritance. More work will be required in order to provide further documentation of this matter.

E. Cowden's Syndrome

Cowden's syndrome was named after a patient[148] who had a wide variety of lesions which included thyroid goiter, fibrocystic disease of the breast, oral fibromas, and multiple trichilemmomas.[149]

During the course of followup on patients with Cowden's syndrome, Brownstein[149] recognized the association between the cutaneous manifestations and breast cancer in women, which included an excess of bilateral breast cancer. Furthermore, these women showed a relatively young age of onset of breast cancer and positive family histories of same. Brownstein also called attention to an association with thyroid goiter, thyroid adenoma or hypothyroidism, and thyroid carcinoma. Gastrointestinal polyps also appear to be relatively common among these patients. Some of the patients also showed anomalies of the female reproductive tract. Starink et al.[150] studied 21 patients with Cowden's syndrome, also referred

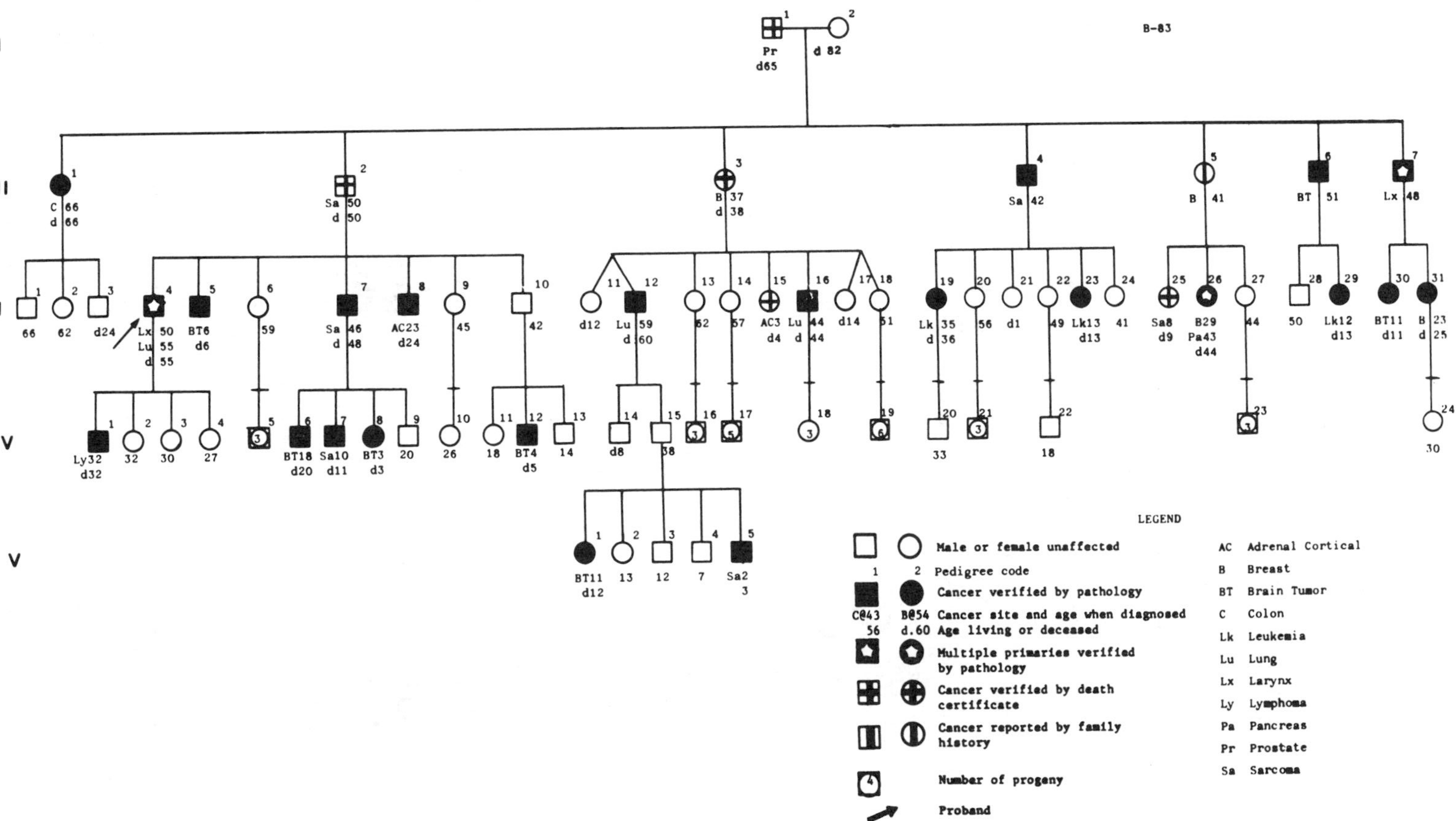

FIGURE 11. Pedigree of an SBLA syndrome kindred. (From Lynch, H. T., Mulcahy, G. M., Harris, R. E., Guirgis, H. A., and Lynch, J. F., *Cancer*, 41, 2055, 1978. With permission.)

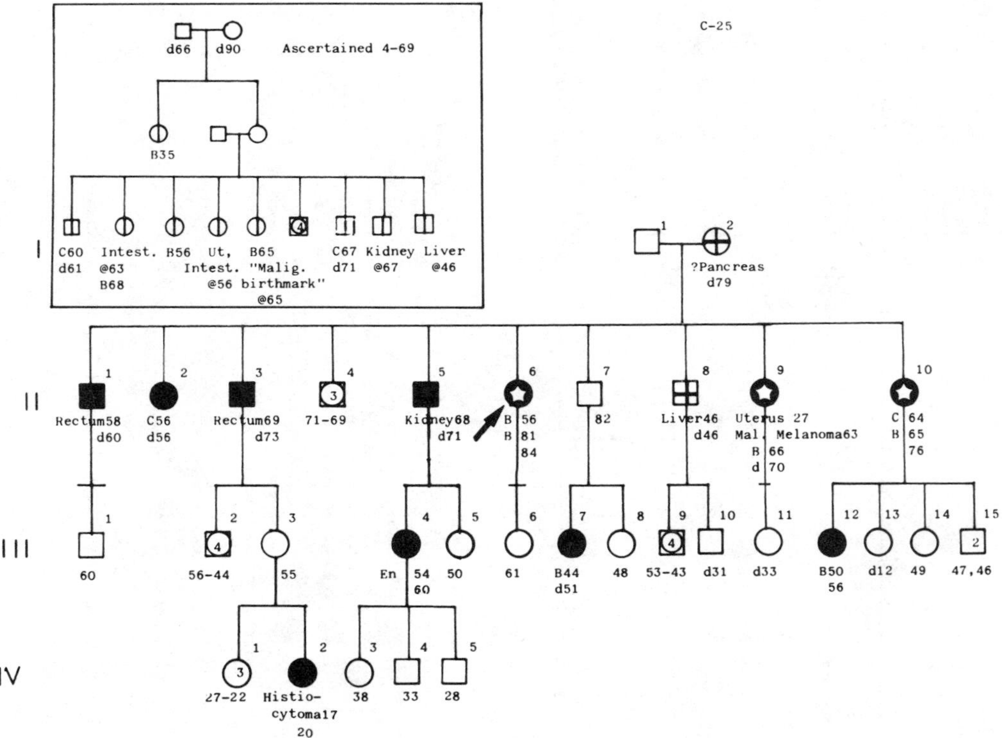

FIGURE 12. Pedigree of a family showing breast cancer in association with tumors seen in hereditary nonpolyposis colon cancer kindreds (Cancer Family Syndrome). (From Lynch, P. M. and Lynch, H. T., *Colon Cancer Genetics*, Van Nostrand Reinhold, Co. New York, 1985. With permission.)

to as multiple hamartoma syndrome. These investigations supported the autosomal dominant mode of inheritance of this disease with high penetrance in both sexes. Mucocutaneous findings were the most constant clinical features (100%) which were almost always manifested by the 2nd decade. Of 18 female patients, 22% manifested breast cancer.

In a review of the literature and clinical experience with this disease, it seems prudent that prophylactic subcutaneous mastectomy should be given priority consideration in the management of women wherein the diagnosis of Cowden's disease is considered to be confirmed. Patients should remain under surveillance for thyroid disease and should also be under a surveillance program for possible development of colonic cancer. With respect to colon cancer, the data is less secure to consider this as an increased risk in Cowden's syndrome. More investigation is required to better delineate cancer association (all sites) in this disease wherein cancer of the breast is an integral lesion.

F. Male Breast Cancer

We have emphasized breast cancer in women throughout this chapter. Our research has not led to any extensive pedigrees with multiple breast cancer-affected males. However, we wish to point out that this subject of "familial breast cancer in males" has been recently reviewed by Kozak et al.[151] In their paper, they described breast cancer in two related males, namely, an uncle and a nephew. In their review of male breast cancer occurring in families, including its association with cancers in other family members, they noted ten such families with males affected, including their own, wherein they believed that sufficient information was given. They stated that six of these families (60%) had females affected with breast cancer and concluded that there are some families wherein males as well as females show an increased risk of developing this disease.

LaRaja et al.[152] reported a family wherein three siblings (a sister and her two brothers) manifested breast cancer. The paternal grandmother of the proband also manifested breast cancer. The sibship was of further interest in that the female sibling had bilateral breast cancer during her premenopausal years and one of her brothers who manifested breast cancer developed this disease at age 41 years. The authors state that their family study is the first one in which a sister and two brothers manifested breast cancer. The family was also noteworthy for other varieties of cancer in that two family members had gastric cancer, one had brain cancer, one had laryngeal cancer, one had a carcinoma of the colon, and one had skin cancer. There was no evidence in the men of clinical features consistent with Klinefelter's syndrome. The authors reviewed the literature for familial breast cancer occurring in male siblings and found only four reports.[153-155]

G. Klinefelter's Syndrome

Patients with Klinefelter's syndrome are at increased risk for breast cancer.[156,157] It is possible that breast cancer risks of XXY males are influenced by genetic variables for cancer diathesis in a manner similar to the breast cancer risk of XX females.[158]

Recently, Evans and Crichlow[159] reviewed the subject of carcinoma of the male breast in Klinefelter's syndrome. They note that the breast cancer risk in men with Klinefelter's syndrome is approximatley 3%. The number of reported patients with breast cancer among Klinefelter's males is only 27 and is too small for meaningful statistical analysis.

Physicians should perform careful breast examination of these high risk XXY males. Screening mammography in such patients should be considered. Prophylactic mastectomy, particularly in the presence of significant gynecomastia, present in most Klinefelter's males, should be considered.

VII. BIOMARKERS AND HEREDITARY BREAST CANCER

Biomarkers may be operationally classified under two major subheadings: (1) histologic, cytogenetic, and other markers in tumor tissue which can be used to divide cancer patients into clinically significant groups and (2) genetic linkage markers which can be used to identify persons with a particular genetic defect. In the case of breast cancer, surprisingly little is known about either of these biomarker subsets in the hereditary form of this disease. However, there is ample reason to believe that given the distinctiveness of hereditary breast cancer, pathology and linkge discriminants should one day be identified.

Lynch et al.[138] reviewed the subject of biomarkers in hereditary breast cancer and have clearly shown that in spite of the importance of this subject to hereditary breast cancer diagnosis, control, and comprehension of pathogenesis, we remain in the dark so far as identification of biomarkers of sufficient sensitivity and specificity for clinical application is concerned. However, some clues have been provided and these are summarized in Table 2.[34,35,102,160-171]

A. Cytogenetics

The cytogenetic evaluation of human solid tumors has received a significantly lesser degree of attention when compared to cytogenetics of the human leukemias.[172] Mitelman[173] in an extensive review of this subject, has shown that less than 10% of the total cytogenetic studies of human cancer pertained to carcinomas. This is of interest in that carcinomas are the most common forms of cancer affecting man. Of these lesions, breast cancer has received greater attention by cytogeneticists when compared to the total number of human solid tumors which have been investigated. Sandberg[174] reported that in the majority of primary and metastatic

Table 2
BIOMARKERS AND BREAST CANCER

Apocrine glands and secretory status — wet ear wax and increased breast secretion positively associated with breast cancer risk[164,166]
Dysplastic epithelial cells in nipple aspirates of premenopausal white women with statistically significant correlation with wet cerumen[169]
gp52 antigen — the envelope glycoprotein (gp52) of the murine mammary tumor virus shows cross-reactivity human breast cancer and with patients showing positive family histories[163]
Endocrine profiles — premenopausal high familial breast cancer risk women
Low urinary estrone and estradiol glucuronides
Plasma adrosterone sulfate significantly low
Genetic risk for breast cancer risk associated with an abnormality in estrogen conjugation[34,35,102]
Glutamic pyruvic transaminase showed a low score of 1.95 at zero recombination[170]
In vitro hyperdiploidy — observed in affected high genetic risk and affecteds[106,162]
Plasminogen activators — malignant transformation of breast and colon appeared to be accompanied by important changes in the production of urokinase-related plasminogen activators and of an inhibitory activity directed against urokinase; the antiurokinase activity was absent in extracts of normal breast or colon tissue[168]
Oncogene research — *ras* activation may be a mechanism by which breast cancer might alter its hormone-dependent phenotype[161]
Natural killer cell activity — elevated natural killer cell activity may be a reaction to the hormonal factors in women with diffuse benign breast syndrome[167] and may be relevent to breast cancer risk; this work is very preliminary
Cytogenetic, regardless of model chromosome number, findings are abnormal in tumor tissue (both primary and metastatic) wherein diploid cells are rare; aneuploid cells and markers are common, particularly involving chromosomes 1, 6, 7, and 11[171]

breast cancer cases, the chromosomal picture, regardless of modal chromosome number, were extremely abnormal. Herein, diploid cells were rare and most of the breast cancers were aneuploid with markers.

Of breast cancer cases investigated by chromosome banding analysis, Trent[171] states that those chromosomes most commonly altered were numbers 1, 6, 7, and 11. Of special interest is that fact that these chromosomes serve as the site for various c-*onc* sequences. For example, three oncogenes have now been mapped to chromosome #1; namely, c-*Blym*-1, c-N-*ras*, and c-*ski*; on chromosome #6, the c-*myb* is on #7, the c-*erb*-B is localized on chromosome 7p, and on chromosome #11, two c-*onc* genes are present; namely, c-H-*ras* (on 11p) and c-*ets* (on 11q).

In the study of hereditary breast cancer kindreds, we have observed an excess of hyperdiploidy in cultured skin fibroblasts, etc.[138] Further investigation of cytogenetics in breast cancer-prone kindreds is clearly indicated given the mentioned preliminary clues identified in this discipline thus far.

Lundberg et al.[175] described loss of heterozygosity in human ductal breast tumors occurring specifically and nonrandomly on chromosome #13. This loss was seen in a small number of cases of ductal carcinoma. These data indicated the possibility that in these cases pathogenesis involved a somatic deletion of genetic material which unmasked a recessive breast cancer predisposing allele.

Ferti-Passantonopoulou and Panani[176] studied the cytogenetics, using G-banding on direct tumor preparations, from five patients with breast cancer. Aberrations in chromosomes, according to frequency, were #1, #11, #3, #6, #5, and #17. In all of the cases, abnormalities of chromosomes #1 and #11 were observed. In each patient, chromosome #1 was involved in at least two different situations. In four of the patients, abnormalities of chromosome #11 showed nonrandom involvement of q22-23. These investigators concluded that "...band 11q22-23, which has been reported to be an inheritable fragile site and is a specific breakpoint in acute leukemia, also may be specific in a group of breast cancer. Thus, correlation of an inheritable fragile site and a malignant disease with familial incidence seems possible."

1. Oncogenes

Oncogenes are an important genetic system which require investigation as potential biomarkers, with attention to germline allele frequency, somatic (tumor) amplifications, deletions, and other mutations, including expression in tumor tissue. The linking of oncogenes to cancer induction or maintenance in humans is primarily circumstantial but very promising and increasingly broad. For example, Slamon et al.[177] have shown that amplification of the HER-2/*neu* gene was a significant predictor of survival in patients with breast cancer. Other examples are cited in a review by Trent,[171] who reported associations between oncogene loci and chromosomal alterations in breast cancers, providing a rationale for priority of linkage search. A review of oncogenes in other cancers was provided by Knudson.[120]

Several oncogenes are frequently genetically altered (amplified, rearranged, deleted) in breast and other cancer. Somatic mutations in breast tumors have been associated with specific aspects of the patient's history, prognosis, or characteristics of the tumor.[177-179] In addition to tumor-specific genetic alterations, the distribution of germ line c-Ha-*ras*-1 restriction fragment length polymorphisms (RFLPs) (alleles) differs significantly from normals in breast,[180] colon, and nonsmall cell lung carcinoma patients.[181] The basis for the C-Ha-*ras*-1 RFLP is a variable tandem repeat (VTR) sequence located 3′ to the coding region of the gene,[182,183] The VTR element is reported to have enhancer activity for the transcription of C-Ha-*ras*-1. These observations suggest that there is a genetic component to these cancers which is due to mutation at the c-Ha-*ras*-1 or at a closely linked locus. It would be prudent to determine whether the frequency of somatic mutations of germ line alleles of c-Ha-*ras*-1 and other cellular oncogenes differs between hereditary breast cancer and nonhereditary breast cancer.

Ras p21, the 21,000-Da protein product of a family of three related cellular oncogenes (Ki-*ras*, Ha-*ras*, N-*ras*), is expressed in the majority of infiltrating ductal breast cancers, but not in benign breast lesions.[184] The enhanced expression likely represents the Ha-*ras*-1 locus. Comparison of *ras* p21 expression in hereditary and nonhereditary breast cancer patients, and study of associations between expression and C-Ha-*ras*-1 genotype, somatic mutations, and other clinicopathologic characteristics is needed.

Our oncogene observations are preliminary and still in progress. However, we believe they are extremely important in that they represent the *first* attempt, so far as we can determine, to perform such studies on a well-defined cohort of hereditary breast cancer-affected patients and their first degree relatives (50% risk for breast cancer). Our findings are restricted to DNA extracted from peripheral blood leukocytes. However, it will now be of extreme importance to perform similar investigations on fresh tumor tissue specimens.

We did not observe any change in *int*-2 or C-Ha-*ras*-1 in DNA from the leukocytes from our hereditary breast cancer patients. There was no evidence for an increased frequency of germline homozygosity at these loci in our hereditary breast cancer patients.

Our findings relevant to *erb*-A-2 showed low frequency of the "a" allele and an increase in the "b" allele. However, there was a lack of discrimination of these alleles among hereditary breast cancer affecteds and hereditary breast cancer at-risk patients. Nevertheless, this entire matter merits further investigation. We stress this point primarily because of the homology of the *erb*-A oncogene with the steroid hormone receptor family,[185,186] which also includes evidence that c-*erb*-A encodes the receptor for thyroid hormone T3.[187,188] Van de Vijver et al.[189] have systematically studied oncogene alterations in a large group of human breast cancer samples. The most frequent alteration which they detected pertained to two linked oncogenes on chromosome#17, c-*erb*-B2 and c-*erb*-A. These investigators concluded that "...the relatively high frequency of *neu* (c-*erb*-B2) points to a functional role in human breast cancer. Coamplification of the *c-erb*-A oncogene could contribute to this disease as well, but is most likely fortuitous." It is important to realize that the breast cancers analyzed in their study[189] were necessarily heterogeneous and most certainly comprised of predominantly sporadic cases. Undoubtedly, they also contained a hereditary subset. However, these investigators did not differentiate the hereditary from the sporadic patients within their sample. Thus, it is possible that a reanalysis of their data relevant to hereditary vs. sporadic might lead to different conclusions and conceivably the c-*erb*-A findings might achieve etiologic significance.

In a study of the HER-2/*neu* oncogene, a member of the *erb*B-like oncogene family, Slamon et al.[177] observed alterations of the gene in 189 primary breast cancers. Furthermore, they noted that HER-2/*neu* was amplified from 2-fold to greater than 20-fold in 30% of the tumors. There was correlation of degress of this gene amplification with several disease parameters. Of particular interest was the finding that fivefold or greater amplification of this gene proved to be a significant predictor of survival as well as time to relapse in the breast cancer affecteds, and it retained its significance when adjustments were made for other prognostic indices. There investigators concluded that "...HER-2/*neu* amplification had greater prognostic value than most currently used prognostic factors, including hormonal-receptor status, in lymph node positive disease. These data indicate that this gene may play a role in the biologic behavior and/or pathogenesis of human breast cancer."

In collaboration with Robert Callahan at the Laboratory of Immunology and Biology of the National Cancer Institute, we attempted to perform studies of H-*ras*-1 allelic deletions on paraffin-embedded tumor tissue using methods of Dubeau et al.,[190] but these efforts have not been successful. We make a plea for archiving fresh breast cancer specimens from patients with hereditary breast cancer. Concurrently, DNA from their blood should be collected. Such efforts as these should significantly expedite our knowledge about these important biomarkers in that highly significant hereditary breast cancer subset of the breast cancer burden.

2. Linkage Studies

Advances in DNA technology, with increasing abundance of polymorphic linkage markers, including RFLPs, have led to significant evidence for linkage in human diseases such as cystic fibrosis,[191,192] in Huntington's chorea,[193] multiple endocrine neoplasia type II,[194] and familial multiple adenomatosis.[195,196] The significance of linkage was recently discussed by White and Lalouel[197] and it has been stressed that the human gene map can be expected to be completely defined in the near future. As this goal nears, the probability of finding a linkage in an adequately designed study approaches 100%.

Within this context, the ultimate objective of research is to localize the deleterious gene at its specific locus on one of the chromosomes. We predict that once gene localization has been accomplished, we will then be in a better position to study the pathogenetic mechanisms which may be responsible for histopathology variance in hereditary breast cancer subsets.

Major advances in biomolecular genetic technology during the past decade have made successful human linkage studies more likely. For example, the growing number of DNA polymorphisms which have become available for genetic linkage studies has enabled the construction of detailed maps of the human genome.[198] These resultant linkage maps are constantly being refined for a variety of chromosome regions.[199] Finding genetic linkage will have immediate relevance to genetic counseling and for the detection of disease heterogeneity. Cancer-prone families will make linkage studies possible; selection of the most informative families will make these research efforts more cost-effective.

The ideal family for linkage investigation would be one in which the phenotype has been clearly defined in the light of the natural history facets of hereditary cancer. Such a family should contain a large number of affected and at-risk subjects who are available for typing, with multiple generations and an extended kindred in which several sibships include affected members.

While advances in the recognition of cancer-prone families through clinical and pedigree analyses have been prodigious during the past 2 decades, there remain many problem areas. Linkage studies of hereditary breast cancer families may be confounded by (1) a sporadic occurrence, (2) incomplete penetrance and variable expressivity of the gene, (3) limited number of at risk women, (4) paternal transmission, (5) deaths of key relatives before the onset of breast cancer, and (6) the occurrence of cancer at nonbreast sites which may be etiologically associated with the breast cancer susceptibility in a given family. It is unclear whether breast cancer-prone families differing in typical age of onset,[124] typical histological type of cancer, or the frequent occurrence of cancer at a particular nonbreast site represent etiologically distinct syndromes, or whether a single major genetic susceptibility defect underlies them.

3. Natural Killer Cell Activity and Enumeration

Evidence increasingly indicates that natural killer (NK) cells are an important effector cell subset in the immunosurveillance of the body against tumors[200-202] as extensively reviewed by Trinchieri and Perussia.[203] In breast cancer studies, Pross et al.[167] did not find any difference in NK activity between women with a family history of breast cancer and normal controls. More recently, however, Strayer et al.[204] did find a difference. In addition to assaying for activity level, it will be important to enumerate NK populations in peripheral blood, using newly developed NK marker antibodies and two-color flow cytometry.

A linkage study of hereditary breast cancer has several benefits beyond its clinical applications. Herein, we are presuming that at least one type of breast cancer is due to a single, major dominant gene. However, breast cancer families are ascertained because they show a dominant pattern of inheritance. Seregation analysis of such biased data cannot provide proof of the single gene hypothesis. On the other hand, linkage is unlikely to be influenced by the bias of family selection. Thus, positive linkage proves that a major gene exists and estimates its location in the genome. If the gene exists, the probability of finding a linkage is fast approaching 100%, as the human linkage map becomes more complete. A corollary of this is the possibility of excluding a gene from the entire genome, thus disproving the single gene hypothesis. While we expect our hypothesis of single gene inheritance for hereditary breast cancer to be proven, the appeal of the linkage approach is that it should provide an answer regardless of our preconceived notions.

VIII. SUMMARY AND CONCLUSIONS

Approximately 8% of breast cancer patients fulfill criteria for hereditary breast cancer. With 135,000 new breast cancer cases expected in 1988,[131] one would then expect 10,500 cases of hereditary breast cancer this year. Each of these hereditary breast cancer cases has between 5 and 10 first degree relatives at risk, putting 54,000 to 108,000 additional individuals per year at risk for hereditary breast cancer.

Currently, we can only differentiate hereditary from nonhereditary breast cancer tentatively, by family history. We cannot identify putative obligate gene carriers until expression of the phenotype (breast cancer). Definition of hereditary breast cancer remains an operational clinicopathologic concept. It may ultimately be segregated from nonhereditary breast cancer cases in a multidimensional space defined by ploidy, oncogene genotype and expression level, NK activity, and the responsible gene(s) may be identified through RFLP technology. Pathology would harbor the potential to supplement family history and allow improved identification of hereditary breast cancer cases in the breast cancer population. Their clinical management could then be improved. More importantly, if we know of closely linked loci, family studies could then identify relatives of those patients who are at inordinately high risk of breast cancer, and contrariwise, those who are not at high risk, so that surveillance programs could then be more highly targeted. Risk markers valid across families, if available, could be used either among members of known hereditary breast cancer families, in the sense of a linked trait, or as a mass screening tool (for those markers which might identify breast cancer in the general population). Environmental interactions could be examined with greater precision when identification of hereditary breast cancer risk factor status is known through biomarker determination.

REFERENCES

1. **Lynch, H. T., Ed.,** *Genetics and Breast Cancer,* Van Nostrand Reinhold, New York, 1981.
2. **Heston, W. E.,** Genetics of cancer, *J. Hered.,* 65, 262, 1974.
3. **Bittner, J. J.,** Relation of nursing to the extra chromosome theory of breast cancer in mice, *Am. J. Cancer,* 97, 90, 1939.
4. **Heston, W. E., Deringer, M. K., and Andervont, H. B.,** Gene-milk agent relationship in mammary tumor development, *J. Natl. Cancer Inst.,* 5, 289, 1945.
5. **Muhlbock, O.,** Note on a new inbred mouse strain GR/A, *Eur. J. Cancer,* 1, 123, 1965.
6. **Bentvelzen, P.,** Hereditary infections with mammary tumor viruses in mice, in *RNA Viruses and Host Genome in Oncogenesis,* Emmelot, P. and Bentvelzen, P., Eds., North-Holland, Amsterdam, 309, 1972.
7. **Huebner, R. J. and Todaro, G. J.,** Oncogenes of RNA tumor viruses as determinants of cancer, *Proc. Natl. Acad. Sci., U.S.A.,* 64, 1087, 1969.
8. **Hollman, K. H.,** Immunologie des tumeurs mammaires, *Ann. Inst. Pasteur,* 122, 809, 1972.
9. **Kouri, R. E., McKinney, C. E., and Henry, T. J.,** Genetic control of breast cancer susceptibility in animals, in *Genetics and Breast Cancer,* Lynch, H. T., Ed., Van Nostrand Reinhold, New York, 14, 1981.
10. **Broca, P. P.,** *Traite' des Tumerus,* Vol. 1 and 2, Asselin, Paris, 1866.
11. **Lynch, H. T., Krush, A. J., Lemon, H. M., et al.,** Tumor variation in families with breast cancer, *JAMA,* 222, 1631, 1972.
12. **Macklin, M. T.,** Comparison of the number of breast cancer patients and the number of expected on the basis of mortality rates, *J. Natl. Cancer Inst.,* 22, 927, 1959.
13. **Dupont, W. D. and Page, D. L.,** Risk factors for breast cancer in women with proliferative breast disease, *N. Engl. J. Med.,* 312, 146, 1985.
14. **Page, D. L. and Dupont, W. D.,** Atypical hyperplastic lesions of the female breast: long-term followup study, *Cancer,* 55, 2698, 1985.
15. Consensus Statement, Is "fibrocystic disease" of the breast precancerous?" *Arch. Pathol. Lab. Med.,* 110, 173, 1986.
16. **Page, D. L.,** Cancer risk assessment in benign breast biopsies, *Hum. Pathol.,* 17, 871, 1986.
17. **Page, D. L., Dupont, W. D., Rogers, L. W., et al.,** Intraductal carcinoma of the breast: followup after biopsy only, *Cancer,* 49, 751, 1982.
18. **Rosen, P. P., Cantrell, B., Mullen, D. L., and DePalo, A.,** Juvenile papillomatosis (Swiss cheese disease) of the breast, *Am. J. Sug. Pathol.,* 4, 3, 1980.
19. **Rosen, P. P., Holmes, G., Lesser, M. L., Kinne, D. W., and Beattie, E. J.,** Juvenile papillomatosis and breast carcinoma, *Cancer,* 55, 1345, 1985.
20. **Page, D. L. and Anderson, T. J.,** *Diagnostic Histopathology of the Breast,* Churchill Livingston, Edinburgh, 1987, 300.
21. **Albano, W. A., Recabaren, J. A., Lynch, H. T., et al.,** Natural history of hereditary cancer of the breast and colon, *Cancer,* 50, 360, 1982.
22. **Mulcahy, G. M. and Platt, R.,** Pathologic aspects of familial carcinoma of breast, in *Genetics and Breast Cancer,* Lynch, H. T., Ed., Van Nostrand Reinhold, New York, 1981, 65.
23. **Lagios, M. D., Rose, M. R., and Margolin, F. R.,** Tubular carcinoma of the breast: association with multicentricity, bilaterality, and family history of mammary carcinoma, *Am. Soc. Clin. Pathol.,* 73, 25, 1980.
24. **Anderson, D. E.,** Genetic study of breast cancer: identification of a high risk group, *Cancer,* 34, 1090, 1974.
25. **Rosen, P. P., Lesser, M. L., Senie, R. T., and Kinne, D. W.,** Epidemiology of breast carcinoma. III. Relationship of family history to tumor type, *Cancer,* 50, 171, 1982.
26. **Marcus, J. N., Page, D. L., Watson, P., Conway, T., and Lynch, H. T.,** High mitotic grade in hereditary breast cancer, *Lab. Invest.,* 58, 61A, 1988.
27. **Azzopardi, J. G., Chepick, O. F., Hartmann, W. J., et al.,** The World Health Organization histological typing of breast tumors, *Am. J. Clin. Pathol.,* 78, 806, 1982.

28. **Ridolfi, R. L., Rosen, P. P., Port, A., et al.,** Medullary carcinoma of the breast: clinicopathologic study with 10-year followup, *Cancer,* 40, 1365, 1977.
29. **Amaku, E. O.,** A review of 40 cases of breast cancer seen in Lagos Teaching Hospital, *West Afr. Med. J.,* 17, 102, 1968.
30. **Templeton, A. C.,** Tumours of the breast, in *Tumours in a Tropical Country: A Survey of Uganda 1964 — 1968,* Templeton, A. C., Ed., Springer-Verlag, New York, 1973, 94.
31. **Rosen, P. P., Ashikari, R., Thaler, H., et al.,** A comparative study of some pathologic features of mammary carcinoma in Tokyo, Japan and New York, U.S.A., *Cancer,* 39, 429, 1977.
32. **Lynch, H. T., Albano, W. A., Layton, M. A., et al.,** Breast cancer, genetics, and age at first pregnancy, *J. Med. Genet.,* 21, 96, 1984.
33. **Woods, K. L., Smith, S. R., and Morrison, J. M.,** Parity and breast cancer: evidence of a dual effect, *Br. Med. J.,* 281, 419, 1980.
34. **Fishman, J., Fukushima, D., O'Connor, J., Rosenfeld, R. S., Lynch, H. T., Lynch, J. F., Guirgis, H., and Maloney, K.,** Plasma hormone profiles of young women at risk for familial breast cancer, *Cancer Res.,* 38, 4006, 1978.
35. **Fishman, J., Fukushima, D. K., O'Connor, J., and Lynch, H. T.,** Low urinary estrogen glucuronides in women at risk for familial breast cancer, *Science,* 204, 1089, 1979.
36. **Moon, R. C.,** Relationship between previous reproductive history and chemically induced mammary cancer in rats, *Int. J. Cancer,* 23, 312, 1969.
37. **Dao, T. L. and Sunderland, H.,** Mammary carcinogenesis by 3-methycholanthrene, I. Hormonal aspects in tumor induction and growth, *J. Natl. Cancer Inst.,* 23, 567, 1959.
38. **McCormick, G. M. and Moon, R. C.,** Effect of pregnancy and lactation on growth of mammary tumors induced by 7,12 DMBA, *Br. J. Cancer,* 19, 160, 1965.
39. **MacMahon, B., Cole, P., and Brown, J.,** Etiology of human breast cancer: a review, *J. Natl. Cancer Inst.,* 50, 21, 1973.
40. **Hirohata, T., Nomura, A. M. Y., Hankin, J. H., Kolonel, L. N., and Lee, J.,** An epidemiologic study on the association between diet and breast cancer, *J. Natl. Cancer Inst.,* 78, 595, 1987.
41. **Chan, P., Head, J. F., Cohen, L. A., et al.,** Influence of dietary fat on the induction of mammary tumors by *N*-nitrosomethylurea: associated hormone changes and differences between Sprague-Dawley and F344 rats, *J. Natl. Cancer Inst.,* 59, 1279, 1977.
42. **Engel, R. W. and Copeland, D. H.,** Influence of diet on the relative incidence of eye, mammary, ear duct, and liver tumors in rats fed 2-acethylaminofluorene, *Cancer Res.,* 11, 180, 1951.
43. **Hopkins, G. J. and West, C. E.,** Effect of dietary polyunsaturated fat on the growth of transplantable adenocarcinoma in C3HAvyfB mice, *J. Natl Cancer Inst.,* 58, 753, 1977.
44. **Hillard, L. A. and Abraham, S.,** Effect of dietary polyunsaturated fatty acids on growth of mammary adenocarcinomas in mice and rats, *Cancer Res.,* 39, 4430, 1969.
45. **Gammal, E. B., Carroll, K. K., and Plunkett, E. R.,** Effects of dietary fat on mammary carcinogenesis by 7,12-dimethylbenz(a)anthracene in rats, *Cancer Res.,* 27, 1737, 1967.
46. **Rao, G. A. and Abraham, S.,** Enhanced growth of transplanted mammary adenocarcinoma induced by C3H mice by dietary linoleate, *J. Natl. Cancer Inst.,* 56, 431, 1976.
47. **Carroll, K. K. and Khor, H. T.,** Effects of level and type of dietary fat on incidence of mammary tumors induced in female Sprague-Dawley rats by 7,12-dimethylbenz(a)anthracene, *Lipids,* 6, 415, 1971.
48. **Carroll, K. K. and Hopkins, G. J.,** Dietary polyunsaturated fat versus saturated fat in relation to mammary carcinogenesis, *Lipids,* 14, 155, 1979.
49. **Drasar, B. S. and Irving, D.,** Environmental factors and cancer of the colon and breast, *Br. J. Cancer,* 27, 167, 1973.
50. **Armstrong, B. and Doll, R.,** Environmental factors and cancer incidence and motality in different countries, with special reference to dietary practices, *Int. J. Cancer,* 15, 617, 1975.
51. **Carroll, K. K.,** Experimental evidence of dietary factors and hormone-dependent cancers, *Cancer Res.,* 35, 3374, 1975.
52. **Miller, A. B., Kelly, A., Choi, N. W., et al.,** A study of diet and breast cancer, *Am. J. Epidemiol.,* 107, 499, 1978.
53. **Graham, S., Marshall, J., Mettlin, C., et al.,** Diet in the epidemiology of breast cancer, *Am. J. Epidemiol,* 116, 68, 1982.
54. **Lubin, J. H., Burns, P. E., Blot, W. J., et al.,** Dietary factors and breast cancer risk, *Int. J. Cancer,* 28, 685, 1981.
55. **Phillips, R. L. and Snowdon, D. A.,** Association of meat and coffee use with cancers of the large bowel, breast, and prostate among Seventh-Day Adventists: preliminary results, *Cancer Res.,* 43, 2403s, 1983.
56. **Hirohata, T., Shigematsu, T., Nomura, A. M., et al.,** Occurrence of breast cancer in relation to diet and reproductive history: a case/control study in Fukuoka, Japan, *Natl. Cancer Inst. Monogr.,* 69, 187, 1985.

57. **Waterhouse, J., Muir, C., Shanmugaratnam, K., et al.,** Cancer incidence in five continents, *IARC Sci. Pub.*, 4, 734, 1982.
58. **Frisch, R. E.,** Dietary fat and risk of breast cancer, *N. Eng. J. Med.*, 317, 165, 1987.
59. **deWaard, F., Cornelis, J. P., and Aoki, M.,** Breast cancer incidence according to weight and height in two cities of the Netherlands and in Aichi prefecture, Japan, *Cancer*, 40, 1269, 1977.
60. **deWaard, F.,** Premenopausal and postmenopausal breast cancer: one disease or two?, *J. Natl. Cancer Inst.*, 63, 549, 1979.
61. **Frisch, R. E., Wyshak, G., Albright, N. L., et al.,** Lower prevalence of breast cancer and cancers of the reproductive system among former college athletes compared to non-athletes, *Br. J. Cancer*, 52, 885, 1985.
62. **Willet, W. C., Stampfer, M. J., Colditz, G. A., et al.,** Dietary fat and the risk of breast cancer, *N. Engl. J. Med.*, 316, 22, 1987.
63. **Apter, D. and Vihko, R.,** Early menarche, a risk factor for breast cancer, indicates early onset of ovulatory cycles, *J. Clin. Endocrinol. Metab.*, 57, 82, 1983.
64. **Miller, A. B. and Bulbrook, R. D.,** The epidemiology and etiology of breast cancer, *N. Engl. J. Med.*, 303, 1246, 1980.
65. **Schatzkin, A., Jones, Y., Hoover, R. N., et al.,** Alcohol consumption and breast cancer in the epidemiologic followup study of the first national health and nutrition examination survey, *N. Engl. J. Med.*, 316, 1169, 1987.
66. **Willet, W. C., Stampfer, M. J., Colditz, G. A., et al.,** Moderate alcohol consumption and the risk of breast cancer, *N. Engl. J. Med.*, 316, 1174, 1987.
67. **Graham, S.,** Alcohol and breast cancer, *N. Engl. J. Med.*, 316, 1211, 1987.
68. **Fraumeni, J. F., Lloyd, J. W., Smith, E. M., and Wagoner, J. K.,** Cancer mortality among nuns: role of martial status in etiology of neoplastic disease in women, *J. Natl. Cancer Inst.*, 42, 455, 1969.
69. **Hertz, R.,** The estrogen-cancer hypothesis with special emphasis on DES, in *Origins of Human Cancer*, Vol. 4, Hiatt, H. H., Watson, J. D., and Winsten, J. A., Eds., Cold Spring Harbor Conference on Cell Proliferation, Cold Spring Harbor Laboratory, Cold Spring Harbor, N.Y., 1977, p1665.
70. **Beatson, G. T.,** On the treatment of inoperable cases of carcinoma of the mammae, *Lancet*, ii, 104, 1896.
71. **Loeb, L.,** Further investigations on the origin of tumors in mice, *J. Med. Res.*, 40, 477, 1919.
72. **Dodds, E. C., Goldberg, L., Lawson, W., and Robinson, R.,** Oestrogenic activity of certain synthetic compounds, *Nature*, 141, 247, 1938.
73. **Dodds, E. C.,** Stilboestrol and after, *Sci. Basis Med. Annu. Rev.*, 1965.
74. **Shimkin, M. B. and Grady, H. G.,** Carcinogenic potency of stilbestrol and estrone in strain C3H mice, *J. Natl. Cancer Inst.*, 1, 119, 1940.
75. **Shimkin, M. B.,** Biologic testing of carcinogens. I. Subcutaneous injection technique, *J. Natl. Cancer Inst.*, 1, 211, 1940.
76. **Gardner, W. U.,** Estrogens in carcinogenesis, *Arch. Pathol.*, 27, 138, 1939.
77. **Lacassagne, A.,** Apparition d'adenocarinomes mammaires chez des souris males traitees par une substance oestrogene synthetique, *C. R. Soc. Biol.*, 129, 641, 1938.
78. **Geschickter, C. T.,** Mammary carcinoma in rat with metastasis induced by estrogen, *Science*, 89, 35, 1939.
79. **Gardner, W. U., Allen, E., Smith, G. M., and Strong, L. C.,** Carcinoma in the cervix of mice receiving estrogens, *JAMA*, 110, 1182, 1938.
80. **Gardner, W. U. and Ferrigno, M.,** Unusual neoplastic lesions of the uterine horns of estrogen-treated mice, *J. Natl. Cancer Inst.*, 17, 601, 1956.
81. **Gardner, W. U.,** Carcinoma of the uterine cervix and upper vagina: induction under experimental conditions in mice, *Ann. N.Y. Acad. Sci.*, 75, 543, 1959.
82. **Loeb, L.,** The significance of hormones in the origin of cancer, *J. Natl. Cancer Inst.*, 1, 169, 1940.
83. **Sartwell, P. E., Arthes, F. G., and Tonascia, J. A.,** Exogeneous hormones, reproductive history, and breast cancer, *J. Natl. Cancer Inst.*, 59, 1589, 1977.
84. **Lemon, H. M., Wotiz, H. H., Parsons, L., and Mozden, P. J.,** Reduced estriol excretion in patients with breast cancer prior to endocrine therapy, *JAMA*, 196, 1128, 1966.
85. **Gross, J., Modan, B., Bertini, B., Spira, O., deWaard, F., Thijssen, J. H., and Vestergaard, P.,** Relationship between steroid excretion patterns and breast cancer incidence in Israeli women origins, *J. Natl. Cancer Inst.*, 59, 7, 1977.
86. **Lemon, H. M.,** Endocrine influence on human mammary cancer formation, *Cancer*, 25, 781, 1969.
87. **Hellman, L., Zumoff, B., Fishman, J., and Gallagher, T. F.,** Peripheral metabolism of 3H-estradiol and the excretion of endogeneous estrone and estriol glucosiduronate in women with breast cancer, *J. Clin. Endocrinol. Metab.*, 33, 138, 1971.
88. **Cole, P., Cramer, D., Yen, S., Paffenbarger, R., MacMahon, B., and Brown, J.,** Estrogen profiles of premenopausal women with breast cancer, *Cancer Res.*, 38, 745, 1978.

89. **Pratt, H. J. and Longcope, C.,** Estriol production rates and breast cancer, *J. Clin. Endocrinol. Metab.*, 46, 44, 1978.
90. **MacFayden, I. J., Forrest, A. P., Prescott, R. J., Golder, M. P., Groom, G. V., Falmy, D. R., and Griffiths, K.,** Circulating hormone concentrations in women with breast cancer, *Lancet,* i, 1100, 1976.
91. **Malarkey, W. B., Schroeder, L. L., Stevens, V. C., James, A. G., and Lanese, R. R.,** Twenty-four hour preoperative endocrine profiles in women with benign and malignant breast disease, *Cancer Res.*, 37, 4655, 1977.
92. **England, P. C., Skinner, L. G., Cottrell, K. M., and Sellwood, R. A.,** Serum estradiol-17 beta in women with benign and malignant breast disease, *Br. J. Cancer,* 30, 571, 1974.
93. **Kirschner, M. A.,** The role of hormones in the etiology of human breast cancer, *Cancer,* 39, 2716, 1977.
94. **Nagasawa, H.,** Prolactin and human breast cancer: a review, *Eur. J. Cancer,* 15, 267, 1979.
95. **Cole, E. N., England, P. C., Sellwood, R. A., and Griffiths, K.,** Serum prolactin concentrations throughout the menstrual cycle of normal women and patients with recent breast cancer, *Eur. J. Cancer,* 13, 677, 1977.
96. **Kwa, H. G., Cleton, F., deJong-Bakker, M., Bulbrook, R. D., Hayward, J. L., and Wang, D. Y.,** Plasma prolactin and its relationship to risk factors in human breast cancer, *Int. J. Cancer,* 17, 441, 1976.
97. **Cole, P. and MacMahon, B.,** Oestrogen fractions during early reproductive life in the etiology of breast cancer, *Lancet,* i, 604, 1969.
98. **Cole, P., MacMahon, B., and Brown, J. B.,** Estrogen profiles of parous and nulliparous women, *Lancet,* ii, 596, 1976.
99. **Pike, M. C., Casagrande, J. T., Brown, J. B., Gerkins, V., and Henderson, B. E.,** Comparison of urinary and plasma hormone levels in daughters of breast cancer patients and controls, *J. Natl. Cancer Inst.*, 59, 1351, 1977.
100. **Morgan, R. W., Vakil, D. V., Brown, J. B., and Elinson, L.,** Estrogen profiles in young women: effect of maternal history of breast cancer, *J. Natl. Cancer Inst.*, 60, 965, 1978.
101. **Henderson, B. R., Gerkins, V., Rosario, I., Casagrande, J., and Pike, M. C.,** Elevated serum levels of estrogen and prolactin in daughters of patients with breast cancer, *N. Engl. J. Med.*, 293, 790, 1975.
102. **Fishman, J., Bradlow, H. L., Fukushima, D., O'Connor, J., Rosenfeld, R., Elston, R., and Lynch, H. T.,** Abnormal estrogen conjugation in women at risk for familial breast cancer is concentrated at the periovulatory stage of the menstrual cycle, *Cancer Res.*, 43, 1884, 1983.
103. **Schneider, J., Kinne, D., Fracchia, A., Pierce, V., Anderson, K. E., Bradlow, H. L., and Fishman, J.,** Abnormal oxidative metabolism of estradiol in women with breast cancer, *Proc. Natl. Acad. Sci. U.S.A.*, 79, 3047, 1982.
104. **Fishman, J. and Martucci, C.,** Biological properties of 16-alpha-hydroxyestrone: implications in estrogen physiology and pathophysiology, *J. Clin. Endocrinol. Metab.*, 51, 611, 1980.
105. **Bucala, R., Fishman, J., and Cerami, A.,** Formation of covalent adducts between cortisol and 16-alpha-hydroxyestrone and protein — possible role in the pathogenesis of cortisol toxicity and systemic lupus erythematosus, *Proc. Natl. Acad. Sci. U.S.A.*, 79, 3320, 1982.
106. **Hobkirk, R., Nilsen, M., and Mori, J.,** 16-hydroxylation of estrone-3-sulfate and estrone in the guinea pig in vivo, *Endocrinology,* 103, 1227, 1978.
107. **Thomas, D. B., Persing, J. P., and Hutchinson, W. B.,** Exogeneous estrogens and other risk factors for breast cancer in women with benign breast diseases, *J. Natl. Cancer Inst.*, 69, 1017, 1982.
108. **Korenman, S. G.,** Oestrogen window hypothesis of the aetiology of breast cancer, *Lancet,* i, 700, 1980.
109. **Bulbrook, R. D. and Hayward, J. L.,** Abnormal urinary steroid excretion and subsequent breast cancer: a prospective study in the Island of Guernsey, *Lancet,* i, 519, 1967.
110. **Bulbrook, R. D., Hayward, J. L., Spicer, C. C., and Thomas, B. S.,** A comparison between the urinary steroid excretion of normal women and women with advanced breast cancer, *Lancet,* ii, 1235, 1962.
111. **Black, M. M. and Zachrau, R. E.,** Family history and hormones in stepwise mammary carcinogenesis, *Ann. N.Y. Acad. Sci.*, 464, 367, 1986.
112. **Black, M. M. and Kwon, C. S.,** Precancerous mastopathie: structural and biological considerations, *Pathol. Res. Pract.*, 166, 491, 1980.
113. **Black, M. M., Kwon, C. S., Leis, H. P., and Barclay, T. H. C.,** Family history and oral contraceptives: unique relationships in breast cancer patients, *Cancer,* 46, 2747, 1980.
114. **Black, M. M., Barclay, T. H. C., Polednak, A., et al.,** Family history, oral contraceptive usage and breast cancer, *Cancer,* 51, 2147, 1983.
115. **Michnovicz, J. J., Hershcopf, R. J., Naganuma, H., Bradlow, H. L., and Fishman, J.,** Increased 2-hydroxylation of estradiol as a possible mechanism for the anti-estrogenic effect of cigarette smoking, *N. Engl. J. Med.*, 315, 1305, 1986.
116. **Lynch, H. T., Fain, P. R., Goldgar, D., et al.,** Familial breast cancer and its recognition in an oncology clinic, *Cancer,* 47, 2730, 1981.
117. **Petrakis, N. L., Ernster, V., and King, M. C.,** Breast cancer, in *Cancer Epidemiology and Prevention,* Schottenfeld, D. S. and Fraumeni, J. F., Eds., W.B. Saunders, Philadelphia, 1981, 855.

118. **Sattin, R. W., Rubin, G. L., Webster, L. A., et al.,** Family history and the risk of breast cancer, *JAMA,* 253, 1908, 1985.
119. **Ottman, R., Pike, M. C., King, M. C., Casagrande, J. T., and Henderson, B. E.,** Familial breast cancer in a population-based series, *Am. J. Epidemiol.,* 123, 15, 1986.
120. **Knudson, A. G.,** Genetics of human cancer, *Annu. Rev. Genet.,* 20, 231, 1986.
121. **Go, R. C. P., King, M.-C., Bailey-Wilson, J., Elston, R. C., and Lynch, H. T.,** Genetic epidemiology of breast cancer and associated cancers in high risk families. I, *J. Natl. Cancer Inst.,* 71, 455, 1983.
122. **Goldstein, A. M., Haile, R. W. C., Marazita, M. L., and Paganini-Hill, A.,** A genetic epidemiologic investigation of breast cancer in families with bilateral breast cancer. I. Segregation analysis, *J. Natl. Cancer Inst.,* 78, 911, 1987.
123. **Lynch, H. T., Guirigs, H. A., Brodkey, F., et al.,** Early age of onset in familial breast cancer: genetic and cancer control implications, *Arch. Surg.,* 111, 126, 1976.
124. **Lynch, H. T., Watson, P., Conway, T., Fitzsimmons, M. L., and Lynch, J. F.,** Breast cancer family history as a risk factor for early onset breast cancer, *Br. Cancer Res. Treat.,* 11, 263, 1988.
125. **Lynch, H. T., Harris, R. E., Guirgis, H. A., et al.,** Early age of onset and familial breast cancer, *Lancet,* ii, 626, 1976.
126. **Morse, D. P.,** Hereditary aspect of breast cancer in a mother and daughter, *Cancer,* 4, 745, 1951.
127. **Colton, T.,** *Statistics in Medicine,* Little, Brown, Boston, 1974, 300.
128. **deWaard, F.,** The epidemiology of breast cancer: review and prospects, *Int. J. Cancer,* 4, 577, 1969.
129. **Williams, R. R.,** Breast and thyroid cancer and malignant melanoma promoted by alcohol-induced pituitary secretion of prolactin TSH and MSH, *Lancet,* i, 996, 1976.
130. **Feber, B., Handy, V. H., Gerhardt, R. P., and Solomon, M.,** Cancer in New York State, Exclusive of New York City, 1941 — 1960, *Bureau of Cancer Control, New York State Department of Health,* Albany, 1962.
131. American Cancer Society, *Cancer-Cancer J. Clin.,* 38, 5, 1988.
132. **Lynch, H. T., Guirgis, H. A., Albert, S., and Brennan, M.,** Familial breast cancer in a normal population, *Cancer,* 34, 1080, 1974.
133. **Penrose, L. S.,** Problem of anticipation in pedigree of dystrophia myotonica, *Ann. Eugen.,* 14, 125, 1948.
134. **Lynch, H. T.,** *Cancer Genetics,* Charles C Thomas, Springfield, IL, 1976, 639.
135. **Lynch, H. T. and Krush, A. J.,** Heredity and breast cancer: implications for cancer detection, *Med. Times,* 94, 599, 1966.
136. **Lynch, H. T.,** *Hereditary Factors In Carcinoma, Recent Results in Cancer Research,* Vol. 12, Springer-Verlag, New York, 1967, 186.
137. **Lynch, H. T., Albano, W. A., Layton, M. A., et al.,** Genetic predisposition to breast cancer, *Cancer,* 53, 612, 1984.
138. **Lynch, H. T., Albano, W. A., Heieck, J. J., et al.,** Genetics, biomarkers, and control of breast cancer: a review, *Cancer Genet. Cytogenet.,* 13, 43, 1984.
139. **Lynch, H. T. and Lynch, J. F.,** Breast cancer genetics in an oncology clinic: 328 consecutive patients, *Cancer Genet. Cytogenet.,* 23, 369, 1986.
140. **Lynch, H. T., Harris, R. E., Guirgis, H. A., et al.,** Familial association of breast/ovarian cancer, *Cancer,* 41, 1543, 1978.
141. **Bottomley, R. H. and Condit, P. T.,** Cancer families, *Cancer Bull.,* 20, 22, 1968.
142. **Bottomley, R. H., Condit, P. T., and Chanes, R. E.,** Cytogenetic studies in familial malignancy, *Clin. Resource,* 15, 334, 1967.
143. **Bottomley, R. H., Trainer, A. L., and Condit, P. T.,** Chromosome studies in a ''cancer family'', *Cancer,* 28, 519, 1971.
144. **Li, F. P. and Fraumeni, J. F.,** Soft-tissue sarcomas, breast cancer, and other neoplasms, *Ann. Intern. Med.,* 71, 747, 1969.
145. **Li, F. P. and Fraumeni, J. F.,** Familial breast cancer, soft-tissue sarcomas, and other neoplasma, *Ann. Intern. Med.,* 83, 833, 1975.
146. **Lynch, H. T., Mulcahy, G. M., Harris, R. E., Guirgis, H. A., and Lynch, J. F.,** Genetic and pathologic findings in a kindred with hereditary sarcoma, breast cancer, brain tumors, leukemia, lung, laryngeal, and adrenal cortical carcinoma, *Cancer,* 41, 2055, 1978.
147. **Birch, J. M., Hartley, A. L., and Marsden, H. B.,** Excess risk of breast cancer in the mothers of children with soft-tissue sarcomas, *Br. J. Cancer,* 49, 325, 1984.
148. **Lloyd, K. M., II. and Dennis, M.,** Cowden's disease: a possible new symptom complex with multiple system involvement, *Ann. Intern. Med.,* 48, 136, 1963.
149. **Brownstein, M. H.,** Breast cancer in Cowden's syndrome, in *Genetics and Breast Cancer,* Lynch, H. T., Ed., Van Nostrand Reinhold, New York, 1981, 187.
150. **Starink, T. M., Van der Veen, J. P., Arwert, F., deWaal, L. P., deLange, G. G., Gille, J. J. P., and Eriksson, A. W.,** The Cowden syndrome: a clinical and genetic study in 21 patients, *Clin. Genet.,* 29, 222, 1986.

151. **Kozak, F. K., Hall, J. G., and Baird, P. A.,** Familial breast cancer in males: a case report and review of the literature, *Cancer,* 58, 736, 1986.

152. **LaRaja, R. D., Pagnozzi, J. A., Rothenberg, R. E., et al.,** Carcinoma of the breast in three siblings, *Cancer,* 55, 2709, 1985.

153. **Everson, P. B., Li, F. P., Fraumeni, J. F., et al.,** Familial male breast cancer, *Lancet,* i, 9, 1976.

154. **Marger, D., Undaneta, N., and Fischer, B.,** Breast cancer in brothers, *Cancer,* 36, 458, 1975.

155. **Teasdale, C., Forbes, J., and Baum, M.,** Familial male breast cancer, *Lancet,* i, 360, 1976.

156. **Jackson, A. W., Muldol, S., Ockey, C. H., and O'Connor, P. J.,** Carcinoma of male breast in association with the Klinefelter syndrome, *Br. Med. J.,* 1, 223, 1965.

157. **Nadel, M. and Koss, L. G.,** Klinefelter's syndrome and male breast cancer, *Lancet,* ii, 366, 1967.

158. **Lynch, H. T., Kaplan, A. R., and Lynch, J. F.,** Klinefelter syndrome and cancer: a family study, *JAMA,* 229, 209, 1974.

159. **Evans, D. B. and Crichlow, R. W.,** Carcinoma of the male breast and Klinefelter's syndrome: is there an association?, *Cancer,* 37, 246, 1987.

160. **Danes, B. S. and Lynch, H. T.,** Increased in vitro tetraploidy in dermal monolayer cultures derived from normals, *Cancer Genet. Cytogenet.,* 8, 81, 1983.

161. **Kasid, A., Lippman, M. E., Papageorge, A. G., Lowy, D. R., and Glemann, E. P.,** Transfection of v-ras$_H$ DNA into MCF-7 human breast cancer cells bypasses dependence on estrogen for tumorigenicity, *Science,* 228, 725, 1985.

162. **Lynch, H. T., Fusaro, R. M., Danes, B. S., Kimberling, W. J., and Lynch, J. F.,** Hereditary malignant melanoma, including biomarkers in the familial atypical multiple mole melanoma syndrome, *Cancer Genet. Cytogenet.,* 8, 325, 1983.

163. **Ohno, T., Mesa-Tejada, R., Keydar, I., Ramanarayanan, M., Bausch, J., and Spiegelman, S.,** Human breast carcinoma antigen is immunologically related to the polypeptide of the group-specific glycoprotein of mouse mammary tumor virus, *Proc. Natl. Acad. Sci. U.S.A.,* 76, 2460, 1979.

164. **Petrakis, N. L.,** Association of genetically determined wet cerumen and breast fluid secretion (abstr.), presented at the 11th Int. Cancer Congress, Florence, Italy, October 20 to 26, 1974, 71.

165. **Petrakis, N. L.,** Physiologic biochemistry and cytologic aspects of nipple aspirate fluids, *Br. Cancer Res. Treat.,* 8, 7, 1986.

166. **Petrakis, N. L., Mason, L., Lee, R., et al.,** Association of race, age, menopausal status, and cerumen type with breast fluid secretion in nonlactating women, as determined by nipple aspiration, *J. Natl. Cancer Inst.,* 54, 829, 1975.

167. **Pross, H. F., Sterns, E., and MacGillis, D. R.,** Natural killer cell activity in women at "high risk" for breast cancer, with and without benign breast syndrome, *Int. J. Cancer,* 34, 303, 1984.

168. **Tissot, J. D., Hauert, J., and Bachmann, F.,** Characterization of plasminogen activators from normal human breast and colon and from breast and colon carcinomas, *Int. J. Cancer,* 34, 295, 1984.

169. **Petrakis, N. L.,** Cerumen phenotype and epithelial dysplasia in nipple aspirates of breast fluid, *Am. J. Phys. Anthropol.,* 62, 115, 1983.

170. **King, M.-C., Go, R. C. P., Lynch, H. T., Elston, R. C., et al.,** Genetic epidemiology of breast cancer associated cancers in high risk families. II, *J. Natl. Cancer Inst.,* 71, 463, 1983.

171. **Trent, J. M.,** Cytogenetic and molecular biologic alterations in human breast cancer: a review, *Br. Cancer Res. Treat.,* 5, 221, 1985.

172. **Trent, J.,** Chromosomal alterations in human solid tumors: implications of the stem cell model to cancer cytogenetics, in *Chromosomes and Oncogenes in Human Cancers,* Vol. 3, Rowley, J. D., Ed., Cancer Surveys, 1984, 395.

173. **Mitelman, F.,** Catalogue of chromosome aberrations in cancer, *Cytogenet. Cell Genet.,* 36, 1, 1983.

174. **Sandberg, A. A.,** *The Chromosomes in Human Cancer and Leukemia,* Elsevier, New York, 1980, 485.

175. **Lundberg, C., Skoog, L., Cavenee, W. K., and Nordenskjold, M.,** Loss of heterozygosity in human ductal breast tumors indicates a recessive mutation on chromosome 13, *Proc. Natl. Acad. Sci. U.S.A.,* 84, 2372, 1987.

176. **Ferti-Passantonopoulou, A. D. and Panani, A. D.,** Common cytogenetic findings in primary breast cancer, *Cancer Genet. Cytogenet.,* 27, 289, 1987.

177. **Slamon, D. J., Clark, G. M., Wong, S. G., et al.,** Human breast cancer: correlation of relapse and survival with amplification of the HER-2/neu oncogene, *Science,* 235, 177, 1987.

178. **Escot, C., Theillet, C., Lidereau, R., et al.,** Genetic alterations of the c-myc proto-oncogene (myc) in human primary breast carcinomas, *Proc. Natl. Acad. Sci. U.S.A.,* 83, 4834, 1986.

179. **Theillet, C., Lidereau, R., Escot, C., et al.,** Loss of a c-H-ras-1 allele and agressive human primary breast carcinomas, *Cancer Res.,* 46, 4776, 1986.

180. **Lidereau, R., Escot, C., Theillet, C., et al.,** High frequency of rare alleles of the human c-Ha-ras-1 proto-oncogene in breast cancer patients, *J. Natl. Cancer Inst.,* 77, 697, 1986.

181. **Heighway, J., Thatcher, N., Cerny, T., and Hasleton, P. S.,** Genetic predisposition to human lung cancer, *Br. J. Cancer,* 53, 453, 1986.

182. **Capon, D. J., Chen, E. Y., Levinson, A. D., et al.,** Complete nucleotide sequences of the T24 human bladder carcinoma oncogene and its normal homologue, *Nature,* 313, 369, 1983.
183. **Krontiris, T. G., DiMartino, N. A., Colb, M., and Parkinson, D. R.,** Unique allelic restriction fragments of the human Ha-ras locus in leukocyte and tumour DNAs of cancer patients, *Nature,* 313, 369, 1985.
184. **Thor, A., Ohuchi, N., Horan-Hand, P., et al.,** Biology of disease: ras gene alterations and enhanced levels of ras p21 expression in a spectrum of benign and malignant human mammary tissues, *Lab. Invest.,* 55, 603, 1986.
185. **Green, S., Walter, P., Kumar, V., et al.,** Human oestrogen receptor cDNA: sequence expression and homology to v-*erb*-a, *Nature,* 320, 134, 1986.
186. **Greene, G. L., Gilna, P., Waterfield, M., et al.,** Sequence and expression of human estrogen receptor complementary DNA, *Science,* 231, 1150, 1986.
187. **Sap, J., Munoz, A., Damm, K., et al.,** The c-*erb*-A protein is a high affinity receptor for thyroid hormone, *Nature,* 324, 635, 1986.
188. **Weinberger, C., Thompson, C. C., Ong, E. S., et al.,** The c-*erb*-A gene encodes a thyroid hormone receptor, *Nature,* 324, 641, 1986.
189. **Van de Vijver, M., van de Bersselaar, R., Devilee, P., et al.,** Amplification of the neu (c-*erb*-B2) oncogene in human mammary tumors is relatively frequent and is often accompanied by amplification of the linked c-*erb*-A oncogene, *Mol. Cell Biol.,* 7, 2019, 1987.
190. **Dubeau, L., Chandler, L. A., Gralow, J. R., et al.,** Southern blot analysis of DNA extracted from formalin-fixed pathology specimens, *Cancer Res.,* 46, 2964, 1986.
191. **Beaudet, A., Bowcock, A., Buchwald, M., et al.,** Linkage of cystic fibrosis to two tightly linked DNA markers: joint report from a collaborative study, *Am. J. Hum. Genet.,* 39, 681, 1986.
192. **Farrall, M., Watson, E., Bates, G., et al.,** Further data supporting linkage between cystic fibrosis and the met oncogene and haplotype analysis with met and pJ3.11, *Am. J. Hum. Genet.,* 39, 713, 1986.
193. **Gusella, J. F., Wexler, N. S., Conneally, P. M., et al.,** A polymorphic DNA marker genetically linked to Huntington disease, *Nature,* 306, 234, 1983.
194. **Mathew, C. G. P., Chin, K. S., Easton, D. F., et al.,** A linked genetic marker for multiple endocrine neoplasia type 2A on chromosome 10, *Nature,* 328, 527, 1987.
195. **Bodmer, W. F., Bailey, C. J., Bodmer, J., et al.,** Localization of the gene for familial adenomatous polyposis on chromosome 5, *Nature,* 328, 614, 1987.
196. **Solomon, E., Voss, R., Hall, V., et al.,** Chromosome 5 allele loss in human colorectal carcinomas, *Nature,* 328, 616, 1987.
197. **White, R. and Lalouel, J.-M.,** Investigation of genetic linkage in human families, *Adv. Hum. Genet.,* 16, 121, 1987.
198. **White, R., Leppert, M., Bishop, D. T., et al.,** Construction of linkage maps with DNA markers for human chromosomes, *Nature,* 313, 101, 1985.
199. **Lathrop, G. M., Lalouel, J. M., and White, R. L.,** Construction of human linkage maps: likelihood calculations for multilocus linkage analysis, *Genet. Epidemiol.,* 3, 39, 1986.
200. **Purtilo, D. T.,** *Immune Deficiency and Cancer,* Plenum Press, New York, 1984.
201. **Hersey, P., Edwards, A., Honeyman, M., and McCarthy, W. H.,** Low natural killer cell activity in familial melanoma patients and their relatives, *Br. J. Cancer,* 40, 113, 1979.
202. **Markowitz, J. F., Alges, H. W., Cunningham-Rundles, S., et al.,** Cancer Family Syndrome: marker studies, *Gastroenterology,* 91, 581, 1986.
203. **Trinchieri, G. and Perussia, B.,** Biology of disease — human NK cells: biologic and pathologic aspects, *Lab. Invest.,* 50, 489, 1984.
204. **Strayer, D. R., Carter, W. A., and Brodsky, I.,** Familial occurrence of breast cancer is associated with reduced natural killer cytotoxicity, *Br. Cancer Res. Treat.,* 7, 187, 1986.

Chapter 19

FAMILIAL MESOTHELIOMA

Henry T. Lynch and Jane F. Lynch

TABLE OF CONTENTS

I. INTRODUCTION

The pioneering efforts of Irving J. Seilikoff, M.D., a pulmonary disease specialist, and his colleagues Jacob Churg, M.D., a pathologist, and E. Cuyler Hammon, D.Sc., a statistician/epidemiologist, did much to provide substantial evidence for the association between asbestos exposure and cancers of the lung, larynx, possibly kidney, and other anatomic sites, including mesothelioma of the pleura and peritoneum.[1]

Asbestos exposure is now believed to be the primary etiologic link to mesothelioma. Other factors have included exposure to radiation, beryllium, and erionite-type zeolite. Cigarette smoking, while showing a synergistic effect with asbestos exposure as the cause of lung cancer, has not been etiologically linked to malignant mesothelioma.

Archeological investigations in Finland have provided evidence of asbestos fibers having been incorporated in pottery in 2500 B.C. During the 5th century, this mineral was used as a wick for lamps. It was used in body armor in the 15th century, and there is evidence that the ancients often wove asbestos with linen. Its commercial use is said to have begun in Italy in 1850 in the production of paper and cloth. Asbestos mining in Canada and South Africa began around 1880 and soon after it apeared in the U.S., Italy, and Russia.

Asbestos has been an extremely useful mineral which has found a vital role in the industrial revolution. For example, production of this mineral in the U.S. increased from approximately 6000 tons in 1900 to more than 650,000 tons in 1975. Asbestos has found commercial use in more than 3000 products.

Its use in pipe insulation and later in brake linings, cement, and protective clothing began in the U.S. and spread worldwide. Its use in ship building flourished in shipyards in the U.S. during the World War II years.[2]

This brief sketch about asbestos clearly identifies the ubiquitous utilization of this mineral, and hence, its potential for widespread exposure to humans. Becklake[2] has provided an excellent historical exposition of the subject of asbestos and its related adverse effect on health. The association between asbestos exposure and its pulmonary sequelae, now referred to as asbestosis, was first recognized in the early 1900s and recorded in the British literature in 1907.

Lynch et al.[3] described a family in which two brothers with prolonged occupational exposure of asbestos manifested malignant pleural mesotheliomas with similar histology. The literature on familial mesothelioma was reviewed. Through permission of the editor and publishers of *Cancer Genetics and Cytogenetics*, much of this report is reproduced herein.

A. Case #1

This 77-year-old white male was born in 1903 (Figure 1, II-1). He was employed as a blacksmith for a railroad for approximately 25 years (1916 to 1941). He had reported extensive exposure to asbestos resulting from welding duties on steam engine boilers. His smoking history was limited to four cigars per day over a 30-year period (1920 to 1950).

In 1981, the patient presented with complaints of shortness of breath and dyspnea on exertion. A thoracentesis and pleural biopsy revealed highly atypical mesothelial cells which were suspicious for mesothelioma. A right thoracotomy and right parietal pleurectomy was performed. Pathological diagnosis was malignant pleural mesothelioma.

The initial right pleural biopsy showed clusters of malignant epithelioid cells which at that time were felt to be highly suggestive of a malignant mesothelioma. The anaplastic cells demonstrated marked pleomorphism with several of the cells demonstrating prominent nucleoli. Numerous mitotic figures were present. Some of the cells demonstrated papillary fronds. No true acinious formation with a central lumen was present. Special stains revealed PAS positivity with partial digestion by diastase reaction. The colloidal iron was weakly

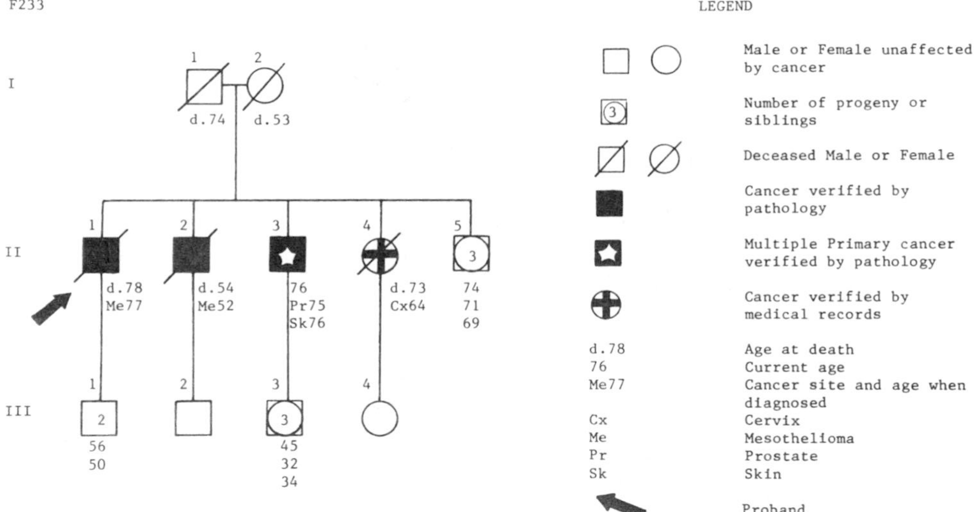

FIGURE 1. Pedigree of family showing mesothelioma in two siblings in conjunction with other cancer incidences. (From Lynch, H. T., Katz, D., and Markvicka, S. E., *Cancer Genet. Cytogenet.*, 15, 25, 1985. With permission.)

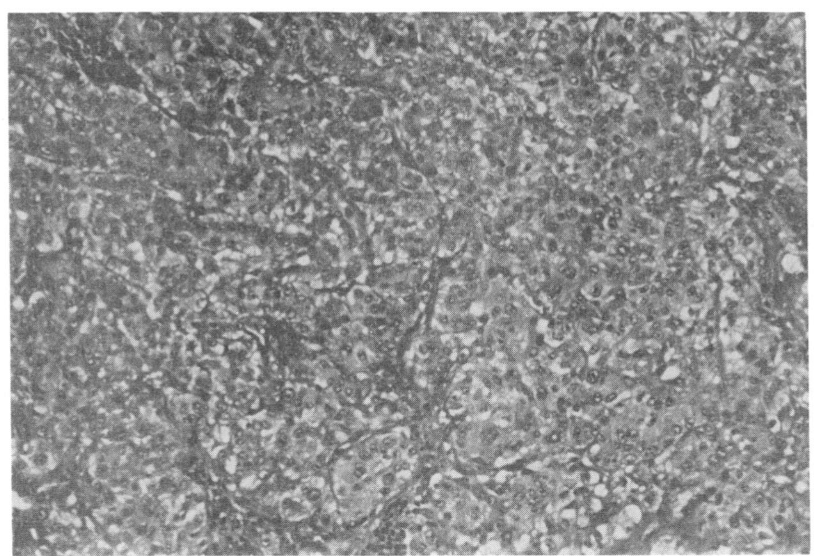

FIGURE 2. Malignant mesothelioma from 77-year-old male showing epithelioid cells arranged in nests and sheets with a thin intervening delicate fibrovascular stroma. (From Lynch, H. T., Katz, D., and Markvicka, S. E., *Cancer Genet. Cytogenet.*, 15, 25, 1985. With permission.)

positive. A mucin stain was negative. Alcian Blue stain showed stronger positivity at a 2.5 pH than at 0.4 pH and this positive reaction was partially removed by hylauronidase.

Approximately 9 d later, pleural tissue from the right lung was submitted. The tissue consisted of sheets of firm, grayish-tan tissue which measured 11.5 × 10.5 × 2.5 cm in aggregate. The individual sheets of tissue were markedly thickened. The microscopic sections (Figures 2 and 3) demonstrated sheets of neoplastic epithelioid cells with increased nuclear-

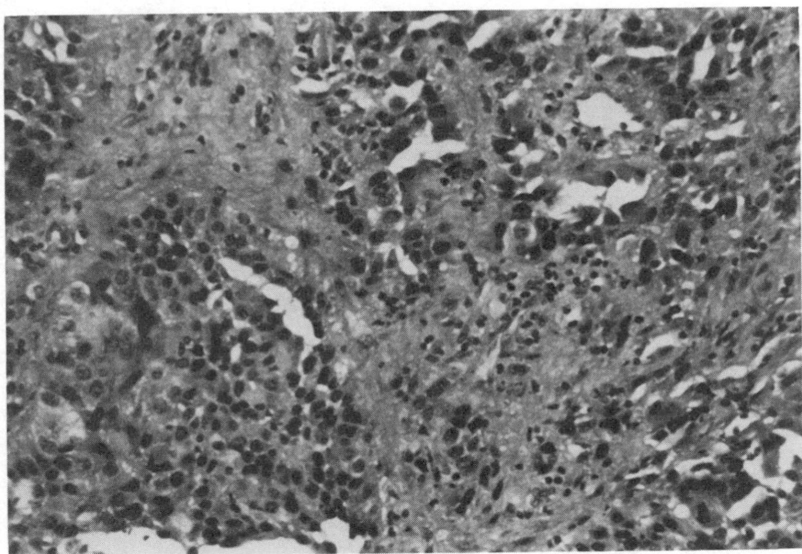

FIGURE 3. Nests of tumor cells forming small tubular structures, mimicking adenocarcinoma. (From Lynch, H. T., Katz, D., and Markvicka, S. E., *Cancer Genet. Cytogenet.*, 15, 25, 1985. With permission.)

cytoplasmic ratio, hyperchromatic nuclei, and eosinophilic cytoplasm. Numerous mitotic figures were present. In areas, the tumor formed tubular structures and in other areas demonstrated a tubopapillary pattern. Again, special stains were consistent with a mesothelioma. Electron microscopy was performed on this tissue revealing long slender microvilli between adjacent cells with glycogen aggregates in the cytoplasm. No junctional complexes were observed. The nuclei were ovoid to indented with small prominent nucleoli. The features were felt to be most consistent with a malignant mesothelioma.

The patient was placed on chemotherapy, but he was unresponsive and expired 87 d later. An autopsy was not performed.

B. Case #2

This 52-year-old white male (Figure 1, II-2) was the brother of patient #1. He was born in 1905 and worked as a steam fitter for approximately 28 years (1928 to 1956). This involved the wrapping of asbestos around steam pipes resulting in continuous and heavy asbestos exposure. Cigarette smoking was confined to less than one pack per day for a decade (1947 to 1957). In 1956, he presented with complaints of dyspnea. A pleural effusion was demonstrated on X-ray. A left pneumonectomy was performed in 1957.

The slides from the left pneumonectomy could not be obtained. However, a copy of the pathology report was reviewed. The diagnosis was a malignant mesothelioma of the left pleura, as well as a tuberculoma of the left upper lobe of the lung. Grossly, the lung showed the pleural surface to be markedly thickened and focally nodular in areas. Microscopically, the tumor was composed of collections of neoplastic cells with hyperchromatic nuclei and eosinophilic cytoplasm. According to the report, the cells were arranged in strands and cords in portions of the tumor, while other areas demonstrated a papillary appearance. Some of the tumor cells were embedded within fibrous stroma, which in areas appeared hyalinized.

The patient expired at age 54 of ''carcinomatosis''. An autopsy was not performed.

C. Case #3

This 76-year-old brother (Figure 1, II-3) of the above patients had worked as a pressman for 45 years (1927 to 1972) and as a shipping coordinator for the current 10 years (1973 to 1983). As far as can be determined, he had never been exposed to asbestos. He admitted smoking cigarettes and cigars for 40 years (1923 to 1963). At age 75, he received a pathological diagnosis of a well-differentiated adenocarcinoma of the prostate. After 1 year, he had a basal cell epithelioma (pathologically verified) of the skin excised.

D. Case #4

The 64-year-old sister (Figure 1, II-4) of the above brothers had been a housewife, was a nonsmoker, and, as far as can be determined, did not have any exposure to asbestos. Her husband's occupational history is unknown. She received a diagnosis of carcinoma of the uterine cervix at age 64 and died of metastases from this lesion at age 73. An autopsy was not performed.

Additional asbestos exposure has been verified within this kinship. The eldest son of the proband, born in 1927 (Figure 1, III-1), reported that from 1942 to 1957, he had received continuous asbestos exposure during his 15-year employment as a foreman in a welding shop. He has been a cigarette smoker (one pack per day) for the past 36 years (1946 to 1983). His 50-year-old brother (Figure 1, III-1) also experienced asbestos exposure over a 10-year period (1947 to 1957). He worked as a welder at the same place of employment as his sibling. This man is a nonsmoker. These two brothers have been approached by a member of our department, but to date, for reasons unknown, have declined cancer surveillance counseling.

No other evidence of cancer has been observed in this family. A nonmalignant uterine tumor was verified in the mother of this sibship (Figure 1, I-2).

Salient findings from reports of familial mesothelioma[4-6] are provided in Table 1. The findings of the family reported by Baris et al.[7] are not listed in the table since pathology descriptions were not available.

II. DISCUSSION

An etiologic link between asbestos exposure and mesothelioma was firmly established in 1960 when Wagner et al.[8] described 33 cases of diffuse pleural mesothelioma from the Northwestern Cape Province of South Africa. There was strong circumstantial evidence that 32 of these patients had contact with asbestos. The type of asbestos mined in this area of South Africa is crocidolite. In 1962, mesothelioma was found to be associated with asbestosis in western Australia,[9] where the crocidolite form of asbestos was also mined.

Selikoff et al.[10] reviewed the relationship between exposure to asbestos and mesothelioma in a study of 307 consecutive deaths (1943 to 1964) among asbestos insulation workers in New York and New Jersey. They found ten deaths due to mesothelioma of the pleura (four cases) or peritoneum (six cases). They concluded that "...mesothelioma must be added to the neoplastic risks of asbestos in insulation showing lung cancer (53 of 307 deaths) and probably cancer of the stomach and colon (34 of 307 deaths) as a significant complication of such industrial exposure in the United States." Family histories, unfortunately, were not reported in any of the above-mentioned studies.[8-11]

Lillington et al.[11] reviewed evidence showing that 23 women who had manifested mesothelioma received only domestic exposure to asbestos, which apparently resulted form residing in the same house as an asbestos worker. In addition, they reported an example of connubial mesothelioma. The husband developed mesothelioma following industrial exposure to asbestos. His wife's mesothelioma was attributed to asbestos exposure which occurred from washing her husband's dusty clothes. Details on the pathology of these lesions was not provided.

Anderson et al.[12] assessed the risk of nonmalignant as well as malignant disease associated

Table 1
FAMILIAL MESOTHELIOMA

						Asbestos Exposure		Smoking history	
Author	**Author number**	**Relation**	**Diagnosis**	**Age at DX**	**Y/N**	**Possible source**	**Duration (years)**	**Type/Amount (per day)**	**Duration (years)**
Smith et al.[2]	a	Brother	Peritoneal mesothelioma (fibromatous type)	54	Y	Direct exposure application of asbestos linings to piles	35	NG/NG	NG
	b	Brother	Peritoneal mesothelioma (fibromatous pattern in some areas and solid epithelial formation in others)	50	Y	Direct exposure insulation of pipes and boilers with asbestos (exposure to asbestos and its dust)	36	NG/NG	NG
Li et al.[3]		Father/ husband	Pulmonary asbestosis; adenocarcinoma of lung	60 71	Y	Direct exposure pipe insulator (1940—1965)	25	Cigarette/1—2 packs	-20
		Mother/	Mesothelioma of right pleura (similar to daughter's tumor)	50	Y	Indirect exposure from husband's clothing	NG	Nonsmoker	
		Daughter	Mesothelioma (mixed pattern of epithelial-type cells with papillary formations)	34	Y	Indirect exposure from father's clothing	NG	Cigarette/2 cigarettes	-15
Risbert et al.[4]	1	Father	Possible "malignant peritoneal mesothelioma"	61	Y	Agricultural worker since "youth" Building worker	NG 8	Cigarette/NG	NG
	2	Son	Tubulopapillary mesothelioma	57	Y	Sawmill worker, builder's laborer for rest of life	2 NG	Cigarette/0.5—1 pack	NG
	3	Son	Tubulopapillary mesothelioma	59	Y	Builder's laborer Paper industry for "rest of life"	2 NG	Cigarette/0.5—3/4 packs	NG
	4	Daughter	Tubulopapillary mesothelioma	50	N			Cigarette/0.5—1 pack	NG
	5	Son	Tubulopapillary tumor with abundant hyaline stroma	48	Y	Building trade	NG	Cigarette/1 pack	NG

Note: NG = not given by author.

From Lynch, H. T., Katz, D., and Markvicka, S. E., *Cancer Genet. Cytogenet.*, 15, 25, 1985. With permission.

with household exposure to work-derived asbestos dust. They investigated a factory wherein well documented asbestos disease had been recorded. In this factory, 1664 workers were employed for variable periods of time, producing amosite asbestos products. Their household contacts, who had lived with them during the time they worked in the factory, were being traced. Two pleural mesothelioma deaths occurred among household contacts. The first occurred in the daughter of a man who had worked with asbestos for more than 13 years. Her household exposure had begun in her early childhood and she died at age 52 from pleural mesothelioma. The second was the daughter of a man with 5 years of asbestos work at the plant. This lady died at age 41 of pleural mesothelioma. Of further interest was a study of 326 otherwise healthy contacts of amosite asbestos workers who were examined 25 to 30 years following onset of presumed household contamination with amosite asbestos. Significantly, 35% had chest X-ray abnormalities (pleural and/or parenchymal) which were characteristic of asbestos exposure. These investigators concluded that household contamination with asbestos from industrial sources can and does occur commonly and that this may lead to characteristic radiologic changes, and in a small fraction, asbestos-related cancer may occur.

Baris et al.[7] discuss endemic malignant pleural mesothelioma in two villages in Turkey; namely, Karain and Tuzkoy. Of 18 deaths in Karain (Urgup Province, Neveshir Region) during 1974, when the population was only 604 inhabitants, 11 were due to malignant pleural mesothelioma.

Clumps of asbestiform fibers were found in the water from the old wells of Karain. Studies in conjunction with the British Medical Research Council Pneumoconiosis Unit and the Department of Mineral Exploitation, University College Kadiv, demonstrated fibers of respirable sizes in rock samples and field soils of Karain. The fibers were found to be erionite-type zeolite through X-ray difraction and analytic transmission electron microscopy studies. These fibers were not found in control villages located 4 and 7 km from Karain.

A very interesting pedigree, referred to as the Sencan family, which included a sister (age 52) and a brother (age 44) with pleural malignant mesothelioma, was described. The brother's spouse had mesothelioma at age 54. Unfortunately, detail on the pathology of these lesions was not provided.

In the second town, namely, Tuzkoy (Gulsehir Province, Nevsehir Region), there were reportedly 1126 individuals over age 25 years (the authors report that the study is still in progress and will be published elsewhere). Endemic cases of calcified plaques and pleural thickening and/or fibrous pleuritis, as well as clustered cases of pleural and peritoneal mesothelioma and other types of cancers were observed. These diseases were not found in a control village 5 km from Tuzkoy. As in the case of Karain, many fibers of repirable sizes were found in the rock samples, street, and field soils which were erionite-type zeolite. Significantly, these fibers were found in the lung tissues of a patient diagnosed as fibrous pleuritis. Finally, the authors call attention to positive family histories of malignant pleural mesothelioma and other neoplastic diseases among residents of Karain and Tuzkoy. However, with the exception of the single pedigree (Sencan family), details on this subject are lacking.

The asbestos contamination of the drinking water in Karain was not considered likely as being etiologic for tumor induction. Asbestos exposure was not observed in Tuzkoy. Rather, erionite, as detected in the soil and rock samples, as well as in the lungs of the subject patient from Tuzkoy with chronic fibrous pleuritis, was considered to be the more likely carcinogen.

A. Pathology of Malignant Mesothelioma

The histology pattern of malignant mesothelioma is quite variable, with some patients demonstrating a purely epithelial or tubulopapillary pattern, while others show a sarcomatous pattern or a mixed epithelial and sarcomatous pattern histologically. According to some authors, approximately half of the malignant mesotheliomas will be of the epithelial or tubulopapillary type, while the other half will demonstrate a mixed epithelial and sarcomatous pattern histologically.[13] Other studies have found 70% of the malignant or diffuse mesotheliomas to be primarily epithelial or a mixed biphasic pattern of epithelial and sarcomatous features.[14]

B. Familial Reports and Pathology

Of interest is the similarity in histology of malignant mesotheliomas within several families. Table 1 provides the salient findings in the only previous identifiable familial accounts of malignant mesothelioma providing descriptive histology of the lesions. The study of Li et al.[5] is of particular interest in that the asbestos exposure to a mother and her daughter was indirect from their husband/father, respectively, who was exposed from 1940 thru 1965 when employed in a shipyard. He manifested pulmonary asbestosis at age 60 and expired from adenocarcinoma of the lung at age 71. Pleural mesotheliomas occurred in the mother and daughter. The daughter's tumor had a biphasic or mixed pattern of epithelial cells with papillary formation and spindle cells while the mother's tumor demonstrated a similar histologic appearance although the fibrosis appeared more extensive.

The family of Smith et al.[4] revealed peritoneal mesotheliomas in two brothers to be of the fibromatous type.

In a family study by Risberg et al.[6] it was significant that four of the five family members with malignant mesothelioma demonstrated a tubulopapillry pattern, although one of the tumors additionally showed abundant hyaline stroma.

In our study of two brothers with malignant mesothelioma (Figure 1), it appears that both tumors were primarily of the epithelial type. The younger brother (Figure 1, II-2) demonstrated papillary structures while his older sibling (Figure 1, II-1) displayed a papillary pattern as well as tubulopapillary structures. The malignant mesothelioma in the younger brother also appeared to demonstrate increased hyalinized fibrous stroma. We therefore postulate that there may possibly be an association between familial malignant mesothelioma and the specific histologic pattern. Needed, however, will be an extensive series of familial vs. nonfamilial mesothelioma patients to clarify this issue. Animal models may also be helpful in resolving this perplexing problem.

The available data on familial mesothelioma are not sufficient to define a genetic mechanism of tumor transmission. However, host factor susceptibility to malignant mesothelioma is suggested and it appears that asbestos exposure or erionite-type zeolite exposure, as in the Turkish experience, is essential for expression of the phenotype (malignant mesothelioma).

The occurrence of additional types of cancer within the familial form of malignant mesothelioma may be a function of a cancer-prone genotype in concert with specific carcinogenic exposures. In the case of the siblings of our mesothelioma-affected brothers, chance is a more likely explanation, particularly since they represent relatively common cancers in our population, i.e., carcinoma of the prostate, skin, and uterine cervix. These patients, so far as we can determine, were never exposed to asbestos. It is conceivable, however, that they may have manifested mesothelioma had they ever received asbestos exposure. For example, Vianna and Polan[15] observed an increased incidence of parental cancer, particularly of the gastrointestinal tract, among 52 women with malignant mesothelioma. Of these females, 15 had known asbestos exposure. The investigators speculated that certain patients with mesotheliomas come from cancer-prone families wherein genetic factors may alter susceptibility to asbestos carcinogenesis.

Familial aggregations of all varieties of cancer, including mesotheliomas, should not be surprising when one considers that the range of susceptibility to many common types of cancer may be as high as 100-fold.[16,17] This reasoning is particularly cogent when considering evidence at the biomolecular level where binding levels of benzo(a)pyrene to DNA vary 50-

to 100-fold in cultured tissues and cells.[18] This enormous variation in carcinogen metabolism in humans may be attributed to the fact that most chemical carcinogens require enzymatic activation, and herein, host factors play a major role in determining variation in such enzyme capability.[19] The sum total of these facts led Harris et al.[20] to postulate that the ratio of metabolic activation to deactivation of carcinogens may determine the individual's cancer risk. This reasoning is in full accord with the concept of ''ecogenetics'', an apt term for describing heritable variation in response to environmental exposures, including carcinogens.[21] In the case of asbestos, there is no enzyme activation required for the expression of its carcinogenic properties.

Why has the significance of host factors in mesothelioma only been recently appreciated? The answer to this is threefold: (1) asbestos exposure has increased remarkably since the turn of the century, as evidenced by its almost ubiquitous employment in many industries, i.e., asbestos production and manufacture, its use in insulation, heating, and building trades, heralded by its use in the rapid expansion of the shipbuilding industries during WWII, (2) there is a remarkably long latent period, with estimates ranging from 20 to 40 years between initial asbestos exposure and the development of mesothelioma. In addition, the amount of asbestos exposure necessary for initiation or promotion of carcinogenesis leading to malignant mesothelioma may be relatively minimal, i.e., handling the clothing of an individual who otherwise has heavy exposure.[5] Hence, we may be only viewing the tip of the iceberg relevant to the future frequency of occurrences of malignant mesothelioma, including its familial form; and finally, (3) documentation of family history has been notoriously ignored in all forms of cancer, including mesothelioma, a disease which heretofore has been considered to be due exclusively to environmental exposure to asbestos.

Our findings, including those several family reports dealing with familial mesothelioma aggregations (Table 1), clearly indicate the need to intensively study the patient's family history in concert with environmental exposures in the search for greater elucidation of the etiology of malignant mesothelioma.

In summary, many epidemiologists predict that the incidence of malignant mesothelioma will increase strikingly within the next decade or two. Nicholson et al.[22] state that approximately 8200 asbestos-related cancer deaths, inclusive of mesothelioma, are now occurring annually. Furthermore, they predict that asbestos-related cancer deaths will rise to 9700 by the year 2000. They also predict that the mortality rate from asbestos exposure will decline, but remain substantial for another 30 years. This reasoning is consonant with the excess exposures to asbestos emanating during WWII and the known prolonged latency interval between asbestos exposure and disease expression. It will therefore be imperative that detailed family histories be obtained on those known to have been exposed to asbestos and to those manifesting mesothelioma, since therapeutic intervention to date has been generally unrewarding. Families at high risk should be subjected to more intensive surveillance, specifically, annual physical examinations, chest X-rays, and attention to early symptomatology, where a high index of suspicion for mesothelioma may be justified.

REFERENCES

1. **Seilikoff, I. J., Churg, J., and Hammond, E. C.,** Asbestos exposure and neoplasia, *JAMA*, 188, 22, 1964.
2. **Becklake, M. R.,** Asbestos-related diseases of the lung and other organs: their epidemiology and implications for clinical practice, *Am. Rev. Respir. Dis.*, 114, 187, 1976.
3. **Lynch, H. T., Katz, D., and Markvicka, S. E.,** Familial mesothelioma: review and family study, *Cancer Genet. Cytogenet.*, 15, 25, 1985.

4. **Smith, P. G., Higgins, P. M., and Park, W. D.,** Peritoneal mesothelioma presenting surgically, *Br. J. Surg.*, 55, 681, 1968.
5. **Li, F. P., et al.,** Familial mesothelioma after intense asbestos exposure at home, *JAMA*, 240, 467, 1978.
6. **Risberg, B., Nickels, J., and Wagermark, J.,** Familial clustering of malignant mesothelioma, *Cancer*, 45, 2422, 1980.
7. **Baris, Y. I., Artvinili, M., and Sahin, A. A.,** Environmental mesothelioma in Turkey, *Ann. N.Y. Acad. Sci.*, 330, 423, 1979.
8. **Wagner, J. C., Sleggs, C. A., and Marchand, P.,** Diffuse pleural mesothelioma and asbestos exposure in North Western Cape Province, *Br. J. Ind. Med.*, 17, 260, 1960.
9. **McNulty, J. C.,** Malignant pleural mesothelioma in asbestos worker, *Med. J. Aust.*, 2, 953, 1962.
10. **Selikoff, I. J., Churg, J., and Hammond, E. C.,** Relation between exposure to asbestos and mesothelioma, *N. Eng. J. Med.*, 272, 560, 1965.
11. **Lillington, G. A., Jamplis, R. W., and Differding, J. R.,** Conjugal malignant mesothelioma, *N. Eng. J. Med.*, 291, 583, 1974.
12. **Anderson, H. A., Lilis, R., Daum, S. M., Fischbein, A. S., and Selikoff, I.,** Household contact asbestos neoplastic risk, *Ann. N.Y. Acad. Sci.*, 270, 311, 1976.
13. **Antman, K.,** Current concepts, malignant mesothelioma, *N. Engl. J. Med.*, 303, 200, 1980.
14. **Carter, D. and Eggleston, J. C.,** Tumors of the Lower Respiratory Tract, Armed Forces Institute of Pathology, Washington, D.C., 328.
15. **Vianna, N. J. and Polan, A. K.,** Nonoccupational exposure to asbestos and malignant mesothelioma in females, *Lancet*, i, 1061, 1978.
16. **Doll, R.,** An epidemiologic perspective of the biology of cancer, *Cancer Res.*, 38, 3573, 1978.
17. **Lynch, H. T.,** *Cancer Genetics*, Charles C Thomas, Springfield, IL, 1976, 639.
18. **Harris, C., Autrup, H., and Stoner, G.,** Metabolism of benzo(a)pyrene by cultured human tissues and cells, in *Polycyclic Hydrocarbons and Cancer: Chemistry, Molecular Biology, and Environment*, Ts'o, P. O. P. and Gelboin, H. V., Eds., Academic Press, New York, 1980, 331.
19. **Kouri, R. E.,** *Genetic Differences in Chemical Carcinogenesis*, CRC Press, Boca Raton, FL, 1978, 223.
20. **Harris, C. C.,** Individual differenes in cancer susceptibility, *Ann. Intern. Med.*, 92, 809, 1980.
21. **Mulvihill, J. J.,** Host factors in human lung tumors: an example of ecogenetics in oncology, *J. Natl. Cancer Inst.*, 57, 3, 1976.
22. **Nicholson, W. J., Perkel, G., and Selikoff, I. J.,** Occupational exposure to asbestos: population at risk and projected mortality — 1980—2030, *Am. J. Ind. Med.*, 3, 259, 1982.

Chapter 20

BIOMOLECULAR GENETICS OF CANCER

Bruce M. Boman

Recent molecular studies have shown that cancer cells carry a number of genetic changes that collectively result in the expression of the malignant phenotype.[1] Numerous oncogenes have been discovered and their characterization reveals that these genes have an important role in normal cellular growth control. Activation or enhanced expression of these genes in tumor cells appears to result in many of their malignant properties. More recently researchers have discovered a different class of genes, tumor- or growth-suppressor genes, which appear to function in normal tissue by inhibiting cellular growth.[2] It is hypothesized that mutations of this type of gene in tumor cells leads to the inactivation of normal growth inhibitory mechanisms.

Several investigators have hypothesized that tumor- or growth-suppressor genes are related to the cancer-predisposing genes in various hereditary cancer syndromes.[1,2] Molecular studies on hereditary cancer syndromes, such as retinoblastoma, suggest that tumors result from at least two genetic changes according to the ''two-hit hypothesis'' proposed by Knudson.[3] In hereditary cases the first hit is proposed to involve an inherited mutation present in the germline and the second hit occurs by a somatic event leading to the loss of the corresponding normal gene on the homologous chromosome. Recent linkage studies using biomolecular markers has led to the chromosome localization of several of these hereditary cancer traits (Table 1).

Further studies suggest that sporadic cancers result from mutations or loss of these same genes through somatic changes.[1-3] It is proposed that in sporadic tumors an initial somatic mutation occurs in one allele followed by loss of the corresponding normal homologue.[3] Studies on retinoblastoma indicate that the second hit in both familial and sporadic forms results from errors occurring during mitosis such as nondisjunction with chromosome loss or recombination. This two-step mechanism probably occurs in many cancers with different loci being involved in different types of tumors. This is supported by numerous studies which show that tumor-specific loss of alleles occurs on different chromosomes depending on the cancer type (Table 1).

Recent studies by several laboratories including ours have studied genetic changes in colorectal carcinomas. Linkage analysis has led to the chromosome localization of some hereditary colon cancer syndromes. The familial polyposis coli (FPC) trait has been mapped to chromosome 5 q21-q22 and the cancer family syndrome (Lynch Syndrome II) is tentatively located on chromosome 18.[14,36] Numerous investigators have studied tumor-specific loss of alleles on different chromosomes in colorectal carcinomas, which show significant loss of genetic material on chromosomes 5, 6, 17, 18, and 22 (Table 2). The loss of alleles on chromosomes 5 and 18 is consistent with Knudson's two-hit hypothesis since loci linked to colon cancer-predisposing genes are located on these chromosomes. The additional loss of genetic material on chromosomes 6, 17, and 22 also appears to be specific because loss of alleles on other chromosomes occurs much less frequently (Table 2).

Further molecular studies on colonic adenomatous polyps from hereditary and sporadic cases reveals that tumor-specific allele loss occurs very infrequently in these premalignant lesions (Table 3). This suggests that the second hit proposed in Knudson's hypothesis involving somatic loss of genetic material occurs during the adenoma to carcinoma transition in this carcinogenic sequence.

A genetic model is proposed on the basis of these studies. It is hypothesized that some

Table 1
CHROMOSOMES SHOWING ALLELE LOSS AND LINKAGE IN SPECIFIC CANCERS

Chorosome	Allele loss	Ref.	Linkage	Ref.
1	Multiple endocrine neoplasia type 2A	4		
2	Uveal melanoma	5		
3	Small cell lung cancer	6, 7, 8, 41		
	Nonsmall cell lung cancer	7, 8, 41		
	Renal cell cancer	9, 10		
5	Colorectal cancer	11—13	Familial polyposis/ Gardner syndrome	14, 15
10			Multiple endocrine neoplasia type 2A	16, 17
11	Wilms' tumor	18, 19	Multiple endocrine neoplasia type 1	24
	Hepatoblastoma	19		
	Rhabdomyosarcoma	19		
	Transitional cell bladder cancer	20		
	Bronchogenic carcinoma	21, 22		
	Breast cancer (nonductal)	23		
	Insulinoma	24		
13	Ductal breast cancer	25	Retinoblastoma	32
	Retinoblastoma	26—29		
	Osteosarcoma	30, 31		
	Small cell lung cancer	41		
	Gastric cancer	42		
17	Colon cancer	13, 33, 34	Neurofibromatosis	35
	Small cell lung cancer	41		
18	Colon cancer	34, 43	Lynch syndrome II	36
22	Acoustic neuroma	37, 38		
	Neurofibromas	37, 38		
	Meningioma	37, 38		

of the mechanisms during colon carcinogenesis involve the gene changes described by Knudson as well as gene activation such as an oncogene. This could occur as follows:

Normal mucosa		**Initiated epithelium**		**Adenoma**		**Malignant cell**		**Cancer**
p+p+	→ Gene loss/ mutation	p−p+	→ Gene activation	p−p+ p−p+ p−p+	→ Gene loss/ mutation	p−	→ Clonal expansion	p− p− p−

In the colon the epithelium may be initiated by inheritance of a cancer-predisposing gene mutation (p−) in which case all the cells in the colon would be initiated. In contrast, a colonic epithelial cell could become initiated in nonhereditary cases secondary to carcinogenic compounds that may be present in the diet, which might result in the loss or mutation of the same gene (p−). In this model it is assumed that this gene loss/mutation involves a tumor- or growth-suppressor gene (p+).

Although a germline mutation is present in all cells of the colon in FPC patients, much of the colonic mucosa is normal appearing. Therefore, another event appears to be necessary in the formation of an adenomatous polyp. Molecular studies support that epithelial cells in adenomas are of clonal origin.[33] Therefore, it is proposed that an initiated cell undergoes another genetic event that leads to activation or enhanced expression of genes signaling

Table 2
CHROMOSOME ALLELE LOSS IN COLORECTAL CARCINOMAS

Chromosome	Marker loci	Losses/ informative	Ref.	Total
1 p	pYNZ2	2/23 (9%)	33	2/34(6%)
p32	L-myc	0/11 (0%)	13	
2 p16-p15	D2S5	0/12 (0%)	12	0/44 (0%)
q32-q36	D2S6	0/11 (0%)	12	
q33-q35	CRYG	0/21 (0%)	13	
3 p14-p21	D3S2	0/15 (0%)	13	0/15 (0%)
5 p	D5S2	0/1 (0%)	13	32/125 (26%)
p	L1.4	6/17 (35%)	11	
p	L1.4	2/5 (40%)	39	
cen-q13	GRL	3/11 (27%)	12	
q21	D5S37	1/15 (7%)	39	
q21-q22	C11p11	4/5 (80%)	13	
q21-q22	C11p11	2/10 (20%)	39	
q22-q31	D5S6	2/7 (29%)	39	
q33.2-q33.3	fms	0/3 (0%)	39	
q34	fms	2/7 (29%)	13	
q34-qter	λMS8	10/44 (23%)	11	
6 q15-q24	myb	2/10 (20%)	13	6/33 (18%)
q15-q24	myb	4/23 (17%)	40	
7	pXg3	3/28 (11%)	33	3/62 (5%)
	D7S22	0/9 (0%)	11	
q21-q22	COL1A2	0/16 (0%)	13	
q22	D7S8	0/9 (0%)	11	
8	D8S8	0/14 (0%)	11	0/14 (0%)
11	D11S16	0/19 (0%)	11	6/81 (7%)
p15	INS	3/25 (12%)	33	
p15	HRAS1	3/19 (16%)	40	
p15	HRAS1	0/18 (0%)	13	
12 pter-p12	D12S2	0/4 (0%)	11	8/84 (10%)
p12.1	KRAS2	0/7 (0%)	12	
p12.1	KRAS2	0/7 (0%)	13	
q14-qter	D12S7	3/21 (14%)	13	
q14-qter	D12S8	4/21 (19%)	13	
q14.3	COL2A1	1/17 (6%)	11	
q22-q24.2	PAH	0/7 (0%)	12	
13 q12-q14	D13S1	0/13 (0%)	11	0/88 (0%)
q22	D13S2	0/24 (0%)	11	
q31	D13S4	0/22 (0%)	11	
q12-q13	p7F12	0/29 (0%)	33	
q21-q22	p9D11			
q21-q22	p1E8			
q32-q33	p9A7			
15 q14-q21	D15S1	1/12 (8%)	13	1/12 (8%)
16 q	p79-2-23	1/27 (4%)	33	1/27 (4%)
17 p	pYNZ22	25/33 (76%)	33	42/98 (43%)
p	MYH2			
p13	D17S1	0/15 (0%)	11	
p13	D17S1	0/6 (0%)	13	
p13	D17S1	9/12 (75%)	34	
q11-q21	ERBA1	0/1 (0%)	11	
q	GH1	8/31 (26%)	33	
q21-q22	TK1			
q	pTHH59			
18	D18S1	0/11 (0%)	13	16/34 (47%)

Table 2 (continued)
CHROMOSOME ALLELE LOSS IN COLORECTAL CARCINOMAS

Chromosome	Marker loci	Losses/ informative	Ref.	Total
	D18S1	12/14 (86%)	34	
	D18S6	4/9 (44%)	43	
19 pter-p13.2	INSR	1/10 (10%)	12	1/25 (4%)
13.1-q13.3	CYP1	0/15 (0%)	12	
20	DOSLC2	0/10 (0%)	33	0/10 (0%)
22 q11	D22S9	5/14 (36%)	13	20/74 (27%)
q11	IGLC	7/24 (29%)	13	
q11	IGLV	4/14 (29%)	13	
q11.1-q11.2	V-Igλ	0/4 (0%)	34	
q11-q13	D22S1	3/15 (20%)	13	
q12-q13	sis	1/3 (33%)	13	

Note: Hereditary and sporadic cases have been pooled.

[a] Percent allelic imbalance.

Table 3
CHROMOSOME ALLELE LOSS IN COLONIC ADENOMATOUS POLYPS

Chromsome	Marker locus	Losses/ informative	Ref.
1 p32	myc	0/7	13
2 q33-q35	CRYG	0/11	13
3 p14-p21	D3S2	0/4	13
5 pter-q35	D5S2	0/2	13
q21-q22	C11p11	0/2	13
q34	fms	0/5	13
q34-qter	λMS8	0/11	11
6 q15-q24	myb	1/7	13
	myb	1/5	40
7 q21-q22	COLIA2	0/5	13
11 p15	HRAS1	0/5	13
	HRAS1	0/7	40
12 p12.1	KRAS2	0/4	13
q14-qter	D12S7	0/11	13
q14-qt34	D12S8	1/9	13
15 q14-q21	D15S1	0/4	13
17 p13-pter	D17S1	0/5	13
p	pYNZ22	1/30	33
18	D18S1	0/7	13
22 q11	D22S9	0/10	13
q11	IGLC	0/11	13
q11	IGLV	0/11	13
q11-q13	D22S1	0/6	13
q12-q13	sis	0/2	13

Note: Hereditary and sporadic cases have been pooled.

cellular growth, such as ras oncogene activation[33] or a gene involving the epidermal growth factor receptor pathway.[46] If cancer-predisposing genes are mutant tumor- or growth-suppressor genes, then the initiated colonic epithelium would probably have borderline growth control ability and be susceptible to environmental factors that promote additional genetic changes leading to a proliferative response and adenomatous polyp formation.

During the progression from an adenoma to a carcinoma, it is proposed that the remaining normal allele of a tumor- or growth-suppressor gene is lost or mutated. This is consistent with the observation of allele loss in carcinomas but rarely in adenomas (Tables 2 and 3). Because adenomas consist of proliferating cells, there is a chance, albeit very small, that a genetic error may occur during mitosis. If an error, such as nondisjunction or mitotic recombination, results in loss of the remaining normal putative tumor- or growth-suppressor gene on the homologous chromosome, then a malignant cell might result. Clonal expansion of this cell would then lead to formation of a colon carcinoma.

Future molecular biologic studies will be important in elucidating the underlying genetic mechanisms involved in colon carcinogenesis.

NOTE ADDED IN PROOF

While this manuscript was in press two important papers were published involving studies on colon tumor samples purified by microdissection or flow cytometry to prevent underscoring of apparent allele loss.[44,45] Both of these large series examined adenomas and carcinomas from hereditary and sporadic cases and reported significant allele loss on chromosomes 5, 17, and 18 (in 19 to 31, 56 to 73, and 52 to 75% of informative cases, respectively). Law et al.[41] observed none of the 33 informative cancer cases to lose alleles on chromosome 22. Subsequent studies in our laboratory failed to demonstrate significant allele loss on chromosome 6 at 3 loci in 22 colorectal carcinomas examined (unpublished data). Therefore, allele losses in colorectal cancer appear to involve chromosomes 5, 17, and 18 more commonly than other chromosomes.

Allelic deletions of chromosome 5q were commonly observed (29%) in class II and III, but not class I sporadic adenomas.[45] An adenoma from a Lynch syndrome patient also showed chromosome 5 allele loss.[44] Adenomas from patients with polyposis failed to show any chromosome 5 allele loss.[44,45] In addition allele loss on chromosome 18 was reported in 47% of class III sporadic adenomas (23 and 18% of class I and II adenomas lost chromosome 18 alleles[45]). This data is consistent with the model proposed in this paper in which inheritence or loss of a tumor-suppressor gene such as on chromosome 5 or 18 creates a selective growth advantage in the colon leading to adenoma formation. Vogelstein et al.[45] also provided further evidence that mutation of a ras oncogene occurs during adenoma formation.

These studies also question whether a two-hit mechanism involving loss/mutation of both alleles at the FPC locus occurs in colorectal carcinomas because chromosome 5 allele loss occurs in only about 25% of sporadic carcinomas (approximately the same percent of sporadic adenomas lose chromosome 5 alleles). In contrast 50% of the FPC colon carcinomas reported to be informative (n = 8) lose chromosome 5 alleles.[13,44] Determination of whether inactivation of both FPC alleles occurs during colon carcinogenesis will probably depend on cloning the FPC gene to analyze FPC gene structure and expression in colorectal carcinomas.

The genetic mechanisms that occur during colon carcinogenesis are probably more complex than the model proposed in this paper because both reports[44,45] and our recent study[43] show allele losses on chromosomes 5, 17, or 18 can occur concurrently. Thus, the genetic alterations that occur in colorectal carcinomas are multiple and may be heterogenous in different carcinomas. However, these genetic changes probably involve a few crucial tumor- or growth-suppressor genes and oncogenes that are involved in normal growth control mechanisms in the colon.[46]

REFERENCES

1. **Friend, S. H., Dryja, T. P., and Weinberg, R. A.,** Oncogenes and tumor-suppressing genes, *N. Engl. J. Med.,* 318, 618, 1988.
2. **Klein, G.,** The approaching era of the tumor suppressor genes, *Science,* 238, 1539, 1987.
3. **Knudson, A. G.,** Retinoblastoma: a prototypic hereditary neoplasm, *Semin Oncol.,* 5, 57, 1978.
4. **Mathew, C. G. P., Smith, B. A., Thorpe, K., Wong, Z., Royle, N. J., Jeffreys, A. J., and Ponder, B. A. J.,** Deletion of genes on chromosome 1 in endocrine neoplasia, *Nature,* 328, 524, 1987.
5. **Mukai, S. and Dryja, T. P.,** Loss of alleles at polymorphic loci on chromosome 2 in uveal melanoma, *Cancer Genet. Cytogenet.,* 22, 45, 1986.
6. **Naylor, S. L., Johnson, B. E., Minna, J. D., and Sakaguchi, A. Y.,** Loss of heterozygosity of chromosome 3p markers in small-cell lung cancer, *Nature,* 329, 451, 1987.
7. **Brauch, H. et al.,** Molecular analysis of the short arm of chromosome 3 in small-cell and non-small cell carcinoma of the lung, *N. Engl. J. Med.,* 317, 1109, 1987.
8. **Kok, K. et al.,** Deletion of a DNA sequence at the chromosomal region 3p21 in all major types of lung cancer, *Nature,* 330, 578, 1987.
9. **Zbar, B., Brauch, H., Talmadge, C., and Linehan, M.,** Loss of alleles of loci on the short arm of chromosome 3 in renal cell carcinoma, *Nature,* 327, 721, 1987.
10. **Kovacs, G., Erlandsson, R., Boldog, F., Ingvarsson, S., Muller-Brechlin, R., Klein, G., and Sumegi, J.,** Consistent chromosome 3p deletion of loss of heterozygosity in renal cell carcinoma, *Proc. Natl. Acad. Sci. U.S.A.,* 85, 1571, 1988.
11. **Solomon, E., Voss, R., Hall, V., Bodmer, W. F., Jass, J. R., Jeffreys, A. J., Lucibello, F. C., Patel, I., and Rider, S. H.,** Chromosome 5 allele loss in human colorectal carcinomas, *Nature,* 328, 161, 1987.
12. **Wildrick, D. M. and Boman, B. M.,** Chromosome 5 allele loss at the glucocorticoid receptor locus in human colorectal carcinomas, *Biochem. Biophys. Res. Commun.,* 150, 591, 1988.
13. **Okamoto, M. et al.,** Loss of constitutional heterozygosity in colon carcinoma from patients with familial polyposis coli, *Nature,* 331, 273, 1988.
14. **Bodmer, W. F., Bailey, C. J., Bodmer, J., Bussey, H. J. R., Ellis, A., Gorman, P., Lucibello, F. C., Murday, V. A., Rider, S. H., Scambler, P., Sheer, D., Solomon, E., and Spurr, N. K.,** Localization of gene for familial adenomatous polyposis on chromosome 5, *Nature,* 328, 614, 1987.
15. **Leppert, M., Dobbs, M., Scrambler, P., O'Connell, P., Nakamura, Y., Stauffer, D., Woodward, S., Burt, R., Hughes, J., Gardner, E., Lathrop, M., Wasmuth, J., Lalouel, J. M., and White, R.,** The gene for familial polyposis coli maps to the long arm of chromosome 5, *Science,* 238, 1411, 987.
16. **Mathew, C. G. P. et al.,** A linked genetic marker for multiple endocrine neoplasia type 2A on chromosome 10, *Nature,* 328, 527, 1987.
17. **Simpson, N. E. et. al.,** Assignment of multiple endocrine neoplasia type 2A on chromosome 10, *Nature,* 328, 528, 1987.
18. **Dao, D. D. et al.,** Genetic mechanisms of tumor-specific loss of 11p DNA sequences in Wilms tumor, *Am. J. Hum. Genet.,* 41, 202, 1987.
19. **Koufos, A., Hansen, M. F., Copeland, N. G., Jenkins, N. A., Lampkin, B. C., and Cavenee, W. K.,** Loss of heterozygosity in three embryonal tumours suggests a common pathogenetic mechanism, *Nature,* 316, 330, 1985.
20. **Fearon, E. R., Feinberg, A. P., Hamilton, S. H., and Vogelstein, B.,** Loss of genes on the short arm of chromosome 11 in bladder cancer, *Nature,* 318, 337, 1985.
21. **Heighway, J., Thatcher, N., Cerny, T., and Hasleton, P. S.,** Genetic predisposition to human lung cancer, *Br. J. Cancer,* 53, 453, 1986.
22. **Willey, J. C., Weston, A., Resau, J., McDowell, E., Trump, B. F., and Harris, C. C.,** Restriction fragment length polymorphism (RFLP) analysis of chromosome 11 in human lung cancers, *Am. J. Hum. Genet.,* 39, A47, 1986.
23. **Ali, I. U., Lidereau, R., Theillet, C., and Callahan, R.,** Reduction to homozygosity of genes on chromosome 11 in human breast neoplasia, *Science,* 238, 185,
24. **Larsson, C., Skogseid, B., Oberg, K., Nakamura, Y., and Nordenskjold, M.,** Multiple endocrine neoplasia type 1 gene maps to chromosome 11 and is lost in insulinoma, *Nature,* 332, 85, 1988.
25. **Lundberg, C., Skoog, L., Cavenee, W. K., and Nordenskjold, M.,** Loss of heterozygosity in human ductal breast tumors indicates a recessive mutation on chromosome 13, *Proc. Natl. Acad. Sci. U.S.A.,* 84, 2372, 1987.
26. **Cavenee, W. K., Hansen, M. F., Nordenskjold, M., Kock, E., Squire, J. A., Phillips, R. A., and Gallie, B. L.,** Genetic origin of mutations predisposing to retinoblastoma, *Science,* 228, 501, 1985.
27. **Dryja, T. P. et al.,** Homozygosity of chromosome 13 in retinoblastoma, *N. Engl. J. Med.,* 310, 550, 1984.

28. **Cavenee, W. K., Dryja, T. P., Phillips, R. A., Benedict, W. F., Godbout, R., Gallie, B. L., Murphree, A. L., Strong, L. C., and White, R. L.,** Expression of recessive alleles by chromosomal mechanisms in retinoblastoma, *Nature,* 305, 779, 1983.
29. **Benedict, W. F., Srivatsan, E. S., Mark, C., Banerjee, A., Sparkes, R. S., and Murphree, A. L.,** Complete or partial homozygosity of chromosome 13 in primary retinoblastoma, *Cancer Res.,* 47, 4189, 1987.
30. **Dryja, T. P., Rapaport, J. M., Epstein, J., Goorin, A. M., Weichselbaum, R., Koufos, A., and Cavenee, W. K.,** Chromosome 13 homozygosity in osteosarcoma without retinoblastoma, *Am. J. Hum. Genet.,* 38, 59, 1986.
31. **Hansen, M. F., Koufos, A., Gallie, B. L., Phillips, R. A., Fodstad, O., Brogger, A., Gedde-Dahl, T., and Cavenee, W. K.,** Osteosarcoma and retinoblastoma: a shared chromosomal mechanism revealing recessive predisposition, *Proc. Natl. Acad. Sci. U.S.A.,* 82, 6216, 1985.
32. **Sparkess, R. S., Murphree, A. L., Lingua, R. W., Sparkes, M. C., Field, L. L., Funderburk, S. J., and Benedict, W. F.,** Gene for hereditary retinoblastoma assigned to human chromosome 13 by linkage to esterase D, *Science,* 219, 971, 1983.
33. **Fearon, E. R., Hamilton, S. R., and Vogelstein, B.,** Clonal analysis of human colorectal tumors, *Science,* 238, 193, 1987.
34. **Monpezat, J.-Ph., Delattre, O., Bernard, A., Grunwald, D., Remvikos, Y., Muleris, M., Salmon, R. J., Frelat, G., Dutrillaux, B., and Thomas, G.,** Loss of alleles on chromosome 18 and on the short arm of chromosome 17 in polyploid colorectal carcinomas, *Int. J. Cancer,* 41, 404, 1988.
35. **Barker, D. et al.,** Gene for von Recklinghausen Neurofibromatosis is in the pericentromeric region of chromosome 17, *Science,* 236, 1100, 1987.
36. **Boman, B. M., Lynch, H. T., Kimberling, W. J., and Wildrick, D. M.,** Letter to the editor: reassignment of a cancer family syndrome gene to chromosome 18, *Cancer Genet. Cytogenet.,* 34, 153, 1988.
37. **Seizinger, B. R., Martuza, R. L., and Gusella, J. F.,** Loss of genes on chromosome 22 in tumorigenesis of human acoustic neuroma, *Nature,* 322, 644, 1986.
38. **Seizinger, B. R., Rouleau, G., Ozelius, L. J., Lane, A. H., St. George-Hyslop, P., Huson, S., Gusella, J. F., and Martuza, R. L.,** Common pathogenetic mechanism for three tumor types in bilateral acoustic neurofibromatosis, *Science,* 236, 317, 1987.
39. **Jhanwar, S., Tops, C., Meera Khan, P., Quanguang, C., Broek, Mvd, Breukel, C., Wijen, J., Vos Jvd, Griffioen, G., Verspaget, H., Lamers, C., and Pearson, P.,** Colon cancer gene(s) on chromosome 5. II. Cytogenetic and molecular marker studies in tumors and cell lines, program of the 40th Annu. Symp. Fundamental Cancer Research, Houston, November 8 to 11, 1987.
40. **Meltzer, S. J., Ahnen, D. J., Battifora, H., Yokota, J., and Cline, M. J.,** Protooncogene abnormalities in colon cancers and adenomatous polyps, *Gastroenterology,* 92, 1174, 1987; **Meltzer, S. J.,** personal communication.
41. **Yokota, J., Wada, M., Shimosata, Y., Terada, M., and Sugimura, T.,** Loss of heterozygosity on chromosome 3, 13, and 17 in small-cell carcinomas and on chromosome 3 in adenocarcinomas of the lung, *Proc. Natl. Acad. Sci. U.S.A.,* 84, 9252, 1987.
42. **Motomura, K., Nishisho, I., Takai, S. I., Tateishi, H., Okazaki, M., Yamamota, M., Miki, T., Honjo, T., and Mori, T.,** Loss of allele at loci on chromosome 13 in human primary gastric cancers, *Genomics,* 2, 180, 1988.
43. **Boman, B. M., Wildrick, D. M., and Alfaro, S.,** Chromosome 18 allele loss at the D18S6 locus in human colorectal carcinomas, *Biochem. Biophys. Res. Commun.,* 155, 463, 1988.
44. **Law, D. J., Olschwang, S., Monpezat, J.-P., Lefrancois, D., Jagelman, D., Petrelli, N. J., Thomas, G., and Feinberg, A. P.,** Concerted nonsyntenic allelic loss in human colorectal carcinoma, *Science,* 241, 961, 1988.
45. **Vogelstein, B., Fearon, E. R., Hamilton, S. R., Kern, S. E., Preisinger, A. C., Leppert, M., Nakamura, Y., White, R., Smits, A. M. M., and Bos, J. L.,** Genetic alterations during colorectal tumor development, *N. Engl. J. Med.,* 319, 525, 1988.
46. **Boman, B. M., Wildrick, D. M., and Lointier, P.,** Growth factors and colon cancer, in Gastrointestinal Cancer: Current Approaches to Diagnosis and Treatment, Annu. Clin. Conf. Cancer, University of Texas M.D. Anderson Cancer Center, Houston, 30, 71, 1988.

INDEX

A

B

D

E

F

G

H

I

J

K

L

M

N

O

S

T

U

V

W

X

Z